# Sports Nutrition

# Sports Nutrition

Yanina Ditamo
Wade Worthen

Kruger Brentt
Publishers
2025

Kruger Brentt Publishers UK. LTD.
Company Number 9728962

Regd. Office: 68 St Margarets Road, Edgware, Middlesex HA8 9UU



ISBN: 978-1-78715-416-2



For information on all our publications visit our website at http://krugerbrentt.com/

# PREFACE

"Sports Nutrition" offers a comprehensive exploration into the science, principles, and practices that underpin optimal nutrition for athletic performance and overall health. This book serves as an essential resource for athletes, coaches, trainers, nutritionists, and anyone interested in understanding the role of nutrition in sports and physical activity.

Nutrition plays a critical role in supporting athletic performance, recovery, and overall well-being. Properly fueling the body with the right nutrients at the right times can enhance endurance, strength, speed, and agility while reducing the risk of injury and illness. Whether you are an elite athlete striving for peak performance or a recreational exerciser looking to maximize your workouts, understanding the fundamentals of sports nutrition is essential for achieving your goals.

As editors of this volume, we have endeavored to compile a diverse array of perspectives, methodologies, and case studies from leading experts and practitioners in the field of sports nutrition. Through a blend of scientific evidence, practical guidance, and real-world examples, this book covers a wide range of topics, including macronutrients and micronutrients, hydration, supplementation, meal planning, and nutrition strategies for specific sports and activities.

Our overarching goal in presenting this book is to provide readers with a comprehensive understanding of the principles and applications of sports nutrition. By offering insights into the latest research, best practices, and evidence-based recommendations in the field, we aim to empower athletes, coaches, trainers, and nutrition professionals to make informed decisions about their dietary choices and optimize their performance, health, and well-being.

We extend our sincere gratitude to all the contributors who have generously shared their expertise, experiences, and insights in the field of sports nutrition. It is our hope that this book will serve as a valuable reference and guide for readers as they strive to achieve their athletic goals and lead healthy, active lifestyles.

**Yanina Ditamo**

**Wade Worthen**

# CONTENTS

# 1 Chapter

# SPORTS NUTRITION: AN INTRODUCTION

Sports nutrition is a rapidly expanding area of scientific investigation and is being driven by high interest from both the academic community and the exercising public [1]. Research into the discipline of sports nutrition is challenging. The interaction of exercise and nutrition is both complex and compelling, with an endless array of potential sports nutrition products, pathways, and hypotheses to be tested. Some proposed sports nutrition strategies and products are innovative while others are based on fanciful conjecture [2].

Research designs for sports nutrition-based studies need to adhere to the highest quality standards to determine efficacy [1,3]. Nutrition dosing regimens are always challenging and, unfortunately, these are often based more on educated guesses and marketing issues than careful science. Many sports nutrition products have blends of macro- and micro-nutrients and phytochemicals that have clinical backing for some of the individual ingredients but not the entire mixture. Few sports nutrition products have been tested for stability, absorption, disposition, metabolism, and excretion.

A "food first" approach for athletes is recommended by most sports nutrition professionals. The problem for some athletes, however, is that they are resistant to adopting dietary patterns that are consistent with published guidelines. For many people that exercise, a healthy dietary pattern is sufficient to supply the nutrients needed to support a healthy response to increased exercise levels [4]. High-level athletes may need extra help beyond the food supply to meet the nutrient demands of stressful exercise workloads, but this is still being debated [1]. Nonetheless, adaptations within a healthy dietary pattern may support both performance and health for even the athletes with the most demanding training programs. For example, recent studies support that fruit and water consumption can complement or even take the place of commercial sports beverages for those exercising intensely for long periods of time [5,6,7].

Sports performance can be measured in many different ways, and nutritional interventions are often evaluated as essential when performance is improved. Some sports nutrition products are targeted for outcomes that are not easily felt by the athlete, including lowered inflammation, immunosuppression, and oxidative stress, and enhanced metabolic recovery [8,9]. This type of benefit is not easily conveyed to the athletes or coach, or in particular, the exercising public.

Advances in measurement technologies are allowing hundreds of metabolites, proteins, lipids, and genes to be measured at one time, improving the capacity to provide accurate and practical guidelines for consumers. Nutrition and exercise have huge effects on nearly every system of the body, both acutely and chronically, and a human systems biology approach, although expensive, is needed to advance scientific understanding [10].

For this Special Issue, research leaders in sports nutrition were approached and invited to submit current reviews in their areas of expertise [11,12,13,14,15,16,17,18,19,20,21] . The topics are novel and wide-ranging, and include updates and insights on protein [11,12], dietary patterns and nutritional interventions to support sleep, older athletes, and sports performance [13,14,15], pre-exercise nutrition [16], supplementation with betaine, iron, and creatine [17,18,19], and sports nutrition research methodologies for body composition and muscle glycogen analysis [20,21]. A major emphasis in all of the papers was a focus on strengths and weaknesses for various sports nutrition strategies, and insights for future research. Kerksick et al. [11] delineated the significance of appropriate dosages of plant proteins in promoting health, environmental sustainability, and responses to exercise training. Chapman et al.'s systematic review and meta-analysis [12] determined that protein supplementation enhances strength and muscle mass under rigorous and prolonged exercise. The narrative review by Gratwicke et al. [13] advised nutritional therapies, including supplementation with tart cherry juice, kiwifruit, 20–40 grams of tryptophan-rich protein, and glycine in the evening, as effective ways for enhancing sleep in athletes. Strasser et al. [14] concentrated on nutritional recommendations for elderly individuals, emphasizing sufficient energy and protein consumption to mitigate declines in bone and muscle mass.

Devrim-Lanpir [15] analyzed five prevalent dietary patterns: vegetarian diets, high-fat ketogenic diets, intermittent fasting diets, gluten-free diets, and low fermentable oligosaccharides, disaccharides, monosaccharides, and polyols (FODMAP) diets. This thorough evaluation encapsulated the advantageous and disadvantageous aspects of each diet concerning athletic performance. Pre-exercise nutrition is a significant and contemporary topic in sports nutrition, with Rothschild et al. [16] offering a comprehensive analysis of how the availability of endogenous and exogenous carbohydrates, fats, and proteins prior to and during exercise can affect adaptations to endurance training.

Betaine (trimethylglycine) can be synthesized endogenously from choline or obtained exogenously from dietary sources such as wheat bran and germ, spinach, and beets. Betaine serves as a methyl donor and assists in regulating intracellular fluid concentrations and cellular volume. Willingham et al. [17] contended that human clinical trials are necessary to ascertain the efficacy of betaine supplementation in enhancing safety and exercise performance in heat, as indicated by animal investigations.

Reduced carbohydrate and energy consumption can adversely affect iron status in athletes, often mediated via hepcidin expression. McKay et al. [18] conducted a thorough narrative assessment that advised athletes to reduce the length of low carbohydrate training phases to mitigate possible impacts on hepcidin and iron control. Creatine is among the most prevalent sports nutrition supplements available, and Arzi et al. [19] provided increasing evidence suggesting that creatine supplementation may mitigate exercise-induced oxidative stress.

Kasper et al. [20] presented a comprehensive review of techniques for assessing body composition. The research group determined that accurately executed skinfold measurements yield valuable data and may be favored over alternative approaches due to their simplicity, cost-effectiveness, minimal influence from lifestyle confounders, and suitability for long-term athlete monitoring. The assessment of muscle glycogen is crucial in sports nutrition research, and Bone et al. [21] warned that high-frequency ultrasound technology for calculating muscle glycogen levels need further advancement.

This Special Issue on sports nutrition presents contemporary updates in various fundamental areas, featuring insights from prominent specialists for future research endeavors. It is anticipated that scientific comprehension will progress as these concepts are transformed into innovative research methodologies and findings.

## REFERENCES

1. Bassaganya-Riera, J.; Berry, E.M.; Blaak, E.E.; Burlingame, B.; le Coutre, J.; van Eden, W.; El-Sohemy, A.; German, J.B.; Knorr, D.; Lacroix, C. Goals in Nutrition Science 2020–2025. *Front. Nutr.* **2021**, 7, 606378. **[Google Scholar]**

2. Burke, L.M.; Castell, L.M.; Casa, D.J.; Close, G.L.; Costa, R.; Desbrow, B.; Halson, S.L.; Lis, D.M.; Melin, A.K.; Peeling, P. International Association of Athletics Federations Consensus Statement 2019: Nutrition for Athletics. *Int. J. Sport Nutr. Exerc. Metab.* **2019**, *29*, 73–84. **[Google Scholar]** **[Green Version]**

3. Maughan, R.J.; Burke, L.M.; Dvorak, J.; Larson-Meyer, D.E.; Peeling, P.; Phillips, S.M.; Rawson, E.S.; Walsh, N.P.; Garthe, I.; Geyer, H. IOC Consensus Statement: Dietary Supplements and the High-Performance Athlete. *Int. J. Sport Nutr. Exerc. Metab.* **2018**, *28*, 104–125. **[Google Scholar]** **[Green Version]**

4. Collins, J.; Maughan, R.J.; Gleeson, M.; Bilsborough, J.; Jeukendrup, A.; Morton, J.P.; Phillips, S.M.; Armstrong, L.; Burke, L.M.; Close, G.L. UEFA Expert Group Statement on Nutrition in Elite Football. Current Evidence to Inform Practical Recommendations and Guide Future Research. *Br. J. Sport Med.* **2021**, *55*, 416. **[Google Scholar]** **[PubMed]**

5. Nieman, D.C.; Gillitt, N.D.; Chen, G.Y.; Zhang, Q.; Sha, W.; Kay, C.D.; Chandra, P.; Kay, K.L.; Lila, M.A. Blueberry and/or Banana Consumption Mitigate Arachidonic, Cytochrome P450 Oxylipin Generation during Recovery from 75-Km Cycling: A Randomized Trial. *Front. Nutr.* **2020**, *7*, 121. **[Google Scholar]** **[PubMed]**

6. Nieman, D.C.; Gillitt, N.D.; Sha, W.; Esposito, D.; Ramamoorthy, S. Metabolic Recovery from Heavy Exertion Following Banana Compared to Sugar Beverage or Water Only Ingestion: A Randomized, Crossover Trial. *PLoS ONE* **2018**, *13*, e0194843. **[Google Scholar]** **[PubMed]** **[Green Version]**

7. Nieman, D.C.; Gillitt, N.D.; Henson, D.A.; Sha, W.; Shanely, R.A.; Knab, A.M.; Cialdella-Kam, L.; Jin, F. Bananas as An Energy Source During Exercise: A Metabolomics Approach. *PLoS ONE* **2021**, *7*, e37479. **[Google Scholar]**

8. Nieman, D.C.; Mitmesser, S.H. Potential Impact of Nutrition on Immune System Recovery from Heavy Exertion: A Metabolomics Perspective. *Nutrients* **2017**, *9*, 513. **[Google Scholar]** **[PubMed]** **[Green Version]**

9. Sorrenti, V.; Fortinguerra, S.; Caudullo, G.; Buriani, A. Deciphering the Role of Polyphenols in Sports Performance: From Nutritional Genomics to the Gut Microbiota toward Phytonutritional Epigenomics. *Nutrients* **2020**, *12*, 1265. **[Google Scholar]**

10. Nieman, D.C.; Lila, M.A.; Gillitt, N.D. Immunometabolism: A Multi-Omics Approach to Interpreting the Influence of Exercise and Diet on the Immune System. *Annu. Rev. Food Sci. Technol.* **2019**, *10*, 341–363. **[Google Scholar]**

11. Kerksick, C.M.; Jagim, A.; Hagele, A.; Jäger, R. Plant Proteins and Exercise: What Role Can Plant Proteins Have in Promoting Adaptations to Exercise? *Nutrients* **2021**, *13*, 1962. **[Google Scholar]**

12. Chapman, S.; Chung, H.C.; Rawcliffe, A.J.; Izard, R.; Smith, L.; Roberts, J.D. Does Protein Supplementation Support Adaptations to Arduous Concurrent Exercise Training? A Systematic Review and Meta-Analysis with Military Based Applications. *Nutrients* **2021**, *13*, 1416. **[Google Scholar]**

13. Gratwicke, M.; Miles, K.H.; Pyne, D.B.; Pumpa, K.L.; Clark, B. Nutritional Interventions to Improve Sleep in Team-Sport Athletes: A Narrative Review. *Nutrients* **2021**, *13*, 1586. **[Google Scholar]**

14. Strasser, B.; Pesta, D.; Rittweger, J.; Burtscher, J.; Burtscher, M. Nutrition for Older Athletes: Focus on Sex-Differences. *Nutrients* **2021**, *13*, 1409. **[Google Scholar]**

15. Devrim-Lanpir, A.; Hill, L.; Knechtle, B. Efficacy of Popular Diets Applied by Endurance Athletes on Sports Performance: Beneficial or Detrimental? A Narrative Review. *Nutrients* **2021**, *13*, 491. **[Google Scholar]**

16. Rothschild, J.A.; Kilding, A.E.; Plews, D.J. What Should I Eat before Exercise? Pre-Exercise Nutrition and the Response to Endurance Exercise: Current Prospective and Future Directions. *Nutrients* **2020**, *12*, 3473. **[Google Scholar]**

17. Willingham, B.D.; Ragland, T.J.; Ormsbee, M.J. Betaine Supplementation May Improve Heat Tolerance: Potential Mechanisms in Humans. *Nutrients* **2020**, *12*, 2939. **[Google Scholar]**

18. McKay, A.K.A.; Pyne, D.B.; Burke, L.M.; Peeling, P. Iron Metabolism: Interactions with Energy and Carbohydrate Availability. *Nutrients* **2020**, *12*, 3692. **[Google Scholar]** **[PubMed]**

19. Arazi, H.; Eghbali, E.; Suzuki, K. Creatine Supplementation, Physical Exercise and Oxidative Stress Markers: A Review of the Mechanisms and Effectiveness. *Nutrients* **2021**, *13*, 869.

20. Kasper, A.M.; Langan-Evans, C.; Hudson, J.F.; Brownlee, T.E.; Harper, L.D.; Naughton, R.J.; Morton, J.P.; Close, G.L. Come Back Skinfolds, All Is Forgiven: A Narrative Review of the Efficacy of Common Body Composition Methods in Applied Sports Practice. *Nutrients* **2021**, *13*, 1075.

21. Bone, J.L.; Ross, M.L.; Tomcik, K.C.; Jeacocke, N.A.; McKay, A.K.A.; Burke, L.M. The Validity of Ultrasound Technology in Providing an Indirect Estimate of Muscle Glycogen Concentrations is Equivocal. *Nutrients* **2021**, *13*, 2371.

# 2 Chapter

# THE EFFICACY OF ULTRASOUND TECHNOLOGY IN DELIVERING AN INDIRECT ASSESSMENT OF MUSCLE GLYCOGEN CONCENTRATIONS IS UNCERTAIN

## 1. INTRODUCTION: AN OVERVIEW

The determination of muscle glycogen content is of key interest in sports nutrition due to its roles as a fuel source in athletic performance and a regulator of muscle metabolism and adaptation [**1**,**2**,**3**]. A technique that could achieve reliable and valid measurements, while being inexpensive, portable, and non-invasive, would have an enormous potential for increasing knowledge and enhancing practice, particularly in work involving elite athletes and field conditions. Therefore, there is understandable excitement around the commercialisation of ultrasound technology aimed at measuring muscle glycogen in both laboratory and field situations [**4**,**5**]. Muscle Sound® (Glendale, CO) uses high-frequency ultrasound technology and image analysis from patented cloud-based software to estimate muscle glycogen content from the echogenicity of the image; this feature is based largely on muscle water content, which is presumed to act as a proxy for glycogen [**4**,**5**,**6**]. It was used in research activities to describe changes in muscle glycogen in response to diet and exercise, as well as being a commercially available tool to guide the preparation and recovery of athletes. Extended applications of Muscle Sound® were more recently proposed, including the monitoring of the glycogen status of critically ill patients in hospital intensive care units as a measure of metabolic health [**7**]. Furthermore, ultrasound techniques are being developed as reliable and valid protocols to monitor subcutaneous fat in athletic populations [**8**]. Nevertheless, this review will focus on the use of Muscle Sound® to assess muscle glycogen within sporting populations and scenarios.

Although validation studies have been published [**4**,**5**], incongruous experiences with the use of this tool [**9**] led us to express concerns about a report on glycogen utilisation during a high-level football match using Muscle Sound® technology [**10**]. We questioned the interpretation of these findings, including acknowledgement of data from our own groups, which refute the validity of the Muscle Sound® technique [**11**]. Rebuttal from the study authors [12], which include co-founders of the technique and commercial company, dismissed our concerns based on assertions that the dissenting studies failed to understand the basis of the use of their tool. Furthermore, they noted that only one contradictory dataset is available in the peer-reviewed literature, while the other study remained an unpublished conference presentation [12].

Considering the numerous applications of muscle glycogen assessments in sports nutrition research (such as exploring methods to improve glycogen storage and gaining insights into post-exercise adaptation strategies) and practice (including advising athletes on optimal fueling for competition or achieving varying levels of carbohydrate availability for training objectives), it is crucial to determine whether the Muscle Sound® technique yields valuable and actionable insights or if it may lead to erroneous research findings and unfounded training and dietary practices. This study aims to analyze the existing research about the application of ultrasound technology for measuring muscle glycogen concentrations in athletic populations. To provide a comprehensive overview, we will incorporate the results of the unpublished project, ensuring complete transparency regarding these data and the reasons for their absence from the literature. This data is significant due to the limited amount of studies on muscle glycogen utilizing Muscle Sound® and the autonomous character of our research. Our study uniquely compares biopsy-derived glycogen measurements with the novel estimated fuel level score from Muscle Sound® technology. The projected fuel level is articulated in a company "position stand" as the criterion by which athletes can receive actionable feedback regarding the appropriateness of their dietary and activity regimens [13]. While the original method for estimating muscle glycogen content in arbitrary units was detailed in two validation studies [4,5], we are not aware of any published research that verifies the reliability and validity of the updated technique, as outlined in company literature, intended for practical applications.The projected fuel level is articulated in a company "position stand" as the criterion by which athletes can receive actionable feedback regarding the appropriateness of their dietary and activity regimens [13].While the original method for estimating muscle glycogen content in arbitrary units was detailed in two validation studies [4,5], we are not aware of any published research that verifies the reliability and validity of the updated technique, as outlined in company literature, intended for practical applications. Considering the numerous applications of muscle glycogen assessments in sports nutrition research (such as exploring methods to improve glycogen storage and gaining insights into post-exercise adaptation strategies) and practice (including advising athletes on optimal fueling for competition or achieving varying levels of carbohydrate availability for training objectives), it is crucial to determine whether the Muscle Sound® technique yields valuable and actionable insights or if it may lead to erroneous research findings and unfounded training and dietary practices. This study aims to analyze the existing research about the application of ultrasound technology for measuring muscle glycogen concentrations in athletic populations. To provide a comprehensive overview, we will incorporate the results of the unpublished project, ensuring complete transparency regarding these data and the reasons for their absence from the literature. This data is significant due to the limited amount of studies on muscle glycogen utilizing Muscle Sound® and the autonomous character of our research. Our study uniquely compares biopsy-derived glycogen measurements with the novel estimated fuel level score from Muscle Sound® technology. The projected fuel level is articulated in a company "position stand" as the criterion by which athletes can receive actionable feedback regarding the appropriateness of their dietary and activity regimens [13]. While the original method for estimating muscle glycogen content in arbitrary units was detailed in two validation studies [4,5], we are not aware of any published research that verifies the reliability and validity of the updated technique, as outlined in company literature, intended for practical applications.

## 2. METHODS TO ASSESS MUSCLE GLYCOGEN

Muscle glycogen is an important fuel store for exercise, as well as a key regulator of metabolism within the muscle cell [**2**]. Indeed, the development of methods to measure its presence and location within the muscle cell provided the first major advances in the science and practice of sports nutrition [**14**]. The first measurements of muscle glycogen were made possible by the introduction of the percutaneous biopsy technique to sports science in the late 1960s [**15,16,17**]. Subsequent modification of the technique included the addition of suction to increase the size of the sample collected [**18**] and movement of the location of the muscle site by 2 cm for subsequent biopsies to avoid the artefact of damage from the first [**19**]. This protocol is still used today, and is considered the "gold standard" for assessment of muscle glycogen stores, while acknowledging the invasiveness of the procedure and its downstream limitations on the subjects and environments in which it might be safely and logistically performed. A muscle sample collected by biopsy (typically 20–200 mg according to the size and type of needle) can be treated with several enzymic, histochemical, or electron microscopy procedures to determine the average glycogen content of mixed muscle, the specific glycogen content of fibre types, or the sub cellular location of glycogen, respectively [**20,21,22**]. In particular, validation studies showed that glycogen measurements from a homogenated muscle sample, freeze-dried to remove variables such as the presence of connective tissue and fluctuating cell water content, provides a reliable measure of the glycogen content of the whole muscle under study [**23**].

Notwithstanding the utility of the biopsy technique in allowing an in-depth analysis of glycogen location within and between different muscle fibres, as well as enabling measurement of a vast host of other muscle metabolites, signalling molecules, and other "omic" interests, there is recognition that other techniques are needed to address the practical and ethical concerns associated with its use. The addition of magnetic resonance spectroscopy (MRS) to magnetic resonance imaging, and the increase in the power of the magnetic fields generated by such equipment, has allowed MRS to become an additional tool to indirectly assess muscle metabolites and fuel stores. This technique uses magnetic fields and radio waves to measure tissue glycogen by monitoring either $^{13}$C natural abundance levels, or $^{13}$C atoms incorporated into glycogen following the administration of a $^{13}$C substrate [**20**]. MRS techniques were shown to provide a reliable assessment of muscle glycogen in healthy and clinical populations [24] and have been applied to assessments of glycogen utilisation or storage in athletic populations [25,26]. Although MRS offers the advantages of providing rapid, non-invasive, and potentially repeated measurements of glycogen in various tissues, its disadvantages include the expense and the need to access specialised facilities and expert technicians.

## 3. MUSCLE SOUND® MEASUREMENTS OF MUSCLE GLYCOGEN

Muscle Sound® is a commercially available tool which uses high-frequency ultrasound and patented software to derive an assessment of muscle glycogen. This technique, utilising a point of care device and cloud-based software, offers features that address the disadvantages of both biopsy and MRS-derived assessments of muscle glycogen; namely, it is a protocol that is non-invasive, relatively cheap, rapid, and portable. The original development of Muscle Sound® was undertaken by researcher-practitioners who noted apparent correlations between ultrasound images and muscle glycogen content. The image greyscale produced on an ultrasound scan is based on the intensity of the ultrasound "echogenicity", or reflection of an ultrasound beam, with the beam being both produced and detected by the transducer forming the ultrasound image [27]. Ultrasound beams are reflected at the boundary between two materials with different acoustic impedances, with strong reflections showing as white on the ultrasound image and weaker echoes being grey [27]. Proprietary information within the Muscle Sound® software aligns a darker image with greater glycogen stores using the principal that greater glycogen, and its associated water content in the muscle fibre, should reflect the lower echo intensity between soft tissue and water [5,27]. Conversely, in instances when glycogen is low and there is less fluid, the echo intensity is greater due to the increased visibility of other tissue boundaries, thus resulting in a brighter image [5,27].

The Muscle Sound® technique, validated in two studies against biopsy-derived measures of muscle glycogen [4,5], produces a glycogen score in arbitrary units (hereafter identified as a.u.), where values are provided in bands of 5, between 0 and 100, with an unknown typical error. However, the assumed relationship between muscle glycogen and water was noted as a technical issue requiring further investigation in one of these foundation studies [5]. Indeed, according to an undated company position stand on the science and application of Muscle Sound® located on the company website [13], further developments of the technique recognised scenarios in which muscle glycogen and water deviated from this relationship, and they provided recommendations for situations in which the use of Muscle Sound® is considered optimal and those that are considered to be sub-optimal (see **Section 6.1**). According to this position stand, the current output from the Muscle Sound® proprietary software provides a muscle energy status, representing the mean of an estimated fuel level and a muscle fuel rating. The company material describes muscle fuel as predominantly glycogen, with contributions from carnitine, creatine, and protein. The estimated fuel level is determined by "placing an image in context of the maximum (100) and minimum (0) points of glycogen obtained from a bank of images captured for a specific participant", with the muscle fuel rating providing a separate rating compared to a large databank of images from many athletes [**13**]. We are unaware of any published validation studies of these new metrics, although the company literature promotes these values for field use in providing athletes with feedback about changes in muscle glycogen resulting from their diet and exercise strategies [**13**].

## 4. THE BONE STUDY OF MUSCLE SOUND®

In 2014, we became aware of the newly launched Muscle Sound® tool and realised both its potential to enhance our work as sports nutrition practitioners and applied researchers, and the opportunity to test its reliability and validity as an additional arm within a pre-existing project investigating interactions between manipulations of muscle glycogen and creatine content [**28**]. Although the main aim of the study was to investigate the effect of creatine and glycogen loading on cycling performance, we embedded a research arm to investigate artefacts in the measurement of lean mass by dual energy X-ray absorptiometry due to changes in muscle water content associated with changes in muscle creatine, glycogen, and water content [**29**]. We invited the Muscle Sound® group to use this opportunity to further test their technology in scenarios that are very common in sports, but outside the conditions under which their own validation studies were conducted [**4,5**]. They were not involved in the study design, funding, or conduct; rather, we funded their visit to Australia to train us in the use of their technique. Although we had intended to use our own ultrasound equipment to capture images, IT security requirements at our workplace prevented us from uploading images to a cloud-based server. Therefore, Muscle Sound® loaned us an ultrasound machine and provided complimentary results of muscle glycogen estimates derived from their proprietary software, using the original algorithm, for the duration of the study. A contract was signed to oversee return of the equipment and, on completion of the study, the contribution of our data towards further development of the proprietary algorithm. Following data collection, the equipment was returned, and a poster presentation was prepared for the 2016 annual meeting of the American College of Sports Medicine (ACSM).

In the days prior to the ACSM meeting, we received a directive from a legal firm engaged by Muscle Sound® to withdraw the poster from the conference. Although we complied, an electronic version of the abstract was included in a review of methods to assess muscle glycogen in sports nutrition activities without our involvement [**20**]. To find a path to our ethical obligation to be transparent with all research outcomes via peer-reviewed publication, we subsequently agreed to allow the company to re-analyse the scans from our study using an updated algorithm and interpretation framework. However, recognising the commercial sensitivity of the two datasets, we decided to delay publication until other studies of the validity of the technique, undertaken by independent research groups, but partially funded by Muscle Sound® [**9**], were released. Although the main results of the current study, that Muscle Sound® failed to provide valid estimates of muscle glycogen, are no longer original, the additional range of scenarios that we have studied (supervised CHO loading, prolonged exercise depletion, and the addition of creatine loading) present novel outcomes. Furthermore, they include the only direct comparison of biopsy-derived glycogen assessments and the Muscle Sound® estimated fuel level score, which is promoted in company material [**13**] as a commercially available use of this tool to provide actionable information to athletes about the suitability of their diet and exercise activities. Once published, we will provide the original data to the Muscle Sound® company.

## 4.1. Study Methods

Twelve competitive male cyclists participated in this study, which was approved by the human research ethics committees of the Australian Institute of Sport (20140612) and the Australian Catholic University (2014 254N). These subjects (32.6 ± 5.1 years; 79.2 ± 9.5 kg; 5.1 ± 0.6 L/min maximum oxygen consumption, and 639 ± 115 W maximum power output) represented a sub-group of a larger cohort who undertook the main project under which this study was performed [**28**]. This study employed a parallel group design to investigate the effect of creatine loading, followed by a within-group cross-over application of carbohydrate loading on muscle substrate, water content, and performance (**Figure 1**). The participants came in for four separate biopsy and ultrasound measurements; baseline (day 0, 6 g carbohydrate/kg body mass (BM)/day for 48 h), glycogen depleted (day 1) and either glycogen loaded or glycogen normal (6 g carbohydrate /kg BM/d for 48 h) with or without creatine supplementation (days 7 and 14). Manipulations of creatine and glycogen stores were achieved by implementing "best practice protocols" of creatine loading (20 g/day for 5 days loading and 3 g/ day for maintenance) [**30**] and glycogen loading (12 g CHO/kg BM/day for 48 h) [**31**] through a standardised pre-packaged diet. Furthermore, a supervised cycling protocol of ~3.5 h was undertaken to deplete muscle glycogen stores. The cycling protocol involved a 120 km time trial, with alternating 1 km and 4 km sprints every 10 km, followed by a ride to exhaustion at 8% gradient and 88% $VO_2$max; further details can be found in [**28**]. Participants consumed 60 g/h CHO during the cycling protocol with post-exercise intake of a low CHO diet (<1 g CHO/kg BM) to restrict the repletion of glycogen stores before a further assessment of muscle glycogen content the following morning. This protocol was chosen to allow us to align our assessment of the depleted glycogen condition with DXA-estimates of body composition assessed according to best practice protocols (overnight fasted and rested conditions [**32**]). This study design provided situations where muscle glycogen was measured under baseline and normalised conditions, a depleted condition, and CHO loaded with or without creatine loading. Four biopsies were conducted over the course of the study, with each being collected from the same leg from an incision that was as least 2 cm from the previously biopsied site [**19**] [**Figure 1**: $Bx_1$–$Bx_4$]. The protocol used for these biopsies, and the determination of glycogen and creatine content in the muscle samples, is described in full elsewhere [**28**].

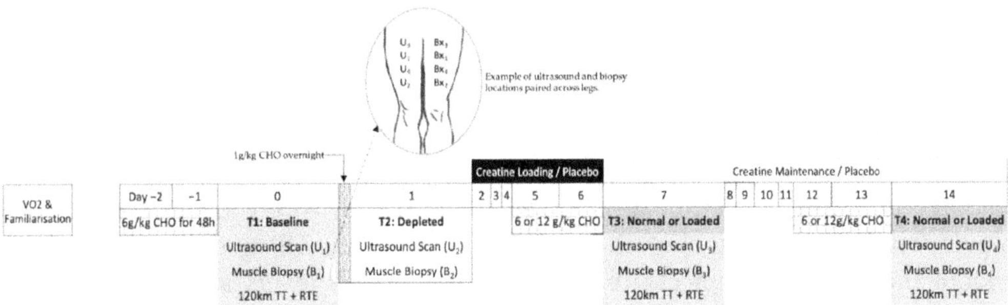


**Figure 1. Overview of study design. (TT, time trial; RTE, ride to exhaustion; ultrasound; and Bx, biopsy).**

## 4.2. Muscle Sound® Score (2015)

Two researchers participating in this study were taught to acquire ultrasound pictures of the vastus lateralis with a portable ultrasound device. The technique was employed to attain satisfactory reliability with repeated pictures, and participants were allocated to the research roster to ensure that each individual was scanned by a single technician during their participation in the study. Thereafter, on each occasion that a muscle biopsy was performed, ultrasound images were captured using the same machine (Terason T3000, TeraTech Corporation, Burlington, MA, USA) and by the same technician. Five ultrasound images were captured at each time-point on the vastus lateralis of the contra-lateral leg, tracking the location of the specific incision on the biopsied leg (**Figure 1**: $U_1$–$U_4$). A further five images were captured on the contra-lateral leg at the site of the original (baseline) assessment (**Figure 1**: $U_1$). The protocol followed Muscle Sound® guidelines with images captured on the transverse plane at a depth of 4 cm and a gain of 45 with the muscle relaxed. The transducer head was manipulated to achieve a bright fascia, which defined the muscle boundary for the region of interest. Images were then uploaded to the Muscle Sound® software (v.2015, Muscle Sound®, LLC, Denver, CO, USA) and processed according to their proprietary protocols. The Muscle Sound® score (0–100) was subsequently provided in arbitrary units (a.u.), noting that such scores were provided in bands of 5 a.u. [**5**]. A single score used in the statistical analysis was obtained by averaging the score from each of the five images at each site.

## 4.3. Estimated Fuel Level (2017)

The ultrasound images were re-analysed by Muscle Sound® using an updated protocol titled "estimated fuel level". Details of this proprietary process were not published, but are described as "placing an image in context of the maximum (100) and minimum (0) points of glycogen obtained from a bank of images captured for a specific participant [**13**]". We have described these values as "points" to distinguish them from the original metrics (described as a.u.).

## 4.4. Statistical Analysis

Agreements between biopsy results and Muscle Sound® projected fuel level scores were evaluated using a 95% intra-class correlation based on a one-way consistency model [33]. Pearson's correlations were employed to ascertain the relationship between site-specific measures. The concentration of muscle glycogen in various stages was evaluated utilizing a general linear mixed model (LMM) with the R package lme4 (R Foundation for Statistical Computing, Vienna, Austria). All models incorporated a random intercept for subjects to account for baseline levels and inter-individual uniformity. Furthermore, creatine dry weight was incorporated as a covariate in all models. Each model was estimated utilizing restricted maximum likelihood, and the statistical significance of the fixed effects was assessed through type II Wald tests employing Kenward–Roger degrees of freedom. Tukey's post hoc comparisons were conducted to identify specific condition differences where substantial fixed effects were observed.

4.5. Results

Figure 2 summarizes the effects of various dietary treatments on biopsy-derived muscle glycogen concentrations, Muscle Sound® scores, predicted fuel level points, and the impact of placebo and creatine supplementation. These data represent measurements taken on one leg using the established protocol to site sequential muscle biopsies ($B_1$–$B_4$), with the Muscle Sound® score being taken on the contra-lateral leg at the corresponding site ($U_1$–$U_4$). There was a significant main effect for the different dietary treatments on biopsy-derived muscle glycogen concentrations ($F(3,29) = 61.2$, $p < 0.001$). Values of biopsy-derived glycogen concentrations for glycogen depletion were lower than baseline, CHO loaded, and normal conditions ($p < 0.001$), while values for carbohydrate loading were significantly greater than normal ($p = 0.013$). Since there were no differences in muscle glycogen between the creatine and placebo groups ($F(1,10) = 0.1$; $p = 0.760$), a combined mean value for the results for each treatment was derived. Nevertheless, creatine dry weight was a significant variable within the model, indicating that higher creatine dry weight values were associated with increased muscle glycogen content ($F(1,33) = 8.6$; $p = 0.006$).

There were no differences in Muscle Sound® scores between dietary treatments ($F(3,27) = 1.1$; $p = 0.384$) or between the placebo and creatine groups ($F(1,10) = 0.3$; $p = 0.627$). Furthermore, no statistically significant differences between dietary treatments ($F(3,28) = 1.1$; $p = 0.352$) or between the placebo and creatine groups ($F(1,10) = 0.2$; $p = 0.701$) were evident for the estimated fuel level points. Finally, creatine dry weight was not associated with either Muscle Sound® ($F(1,28) = 2.04$; $p = 0.165$) or estimated fuel level points ($F(1,37) = 3.07$; $p = 0.088$). An ICC of −0.75 (95% CI −0.85, −0.59) was apparent in the relationship between biopsy-derived muscle glycogen content and Muscle Sound® scores, with a similarly unclear relationship between biopsy-derived muscle glycogen content and estimated fuel level points (ICC of −0.72 (95% CI −0.83, −0.55)). The estimated fuel level points were quantitatively higher than the Muscle

Sound® score, reflecting an amplification of the original values from an absolute value to a relative range.

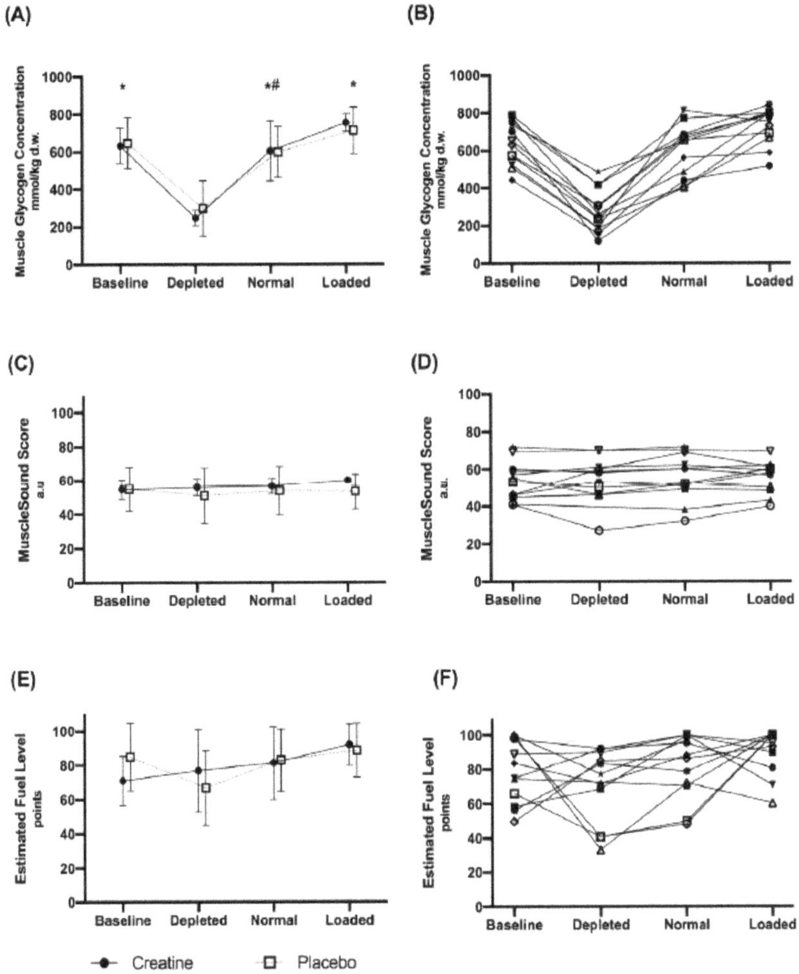


**Figure 2. Biopsy-derived muscle glycogen concentrations (A,B) Muscle Sound® scores in arbitrary units (C,D) and estimated fuel level points (E,F) for the creatine and placebo conditions during each dietary treatment: baseline, glycogen depleted, normal and carbohydrate loaded. Values are mean ± SD in panels A, C and E with individual data shown in panels B, D and F. * Indicates a significant difference to depleted. # Indicates a significant difference to loaded.**

There were no differences between the Muscle Sound® score values collected from the site on the contra-lateral leg corresponding to the biopsy site ($U_1$–$U_4$) and the measurements taken on a static site of the leg ($U_1$) for each treatment. Indeed, there was a significant correlation ($r = 0.87$ (95% CI: 0.78–0.93); $p < 0.001$) between the values from the two different sites (**Figure** 3A). Likewise, there were no between-site differences in the values of estimated fuel level points for each treatment, but the correlation between these values was lower (**Figure** 3B; ($r = 0.63$ (0.42–0.78); $p < 0.001$)). A separate examination of the results of Muscle Sound® scores taken at the same site (U1) showed a small but significant ($p$ = 0.024) difference between depleted (53 ± 13 a.u.) and loaded treatments (57 ± 10 a.u.). However, these did not differ from baseline (56 ± 3 a.u.) or normal (57 ±12 a.u.) values. Furthermore, the numerical difference between the mean values was smaller than the gradation (bands of 5 a.u.) between sequential results. The estimated fuel level points mirrored these outcomes with an increased spread in both the mean values and SD. Differences were detected between depleted (59 ± 30) and loaded (91 ± 14) treatments ($p$ = 0.026), but neither of these differed from the baseline (78 ± 19) or normal (77 ± 22) values.

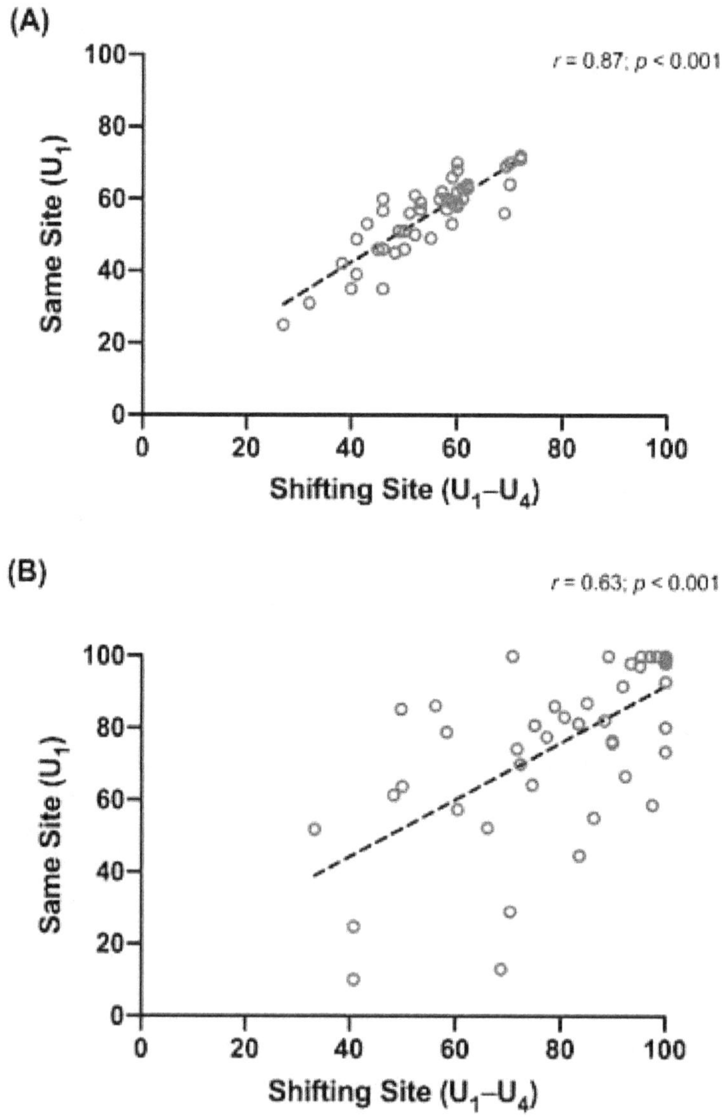


**Figure 3. Correlation between values for Muscle Sound® score (A) and the estimated fuel level (B) measured at the same site ($U_1$) and at the shifting site ($U1_1$–$U_4$) corresponding to the muscle biopsy.**

## 5. THE LITERATURE PERTAINING TO MUSCLE SOUND® EVALUATION OF MUSCLE GLYCOGEN

Table 1 presents a summary of the existing literature utilizing Muscle Sound® technology to evaluate alterations in muscle glycogen levels due to food and exercise treatments. This encompasses the validation studies that initially established Muscle Sound® as a surrogate for biopsy-derived muscle glycogen measurements [4,5], two additional datasets where muscle glycogen levels and their variations were evaluated through ultrasound and chemical methods [9], the Bone data presented herein, and a recently published investigation that utilized Muscle Sound® exclusively to monitor alterations in muscle glycogen content during an exercise session [10]. The final publication utilizing the newly estimated fuel level metric is absent from this table due to variations in focus and approach; nevertheless, it is incorporated in the discussions.

M, male; a.u., arbitrary units; Bx, biopsy; U, Ultrasound scan; ASIS, anterior superior iliac spine; @, at; CHO, carbohydrates; $VO_2max$, maximal oxygen capacity; NA, not available; PPO, peak power output; NS, not significant; and EFL, estimated fuel level; * All biopsy-derived glycogen values presented as mmol/kg dry weight (dw), with conversion from mmol/L wet weight (ww) involving multiplication by 4.28 [**34**].

Although laboratory-based cycling protocols represent the most frequently investigated mode of exercise, several studies have included real-world competition involving field-based team sports (see **Table 1**). Dietary manipulations include low, moderate, and high CHO intakes, as well as creatine loading. Muscle and body water content, although not directly measured in any of these studies, is likely to be altered by the acute effects of exercise as well as exercise-associated dehydration. Although vastus lateralis was the muscle investigated in the majority of studies, differences in study protocols around the Muscle Sound® assessment included muscle tension (relaxed vs. contracted), whether the same or contra-lateral leg was used between or within glycogen-assessment protocols, whether the scan was meant to represent the same or a related muscle site, and how many scans were used to derive the Muscle Sound® outcome.

**Table 1. Studies involving ultrasound (Muscle Sound®) measurements of muscle glycogen, including comparison to biopsy-derived chemical assessments of glycogen.**

| | Hill & San-Millan 2014 | Nieman et al., 2015 | Routledge et al., 2019a | Routledge et al., 2019b | San-Millan et al., 2020 | Bone et al., 2020 |
|---|---|---|---|---|---|---|
| Study population | 22 M cyclists (competitive: professional and amateur: category 1–4) | 20 M cyclists (regular competitors in road and TT: $VO_2$max: 47.9 ± 7.8 mL/kg/min) | 14 M rugby league players (professional) | 16 M recreationally active VO2max 49.9 ± 7.5 mL/kg/min | 9 M soccer players: (professional: U.S. major soccer league) | 12 M cyclists/triathletes (well-trained: VO2max 64.5 ± 7.6 mL/kg/min) |
| Scenarios of glycogen measurement | Pre-exercise: CHO loaded<br>Post exercise depletion (endurance cycling) | Pre-exercise: normalised glycogen?<br>Post exercise depletion (endurance cycling) | Pre-exercise: normalised glycogen?<br>Post-exercise depletion (field: team sport) | Pre-exercise: normalised glycogen<br>Post-exercise: substantial depletion<br>CHO loaded | Pre-exercise: normalised glycogen?<br>Post exercise depletion (field: team sport) | Pre-exercise: normalised CHO<br>Pre-exercise: maximally CHO loaded<br>Pre-exercise: normalised CHO + creatine loaded<br>Pre-exercise: CHO loaded and creatine loaded<br>Post-exercise: substantial deletion |
| Dietary protocols (CHO intake) | Glycogen preparation: "optimized" via 3 days @ 8 g/kg<br>Pre-exercise meal: NA<br>During exercise: NA (self-managed with instructions) | Glycogen preparation: NA<br>Pre-exercise meal: NA<br>During exercise: water only | Glycogen preparation: NA<br>Pre-exercise: NA<br>During exercise: water only | Supervised exercise depletion followed by either 36 h of low CHO (2 g/kg) or high CHO (8 g/kg) | Glycogen preparation: "24 h team nutrition protocols"; pre-exercise meal: "team nutrition"; during exercise: 40 g at warm up and 65 g at half time | Glycogen preparation: Normalised: 48 h @ 6 g/kg CHO loaded: 48 h @ 12 g/kg Pre-exercise meal: 2 g/kg During exercise: 60 g/h Depletion: 18 h @ 1 g/kg |

| | Hill & San-Millan 2014 | Nieman et al., 2015 | Routledge et al., 2019a | Routledge et al., 2019b | San-Millan et al., 2020 | Bone et al., 2020 |
|---|---|---|---|---|---|---|
| Exercise protocol | 90 min cycling on lode ergometer at "moderate-high intensity eliciting CHO oxidation rates of 2–3 g/min." | 75 km (~168 min) TT on own bike mounted on ergometer | 80 min rugby league match | Glycogen depletion cycling protocol: 90%/50% PPO and 80%/60% PPO until exhaustion (* low CHO trial: extra 45 min at 60% PPO). | 90 min soccer match. | 120 km TT (alternating 1 and 4 km sprints every 10 km) + TTE on cycle at 8% gradient and 88% $VO_2$max. |
| Timing of glycogen measure-ments | Baseline: immediately before exercise Post-exercise: NA | Baseline: NA Post-exercise: within 20–30 min | Baseline: 60 min pre-match. Post-exercise: within 40 min. | Post-exercise: NA Depleted: 36 h after exercise + low CHO CHO loaded: 36 h after exercise + high CHO | Baseline: 10 min before warm-up. Post-exercise: within 5–10 min | Pre-exercise: 2 h prior to exercise (e.g., before pre-exercise meal) Depleted ~18 h post exercise + low CHO |
| Muscle assessed | Rectus Femoris (U and Bx)<br>U on Vastus lateralis: (data not provided) | Vastus lateralis<br>Rectus Femoris | Vastus lateralis | Vastus lateralis | Rectus femoris (U only) | Vastus lateralis |
| Muscle state | Contracted | Not advised | Relaxed | Relaxed | NA | Relaxed |
| Muscle biopsy location | Baseline Bx on right leg. Post-exercise Bx on left leg. Mid-point between ASIS to superior patellar. Same location as ultra-sound | Baseline and post-exercise Bx on same leg 2 cm apart Same location as ultrasound | Baseline and post-exercise Bx on same leg 2 cm apart | Bx for low and high CHO dietary conditions on same leg 1–2 cm apart | Nil | Bx on same leg. Mid-point between ASIS and anterior superior aspect of patella. Four sites 2 cm apart (see **Figure 1**) |

| | Hill & San-Millan 2014 | Nieman et al., 2015 | Routledge et al., 2019a | Routledge et al., 2019b | San-Millan et al., 2020 | Bone et al., 2020 |
|---|---|---|---|---|---|---|
| Ultrasound location | Same leg as Bx. Baseline U on right leg. Post-exercise U on left leg | Same leg as Bx | Same leg as Bx. 50% of length and width of VL determined by U | Same leg and same site as Bx. 50% of length and width of VL determined by U | NA—same leg used for pre- and post-U scans? | U on contralateral leg (1) at corresponding location to muscle biopsy (at each of 4 sites—**Figure 1**) |
| Ultrasound Scan protocol | NA | Mean of 3 scans | NA | NA | Mean of 2 scans | Mean of 5 scans |
| Glycogen data * | Bx: Glycogen (mmol/kg dw) reduced from 416 ± 146 to 267 ± 98 by exercise ($p < 0.001$). U: Muscle Sound® score (a.u.) reduced from 59.8 ± 15.9 to 39.8 ± 13.9 post-exercise ($p < 0.0001$) | Bx: Glycogen (mmol/kg dw) showed mean change of 306 ± 99 * due to exercise (~407 to 101) ($p < 0.001$). U: baseline and post-exercise glycogen score data not provided | Bx: Glycogen (mmol/kg dw) reduced from 443 ± 65 to 271 ± 94 ($p < 0.0001$) by exercise. U: no change in Muscle Sound® score from baseline (47 ± 6 a.u.) to post-exercise (49 ± 8 a.u.; $p = 0.4$) | Bx: Glycogen (mmol/kg dw) with high dietary CHO: 531 ± 129 vs. low CHO dietary intake: 252 ± 64 ($p < 0.001$). U: Muscle Sound® score (a.u.) with high dietary CHO: 56 ± 7 vs. low dietary CHO intake: 54 ± 6 ($p = 0.3$) | Bx: No biopsy conducted. U: Muscle Sound® score ("points") decreased from 80 ± 8.6 to 63.9 ± 10.2. ($p = 0.005$) | Bx: Glycogen (mmol/kg dw) reduced from 639 ± 115 to 276 ± 115 with depletion and increased with CHO loading to: 730 ± 98 ($p < 0.05$) U: Muscle Sound® score (a.u.): 55 ± 10 (baseline); 52 ± 13 (depletion) and 56 ± 8 (CHO loaded), NS. U: EFL (points): 79 ± 18 (baseline); 70 ± 22 (depletion) and 90 ± 14 points (CHO loading), NS. |

The first two publications involving Muscle Sound® were designed to directly validate its use for indirect assessment of muscle glycogen concentrations, measuring glycogen content before and after a 90 min steady-state [**4**] or ~158 min time-trial cycling protocol [**5**] at the same or a similar site in the chosen muscle. In both studies, the ultrasound scan and subsequent biopsy were undertaken at the same site, with the ultrasound being conducted first, followed by the collection of the biopsy, guided by the ultrasound. In the first study [**4**], one leg was used for the pre-exercise assessment, while the contra-lateral leg was used in the same manner for the post-exercise assessment to avoid the effect of the muscle biopsy on subsequent glycogen storage at that muscle site [**19**]. In the second study, the same leg was used for both assessments, but the second biopsy was taken at a site 2 cm from the first; this is sufficient to avoid the effects of such muscle damage on glycogen content, at least by the biopsy technique [**19**]. With the longer cycling protocol, Nieman et al. reported significant correlations between the two measurement techniques for pre- (0.92, $p < 0.001$), post- (0.90, $p < 0.001$), and exercise-associated changes (0.92, $p < 0.001$) in glycogen concentrations in the vastus lateralis muscle [**5**]. Here, the chemical method showed a reduction in muscle glycogen content by 77 ± 17%, representing an absolute change of ~71 mmol/kg ww (~306 mmol/kg dw) glycogen; the absolute scores on the Muscle Sound® 0–100 a.u. rating were not provided [**5**]. These data represent a more practical and representative examination of glycogen utilisation during a prolonged endurance sport than the earlier study of Hill and San Millan [**4**], which employed a 90 min cycling protocol and biopsy collection from the infrequently studied rectus femoris muscle. Indeed, in the earlier study, absolute glycogen values achieved by the dietary preparation protocol and their subsequent utilisation during exercise were lower, with muscle glycogen being reduced by 36% according to chemical analysis and a Muscle Sound® change score of ~60 to ~40 a.u. (33% decrease). Nevertheless, correlations between the chemical and ultrasound-mediated assessments of muscle glycogen concentration had pre- (0.92, $p < 0.001$), post- (0.90, $p < 0.001$), and exercise-associated changes (0.92, $p < 0.001$) [**4**].

In contrast to these earlier reports, an investigation of two separate exercise scenarios by another research group failed to find consistency between the Muscle Sound® scores and biopsy-derived assessments of muscle glycogen changes due to exercise and diet [**9**]. In these studies, which involved cycling and a rugby league match, measurements were made on the same leg, with the biopsy sites 2 cm apart [**9**]. Although the muscle biopsy protocol identified a ~40% reduction in glycogen content as a result of match play in a real-world rugby league competition (pre-game: 443 ± 65 and post-game: 271 ± 94 mmol/kg dry weight (dw), $p < 0.001$), there were no changes in the Muscle Sound ® scores (47 ± 6 vs. 49 ± 7, $p = 0.4$).

A separate study, involving a cycling protocol, was undertaken to remove any potential confounding effects associated with the characteristics of rugby play (i.e., intermittent nature and the magnitude of the muscle contractile forces) that might interfere with the ultrasound image and explain the discrepant results. This second investigation involved an exercise-depletion protocol after which either a low carbohydrate diet or a carbohydrate loading regimen was implemented for 36 h [**9**]. Although biopsy-derived muscle glycogen concentrations after the carbohydrate loading diet were more than doubled in comparison to 36 h of low carbohydrate recovery (~531 vs. 252 mmol/kg dw, **Table 1**), there were no differences ($p = 0.9$) in corresponding Muscle Sound® scores (56 ± 7 vs. 54 ± 6 a.u.). In summary, two separate studies of different types of exercise failed to find significant correlations between changes in muscle glycogen concentration and changes in Muscle Sound® scores, and, in both protocols, the ultrasound results failed to detect what could be considered predicable changes in glycogen stores.

The results of the Bone study, presented in this paper, are in agreement with the latter two datasets in finding that the Muscle Sound® technique failed to provide meaningful information about muscle glycogen concentrations in athletes. The mean values for muscle glycogen derived from chemical analysis of mixed muscle samples showed larger ranges than reported in the comparative literature, with pre-exercise values after a glycogen loading technique of ~730 mmol/kg wet weight (ww) and a post-exercise reduction of ~364 mmol/kg ww. These values reflect the more aggressive CHO loading regimen and the demanding nature of the exercise protocol. Despite a greater opportunity to detect differences in muscle glycogen, we found that the original Muscle Sound® technique generally failed to track the results achieved by chemical analysis of mixed muscle biopsy samples across a range of diet and exercise manipulations, and failed to show the expected significant changes in glycogen concentrations. Individual data showed a range of responses, both in magnitude and direction, in response to each treatment (**Figure 2**). The only Muscle Sound® comparison that yielded a statistically significant difference involved measurements taken from the same site between the depleted and loaded treatments. However, in the case of the original scoring system, the difference was numerically small (53 ± 13 vs. 57 ± 10 a.u.) and was less than the band (5 a.u.) by which results were provided, rendering it of minimal clinical value. Furthermore, this analysis failed to detect differences between the normal glycogen stores and treatments that either increased or decreased these. The estimated fuel level, an updated Muscle Sound® metric representing results relative to the lowest and highest scores for the individual athlete, mirrored these results. Although this metric amplified the numerical value of the original score results, and created a greater difference between the mean values, it also increased the range of the results. Therefore, it failed to change the ability of the protocol to detect differences between most treatments.

Two additional publications, which involved the use of Muscle Sound® to investigate changes in muscle glycogen in scenarios of real-life sports without alternative confirmation of glycogen stores, are available. One study [**10**] involved an investigation of changes in muscle glycogen during a football (soccer) match in a professional American league (**Table 1**). Players followed their typical nutrition practices before and during the match, while the Muscle Sound® technique was used to assess glycogen stores pre- and post-game. From the methodology described in the paper, we assumed this protocol involved the traditional Muscle Sound® score technique, albeit with results presented as "points", rather than the new metrics described in the company's position stand [13]. There was no confirmation of these results with an independent chemical measurement of glycogen, nor was the hydration status of the players measured before or after the match. Nevertheless, the study reported a mean decline in Muscle Sound® glycogen scores of 20% over the course of the match, with inter-individual ranges of 6% to 44%, and some variability in the size of the pre-game stores. As predicted, but not verified by information on individual workload characteristics of the specific game, the decline in muscle glycogen points was numerically greater in midfield and forward players than defence players, and was lowest in the goal keeper. Although these results appear unremarkable, the authors suggested that the protocol identified players who had not adequately fuelled prior to the game, as well as players who might undertake more aggressive fuelling strategies during the game. Here, we note that if within-game fuelling provides an additional exogenous fuel source as glycogen stores become depleted, rather than substantially changing patterns of glycogen depletion during the match, the pre- and post-measurement of glycogen by any technique may provide confusing results.

The final publication involved the use of Muscle Sound® to monitor resting levels of glycogen in U.S. Division 1 collegiate female volleyball players on each morning of a 9 day pre-season training camp [35]. The Muscle Sound® information was provided in the form of muscle fuel rating, which, as previously noted, remains unvalidated in a peer-reviewed published format. This investigation focused on bilateral asymmetries in the glycogen stores in the rectus femoris in these athletes prior to each morning's training session. The study reported an increase in muscle fuel ratings from the first to second day, with a sustained elevation over the rest of the camp and a 58% difference (higher level) between ratings for the dominant versus non-dominant leg. Although the temporal changes did not track with the training load over the camp (higher in the first days), the authors noted that no dietary control or assessment was implemented. The difference in fuel ratings between legs was attributed to faster rates of glycogen storage in "the more conditioned" dominant leg. Although endurance-trained muscle is known to have higher resting glycogen stores than non-trained muscle (e.g., 500 vs. 350 mmol/kg dw [36]), it is difficult to imagine that the magnitude of difference between legs within the same well-trained athlete would be as large as reported, albeit with a different assessment metric (muscle fuel rating of 52 vs. 33 points). The authors suggested that bilateral asymmetries in glycogen content in volleyball athletes might be used to assess for injury risk, noting that large asymmetries and bilateral deficits in muscle strength are sometimes linked to injuries in athletes [35]. Although this would be a potentially valuable application, there is presently no validation of either the muscle fuel rating score as a measure of muscle glycogen, whether glycogen utilisation patterns are sufficiently different between limbs across a range of symmetrical and asymmetrical exercise activities detected by any technique, nor whether this is associated with injury risk or patterns.

In conclusion, the evidence endorsing the efficacy of ultrasound technology, namely the Muscle Sound® patented approach, as a reliable indicator of muscle glycogen levels is inconclusive. As a research instrument, two data sets from laboratory cycling protocols confirmed a correlation with glycogen content measurements from a biopsy-derived mixed muscle sample, yielding muscle glycogen levels ranging from 0 to 100 in arbitrary units under controlled conditions. Moreover, the alterations in muscle glycogen reserves aligned with the anticipated results of diverse dietary and exercise regimens. A separate data set obtained in a field situation yielded glycogen score results that were coherent, however not independently validated. Three other data sets pertaining to laboratory and field applications, however, contradict these conclusions. Two studies conducted under controlled laboratory circumstances in cycling models, together with another conducted during an actual team sport competition, did not reveal connections between the two sources of data regarding glycogen storage. Crucially, none of these data sets reliably identified variations in Muscle Sound® scores, despite controlled alterations in food and exercise that are recognized to produce significant changes. In one of these investigations, a novel method for presenting Muscle Sound® results, outlined in a company-issued position statement and assumed to reflect its current commercial applicability, likewise failed to identify outcomes anticipated by the study interventions. This transpired despite adherence to standardized protocols (e.g., employing a singular trained tester, maintaining laboratory conditions, and averaging five distinct scans) that may not be feasible in the real-world scenarios for which it is advocated. Two primary concerns about the validity and reliability of the Muscle Sound® approach have been identified for examination.

## 6. VALIDITY OF THE MUSCLE SOUND® TECHNIQUE: THE GLYCOGEN: WATER RATIO

### 6.1. General Principles

The Muscle Sound® technique is based on the principle that the echogenicity or brightness of an ultrasound image reflects the speed of the sound waves reflected by scanned tissues, and in turn, their water content [**10,12**]. Water, which provides little resistance, produces a dark (hypoechoic) image that can be quantified via the pixel intensity of the image on the scan image [**10,12**]. In turn, muscle glycogen is quantified by the assumption of a constant relationship with bound water of 1:3 [**10,12**]. Such calculations are achieved when an image captured by a high-frequency ultrasound is examined by the cloud-based proprietary software of the Muscle Sound® company.

Although it is well accepted that fluid is stored when glycogen is formed, the persistence of a fixed relationship over a range of glycogen concentrations has been challenged both in the general literature and in relation to the Muscle Sound® protocol [**9,10,11,12,37,38**]. The first validation study of Muscle Sound® [**4**] did not identify the water to muscle glycogen ratio as an underpinning principle of the ultrasound technique; this explanation was provided in the subsequent validation study. Here, although a tight correlation between ultrasound and biopsy-derived measures of muscle glycogen was reported, the authors noted that "additional research is needed to determine how exercise-induced changes in muscle water content influence this relationship". Indeed, knowledge of factors that change the muscle glycogen to water ratio, or muscle water content, formed the basis of our recent letter expressing concerns around the Muscle Sound® technology **[11]**, wherein we noted that these can change in variable directions as a result of diet-exercise manipulations. The literature on this issue will now be summarised.

Studies on the relationship between tissue water and glycogen content were undertaken in both the liver and muscle in humans and rodents. In the latter case, direct chemical analysis of whole tissues was used to calculate a glycogen:water ratio of 1:2.7 in rat livers under conditions where non-glycogen solids remained constant **[6]**. However, Sherman et al. **[37]** failed to find a consistent ratio of glycogen and water in rat skeletal muscle when manipulations to both increase and decrease glycogen content were undertaken. Meanwhile, studies on human subjects are limited to protocols using indirect or sampling measurements. An early investigation of carbohydrate loading **[38]** measured muscle glycogen concentrations in arm and leg biopsy samples, while using changes in body mass, body water derived from a tritium dilution, and muscle mass derived from potassium measurements to estimate a glycogen to water ratio ranging from 1:3 to 1:5. Caveats noted by the authors included the uncertainties of the measurements and the inability to measure the site of the water storage **[38]**. An updated version of this study, using bio-electric impedance (BIS) to measure body water and MRS to measure muscle glycogen, calculated an increase in intra-cellular water that aligned with a 1:4 ratio **[39]**. Despite modern techniques, issues related to the precision of measurement and the nature of the increase in body water remain. Furthermore, these studies have involved conditions in which fluid availability was optimised while muscle glycogen stores were manipulated.

Various scenarios can occur in which tissue water changes independently of changes in glycogen stores. Indeed, ultrasound technology was proposed as a technique to monitor tissue hydration in athletes **[40]**, particularly as a marker of dehydration in athletes in weight-making sports **[41]**. Early understandings of muscle glycogen synthesis theorised that the associated water storage might play a regulatory role in this process. However, a study of post-exercise muscle restoration over a 15 h period found that cyclists who were dehydrated by ~5% BM or 8% body water had similar glycogen synthesis, but lower muscle water content than the trial in which they were euhydrated during recovery **[42]**. Meanwhile, Fernandez-Elias et al. investigated changes in the glycogen and water content of muscle samples collected over 4 h of recovery from strenuous exercise, reporting a ratio of 1:3 when the subjects were dehydrated (replacing only 400 mL fluid) and 1:17 when a volume equal to the total fluid deficit (~3170 mL) was consumed **[43]**. It was noted that these calculations included all water in the muscle rather than that bound to the glycogen.

Other muscle solutes, including elements that can be acutely changed, contribute to its osmotic environment. It is well documented that rapid creatine supplementation protocols are associated with an increase (~1 kg) in body mass that is largely attributed to a gain in body water [44,45,46]. Results from the larger study from which the Bone Muscle Sound® data were collected included a 6% increase in muscle creatine concentrations and a 22% increase in muscle glycogen when their respective loading protocols were undertaken according to best practice principles [29]. The corresponding changes in total body water and intracellular water, measured via BIS, were 1.3% and 1.4% (creatine loaded), and 2.3% and 2.2% (glycogen loaded), respectively [29]. It is possible, therefore, that changes in muscle creatine, and its associated effect on muscle water, contributed to failure of the Muscle Sound® to accurately track the changes in muscle glycogen stores. Indeed, we showed that these changes in muscle water, creatine, and glycogen confounded the measurement of body composition via dual X-ray absorptiometry in this study, due to a violation of the assumptions of normal relationships between these body characteristics [29].

The existence of a stable correlation between muscle glycogen and water is not substantiated, as ample research indicates that numerous conditions, commonly encountered in sports, can independently influence one or both variables. Theoretically, even if the Muscle Sound® approach is accurately calibrated to assess muscle glycogen based on a specific glycogen:water ratio under certain conditions, it will be rendered worthless in scenarios where this precise ratio is absent. While additional research addressing these varying conditions may improve the algorithms connecting ultrasound images to glycogen measurements, the extensive array of potential scenarios necessitating examination is likely to complicate the achievement and integration of this process into calculations. Without such knowledge, it is challenging to accurately ascertain the conditions in which the assumptions underpinning the present Muscle Sound® approach may hold true. While these criteria were not explicitly examined or recognized in the published research about the Muscle Sound® approach, the position statement on the company's website delineates the circumstances in which its application is optimal and sub-optimal (Table 2). These situations seem to intersect and encompass certain, but not all, of the scenarios previously recognized in which glycogen-to-water ratios may be modified.

**Table 2. Scenarios of use of Muscle Sound® measurement of muscle glycogen *.**

| Optimal Scenarios | Sub-Optimal Scenarios |
|---|---|
| • Pre and immediately post-exercise<br>• Several hours after the end of moderate to high intensity/long duration exercise (such as cycling that does not involve extensive eccentric contractions)<br>• One to two days or more after high intensity/long duration sports such as soccer, football, rugby, and basketball<br>• One to two days before a competition | • Within several hours of the end of moderate to high intensity/moderate duration steady state exercise<br>• The day after high intensity/long duration competition in sports such as soccer, football, rugby, and basketball |

* Information taken from Muscle Sound® position stand on Science and Application [13].

## 6.2. Targeted Critique of Research Lacking Evidence for the Validity of Muscle Sound®

Data sets where a Muscle Sound® evaluation of muscle glycogen content did not align with measurements obtained from chemical analysis of biopsy-derived muscle were criticized for introducing variables that disrupted the muscles' water balance. Concerns were expressed about the rugby league match study, highlighting that the methodology indicated data collecting took place "within 40 minutes of the game's conclusion." It was claimed that this interval could have facilitated the occurrence of artifacts, including muscle microtrauma resulting from physical activities, post-exercise glycogen synthesis from lactate, and inadequate regulation of fluid intake during recovery. [**12**]. Support for these statements was provided from studies which observed fluid shifts when >3 L of fluid was consumed over 4 h of recovery [**43**], or low rates of glycogen synthesis (1–2 mmol/kg ww/h) in recovery from high-intensity exercise in the absence of carbohydrate intake [**47**]. However, it was also noted that the recently published study of glycogen use in a soccer match failed to describe the post-exercise assessment, other than that it was "immediately" after the game. No information was provided about hydration status prior to the match nor fluid intake during the match in this study, although other investigations of elite soccer players have noted that individual players may commence a match in various states of fluid balance, including significant dehydration, and incur variable rates of sweat loss during a match [**48,49**]. Therefore, it is curious to propose differences in tolerances to such potentially confounding factors between essentially similar studies. Although the presence of some confounding factors was acknowledged in both studies, it was noted that if the Muscle Sound® technique was to be promoted for use in real-life sport, it needs to be sufficiently robust to tolerate the practical conditions of use (a likely short interval between the cessation of exercise and access to each athlete to undertake assessments).

The cycling procedures utilized in the Bone study and the research conducted by Routledge et al. [9] conformed to the ideal conditions for employing Muscle Sound® assessments, incorporating regulation of fluid intake and hydration status.We determined that creatine supplementation may alter glycogen reserves and muscle hydration; this prompted our interest in investigating Muscle Sound® under these settings.This technique did not identify any differences in glycogen assessments between the creatine and placebo groups across all treatments, nor did it reveal differences between baseline and depleted treatments for the entire participant cohort prior to the initiation of creatine supplementation.Consequently, it does not seem to offer a singular or primary artifact elucidating the inadequacy of the Muscle Sound® technique in evaluating muscle glycogen content in our investigation.

# 7. VALIDITY OF THE MUSCLE SOUND® TECHNIQUE: LOCATION OF THE MUSCLE SITE

## *7.1. General Principles*

The two original validation studies of the Muscle Sound® technique [**4,5**] used protocols that allowed the biopsy to be taken from the identical site on which the image was captured. Meanwhile, as previously identified (**Table 1**), the outlying studies ([**9**] and the Bone study presented here) took care to standardise the sites from which both ultrasound images and biopsy samples were collected, but used different sites from the same muscle between and within treatments to accommodate best practice associated with the collection of sequential muscle biopsies. A key premise of the Muscle Sound® protocol, at least in research scenarios, was that the location of the image for sequential assessments or comparison with biopsy assessments must be identical. However, much of the extended commentary about the protocol [**10**], and the specific criticisms of studies which found it did not provide a valid assessment of muscle glycogen [**12**], misunderstood or misrepresented the larger literature on the assessment of muscle glycogen. Specifically, comments about the variability of glycogen within muscle [**10,12**] demonstrated a failure to understand the capability of various assessments techniques.

This review has identified that all studies of muscle glycogen in humans utilised indirect and sampling techniques. The basis of such sampling, which occurred in both of the original Muscle Sound® validation studies, is that a small piece of muscle collected in a biopsy needle or captured in an ultrasound image includes sufficient muscle fibres to represent the aggregated features of individual fibres. Indeed, both the Muscle Sound® score and the chemical analysis of a biopsy sample represent the characteristics of "mixed muscle". Enhanced techniques of analysing biopsy samples include histochemical staining techniques to identify differences in the storage and utilisation of glycogen between different types of muscle fibres [**50**], and, more recently, electron microscopy of single fibres identified different sub-cellular locations of glycogen particles [**21,22,51,52**]. Such techniques have helped to understand exercise metabolism and mechanisms of fatigue during exercise. However, ultrasound techniques, just like chemical assessments of homogenates or mixed muscle samples, cannot achieve such a granular assessment. Rather, they provide an overarching, yet still valuable, perspective of muscle fuel stores. In the case of muscle biopsies, there is a specific reason to require and validate the use of different sites for sequential biopsy samples; subsequent biopsies need to be taken from muscle that has not had its glycogen storage capacity impaired by trauma from the first biopsy [**19**]. However, it was shown that differences in the glycogen content of mixed muscle samples, representing the average of a large number of individual muscle fibres from a number of individual sites across a muscle, are minor [**23**]. We acknowledge that the collection of biopsy samples from adjacent, but non-identical sites, or sites from contra-lateral limbs in scenarios involving symmetrical exercise protocols, may contribute to the technical error of measurement involved with chemical determination of muscle glycogen stores. Nevertheless, it is the basis of a robust literature involving many hundreds of studies, which have determined resting muscle glycogen concentrations in different populations [**36**], glycogen utilisation during exercise [**1,53**], and glycogen synthesis in response to diet [**19,54,55**].

Although the size of a biopsy sample can be measured (typically, 20–200 mg), the size and location of the actual site captured in the ultrasound image is uncertain. Since the analysis of the scan is undertaken via proprietary cloud-based software, the precise size and location of the sample and site, and its ability to represent the total muscle, ultimately lies with the company software, rather than the scan technician. Nevertheless, even if there are concerns about the validity of Muscle Sound® glycogen assessments, there is some evidence of its reliability in estimating glycogen content across a muscle site. Indeed, the first study of the technique noted a significant correlation between the Muscle Sound® glycogen content and its changes due to an exercise bout between two *separate* muscles. Here the correlation between glycogen stores of the rectus femoris and vastus lateralis were $r = 0.93$ ($p < 0.0001$), $r = 0.91$ ($p < 0.0001$), and $r = 0.76$ ($p < 0.0001$) for the pre-exercise, post-exercise, and exercise change scores, respectively [**4**]. Furthermore, in the Bone study reported in this review, we found a significant correlation between Muscle Sound® scores at a single site and a shifting site within the same muscle, across a range of treatments (**Figure 3**). Therefore, in theory and in practice, there is evidence that in the absence of muscle damage, changes in glycogen in response to diet and exercise are similarly expressed across the gross aspect of a muscle.

## 7.2. Specific Criticism of Studies That Fail to Support the Muscle Sound® Technique

The major rebuttal of data sets that have found that the Muscle Sound® technique was unable to provide a valid measurement of muscle glycogen [**10,12**] is that "since glycogen is stored in different pools within a same muscle and therefore not uniformly stored, technically it is not possible to correlate the glycogen content from a very small portion of a muscle (1–2 $cm^2$) with the glycogen content of an entire muscle" [**10**]. We have identified that this criticism of mixed muscle samples was confused with findings of sub-pools of glycogen within a single muscle fibre or between fibre types, and does not provide a legitimate understanding of broader muscle glycogen assessment. It is not necessary to make further comment on this issue. Nevertheless, if differences in the glycogen content of different sites within the same muscle do exist, this might provide an explanation for the lack of correlation between the biopsy site and ultrasound site in the dissenting studies discussed within this review. However, it fails to explain the failure of the Muscle Sound® protocol to detect changes in its glycogen assessment metrics when across ultrasound scans taken at the same site on subsequent occasions. That such differences were both logical, based on knowledge of supervised diet and exercise treatments, and easily detected from chemical analysis of biopsy samples creates legitimate concern about the validity of the Muscle Sound® technique.

## 8. CONCISE SUMMARY

We recognize the promising potential and significance of a cost-effective, portable, and non-invasive technique for assessing muscle glycogen in sports nutrition research and application. Moreover, ultrasonic techniques may offer novel applications in sports nutrition, particularly in evaluating body composition. Nonetheless, a meticulous examination of the literature, incorporating previously unpublished findings from our own research, does not yield unequivocal evidence endorsing the application of the ultrasound technology (Muscle Sound®) for assessing muscle glycogen levels or their variations resulting from supervised exercise and dietary interventions. This may be a problem with the fundamental principles of the technique, as well as the inadequacy of existing algorithms to accommodate a broader spectrum of variations in muscle glycogen or other alterations in muscle solutes and water commonly observed in sports nutrition practice. We recognize that two validation studies have indicated the apparent efficacy of this technique in evaluating alterations in muscle glycogen under comparable dietary and exercise conditions. Despite these observations, the efficacy of this approach for evaluating muscle glycogen, particularly in field applications where conditions and treatments may be less regulated than in research settings, should be regarded as uncertain. Additional independent research is necessary and should encompass several scenarios in which muscle glycogen levels are altered across the spectrum of concentrations often observed in athletes, regardless of variations in muscle water and solute content. Laboratory and real-world scenario investigations should be incorporated to assess the method's tolerance to variations in logistics and data capture rigor.

## AT A GLANCE

Researchers and practitioners in sports nutrition would significantly benefit from a swift, portable, and non-invasive method for assessing muscle glycogen, applicable in both laboratory and field settings. This elucidates the fascination with Muscle Sound®, the inaugural commercial device employing high-frequency ultrasound technology and image processing via patented cloud-based software to assess muscle glycogen levels based on the echogenicity of the ultrasound image. This approach primarily relies on muscle water content, which is assumed to provide as an indicator of glycogen levels. Notwithstanding the initial validation studies' promise, subsequent research from independent entities revealed inconsistent findings, as Muscle Sound® scores did not correlate with glycogen levels in biopsy-derived mixed muscle samples nor exhibit the anticipated variations in muscle glycogen linked to different dietary and exercise regimens. The elucidation of difficulties pertaining to the assessment site fails to address these differences, and there are significant concerns regarding the assumption that the glycogen-to-water ratio in muscle remains constant. While additional research on this technique is necessary, the existing evidence regarding Muscle Sound® technology's ability to deliver valid and relevant insights into muscle glycogen levels is, at best, ambiguous.

## REFERENCES


1. Areta, J.L.; Hopkins, W.G. Skeletal Muscle Glycogen Content at Rest and During Endurance Exercise in Humans: A Meta-Analysis. *Sports Med.* **2018**, *48*, 2091–2102. **[Google Scholar]**
2. Philp, A.; Hargreaves, M.; Baar, K. More than a store: Regulatory roles for glycogen in skeletal muscle adaptation to exercise. *Am. J. Physiol. Endocrinol. Metab.* **2012**, *302*, E1343–E1351. **[Google Scholar] [Green Version]**
3. Impey, S.G.; Hearris, M.A.; Hammond, K.M.; Bartlett, J.D.; Louis, J.; Close, G.L.; Morton, J.P. Fuel for the Work Required: A Theoretical Framework for Carbohydrate Periodization and the Glycogen Threshold Hypothesis. *Sports Med.* **2018**, *48*, 1031–1048. **[Google Scholar] [PubMed] [Green Version]**
4. Hill, J.C.; Millan, I.S. Validation of musculoskeletal ultrasound to assess and quantify muscle glycogen content. A novel approach. *Phys. Sportsmed.* **2014**, *42*, 45–52. **[Google Scholar] [PubMed]**
5. Nieman, D.C.; Shanely, R.A.; Zwetsloot, K.A.; Meaney, M.P.; Farris, G.E. Ultrasonic assessment of exercise-induced change in skeletal muscle glycogen content. *BMC Sports Sci. Med. Rehabil.* **2015**, *7*, 9. **[Google Scholar] [PubMed] [Green Version]**
6. McBride, J.J.; Guest, M.M.; Scott, E.L. The storage of the major liver components; emphasizing the relationship of glycogen to water in the liver and the hydration of glycogen. *J. Biol. Chem.* **1941**, *139*, 943–952. **[Google Scholar]**
7. Wischmeyer, P.E.; San-Millan, I. Winning the war against ICU-acquired weakness: New innovations in nutrition and exercise physiology. *Crit. Care* **2015**, *19* (Suppl. 3), S6. **[Google Scholar] [PubMed] [Green Version]**
8. Muller, W.; Furhapter-Rieger, A.; Ahammer, H.; Lohman, T.G.; Meyer, N.L.; Sardinha, L.B.; Stewart, A.D.; Maughan, R.J.; Sundgot-Borgen, J.; Muller, T.; et al. Relative Body Weight and Standardised Brightness-Mode Ultrasound Measurement of Subcutaneous Fat in Athletes: An International Multicentre Reliability Study, Under the Auspices of the IOC Medical Commission. *Sports Med.* **2020**, *50*, 597–614. **[Google Scholar] [Green Version]**
9. Routledge, H.E.; Bradley, W.J.; Shepherd, S.O.; Cocks, M.; Erskine, R.M.; Close, G.L.; Morton, J.P. Ultrasound Does Not Detect Acute Changes in Glycogen in Vastus Lateralis of Man. *Med. Sci. Sports Exerc.* **2019**. **[Google Scholar] [PubMed]**
10. San-Millan, I.; Hill, J.C.; Calleja-Gonzalez, J. Indirect Assessment of Skeletal Muscle Glycogen Content in Professional Soccer Players before and after a Match through a Non-Invasive Ultrasound Technology. *Nutrients* **2020**, *12*, 971. **[Google Scholar] [PubMed] [Green Version]**
11. Ortenblad, N.; Nielsen, J.; Gejl, K.D.; Routledge, H.E.; Morton, J.P.; Close, G.L.; Niemann, D.C.; Bone, J.L.; Burke, L.M. Comment on: "Changes in Skeletal Muscle Glycogen Content in Professional Soccer Players before and after a Match by a NonInvasive Muscle Sound((R)) Technology. A Cross Sectional Pilot Study Nutrients 2020, 12(4), 971". *Nutrients* **2020**, *12*, 2070. **[Google Scholar]**
12. San-Millan, I.; Hill, J.C.; Calleja-Gonzalez, J. Reply to Comment on: "Changes in Skeletal Muscle Glycogen Content in Professional Soccer Players before and after a Match by a Non-Invasive Muscle Sound((R)) Technology. A Cross Sectional Pilot Study Nutrients 2020, 12(4), 971". *Nutrients* **2020**, *12*, 2066. **[Google Scholar] [PubMed]**
13. The Muscle Sound Company. Position Stand. *Science and Application (of Muscle Sound).* The Muscle Sound Company: Denver Colorado, CO, USA. Available online: **http://www.Muscle Sound.com/wp-content/uploads/2018/02/Position-Stand-2018.pdf** (accessed on 24 February 2021).
14. Burke, L.M.; Hawley, J.A. Swifter, higher, stronger: What's on the menu? *Science* **2018**, *362*, 781–787. **[Google Scholar] [PubMed] [Green Version]**
15. Bergstrom, J.; Hermansen, L.; Hultman, E.; Saltin, B. Diet, muscle glycogen and physical performance. *Acta Physiol. Scand.* **1967**, *71*, 140–150. **[Google Scholar] [PubMed]**

16. Hermansen, L.; Hultman, E.; Saltin, B. Muscle glycogen during prolonged severe exercise. *Acta Physiol. Scand.* **1967**, *71*, 129–139. **[Google Scholar]**

17. Bergstrom, J.; Hultman, E. Muscle glycogen synthesis after exercise: An enhancing factor localized to the muscle cells in man. *Nature* **1966**, *210*, 309–310. **[Google Scholar]**

18. Evans, W.J.; Phinney, S.D.; Young, V.R. Suction applied to a muscle biopsy maximizes sample size. *Med. Sci. Sports Exerc.* **1982**, *14*, 101–102. **[Google Scholar] [PubMed]**

19. Costill, D.L.; Pearson, D.R.; Fink, W.J. Impaired muscle glycogen storage after muscle biopsy. *J. Appl. Physiol.* **1988**, *64*, 2245–2248. **[Google Scholar]**

20. Greene, J.; Louis, J.; Korostynska, O.; Mason, A. State-of-the-Art Methods for Skeletal Muscle Glycogen Analysis in Athletes-The Need for Novel Non-Invasive Techniques. *Biosensors* **2017**, *7*, 11. **[Google Scholar] [Green Version]**

21. Jensen, R.; Ortenblad, N.; Stausholm, M.H.; Skjaerbaek, M.C.; Larsen, D.N.; Hansen, M.; Holmberg, H.C.; Plomgaard, P.; Nielsen, J. Heterogeneity in subcellular muscle glycogen utilisation during exercise impacts endurance capacity in men. *J. Physiol.* **2020**. **[Google Scholar]**

22. Ørtenblad, N.; Nielsen, J. Muscle glycogen and cell function—Location, location, location. *Scand. J. Med. Sci. Sports* **2015**, *25*, 34–40. **[Google Scholar]**

23. Harris, R.C.; Hultman, E.; Nordesjö, L.O. Glycogen, Glycolytic Intermediates and High-Energy Phosphates Determined in Biopsy Samples of Musculus Quadriceps Femoris of Man at Rest. Methods and Variance of Values. *Scand. J. Clin. Lab. Investig.* **1974**, *33*, 109–120. **[Google Scholar]**

24. Heinicke, K.; Dimitrov, I.E.; Romain, N.; Cheshkov, S.; Ren, J.; Malloy, C.R.; Haller, R.G. Reproducibility and absolute quantification of muscle glycogen in patients with glycogen storage disease by 13C NMR spectroscopy at 7 Tesla. *PLoS ONE* **2014**, *9*, e108706. **[Google Scholar]**

25. Rico-Sanz, J.; Zehnder, M.; Buchli, R.; Dambach, M.; Boutellier, U. Muscle glycogen degradation during simulation of a fatiguing soccer match in elite soccer players examined noninvasively by 13C-MRS. *Med. Sci. Sports Exerc.* **1999**, *31*, 1587–1593. **[Google Scholar] [PubMed]**

26. Zehnder, M.; Rico-Sanz, J.; Kuhne, G.; Boutellier, U. Resynthesis of muscle glycogen after soccer specific performance examined by 13C-magnetic resonance spectroscopy in elite players. *Eur. J. Appl. Physiol.* **2001**, *84*, 443–447. **[Google Scholar] [PubMed]**

27. Aldrich, J.E. Basic physics of ultrasound imaging. *Crit. Care Med.* **2007**, *35*, S131–S137. **[Google Scholar] [PubMed]**

28. Tomcik, K.A.; Camera, D.M.; Bone, J.L.; Ross, M.L.; Jeacocke, N.A.; Tachtsis, B.; Senden, J.; LJC, V.A.N.L.; Hawley, J.A.; Burke, L.M. Effects of Creatine and Carbohydrate Loading on Cycling Time Trial Performance. *Med. Sci. Sports Exerc.* **2018**, *50*, 141–150. **[Google Scholar]**

29. Bone, J.L.; Ross, M.L.; Tomcik, K.A.; Jeacocke, N.A.; Hopkins, W.G.; Burke, L.M. Manipulation of Muscle Creatine and Glycogen Changes Dual X-ray Absorptiometry Estimates of Body Composition. *Med. Sci. Sports. Exerc.* **2017**, *49*, 1029–1035. **[Google Scholar] [PubMed] [Green Version]**

30. Harris, R.C.; Soderlund, K.; Hultman, E. Elevation of creatine in resting and exercised muscle of normal subjects by creatine supplementation. *Clin. Sci.* **1992**, *83*, 367–374. **[Google Scholar] [Green Version]**

31. Burke, L.M.; Hawley, J.A.; Wong, S.H.; Jeukendrup, A.E. Carbohydrates for training and competition. *J. Sports Sci.* **2011**, *29* (Suppl. 1), S17–S27. **[Google Scholar] [PubMed]**

32. Nana, A.; Slater, G.J.; Stewart, A.D.; Burke, L.M. Methodology review: Using dual-energy X-ray absorptiometry (DXA) for the assessment of body composition in athletes and active people. *Int. J. Sport Nutr. Exerc. Metab.* **2015**, *25*, 198–215. **[Google Scholar]**

33. Koo, T.K.; Li, M.Y. A Guideline of Selecting and Reporting Intraclass Correlation Coefficients for Reliability Research. *J. Chiropr. Med.* **2016**, *15*, 155–163. **[Google Scholar] [Green Version]**

34. Hawley, J.A.; Schabort, E.J.; Noakes, T.D.; Dennis, S.C. Carbohydrate-loading and exercise performance. An update. *Sports Med.* **1997**, *24*, 73–81. **[Google Scholar]**

35. Sanders, G.; Boos, B.; Shipley, F.; Peacock, C. Bilateral Asymmetries in Ultrasound Assessments of the Rectus Femoris throughout an NCAA Division I Volleyball Preseason. *Sports* **2018**, *6*, 94. **[Google Scholar] [PubMed] [Green Version]**

36. Hearris, M.A.; Hammond, K.M.; Fell, J.M.; Morton, J.P. Regulation of Muscle Glycogen Metabolism during Exercise: Implications for Endurance Performance and Training Adaptations. *Nutrients* **2018**, *10*, 298. **[Google Scholar] [Green Version]**

37. Sherman, W.M.; Plyley, M.J.; Sharp, R.L.; Van Handel, P.J.; McAllister, R.M.; Fink, W.J.; Costill, D.L. Muscle glycogen storage and its relationship with water. *Int. J. Sports Med.* **1982**, 3, 22–24. **[Google Scholar] [PubMed]**

38. Olsson, K.E.; Saltin, B. Variation in total body water with muscle glycogen changes in man. *Acta Physiol. Scand.* **1970**, *80*, 11–18. **[Google Scholar] [PubMed]**

39. Shiose, K.; Yamada, Y.; Motonaga, K.; Sagayama, H.; Higaki, Y.; Tanaka, H.; Takahashi, H. Segmental extracellular and intracellular water distribution and muscle glycogen after 72-h carbohydrate loading using spectroscopic techniques. *J. Appl. Physiol (1985)* **2016**, *121*, 205–211. **[Google Scholar] [PubMed] [Green Version]**

40. Sarvazyan, A.; Tatarinov, A.; Sarvazyan, N. Ultrasonic assessment of tissue hydration status. *Ultrasonics* **2005**, *43*, 661–671. **[Google Scholar]**

41. Utter, A.C.; McAnulty, S.R.; Sarvazyan, A.; Query, M.C.; Landram, M.J. Evaluation of ultrasound velocity to assess the hydration status of wrestlers. *J. Strength Cond. Res.* **2010**, *24*, 1451–1457. **[Google Scholar] [PubMed]**

42. Neufer, P.D.; Sawka, M.N.; Young, A.J.; Quigley, M.D.; Latzka, W.A.; Levine, L. Hypohydration does not impair skeletal muscle glycogen resynthesis after exercise. *J. Appl. Physiol.* **1991**, *70*, 1490–1494. **[Google Scholar] [PubMed] [Green Version]**

43. Fernandez-Elias, V.E.; Ortega, J.F.; Nelson, R.K.; Mora-Rodriguez, R. Relationship between muscle water and glycogen recovery after prolonged exercise in the heat in humans. *Eur. J. Appl. Physiol.* **2015**, *115*, 1919–1926. **[Google Scholar] [PubMed] [Green Version]**

44. Dalbo, V.J.; Roberts, M.D.; Stout, J.R.; Kerksick, C.M. Putting to rest the myth of creatine supplementation leading to muscle cramps and dehydration. *Br. J. Sports Med.* **2008**, *42*, 567–573. **[Google Scholar] [PubMed]**

45. Deminice, R.; Rosa, F.T.; Pfrimer, K.; Ferrioli, E.; Jordao, A.A.; Freitas, E. Creatine Supplementation Increases Total Body Water in Soccer Players: A Deuterium Oxide Dilution Study. *Int. J. Sports Med.* **2016**, *37*, 149–153. **[Google Scholar] [PubMed]**

46. Powers, M.E.; Arnold, B.L.; Weltman, A.L.; Perrin, D.H.; Mistry, D.; Kahler, D.M.; Kraemer, W.; Volek, J. Creatine Supplementation Increases Total Body Water Without Altering Fluid Distribution. *J. Athl. Train.* **2003**, *38*, 44–50. **[Google Scholar] [PubMed]**

47. Hermansen, L.; Vaage, O. Lactate disappearance and glycogen synthesis in human muscle after maximal exercise. *Am. J. Physiol. Endocrinol. Metab.* **1977**, *233*, E422–E429. **[Google Scholar]**

48. Aragón-Vargas, L.F.; Moncada-Jiménez, J.; Hernández-Elizondo, J.; Barrenechea, A.; Monge-Alvarado, M. Evaluation of pre-game hydration status, heat stress, and fluid balance during professional soccer competition in the heat. *Eur. J. Sport Sci.* **2009**, *9*, 269–276. **[Google Scholar] [Green Version]**

49. Castro-Sepulveda, M.; Astudillo, J.; Letelier, P.; Zbinden-Foncea, H. Prevalence of Dehydration Before Training Sessions, Friendly and Official Matches in Elite Female Soccer Players. *J. Hum. Kinet.* **2016**, *50*, 79–84. **[Google Scholar]**

50. Vollestad, N.K.; Vaage, O.; Hermansen, L. Muscle glycogen depletion patterns in type I and subgroups of type II fibres during prolonged severe exercise in man. *Acta. Physiol. Scand.* **1984**, *122*, 433–441. **[Google Scholar]**

51. Gejl, K.D.; Hvid, L.G.; Frandsen, U.; Jensen, K.; Sahlin, K.; Ørtenblad, N. Muscle glycogen content modifies SR Ca2+ release rate in elite endurance athletes. *Med. Sci. Sports Exerc.* **2014**, *46*, 496–505. **[Google Scholar] [Green Version]**

52. Ortenblad, N.; Nielsen, J.; Saltin, B.; Holmberg, H.C. Role of glycogen availability in sarcoplasmic reticulum Ca2+ kinetics in human skeletal muscle. *J. Physiol.* **2011**, *589*, 711–725. **[Google Scholar] [PubMed]**

53. Impey, S.G.; Hammond, K.M.; Shepherd, S.O.; Sharples, A.P.; Stewart, C.; Limb, M.; Smith, K.; Philp, A.; Jeromson, S.; Hamilton, D.L.; et al. Fuel for the work required: A practical approach to amalgamating train-low paradigms for endurance athletes. *Physiol. Rep.* **2016**, *4*. **[Google Scholar] [PubMed]**

54. Betts, J.; Williams, C.; Duffy, K.; Gunner, F. The influence of carbohydrate and protein ingestion during recovery from prolonged exercise on subsequent endurance performance. *J. Sports Sci.* **2007**, *25*, 1449–1460. **[Google Scholar] [PubMed]**

55. Margolis, L.M.; Allen, J.T.; Hatch-McChesney, A.; Pasiakos, S.M. Coingestion of Carbohydrate and Protein on Muscle Glycogen Synthesis after Exercise: A Meta-analysis. *Med. Sci. Sports Exerc.* **2021**, *53*, 384–393. **[Google Scholar] [PubMed]**

# 3 Chapter

# THE ROLE OF PLANT PROTEINS IN FACILITATING EXERCISE ADAPTATIONS

## 1. INTRODUCTION: AN OVERVIEW

Plant proteins have gained increasing attention for their potential to support exercise adaptations, particularly as more individuals adopt plant-based diets. Unlike animal proteins, which are often lauded for their complete amino acid profiles, plant proteins provide unique advantages that can enhance muscle recovery, growth, and overall performance. Rich in essential amino acids, vitamins, and minerals, these proteins not only contribute to muscle synthesis but also play a crucial role in reducing inflammation and promoting overall health. As research continues to unveil the benefits of plant-based nutrition, understanding the specific mechanisms by which plant proteins facilitate exercise adaptations becomes essential for athletes and fitness enthusiasts alike. This exploration reveals not only the nutritional value of plant proteins but also their potential to optimize athletic performance and support long-term health goals.

### 1.1. Muscle Protein Metabolism and Skeletal Muscle

The maintenance of and optimizing the accretion of skeletal muscle mass are critical outcomes for athletic-minded individuals, whether the goal is increased performance, improved muscularity, or enhanced recovery. Furthermore, while skeletal muscle mass accretion is often a goal of active individuals, there are direct clinical applications and benefits for the general public as well, especially for aging adults. Skeletal muscle is regulated through a near-continual ebb and flow between rates of muscle protein synthesis (MPS) and breakdown [**1**]. Muscle mass loss occurs during a net negative balance (breakdown > synthesis) while muscle gain occurs when synthesis rates outweigh breakdown. Rates of MPS and muscle protein breakdown are highly sensitive to physical activity and dietary intake, namely protein and essential amino acid intake [**2**], with evidence available indicating that rates of MPS are more sensitive to changes in exercise status and dietary intake [**3**]. As a result, observed changes in MPS rates are viewed to be primarily responsible for the changes in muscle mass in response to exercise and nutrition experienced over time [**4**].

## 1.2. The Importance of Added Protein to Optimize Exercise Training Adaptations

Supplementing the diet with added protein beyond the recommended dietary allowance (RDA) has long been a well-supported tactic for exercising athletes to optimize exercise training adaptations. In this respect, multiple review articles and position stands have advocated for a greater intake of dietary protein to support increased physical training volumes, heighten exercise training adaptations, and promote health and recovery [**5**,**6**,**7**,**8**,**9**]. Previously, Cermak and colleagues [**10**] completed a meta-analysis of studies that employed some form of protein supplementation while completing resistance training. Results from this analysis included data from over 680 subjects and concluded that protein supplementation led to a significantly greater increase in fat-free mass (mean difference: 0.69 kg, 95% CI: 0.47–0.91 kg, $p < 0.001$) and maximal lower-body strength (mean difference: 13.5 kg, 95% CI: 6.4–20.7 kg, $p < 0.005$) when compared to a placebo. These results were extended by Morton and investigators [**7**] who used a meta-analysis and meta-regression approach to establish the efficacy of protein supplementation while also identifying the minimum amount of daily protein needed to maximize efficacy. In this study, 49 studies were included that represented 1863 participants and the authors reported that protein supplementation was responsible for significant increases in strength (1 RM), fat-free mass, and muscle cross-sectional area. Moreover, results from this study highlighted that a daily protein intake beyond 1.62 g/kg/day offered no further impact in facilitating improvements in fat-free mass. It is important to note, this is well above (~2×) the RDA for protein, indicating that active individuals benefit from consuming greater amounts of protein. Whether or not higher amounts facilitate improvements in other outcomes such as strength, recovery, mitigation of fat-free mass loss seen while dieting was not identified in their analysis. Notably, this amount of protein is consistent with the protein recommendation set forth by Jäger and colleagues [**5**] in the position stand published by the International Society of Sports Nutrition as well as the position stand endorsed by the American College of Sports Medicine, Dietitians of Canada and Academy of Nutrition and Dietetics (the former American Dietetic Association) [**11**]. Dietary proteins are well known to serve as the primary supplier of amino acids that can be used as building blocks to make larger proteins, such as those produced during MPS. Previous studies have highlighted the importance of the essential amino acids [**12**,**13**] at stimulating rates of MPS. In addition, extensive research continues to explore the role of leucine in its ability to stimulate the initiation of protein translation [**14**,**15**]. All things considered, exercising individuals require greater amounts of dietary protein to support their training needs, which creates a need for these individuals to purposefully include various sources of protein that deliver optimal amounts of the essential amino acids.

## 1.3. The Case for Plant Proteins

Many sources of protein are available for consumption in the human diet. For years, heavy emphasis was placed on consuming complete protein sources, or any protein source that provides all of the essential amino acids in both the needed amount and in adequate proportion to support cellular needs across the body as well as production of nonessential amino acids [8]. Consequently, great focus has been placed on consuming animal protein sources, namely because of their high amino acid contents and favorable protein quality ratings [16]. At the same time, plant proteins were deemed inferior for these outcomes and not until recently has interest in plant proteins begun to accelerate. Several reasons are commonly associated with consuming greater amounts of plant proteins. Most commonly, plant-based diets are routinely linked with reductions in the risk of developing cancers, type 2 diabetes, and cardiovascular diseases [17]. In addition, many plant protein advocates highlight a greater level of economic sustainability than what is observed with diets that are predominantly animal protein. Finally, approximately 60% of dietary proteins consumed worldwide come from plant sources with an estimated 4 billion people across the globe consuming a primarily plant-based diet [18]. While such health considerations are unquestionably important, the aim of this review will center upon the implications of plant protein consumption and plant-based diets on outcomes linked to exercise performance, associated exercise training adaptations, and recovery.

## 1.4. Quality Considerations for Both Animal and Plant-Based Protein

Many factors contribute to the anabolic potential of a protein source, which often include the amounts of total amino acids, essential amino acids, and branched-chain amino acids, respectively in addition to the protein's digestibility, digestion rate, and kinetics observed during absorption. In this respect, dietary protein quality is commonly assessed based upon the essential amino acid composition provided by the protein source as it relates to human needs, against the ability of the protein to be digested, absorbed, and assimilated by various tissues in the body [19]. Several approaches have been used to assess protein quality including biological value, net protein utilization, and protein digestibility corrected amino acid scores (PDCAAS) [20], while digestible indispensable amino acid score (DIAAS) have been more recently proposed. As seen in an excellent review by Berrazaga et al. [16], biological values for common plant sources range from 56–74 while ranges of 77–104 are reported for various animal sources on theoretical 100-point scales. A similar dichotomy is observed for net protein utilization values, whereby plant sources range from 53–67 while animal sources range from 73–94 on a 100-point scale. One of the most commonly used quality comparators is that of Protein Digestibility Corrected Amino Acid Scores (PDCAAS) [21]. When using this approach, a score of 100 suggests that after considering its fecal digestibility, a given protein source can fully deliver all of the essential amino acids required by the body. In this respect, animal protein sources such as casein, whey, milk, and eggs all have scores of 100 while red meat has a score of 92. In contrast, all other common sources of plant proteins have PDCAAS values below 100 (commonly reported range of 45–75 per Barrazaga et al. [16]), with soy protein being the only exception, which has a score of 100. Similarly, if the DIAAS approach is used to assess protein quality, a similar trend is observed in that animal sources are commonly above

100 while nearly all plant sources are below 100. In this respect, Gorissen et al. [**22**] compared the amino acid contents of various sources of plant-based isolates against common sources of animal proteins and human skeletal muscle samples. Again, it was illustrated that many plant protein sources have inadequate amounts of certain amino acids (e.g., lysine, methionine) while also consistently having lower amounts of the essential and branched-chain amino acids, particularly when compared to animal protein sources as well as the amino acid content found in human skeletal muscle. To further reiterate this point, van Vliet and colleagues [**23**] have indicated previously that essential amino acid composition of a protein source was predictive of skeletal muscle's anabolic potential and that all essential amino acids should be present in optimal amounts. For these reasons, higher quality sources of protein (at least when viewed in the context of amino acid profiles) should serve as more effective protein sources in terms of anabolic potential and its innate ability to facilitate skeletal muscle accretion and promote other desired adaptations. Finally, leucine content of a protein source continues to get interest for its role in initiating the translation of muscle proteins [**14,15**]. Towards this end, a general acceptance has suggested the leucine content of a protein source functions as a vital and reliable predictor of MPS rates. When leucine contents are compared across different protein sources, whey protein is the highest (~12–14%) [**22**], which aligns with whey protein's superior ability to stimulate MPS rates when compared to isocaloric and isonitrogenous amounts of other protein sources [**24**]. Moreover, animal protein sources generally have higher amounts of leucine (8–9% for non-dairy animal sources) and >10% for dairy protein sources while plant sources routinely have a leucine content of 6–8% [**22,23**].

Beyond amino acid content, digestibility and absorption kinetics can also influence the value of a protein. In terms of digestibility, it is well documented that the digestibility of many sources of plants is much lower (45–80%) than what is observed with various animal proteins (>90%) [**25**]. While somewhat beyond the scope of this review, the observed differences in digestibility are largely thought to be due to structural differences that exist within the actual protein molecule found in many plant and animal proteins. For example, many sources of plants have compounds (i.e., anti-nutritional factors such as phytic acid, protease inhibitors, tannins, etc.) that compromise their digestibility. Another key factor related to the impact of consuming different sources of protein is the absorption of amino acids in plasma followed by the utilization rates exhibited by various proteins. In this respect, several studies have illustrated divergent utilization rates when comparing animal to plant sources of protein. For example, the classic work of Boirie [**26,27**] and Dangin [**28,29**] clearly demonstrated different absorption and utilization rates for two milk proteins, whey and casein. Moreover, the observed differences in rates of muscle protein metabolism have been shown to be inextricably linked to differences in utilization rates whereby whey absorbs faster and robustly stimulates rates of MPS while casein absorbs at a slower rate and consequently functions more to attenuate protein breakdown. When considering differences observed for various plant proteins, previous work has shown that soy ingestion is absorbed at a slower rate than what is observed from whey [**24,30**], which helps to explain the lower rates of myofibrillar protein synthesis observed by Yang and colleagues [**4**] after graded doses (0–40 g) of soy isolate at rest and after exercise in elderly men. While rates of myofibrillar protein synthesis were observed to increase with an increase in the dose of soy protein, the observed rates were less than what had been previously observed with equivalent doses of whey [**24**]. Additional research involving wheat proteins demonstrated them to have higher deamination rates when compared to milk proteins (25% vs. 16%, respectively) [**31,32,33**]. These differences are important as they are thought to be directly related to the lower observed net protein utilization rates between wheat (66%) when compared to milk (80%) proteins. Furthermore, other studies have illustrated a greater degradation of amino acids from soy protein when compared to degradation rates observed for casein and whey [**24,30,34,35**]. Towards this end, measured nitrogen losses (either via deamination or intestinal loss) and splanchnic nitrogen retention are higher when plant proteins are consumed when compared to ingestion of animal proteins. In effect, these outcomes illustrate that the availability of amino acids to peripheral tissues and locations from plant proteins is lower than that of animal protein [**36,37**] and these differences are thought to be key drivers to the post-prandial protein synthetic response observed in various tissues. Importantly, the reader should understand that these reasons effectively function as the basis for why different sources of protein exhibit varying degrees of anabolic potential, in regards to stimulating muscle protein accretion and promotion of exercise training adaptations over time.

## 2. METHODS

This article was prepared using a narrative approach. The purpose of the review was to evaluate and review the current literature that has examined the potential impact of various plant proteins on exercise training adaptations and recovery. A range of databases, including PubMed, Medline, Google Scholar, EBSCO-host were used to search for articles for this review paper and were last accessed on 4/10/21. Inclusion criteria consisted of those studies that involved human research participants and use of at least one source of plant protein as a primary investigative agent in the study. Studies involving both acute and prolonged models were included with the majority of acute studies focusing on changes in amino acid concentration and rates of muscle protein metabolism. Prolonged studies commonly highlighted outcomes related to strength, performance, recovery, and fat-free mass. Key words routinely used to search for articles were as follows: protein, exercise, plant, oat, potato, wheat, soy, rice, pea, animal, whey, casein, beef, resistance training, strength, body composition, and MPS. Articles were chosen for inclusion based on the information they outlined and were incorporated throughout this paper.

## 3. ACUTE INVESTIGATIONS INVOLVING PLANT PROTEINS AND PHYSICAL ACTIVITY

The acute post-prandial anabolic response of an ingested protein is largely mediated by its amino acid content, with essential amino acid content, leucine, in particular, being a key driving force [**8**,**9**]. While preferences for certain protein sources may be influenced by moral beliefs, environmental considerations, dietary preferences, or assumptions regarding subsequent health outcomes, differences in amino acid content across protein sources dictate the anabolic properties of the protein. Moreover, consistent increases in MPS throughout the day have been shown to be advantageous for maximizing skeletal muscle protein accretion over time [**38**]. As such, it has long been suggested that higher quality sources of dietary protein confer a greater potential to increase skeletal muscle accretion compared to lower quality sources of protein.

Animal and plant-based proteins are commonly characterized by their ability to influence postprandial amino acid profiles and in their capacity to modulate rates of MPS post-ingestion. When one considers the substantial growth in popularity of plant-based diets, a number of studies have therefore examined the acute responses to a bolus ingestion of protein from varying plant-based sources [**4**,**24**,**30**,**34**,**39**,**40**,**41**,**42**,**43**,**44**], either compared to isonitrogenous animal-derived protein sources or when consumed at higher doses of total protein. Moreover, these studies often examine differences in anabolic properties both at rest or post-resistance exercise to further examine the anabolic potential or synergistic benefits when combined with exercise modalities [**4**,**24**,**42**]. For example, Wilkinson et al. [**39**] noted greater net balance in protein levels after milk ingestion compared to an isonitrogenous soy beverage, which also equated to a greater increase in fractional synthetic rate (0.10 ± 0.01 vs. 0.07 ± 0.01%/h; $p < 0.05$). Similarly, Tang et al. [**24**] observed a greater increase in blood EAA, branch-chained amino acid and leucine concentrations following ingestion of a whey protein hydrolysate compared to both micellar casein and soy protein isolate. Subsequently, MPS was 93% greater after consumption of whey protein compared to casein, and 18% greater than soy after exercise. These results indicated that, at rest, whey protein may elicit a more robust anabolic response immediately post-ingestion compared to casein and soy. In response to exercise, whey protein again stimulated MPS rates that were greater than both soy and casein protein, while soy was found to be greater than casein. Using a short-term supplementation protocol of 14 days, Kraemer and investigators [**40**] reported an attenuation of post-exercise increases in testosterone following ingestion of soy protein compared to whey protein while whey protein blunted the release of cortisol post-exercise in resistance trained males. Yang et al. [**4**] extended these findings and determined that a 20-g dose of soy protein isolate elicited a myofibrillar protein synthetic response that was significantly less than an equivalent dose of whey protein, but more importantly that the rates observed from a 20-g dose of soy protein were not significantly increased from consuming no protein. When the dose of protein was increased to 40 g, whey protein elicited significantly greater rates of myofibrillar protein synthesis when compared to rates observed from soy ingestion at the same dose. Finally, the 40-g dose of soy was able to demonstrate significantly greater rates of MPS when compared to when no protein was ingested. Collectively, results from these studies highlight the superiority of animal proteins (milk, whey, and casein) at stimulating acute increases in MPS rates both at rest and after exercise when compared to soy ingestion.

To accommodate the growing demand for plant-based diets, several plant protein sources have appeared in the marketplace. In this respect, acute amino acid absorption responses to a rice protein isolate identified a 6.8% lower total amino acid concentration area under the curve in rice protein isolate when compared to a whey protein isolate, but this difference was not statistically significant. Additionally, area under the curve values for essential and nonessential amino acids were not different between the two protein conditions. The time to reach peak concentration was faster with whey protein ingestion for the essential amino acids, non-essential amino acids, and total amino acids. Interestingly, however, the time to reach peak concentration for leucine was faster for rice protein isolate ingestion versus whey protein isolate ingestion [**44**].

In addition to this work, several studies have also assessed acute changes in MPS rates in addition to amino acid absorption to acute doses of oat, potato, peanut, and wheat protein [**41,42,43,44,45,46**]. For example, Lamb et al. [**46**] did not observe a difference in 24-h myofibrillar protein synthetic rates in subjects who received a peanut protein powder supplement versus those who received no supplement, following a bout of resistance training in older adults (59 ± 8 years). It is possible that a greater amount of peanut protein may be required in older adults to elicit meaningful post-prandial anabolic properties. In a similar manner, Gorissen et al. [**43**] observed greater increases in post-prandial plasma essential amino acid concentrations after whey protein ingestion (2.23 ± 0.07 mM) compared to casein (1.53 ± 0.08 mM) and wheat protein (1.50 ± 0.04 mM) ($p < 0.01$). Further, a greater increase in myofibrillar protein synthesis rate was observed after casein protein ingestion compared to whey protein (0.050% ± 0.005%/h vs. 0.032% ± 0.004%/h) ($p = 0.003$). Interestingly, post-prandial increases in plasma leucine concentrations were greater after whey protein ingestion compared to more than double the amount (60 g) of wheat protein (peak value: 580 ± 18 compared with 378 ± 10 mM, respectively; $p < 0.01$), despite comparable leucine concentrations per serving (~4 g). Another plant-based source of protein, potato protein, has a relatively high essential amino content compared to other protein sources [**22**], when expressed as a percent of total protein. A recent study by Oikawa et al. [**42**] indicated that consumption of 25 g of potato protein twice daily (1.6 g/kg/day total protein) increased myofibrillar protein synthesis at rest and in an exercised limb beyond that observed following consumption of a control diet (0.8 g/kg/day total protein) in young women (20.5 ± 3 years). Most recently, Pinckaers et al. [**41**] reported similar increases in post-prandial myofibrillar protein synthesis rates following consumption of a 400 mL beverage containing either 30 g of milk protein concentrate, 30 g of wheat protein hydrolysate, or 15 g of wheat protein hydrolysate plus 15 g of milk protein concentrate in young males (23 ± 3 years). Thereby indicating that wheat protein can elicit comparable anabolic properties as milk protein, when consumed in equal amounts. Collectively, these studies indicate that while several plant-based protein sources may elicit post-prandial increases in essential amino acid concentrations and subsequent increases in myofibrillar protein synthesis rates, these effects are likely to be less than or equal to what is observed following ingestion of comparable amounts of whey or casein protein. However, more research is warranted to investigate some of the newer formulations of plant-derived protein powders, such as rice, oat and potato protein and how their acute anabolic properties may influence adaptations over time; particularly when consumed in conjunction with other nutrients or exercise regimens. Overall, recent evidence indicates that when quantifying the anabolic efficiency (net protein balance/caloric intake), beef displayed greater efficiency values compared to eggs, pork loin, tofu, kidney beans, peanut butter and mixed nuts [**47**]. As such, animal-based sources of protein may serve as a more efficient protein source, when taking into consideration the overall energy content of a food item or meal. As a result, there has also been an interest in the development of strategies to augment the anabolic properties of plant proteins to compensate for a lower anabolic potential, a topic which will be discussed later in this review. A summary of studies to date that have examined differences in the acute anabolic response to animal and plant-based sources of protein is presented in **Table 1**.

**Table 1. Summary Table of Acute Responses to Plant Protein Ingestion.**

| Reference | Participants | Design | Study Duration | Dosing Protocol | Exercise Program | Primary Variables | Key Findings |
|---|---|---|---|---|---|---|---|
| Wilkinson et al. 2007 [39] | 8 healthy males (21.6 ± 0.3 years.) | RCT, crossover (2 groups) Milk (*n* = 8) Soy (*n* = 8) | 1 trial visit per condition 7-day washout | Macronutrient -matched soy or milk beverages (18 g protein) | Lower body exercise bout | Protein kinetics Net muscle protein balance | ↓ Net balance (AUC) after soy ingestion vs. milk<br>↓ Fractional synthesis rate in muscle after soy consumption vs. milk |
| Tang et al. 2009 [24] | 6 healthy young men (22.8 ± 3.9 years.) | RCT, crossover (3 groups) Whey (*n* = 6) Casein (*n* = 6) Soy (*n* = 6) | | 10 g of EAA in the form of: Whey, casein and soy protein | Unilateral lower-body exercise | Mixed muscle protein fractional synthetic rate (FSR) Blood EAA | ↓ Blood EAA, BCAA, and leucine concentrations following soy ingestion compared to whey ↓ MPS (~18%) after soy consumption vs. whey after exercise<br>↑ MPS (~64%) with soy consumption at rest and following resistance exercise (69%) vs. casein |
| Yang et al. 2012 [4] | 30 elderly men (71 ± 5 years.) | RCT (3 groups) Control Soy 20 g Soy 40 g | 1 trial visit per group 4 h post-protein consumption | 20 g or 40 g of soy protein isolate Compared to previous responses from similarly aged men who had ingested 20 g and 40 g of whey protein isolate | Acute bout of unilateral knee-extensor resistance exercise prior to ingesting no protein | Myofibrillar protein synthesis (MPS) | ↑ Whole-body leucine oxidation for S20 vs. W20 ↔ in both exercised and non-exercised leg muscles for S20 vs. 0 g<br>↓ MPS post S40 under both rested and post-exercise conditions vs. W40<br>↑ MPS post S40 than 0 g under post-exercise conditions |

| Reference | Participants | Design | Study Duration | Dosing Protocol | Exercise Program | Primary Variables | Key Findings |
|---|---|---|---|---|---|---|---|
| Kraemer et al. 2013 [40] | 10 resistance trained males (21.7 ± 2.8 years.) | RCT, crossover (3 groups) Whey protein isolate Soy protein isolate Maltodextrin | 14 days | 20 g | Acute heavy resistance exercise test consisting of 6 sets of 10 repetitions in the squat exercise at 80% of the subject's 1 RM | Sex hormones post resistance training | ↓ Testosterone responses following supplementation with soy protein<br>↔ SHBG concentrations between experimental treatments<br>↔ in estradiol concentrations between groups |
| Purpura et al. 2014 [44] | 10 trained male subjects (22.2 ± 4.2 years.) | RCT, crossover (2 groups) Rice protein Whey protein | 2 trial visits per condition (7-day washout) | 48 g isonitrogenous and isocaloric | N/A | Plasma concentrations of amino acids | ↑ Tmax for RPI for EAA, non-EAA, and total amino acids<br>↔ For AUC between conditions<br>↔ for Cmax between conditions<br>↑ Cmax faster for leucine in the RPI group. |
| Gorissen et al. 2016 [43] | 60 healthy older men (71 ± 1 years.) | RCT (5 groups) Wheat ($n$ = 12) WPH35 g ($n$ = 12) Casein ($n$ = 12) Whey ($n$ = 12) WPH60 g ($n$ = 12) | 1 trial visit per group. 240 min | 35 g or 60 g | N/A | Postprandial increase in plasma EAA concentrations | ↓ Postprandial increase in plasma EAA concentration after ingesting WPH-35 vs. Whey-35 ↓ Myofibrillar protein synthesis rates after ingesting WPH-35 vs. MCas-35<br>↓ Postprandial increase in plasma leucine concentrations after ingesting WPH-60 vs. Whey-35 |

| Reference | Participants | Design | Study Duration | Dosing Protocol | Exercise Program | Primary Variables | Key Findings |
|---|---|---|---|---|---|---|---|
| Oikawa et al. 2020 [**42**] | 24 healthy young women (21 ± 3 years.) | RCT, single blind (2 groups)<br>PP (*n* = 12)<br>Control (*n* = 12) | | 25 g of potato protein (PP) twice daily (1.6 g/kg/d total protein)<br>(CON) (0.8 g/kg/d total protein) for 2 weeks. | Unilateral RE (~30% of maximal strength to failure) was performed thrice weekly with the opposite limb serving as a non-exercised control (Rest) | Myofibrillar protein synthesis | ↑ MPS at Rest, and in the Exercise limb following PP ingestion<br>↑ MPS in CON vs. baseline after Exercise only. |
| Pinckaers et al. 2021 [**41**] | 36 males (23 ± 3 years.) | RCT, parallel-group design<br>3 groups (*n* = 12/group) | | 30 g milk protein (MILK)<br>30 g wheat protein (WHEAT)<br>30 g blend combining 15 g wheat plus 15 g milk protein (WHEAT +MILK). | N/A | Post-prandial plasma amino acid profiles<br>Myofibrillar protein synthesis rates | ↓ Post-prandial plasma EAA concentration post WHEAT vs. MILK<br>↔ Post-prandial plasma EAA concentration post MILK and WHEAT+MILK<br>↔ Post-prandial myofibrillar protein synthesis rates between MILK vs WHEAT<br>↔ Post-prandial myofibrillar protein synthesis rates between MILK vs WHEAT+MILK |

↔ = No difference ($p > 0.05$) change; ↑ = Greater increase ($p < 0.05$) over control or other condition/intervention. ↓ = Lesser or decrease ($p < 0.05$) over control or other condition/intervention. AUC = area under the curve; MILK = Milk protein; MCas = Micellar casein; WPH = wheat protein hydrolysate; RPI = Rice protein isolate; WPI = Whey protein isolate; EAA = Essential amino acid; NEAA = non-essential amino acid; TAA = total amino acid; AUC = Area under the curve; $C_{max}$ = maximum concentration; $t_{max}$ = time at which maximum concentration was reached. Nmol/mL = nanomole/milliliter; PP = Potato protein. 1 RM = one repetition maximum. N/A = Not applicable as no exercise protocol was used.

## 4. EXTENDED RESEARCH ON PLANT PROTEINS AND PHYSICAL ACTIVITY

Up until 2013, the only research involving plant protein ingestion and regular resistance training across several weeks was completed using soy [**48,49,50,51,52**]. A summary table of the results of all studies which have compared a plant protein to an animal protein source (usually whey) over several weeks while completing resistance training can be found in **Table 2.** Brown and colleagues [**48**] had 27 college-aged males who were enrolled in a university weight training class consume, in a double-blind fashion, a protein bar containing either 33 g of whey or soy protein while a third group completed the training, but did not consume either bar. Over nine weeks all participants completed the resistance-training program that consisted of 3 sets of 4–6 repetitions two days per week and incorporated 14 different exercises that targeted all major muscle groups. The two protein groups gained similar amounts of lean body mass while the group that only completed the resistance training did not gain any lean mass. Candow et al. [**49**] used a similar study approach whereby 27 untrained healthy men and women supplemented with isocaloric doses of either whey or soy protein while following a whole-body, 4 days per week resistance training program for six weeks. Each protein source was delivered in two equal doses on training days before and after each workout while on non-training days, three equal doses were taken and spread evenly across the day. The total daily protein dose was 1.2 g/kg/day. Thus, a 70-kg individual would have consumed 84 total grams of protein per day or an estimated 28–42 g per dose. Each exercise was performed in 4–5 sets of 6–12 repetitions at an intensity of 60–90% 1 RM. Again, both sources of protein supplementation increased strength gains and accretion of lean tissue when compared to the carbohydrate control group, but no differences were identified between the plant (soy) and animal (whey) source of protein. Hartman et al. [**51**] had young men complete a weekly resistance training program for 12 weeks while consuming either a soy or skimmed milk beverage immediately and one hour after each workout (delivering 35 g of protein for each condition) and found that greater gains ($p < 0.05$) in fat-bone-free mass occurred with the skimmed milk group (3.9 kg, 6.2%) than what was observed in the soy group (2.8 kg, 4.4%). In 2009, Denysschen et al. [**50**] supplemented 28 overweight male subjects (body mass index of 25–30 kg/m$^2$), all with total serum cholesterol > 200 mg/dL with either a placebo, soy, or whey protein. The whey, soy, and carbohydrate (placebo) all contained approximately 26 g and were administered in a randomized, double-blind fashion while each participant completed a 12-week supervised resistance training program. In accordance with the Brown and Candow studies, all three groups experienced significant increases in strength and fat-free mass. In addition, this study also illustrated similar decreases in percent body fat, waist-to-hip ratio, and total cholesterol in all three groups.

**Table 2. Summary Table of Prolonged (Training) Examining Exercise Training Adaptations Using Plant Protein Sources.**

| Reference | Participants (Age) | Design | Study Duration | Dosing Protocol (Timing) | Exercise Program | Primary Variables | Key Findings |
|---|---|---|---|---|---|---|---|
| Babault et al. [56] | 161 males (18–25 years) | RCT (3 groups)<br>Control ($n$ = 54)<br>Whey ($n$ = 53)<br>Pea ($n$ = 53) | 12 weeks | 50 g pea/day (two 25 g doses) | RT 3×/week | Muscle thickness<br>Strength | ↑ Bicep thickness<br>↑ 1-RM Strength |
| Brown et al. [48] | 27 healthy, college-aged males (19–25 years) | RCT (3 groups)<br>Control ($n$ = 9)<br>Whey ($n$ = 9)<br>Soy ($n$ = 9) | 9 weeks | 33 g soy/day (11 g dose 3x/d) | RT 2×/week | Body comp | ↑ Fat-free mass<br>↓ Percent body fat |
| Candow et al. [49] | 27 non-active males and females (18–35 years) | RCT (3 groups)<br>Control ($n$ = 9)<br>Whey ($n$ = 9)<br>Soy ($n$ = 9) | 6 weeks | 1.2 g soy/day (3 daily doses) | RT 4×/week | Body comp<br>Strength | ↑ Fat-free mass<br>↑ Strength |
| DeNysschen et al. [50] | 28 overweight males (21–50 years) | RCT (3 groups)<br>Control ($n$ = 9)<br>Whey ($n$ = 10)<br>Soy ($n$ = 9) | 12 weeks | 26 g soy/day(Post-workout) | RT 3×/week | Body comp<br>Strength<br>Anthropometrics | ↑ Fat free mass<br>↓ Percent body fat<br>↑ Strength<br>↓ Waist-to-hip ratio |
| Hartman et al. [51] | 57 healthy males(18–30 years) | RCT (3 groups)<br>Control ($n$ = 19)<br>Milk ($n$ = 18)<br>Soy ($n$ = 19) | 12 weeks | 17.5 g soy/day (Post-workout) | RT 5×/week | Body comp<br>Strength<br>Muscle fiber size | ↑ Fat-free mass<br>↔ Strength<br>↑Muscle fiber area |
| Hevia-Larrain et al. [60] | 38 untrained young males (18–35) | RCT (2 groups)<br>Vegans ($n$ = 19)<br>Ominivores ($n$ = 19) | 12 weeks | 1.6 g/kg/day (Soy or Whey) | RT 2×/week | Leg muscle mass<br>Muscle mass<br>Muscle fiber size<br>Strength | ↑ Leg muscle mass<br>↑ Lean body mass<br>↑ VL CSA<br>↑ Leg press 1-RM |

| Reference | Participants (Age) | Design | Study Duration | Dosing Protocol (Timing) | Exercise Program | Primary Variables | Key Findings |
|---|---|---|---|---|---|---|---|
| Joy et al. [**53**] | 24 healthy males (18–30) | RCT (2 groups)<br>Rice (*n* = 12)<br>Whey (*n* = 12) | 8 weeks | 48 g rice/day (Post-workout) | RT 3×/week | Body comp<br>Strength<br>Power | ↑ Fat-free mass<br>↑ Strength<br>↑ Wingate power |
| Lamb et al. 2020 [**46**] | 39 non-active older males and females (50–80 years) | RCT (2 groups)<br>Control (*n* = 19)<br>Peanut protein (*n* = 20) | 10 weeks | 30 g peanut/day (1x/d) | RT 2×/week | Body comp<br>Muscle thickness<br>Knee flexion torque | ↔ Body comp<br>↑ VL thickness<br>↑ Knee flexion torque |
| Lynch et al. [**59**] | 48 non-active males and females (18–35 years) | RCT (2 groups<br>Whey (*n* = 26)<br>Soy (*n* = 22) | 12 weeks | 19 g whey or 26 g soy/day (post-workout) | RT 3×/week | Body mass<br>Body comp<br>Muscle thickness<br>Knee flexion and extension torque | ↑ Body mass<br>↑ Fat-free mass<br>↔ VL thickness<br>↑ Peak torque |
| Mobley et al. [**58**] | 75 healthy, untrained males (19–23 years) | RCT (5 groups)<br>Control (*n* = 15)<br>Leucine (*n* = 14)<br>WPC (*n* = 17)<br>WPH (*n* = 14)<br>Soy (*n* = 15) | 12 weeks | 39.2 g soy/day (post-workout and pre-sleep) | RT 3×/week | Strength<br>Body mass<br>Body comp<br>Muscle fiber CSA | ↔ Strength<br>↔ Body mass<br>↑ Muscle Mass<br>↑ Type I/II CSA |
| Moon et al. [**54**] | 24 healthy, trained males (18–50 years) | RCT (2 groups)<br>Whey (*n* = 12)<br>Rice (*n* = 12) | 8 weeks | 24 g rice or whey/day (post-workout) | RT 4×/week | Body comp<br>Muscular strength<br>Muscular Endurance<br>Anaerobic Capacity | ↑ Body comp<br>↑ 1-RM strength<br>↑ Rep to fatigue<br>↑ Wingate power |

| Reference | Participants (Age) | Design | Study Duration | Dosing Protocol (Timing) | Exercise Program | Primary Variables | Key Findings |
|---|---|---|---|---|---|---|---|
| Reidy et al. [57] | 67 healthy males (18–35 years) | RCT (3 groups)<br>Control ($n = 23$)<br>Whey ($n = 22$)<br>Soy ($n = 23$) | 12 weeks | 22 g soy or whey/day (post-workout) | RT 3×/week | Body comp<br>Strength<br>mCSA<br>Muscle thickness | ↑ Lean body mass<br>↔ 1RM strength<br>↔ mCSA<br>↔ Muscle thickness |
| Thomson et al. [61] | 83 older adults (50–79 years) | RCT (3 groups)<br>Control ($n = 23$)<br>MILK ($n = 34$)<br>Soy ($n = 26$) | 12 weeks | 27 g soy/day (post-workout) | RT 3x/week | Strength<br>Body comp<br>Physical function | ↔ Strength<br>↑ Lean mass<br>↑ Physical function |
| Volek et al. [52] | 63 untrained males and females (18–35 years) | RCT (3 groups)<br>Control ($n = 22$)<br>Whey ($n = 19$)<br>Soy ($n = 22$) | 9 months | 24 g soy protein (Post-workout) | RT 3 ×/week | Body comp | ↑ Lean body mass<br>↔ Fat mass |

↔ = No difference ($p > 0.05$) change; ↑ = Greater increase ($p < 0.05$) over control or other condition/intervention. ↓ = Lesser or decrease ($p < 0.05$) over control or other condition/intervention. WPC = whey protein concentrate; WPH = whey protein hydrolysate; MILK = milk protein; mCSA = muscle cross-sectional area; 1 RM = one repetition maximum.

Volek and investigators [52] randomized non-resistance trained men and women to consume either 24 g of whey protein, 24 g of soy protein, or 24 g of a carbohydrate control while completing a supervised and periodized resistance training program over a nine-month period. Lean body mass gains in the individuals consuming whey protein were found to be significantly greater (~3.3 kg) than what was observed in the soy (~1.8 kg) and carbohydrate (~2.3 kg) groups.

In 2013, Joy and colleagues [53] were the first to examine the impact of rice protein for its ability to impact resistance training adaptations and this was also one of the first times a plant protein source other than soy was assessed for its potential to impact resistance training adaptations. This study randomized 24 healthy males in a double-blind fashion to ingest either 48 g of whey protein or rice protein isolate. The participants supplemented for eight weeks and followed a three day per week resistance training program. Significant increases in fat-free mass, maximal strength, and lower-body power occurred in both protein groups, but no differences in changes were observed between the two protein sources. The protein dose in this study (48 g) was chosen to ensure that adequate amounts of leucine were being delivered in both the rice and whey protein groups. Results of the study revealed similar outcomes as seen previously with soy, whereby similar short-term changes in resistance training adaptations were observed between plant and animal protein sources. As a follow-up, Moon and colleagues [54] had 24 healthy, resistance-trained males perform a four days per week split-body, linearly periodized resistance training program (3–4 sets of 6–10 RM loads) for ten weeks. In a randomized, double-blind fashion, participants began supplementing daily after completing two weeks of resistance training with 24-g doses of either a rice or whey protein concentrate. The chosen dose in this study was intended to deliver a dose of rice protein that just met what has been considered by many to be the minimum amount of leucine (~2.0 g) to stimulate protein translation [5,55]. As seen previously, significant increases in body mass, total body water, lean mass, fat-free mass, maximal upper body strength, upper body volume, and maximal lower-body strength were observed throughout the study in both groups. No differences between the two protein groups were observed for any of these outcomes, leading the authors to conclude that the observed resistance training outcomes were similar between the two protein conditions. These results are significant in the sense that this was one of the first studies to illustrate similar potential of a plant protein source to elicit changes in strength and body composition, using a smaller dose of a plant-based protein over a short period of exercise training and supplementation. Moreover, the findings also support the notion that as long as an efficacious dose of leucine and essential amino acids are ingested, that favorable exercise training adaptations can result from a plant protein source.

In 2015, Babault and colleagues [56] investigated the impact of a pea protein on changes in exercise training adaptations. Over 12 weeks, 161 males between the ages of 18–35 years completed upper body resistance training while supplementing with either pea protein, whey protein, or placebo. The total protein dose was 50 g per day that was divided up into two 25-g doses each day. Increases in muscle thickness tended ($p = 0.09$) to be greater in the pea protein group when compared to changes observed in the whey and placebo groups. Interestingly, when a sub-analysis was completed of those participants who had the lowest strength levels to start the study, pea protein supplementation exhibited a greater ability to increase muscle thickness levels. These results led the authors to conclude that a pea protein supplement could serve as an alternative to whey protein. Reidy and investigators [57] were the first to investigate the ability of a blend of soy and dairy proteins to increase strength and body composition. In randomized, double blind fashion, 58 participants consumed a 22-g dose of a soy-dairy protein balance, 22 g of whey protein isolate or an isocaloric carbohydrate placebo. Participants supplemented for 12 weeks while completing a resistance-training program. All groups experienced increases in lean mass, with the changes observed in the soy-dairy protein tending to be greater than what was seen in carbohydrate ($p = 0.09$), with no differences being observed between the whey protein isolate ($p = 0.55$). Changes in strength were similar between all groups. Muscle thickness was significantly increased in all participants with a trend being observed for differences between groups (Mean: 0.92 kg, 95% CI: –0.12, 1.95 kg, $p = 0.09$). In 2017, Mobley et al. [58] reported no differences between groups for the observed changes in strength, body composition or various tissue attributes of skeletal muscle or adipose tissue after supplementing and resistance training for 12 weeks. In this study, 75 untrained college-aged males were randomly assigned to consume a carbohydrate placebo, whey protein hydrolysate, whey protein concentrate, or a soy protein concentrate. A similar outcome was reported for Lynch and colleagues [59] who randomly supplemented 48 untrained men and women for 12 weeks with either 19 g of whey protein isolate or 26 g of soy protein isolate; protein dose amounts that both delivered 2 g of leucine. In both protein groups, body mass, lean mass, peak extension and flexion torques all increased significantly in both groups while muscle thickness tended to increase after 12 weeks of resistance. As seen in previous studies, no differences between the two protein groups were observed for the measured outcomes.

Hevia-Larrain and colleagues [60] have been one of the only research groups to examine the impact of habitually consuming a plant-based versus an omnivorous diet. This project examined the impact of protein-matched diets on resistance training adaptations in 38 young men who were physically active, but naïve to resistance training. Habitual (longer than 12 months) vegans or omnivores were assigned to a protein group and were given supplemental protein (in the form of soy protein for vegans and whey protein for omnivores) to achieve a daily protein intake of 1.6 g/kg/day. For 12 weeks, each participant resistance trained their lower-body musculature two times per week and has strength, muscle mass and cross-sectional area assessed. All measured outcomes improved in both groups across the 12-week study protocol, but there were no differences between the two protein groups. These outcomes support previous work that indicates that plant proteins, when provided as part of daily protein intake that meets daily needs, can lead to comparable improvements in strength and body composition outcomes when compared to animal proteins.

In summary, a growing number of studies have evaluated the ability of plant protein sources to stimulate resistance-training adaptations in comparison to the adaptations seen with an animal source of protein. When viewed collectively, the majority of published studies, as designed, consistently indicate that plant proteins can deliver similar changes in strength and body composition when strategies are taken to either equate the amount of leucine being delivered or ensuring that enough leucine and the other essential amino acids are being delivered. The majority of studies completed thus far have been 8–12 weeks in duration and this may function as an important consideration when interpreting this literature. A key exception to this was seen with Volek et al. [**52**] who reported more favorable adaptations after whey protein ingestion when compared to an identical dose of soy protein after 9 months of training. Thus, it remains quite possible that while studies performed of shorter durations are reporting equivalence within these established delimitations that if future studies are performed for longer time periods (4–6 months or longer) that different outcomes may result. To support this notion, the Moon et al. [**54**] study reported no differences in strength and body composition changes after eight weeks of supplementing with a 24-g dose of either rice or whey protein with a total daily protein intake of 1.4–2.0 g/kg/day, however, the largest mean changes from baseline were observed in the whey protein group.

## 5. CONSIDERATIONS FOR THE RECOVERY OF PLANT PROTEIN SOURCES

Additional research has examined the ability of various plant-based proteins for their ability to influence post-exercise protein kinetics and recovery [**62,63,64,65**]. For example, Kritikos et al. [**62**] recently examined differences in recovery kinetics following speed endurance training in male soccer players after ingesting whey or soy protein. The authors concluded that both whey and soy protein were able to mitigate reductions in field-based performance during successive speed-endurance training sessions, with neither protein source appearing to have an effect on exercise-induced muscle damage or markers of oxidative stress. Using an eccentric muscle damage model, Nieman and investigators [**64**] compared the ability of whey or pea protein to mitigate decrements in force production and increases in markers of swelling, muscle damage, and inflammation. A 90-min bout of eccentric exercise in 92 untrained, non-obese males was used to invoke muscle damage. The participants were divided into three groups: placebo (water), whey protein (0.9 g/kg divided into three doses per day), and pea protein (0.9 g protein/kg divided into three doses per day) and changes in force production, power, and blood markers were assessed each day for five consecutive days. Following muscle damage, Whey protein significantly attenuated increases in blood-based markers of muscle damage while the changes observed in pea protein were not significantly different than what was observed in the water condition. No differences, however, were identified between the magnitudes of differences observed in the two protein groups. Xia et al. [**63**] examined the effects of oat protein supplementation on markers of muscle damage and inflammation in addition to measures of performance following downhill running. After 14 days of supplementation with 25 g per day of oat protein, an attenuation of the observed increases in eccentric exercise-induced muscle soreness and serum concentrations of IL-6, creatine kinase, myoglobin, and C-reactive protein were observed. A marked reduction in lower limb edema, in addition to a lesser reduction in muscle strength, knee-joint range of motion and vertical jump performance was observed following oat protein supplementation when compared to placebo.

In contrast with the previous findings that suggested a favorable ability of protein to promote recovery, Saracino and researchers [**65**] had 27 recreationally active, middle-aged men complete 5 sets of 15 repetitions using eccentric contractions the knee extensors and flexors. Starting the same day as which muscle damage occurred, participants ingested equivalent doses (40 g) of whey protein hydrolysate, whey isolate, or a rice and pea protein combination in addition to a placebo group 30 min prior to going to sleep and did this supplementation regimen again for the next two nights. Nutrient intake was standardized to ensure adequate daily protein and a series of circumference, soreness, muscle damage markers and strength measures were taken for 72 h after completion of the exercise bout. While widespread and predictable changes in the measured outcomes occurred in response to the exercise bout, no differences were identified between any of the supplementation groups. As such, the authors concluded that pre-sleep supplementation protein ingestion, regardless of protein source, did not aid in muscle recovery from muscle-damaging exercise. The results from the Saracino study align with previous indications by Pasiakos et al. [**66**], who concluded in their meta-analysis that added protein may exert limited benefit in terms of promoting recovery and reducing muscle damage and soreness. In this respect, it is difficult to draw conclusions across studies that investigated the effects of only plant or animal-based proteins in isolation, rather than comparing multiple protein sources within the same study.

**Table 3. Summary Table of Studies Examining Exercise Recovery Outcomes Using Plant Protein Sources.**

| Author (Year) | Participants (Age) | Design | Study Duration | Dosing Protocol (Timing) | Exercise Program | Primary Variables | Key Findings |
|---|---|---|---|---|---|---|---|
| Nieman et al. [64] | 92 healthy, untrained males(18–55 years) | RCT (3 groups) Control ($n$ = 30) Whey ($n$ = 31) Pea ($n$ = 31) | 5 days | 0.3 g/kg/d pea or whey/day (Pre-workout) | 90 min eccentric exercise bout | Strength Vertical jump Anaerobic power Muscle soreness | ↔ 1 RM strength ↔ Vertical jump ↔ Wingate power ↑ Muscle soreness |
| Saracino et al. [65] | 27 active, middle-aged males(40–64 years) | RCT (4 groups) Control ($n$ = 6) WPH ($n$ = 9) WPI ($n$ = 6) Rice/pea ($n$ = 6) | 3 days | 40 g rice/Pea blend/day (pre-sleep) | Lower body muscle-sdamaging exercise | MVC Muscle soreness Thigh circumference | ↓ MVC ↔ Muscle soreness ↔ Thigh circumference |
| Kritikos et al. [62] | 10 well-trained soccer players ($n$ = 10) | RCT, crossover | 3 days | 1.5 g/kg/day whey or soy | Field-based speed training sessions | Performance Isokinetic strength MVC Lower body power Muscle damage Creatine kinase Muscle soreness | ↓ Isokinetic leg strength ↓ MVC ↓ Speed ↓CMJ ↑ CK ↑ DOMS |
| Xia et al. [63] | 16 healthy, non-active males (19.7 ± 1.1 years) | RCT (2 groups) Control ($n$ = 8) Oat ($n$ = 8) | 19 days | 25 g oat/day (post-workout) | Downhill running | Muscle soreness IL-6 Creatine kinase Leg strength Vertical jump | ↓ Muscle soreness ↓ IL-6 ↓ CK ↑ 1 RM strength ↑ Vertical jump |

↔ = No difference ($p > 0.05$) change; ↑ = Greater increase ($p < 0.05$) over control or other condition/intervention. ↓ = Lesser or decrease ($p < 0.05$) over control or other condition/intervention. WPC = whey protein concentrate; WPH = whey protein hydrolysate; WPI = whey protein isolate; MILK = milk protein; DOMS = delayed onset muscle soreness; CK = creatine kinase; IL-6 = interleukin-6; MVC = maximal voluntary contraction; 1 RM = one repetition maximum.

As such, contextual factors such as exercise modalities, differences in protein metabolism assessment techniques and subject characteristics may confound any further ability to draw conclusions across the literature regarding a superior effect of one protein sources over the other. Consequently, more studies are needed that examine the potential of single or blended sources of plant protein in comparison to animal sources for their ability to differentially impact performance or various recovery metrics in response to challenging doses of exercise. A summary table of all studies which have compared some aspect of exercise recovery between a plant and animal source of protein can be found in **Table 3**.

## 6. FACTORS FOR SENIOR INDIVIDUALS

It is well-established that as individuals age their rate of muscle mass loss (i.e., sarcopenia) [**67**,**68**] and muscle strength and function loss (e.g., dynapenia) [**69**] both increase. Accepted countermeasures for these changes are an increase in weight-bearing (resistance) exercise and an adequate delivery of protein and amino acids. In this respect, several studies are now available that have examined the impact of protein ingestion in older populations. For example, post-prandial MPS rates after ingesting 24 g of soy protein have been shown to be lower in older adults when compared to beef protein ingestion [**70**]. Moreover, Yang and colleagues [**4**] examined the dose-response impact of soy protein ingestion in older adults and found that doses of up to 40 g of soy protein failed to elevate MPS rates from basal (fasting) levels. In consideration of soy ingestion, these results are important as they seemingly suggest that even a large dose (40 g) may fail to appropriately stimulate MPS rates. Other studies have examined the impact of plant-based foods in elderly women [**71**] and concluded that net protein synthesis was lower during a high vegetable protein diet versus a high animal protein diet. Moreover, Gorissen et al. [**43**] had 60 healthy older men consume one of four sources of protein in a 35-g dose: whey, micellar casein, wheat, or wheat protein hydrolysate or a 60-g dose of wheat protein hydrolysate (an amount that deliver equivalent amounts of leucine as in the 35 g dose of whey). Postprandial increases in plasma leucine were highest after ingesting whey while myofibrillar protein synthesis increases were greater in whey and casein while the 60-g dose of wheat matched rates of myofibrillar protein synthesis. When viewed in concert with the findings of Yang et al. [**4**], these outcomes highlight the need for older individuals to either consume larger doses of plant proteins or for strategies to be implemented that increase the anabolic potential of the plant protein dose. Practically speaking, these results are troubling and seemingly work against the age-related loss of appetite and enjoyment from food that occurs with advancing age [**72**].

Finally, two studies have examined the impact of combining different sources of plant proteins in combination with resistance training in older adults to identify the impact that plant protein consumption may have on changes in strength and body composition. Briefly, Thomson et al. [**61**] compared changes in strength and body composition in both soy protein and dairy protein (both consumed in dosages of 27 g/day and a total protein intake of 1.2 g/kg/day) in a group of older (61.5 ± 7.4 years) adults. After 12 weeks, both groups experienced increases in strength and fat-free mass, but no differences between the two protein sources were found. Similarly, Lamb and colleagues [**46**] randomized 39 older (58 ± 8 years), untrained men and women to consumed either a defatted peanut protein powder (30 g protein, 9 g essential amino acids) or no supplement at all. Hypertrophy and performance were assessed six and ten weeks after supplementation and no changes in fat mass, lean, or percent body fat were found between the groups. An increase in vastus lateralis thickness was observed in the peanut protein group when compared to the no-supplement controls and peak power increased in the peanut powder group. The authors concluded that a defatted peanut protein powder may positively impact resistance training adaptations seen in a group of healthy, older previously untrained men and women. More research is needed to help identify what differential impact, if any, plant protein sources may hold over animal sources of protein.

## 7. AUGMENTING THE ANABOLIC POTENTIAL OF PLANT SOURCES

Multiple techniques are available to enhance the anabolic capacity of different protein sources. These tactics encompass, but are not limited to, augmenting daily protein consumption, co-ingesting plant proteins with amino acids or other nutrients, supplementing plant sources with amino acids identified as deficient or limiting, and amalgamating diverse protein sources. Certainly, the easiest solution to overcome the lower levels of amino acids and digestibility is to increase the size of protein dose. In this respect, studies in younger subjects [**15,73**] illustrate that a dose of 20–25 g of protein (0.25 g/kg body/dose) can maximize MPS using animal sources. When using plant protein sources, as highlighted by other studies [**4,43**], larger doses are likely needed to maximize the MPS response. While accepted to be a simple recommendation, pragmatic aspects must be considered as sometimes larger doses might be challenging for people to consume due to larger volume of fluid, higher fiber intakes (common in plant-based foods), or food being needed to ingest, particularly for older individuals.

Another strategy that needs further exploration involves the co-ingestion of plant proteins with various nutrients to help increase the anabolic potential of plant protein, particularly in those populations that need more protein and/or may not be consuming enough protein. Towards this end, previous research has indicated that consuming omega-3 fatty acids with an amino acid infusion surrounding resistance exercise can heighten anabolic sensitivity of skeletal muscle and increase rates of MPS [**74,75**]. This practice, however, has yet to be evaluated in an exercise training model in combination with plant protein consumption. Nonetheless, these results are of great interest and future research should seek to explore this approach with plant sources of protein to determine if the increased anabolic sensitivity also occurs with intact plant ingestion and then if this translates to greater gains in health and resistance training adaptations.

As highlighted earlier, the leucine content of feeding has been shown to be of critical importance in terms of stimulating MPS [**14,15**]. In this respect and on a per gram basis, plant sources have lower amounts of leucine as well as many of the essential amino acids [22]. To overcome these shortcomings, researchers have explored the impact of consuming smaller doses of protein but fortifying the dose with added leucine or other limiting amino acids. For example, Churchward-Venne and colleagues [76] added leucine to a small dose (6.25 g) of whey protein to match the leucine that was delivered in a 25-g dose of whey protein. They demonstrated this approach was effective at stimulating fed rates of MPS, but the 25-g dose of whey protein better sustained exercise-induced rates of MPS. While the approach has yet to be examined using a plant protein sources, previous studies [77,78] that combined plant proteins with leucine or all three branched-chain amino acids have illustrated favorable changes in MPS and how certain amino acids are metabolized inside various tissues. Future work should build upon these approaches to examine their efficacy at promoting favorable adaptations to exercise training.

A commonly proposed solution to overcoming the shortcomings associated with plant protein intake center upon mixing the plant source with an animal source or another plant source [79]. Using this approach, acute MPS responses were assessed after ingesting a protein blend of 25% whey protein, 25% soy protein, and 50% casein protein and completion of a single bout of lower-body resistance exercise. When compared to an isonitrogenous dose of whey protein in young, healthy males, the protein blend increased mixed MPS rates to a similar magnitude as what was observed with whey protein consumption [80]. This acute study was followed up using a 12-week resistance-training model whereby Reidy and colleagues [57] supplemented 68 young, healthy males daily with 22-g doses of either a blend of soy and dairy proteins, an isocaloric carbohydrate control, or a protein-equated whey protein group while performing a supervised resistance training program three days per week. When compared to a carbohydrate control, the protein blend tended to increase lean mass while no change was observed in the whey protein group. The authors concluded that the intake of a protein blend marginally improved whole-body and arm lean mass growth, whereas strength alterations were comparable between groups. For numerous individuals, a protein mixture including merely 25% soy protein and 75% animal protein will be unacceptable. Consequently, based on the fundamental rationale for solely opting for plant-based protein sources, it may be impractical for humans to amalgamate plant- and animal-based proteins. In this context, the amalgamation of several plant protein sources has been investigated to optimize amino acid provision while ensuring the blend is entirely plant-based. At now, there is no data utilizing this method to detect acute alterations in muscle protein synthesis responses or modifications in resistance training adaptations following several weeks of treatment. Further investigation in this domain should be contemplated.

Another technique to enhance the possible effects of plant protein consumption may focus on the time or closeness of nutrient intake in relation to exercise. The concept of nutritional timing is not novel, and the current stance on the subject has extensively examined the literature regarding its effectiveness [81]. As previously noted, resistance training triggers a sensitization phase in skeletal muscle that amplifies the anabolic effects of protein consumption [82]. Consequently, a larger proportion of amino acids obtained from dietary sources is allocated to peripheral tissues rather than splanchnic extraction, hence promoting enhanced rates of muscle protein synthesis (MPS) [83]. This increased sensitivity has been demonstrated to endure for up to 24 hours following the conclusion of an exercise session [82]. Thus, when plant protein feedings are administered, which may yield a reduced bolus of amino acids due to various factors discussed in this paper, they can still elicit significant increases in muscle protein synthesis rates if consumed during this phase of heightened sensitivity. No research has yet investigated the time of plant protein administration, and future studies should aim to ascertain the degree to which these tactics may enhance adaptations typically observed from resistance training. Recent studies by Stecker [84] and Jäger [85] have demonstrated that the incorporation of different probiotic strains into animal and plant protein sources may positively influence the absorption of various amino acids into the bloodstream when consumed concurrently with protein.

## 8. CONCISE SUMMARY

The popularity of plant proteins has grown substantially in recent years. Initial research that examined the acute impact of various sources of protein at stimulating MPS clearly points towards an advantage for the highest quality protein sources, which are viewed to be those that are derived from animal sources. As such, animal proteins were strongly advocated for health and performance outcomes while plant sources of protein were viewed to be inferior at helping exercising individuals achieve their exercise training goals. Only recently have studies begun to appear that have compared the ability of various animal and plant protein sources regarding facilitating increases in strength, endurance, power, fat-free mass accretion, and recovery over the course of several weeks of exercise training and supplementation. From this prolonged data, a consistent pattern has appeared which suggests that when total daily protein intake is achieved at levels recommended for exercising athletes (1.4–2.0 g/kg/day) [**5**,**7**,**11**], the source of protein does not function as a determining factor in the observed outcomes.

Two key considerations stemming from this conclusion, however, must be considered. First, only one study to date [**60**] has made such comparisons in study participants who were habitually consuming either plant or animal sources of protein. This point is not made to detract from the significance of the other published findings, but the majority of studies that have provided a daily dose of a plant protein have done so with individuals consuming diets mixed with various animal protein sources. Thus, for a 180-pound (81.7 kg) individual who is consuming 1.5 g/kg/day of protein, a daily 25-g dose of plant protein represents approximately 20% of that individual's daily protein intake and one can reasonably question how much impact changing the source of just 20% of the daily protein delivered will impact overall outcomes. Second, nearly all studies (acute and prolonged) have utilized free amino acid mixtures or isolated protein powders while the majority of nearly all dietary protein is consumed as some form of mixture of macro- and micronutrients. More research needs to continue to explore how the matrix of nutrients found in single foods and meals impacts these outcomes. The future is bright, however, for plant proteins, as strategies have been articulated in this paper and others [**16**,**23**] regarding various strategies that can be considered to help increase the quality of each plant protein feeding. In this respect, more research is needed to identify if co-ingestion of plant proteins with various nutrients can heighten desired physiological adaptations by exercising individuals. Furthermore, research should explore how changes in plant protein manufacturing (hydrolyzing, heat treatment, etc.) as well as the timing or pattern of how the protein is administered, particularly in reference to completion of resistance exercise, may confer certain advantages.

## AT A GLANCE

Insufficient dietary protein is crucial for various health aspects, with current studies indicating that physically active adults require higher protein intake. Animal protein sources consistently rank among the greatest in quality, mostly due to their elevated concentrations of key amino acids and superior digestion and absorption characteristics. In recent years, the incorporation of plant protein sources into the diet has increased, and evidence continues to mount regarding the comparison of various plant protein sources with animal protein sources in their capacity to stimulate muscle protein synthesis (MPS), enhance exercise training adaptations, and promote recovery from exercise. The most substantial increases in muscle protein synthesis (MPS) arise from effective dosages of whey protein isolate; nevertheless, other studies have demonstrated that diverse plant sources can also significantly enhance resting MPS rates. Research has demonstrated that a sufficient quantity of plant protein, including adequate essential amino acids, particularly leucine, taken over a duration of 8–12 weeks, can elicit adaptations to exercise training comparable to those achieved with animal protein sources. Further investigation is required to determine whether extended supplementation durations preserve equivalency across the protein sources. Various methods are available to enhance the anabolic potential of plant protein sources, and further research is required to ascertain which method, if any, provides significant benefits. In conclusion, given the beneficial health effects of augmenting plant consumption and environmental sustainability, the inclination towards increased plant protein consumption will persist. The evidence supporting plant proteins for exercising individuals has significantly expanded, with numerous findings suggesting that the intake of a plant protein source in an effective dosage (generally exceeding that of animal protein) can elicit comparable and beneficial effects on amino acid uptake, muscle protein synthesis rates, and adaptations to exercise training, including strength, body composition, and recovery.

## REFERENCES

1. Burd, N.A.; Tang, J.E.; Moore, D.R.; Phillips, S.M. Exercise training and protein metabolism: Influences of contraction, protein intake, and sex-based differences. *J. Appl. Physiol.* **2009**, *106*, 1692–1701. [**Google Scholar**] [**PubMed**]

2. Koopman, R.; van Loon, L.J. Aging, exercise, and muscle protein metabolism. *J. Appl. Physiol.* **2009**, *106*, 2040–2048. **[Google Scholar]**

3. Biolo, G.; Tipton, K.D.; Klein, S.; Wolfe, R.R. An abundant supply of amino acids enhances the metabolic effect of exercise on muscle protein. *Am. J. Physiol.* **1997**, *273*, E122–E129. **[Google Scholar] [PubMed]**

4. Yang, Y.; Churchward-Venne, T.A.; Burd, N.A.; Breen, L.; Tarnopolsky, M.A.; Phillips, S.M. Myofibrillar protein synthesis following ingestion of soy protein isolate at rest and after resistance exercise in elderly men. *Nutr. Metab.* **2012**, *9*, 57. **[Google Scholar] [PubMed] [Green Version]**

5. Jäger, R.; Kerksick, C.M.; Campbell, B.I.; Cribb, P.J.; Wells, S.D.; Skwiat, T.M.; Purpura, M.; Ziegenfuss, T.N.; Ferrando, A.A.; Arent, S.M.; et al. International Society of Sports Nutrition Position Stand: Protein and exercise. *J. Int. Soc. Sports Nutr.* **2017**, *14*, 20. **[Google Scholar] [PubMed] [Green Version]**

6. Phillips, S.M. A brief review of higher dietary protein diets in weight loss: A focus on athletes. *Sports Med.* **2014**, *44* (Suppl S2), S149–S153. **[Google Scholar] [Green Version]**

7. Morton, R.W.; Murphy, K.T.; McKellar, S.R.; Schoenfeld, B.J.; Henselmans, M.; Helms, E.; Aragon, A.A.; Devries, M.C.; Banfield, L.; Krieger, J.W.; et al. A systematic review, meta-analysis and meta-regression of the effect of protein supplementation on resistance training-induced gains in muscle mass and strength in healthy adults. *Br. J. Sports Med.* **2018**, *52*, 376–384. **[Google Scholar]**

8. Phillips, S.M.; Chevalier, S.; Leidy, H.J. Protein "requirements" beyond the RDA: Implications for optimizing health. *Appl. Physiol. Nutr. Metab.* **2016**, *41*, 565–572. **[Google Scholar] [Green Version]**

9. Phillips, S.M.; Van Loon, L.J.C. Dietary protein for athletes: From requirements to optimum adaptation. *J. Sports Sci.* **2011**, *29* (Suppl S1), S29–S38. **[Google Scholar]**

10. Cermak, N.M.; Res, P.T.; de Groot, L.C.; Saris, W.H.; van Loon, L.J. Protein supplementation augments the adaptive response of skeletal muscle to resistance-type exercise training: A meta-analysis. *Am. J. Clin. Nutr.* **2012**, *96*, 1454–1464. **[Google Scholar] [Green Version]**

11. Rodriguez, N.R.; DiMarco, N.M.; Langley, S.; American Dietetic Association; Dietitians of Canada; American College of Sports Medicine: Nutrition and Athletic Performance. Position of the American Dietetic Association, Dietitians of Canada, and the American College of Sports Medicine: Nutrition and athletic performance. *J. Am. Diet. Assoc.* **2009**, *109*, 509–527. **[Google Scholar]**

12. Tipton, K.D.; Gurkin, B.E.; Matin, S.; Wolfe, R.R. Nonessential amino acids are not necessary to stimulate net muscle protein synthesis in healthy volunteers. *J. Nutr. Biochem.* **1999**, *10*, 89–95. **[Google Scholar]**

13. Volpi, E.; Kobayashi, H.; Sheffield-Moore, M.; Mittendorfer, B.; Wolfe, R.R. Essential amino acids are primarily responsible for the amino acid stimulation of muscle protein anabolism in healthy elderly adults. *Am. J. Clin. Nutr.* **2003**, *78*, 250–258. **[Google Scholar]**

14. Drummond, M.J.; Rasmussen, B.B. Leucine-enriched nutrients and the regulation of mammalian target of rapamycin signalling and human skeletal muscle protein synthesis. *Curr. Opin. Clin. Nutr. Metab. Care* **2008**, *11*, 222–226. **[Google Scholar]**

15. Witard, O.C.; Jackman, S.R.; Breen, L.; Smith, K.; Selby, A.; Tipton, K.D. Myofibrillar muscle protein synthesis rates subsequent to a meal in response to increasing doses of whey protein at rest and after resistance exercise. *Am. J. Clin. Nutr.* **2014**, *99*, 86–95. **[Google Scholar] [PubMed] [Green Version]**

16. Berrazaga, I.; Micard, V.; Gueugneau, M.; Walrand, S. The Role of the Anabolic Properties of Plant- versus Animal-Based Protein Sources in Supporting Muscle Mass Maintenance: A Critical Review. *Nutrients* **2019**, *11*, 1825. **[Google Scholar] [PubMed] [Green Version]**

17. Lynch, H.; Johnston, C.; Wharton, C. Plant-Based Diets: Considerations for Environmental Impact, Protein Quality, and Exercise Performance. *Nutrients* **2018**, *10*, 1841. **[Google Scholar] [PubMed] [Green Version]**

18. FAOSTAT. *Food Balance Sheets*; Food and Agriculture Organization of the United Nations Statistics Division: Rome, Italy, 2013. **[Google Scholar]**

19. Moore, D.R.; Soeters, P.B. The Biological Value of Protein. *Nestle Nutr. Inst. Workshop Ser.* **2015**, *82*, 39–51. **[Google Scholar] [PubMed]**

20. Eggum, B. Comments on report of a joint FAO/WHO expert consultation on protein quality evaluation, Rome 1990. *Z. Ernahr.* **1991**, *30*, 81–88. **[Google Scholar] [PubMed]**

21. Schaafsma, G. The protein digestibility-corrected amino acid score. *J. Nutr.* **2000**, *130*, 1865S–1867S. **[Google Scholar] [PubMed] [Green Version]**

22. Gorissen, S.H.M.; Crombag, J.J.R.; Senden, J.M.G.; Waterval, W.A.H.; Bierau, J.; Verdijk, L.B.; van Loon, L.J.C. Protein content and amino acid composition of commercially available plant-based protein isolates. *Amino Acids* **2018**, *50*, 1685–1695. **[Google Scholar] [Green Version]**

23. van Vliet, S.; Burd, N.A.; van Loon, L.J. The Skeletal Muscle Anabolic Response to Plant-versus Animal-Based Protein Consumption. *J. Nutr.* **2015**, *145*, 1981–1991. **[Google Scholar] [Green Version]**

24. Tang, J.E.; Moore, D.R.; Kujbida, G.W.; Tarnopolsky, M.A.; Phillips, S.M. Ingestion of whey hydrolysate, casein, or soy protein isolate: Effects on mixed muscle protein synthesis at rest and following resistance exercise in young men. *J. Appl. Physiol.* **2009**, *107*, 987–992. **[Google Scholar] [PubMed]**

25. FAO/WHO. Dietary protein quality evaluation in human nutrition. Report of an FAQ Expert Consultation. *FAO Food Nutr. Pap.* **2013**, *92*, 1–66. **[Google Scholar]**

26. Boirie, Y.; Dangin, M.; Gachon, P.; Vasson, M.P.; Maubois, J.L.; Beaufrere, B. Slow and fast dietary proteins differently modulate postprandial protein accretion. *Proc. Natl. Acad. Sci. USA* **1997**, *94*, 14930–14935. **[Google Scholar] [PubMed] [Green Version]**

27. Boirie, Y.; Gachon, P.; Corny, S.; Fauquant, J.; Maubois, J.L.; Beaufrere, B. Acute postprandial changes in leucine metabolism as assessed with an intrinsically labeled milk protein. *Am. J. Physiol.* **1996**, *271*, E1083–E1091. **[Google Scholar]**

28. Dangin, M.; Boirie, Y.; Garcia-Rodenas, C.; Gachon, P.; Fauquant, J.; Callier, P.; Ballevre, O.; Beaufrere, B. The digestion rate of protein is an independent regulating factor of postprandial protein retention. *Am. J. Physiol. Endocrinol. Metab.* **2001**, *280*, E340–E348. **[Google Scholar] [Green Version]**

29. Dangin, M.; Boirie, Y.; Guillet, C.; Beaufrere, B. Influence of the protein digestion rate on protein turnover in young and elderly subjects. *J. Nutr.* **2002**, *132*, 3228S–3233S. **[Google Scholar]**

30. Bos, C.; Metges, C.C.; Gaudichon, C.; Petzke, K.J.; Pueyo, M.E.; Morens, C.; Everwand, J.; Benamouzig, R.; Tome, D. Postprandial kinetics of dietary amino acids are the main determinant of their metabolism after soy or milk protein ingestion in humans. *J. Nutr.* **2003**, *133*, 1308–1315. **[Google Scholar] [PubMed]**

31. Mariotti, F.; Mahe, S.; Benamouzig, R.; Luengo, C.; Dare, S.; Gaudichon, C.; Tome, D. Nutritional value of [15N]-soy protein isolate assessed from ileal digestibility and postprandial protein utilization in humans. *J. Nutr.* **1999**, *129*, 1992–1997. **[Google Scholar] [PubMed]**

32. Gaudichon, C.; Mahe, S.; Benamouzig, R.; Luengo, C.; Fouillet, H.; Dare, S.; Van Oycke, M.; Ferriere, F.; Rautureau, J.; Tome, D. Net postprandial utilization of [15N]-labeled milk protein nitrogen is influenced by diet composition in humans. *J. Nutr.* **1999**, *129*, 890–895. **[Google Scholar]**

33. Bos, C.; Juillet, B.; Fouillet, H.; Turlan, L.; Dare, S.; Luengo, C.; N'Tounda, R.; Benamouzig, R.; Gausseres, N.; Tome, D.; et al. Postprandial metabolic utilization of wheat protein in humans. *Am. J. Clin. Nutr.* **2005**, *81*, 87–94. **[Google Scholar] [Green Version]**

34. Luiking, Y.C.; Deutz, N.E.; Jakel, M.; Soeters, P.B. Casein and soy protein meals differentially affect whole-body and splanchnic protein metabolism in healthy humans. *J. Nutr.* **2005**, *135*, 1080–1087. **[Google Scholar] [PubMed] [Green Version]**

35. Lohrke, B.; Saggau, E.; Schadereit, R.; Beyer, M.; Bellmann, O.; Kuhla, S.; Hagemeister, H. Activation of skeletal muscle protein breakdown following consumption of soyabean protein in pigs. *Br. J. Nutr.* **2001**, *85*, 447–457. **[Google Scholar] [PubMed] [Green Version]**

36. Fouillet, H.; Bos, C.; Gaudichon, C.; Tome, D. Approaches to quantifying protein metabolism in response to nutrient ingestion. *J. Nutr.* **2002**, *132*, 3208S–3218S. **[Google Scholar] [Green Version]**

37. Millward, D.J.; Fereday, A.; Gibson, N.R.; Cox, M.C.; Pacy, P.J. Efficiency of utilization of wheat and milk protein in healthy adults and apparent lysine requirements determined by a single-meal [1-13C]leucine balance protocol. *Am. J. Clin. Nutr.* **2002**, *76*, 1326–1334. **[Google Scholar]**

38. Areta, J.L.; Burke, L.M.; Ross, M.L.; Camera, D.M.; West, D.W.; Broad, E.M.; Jeacocke, N.A.; Moore, D.R.; Stellingwerff, T.; Phillips, S.M.; et al. Timing and distribution of protein ingestion during prolonged recovery from resistance exercise alters myofibrillar protein synthesis. *J. Physiol.* **2013**, *591*, 2319–2331. **[Google Scholar]**

39. Wilkinson, S.B.; Tarnopolsky, M.A.; Macdonald, M.J.; Macdonald, J.R.; Armstrong, D.; Phillips, S.M. Consumption of fluid skim milk promotes greater muscle protein accretion after resistance exercise than does consumption of an isonitrogenous and isoenergetic soy-protein beverage. *Am. J. Clin. Nutr.* **2007**, *85*, 1031–1040. **[Google Scholar] [PubMed]**

40. Kraemer, W.J.; Solomon-Hill, G.; Volk, B.M.; Kupchak, B.R.; Looney, D.P.; Dunn-Lewis, C.; Comstock, B.A.; Szivak, T.K.; Hooper, D.R.; Flanagan, S.D.; et al. The effects of soy and whey protein supplementation on acute hormonal reponses to resistance exercise in men. *J. Am. Coll. Nutr.* **2013**, *32*, 66–74. **[Google Scholar]**

41. Pinckaers, P.J.M.; Kouw, I.W.K.; Hendriks, F.K.; van Kranenburg, J.M.X.; de Groot, L.; Verdijk, L.B.; Snijders, T.; van Loon, L.J.C. No differences in muscle protein synthesis rates following ingestion of wheat protein, milk protein, and their protein blend in healthy, young males. *Br. J. Nutr.* **2021**, 1–38. **[Google Scholar]**

42. Oikawa, S.Y.; Bahniwal, R.; Holloway, T.M.; Lim, C.; McLeod, J.C.; McGlory, C.; Baker, S.K.; Phillips, S.M. Potato Protein Isolate Stimulates Muscle Protein Synthesis at Rest and with Resistance Exercise in Young Women. *Nutrients* **2020**, *12*, 1235. **[Google Scholar]**

43. Gorissen, S.H.; Horstman, A.M.; Franssen, R.; Crombag, J.J.; Langer, H.; Bierau, J.; Respondek, F.; van Loon, L.J. Ingestion of Wheat Protein Increases In Vivo Muscle Protein Synthesis Rates in Healthy Older Men in a Randomized Trial. *J. Nutr.* **2016**, *146*, 1651–1659. **[Google Scholar]**

44. Purpura, M.; Lowery, R.P.; Joy, J.M.; De Souza, E.O.; Kalman, D. A comparison of blood amino acid concentrations following ingestion of rice and whey protein isolate: A double-blind, crossover study. *J. Nutr. Health Sci.* **2014**, *1*, 306. **[Google Scholar]**

45. Arya, S.S.; Salve, A.R.; Chauhan, S. Peanuts as functional food: A review. *J. Food Sci. Technol.* **2016**, *53*, 31–41. **[Google Scholar] [Green Version]**

46. Lamb, D.A.; Moore, J.H.; Smith, M.A.; Vann, C.G.; Osburn, S.C.; Ruple, B.A.; Fox, C.D.; Smith, K.S.; Altonji, O.M.; Power, Z.M.; et al. The effects of resistance training with or without peanut protein supplementation on skeletal muscle and strength adaptations in older individuals. *J. Int. Soc. Sports Nutr.* **2020**, *17*, 66. **[Google Scholar] [PubMed]**

47. Park, S.; Church, D.D.; Schutzler, S.E.; Azhar, G.; Kim, I.Y.; Ferrando, A.A.; Wolfe, R.R. Metabolic Evaluation of the Dietary Guidelines' Ounce Equivalents of Protein Food Sources in Young Adults: A Randomized Controlled Trial. *J. Nutr.* **2021**. **[Google Scholar] [PubMed]**

48. Brown, E.C.; DiSilvestro, R.A.; Babaknia, A.; Devor, S.T. Soy versus whey protein bars: Effects on exercise training impact on lean body mass and antioxidant status. *Nutr. J.* **2004**, 3, 22. **[Google Scholar] [PubMed]**

49. Candow, D.G.; Burke, N.C.; Smith-Palmer, T.; Burke, D.G. Effect of whey and soy protein supplementation combined with resistance training in young adults. *Int. J. Sport Nutr. Exerc. Metab.* **2006**, *16*, 233–244. **[Google Scholar]**

50. Denysschen, C.A.; Burton, H.W.; Horvath, P.J.; Leddy, J.J.; Browne, R.W. Resistance training with soy vs whey protein supplements in hyperlipidemic males. *J. Int. Soc. Sports Nutr.* **2009**, *6*, 8. **[Google Scholar] [PubMed] [Green Version]**

51. Hartman, J.W.; Tang, J.E.; Wilkinson, S.B.; Tarnopolsky, M.A.; Lawrence, R.L.; Fullerton, A.V.; Phillips, S.M. Consumption of fat-free fluid milk after resistance exercise promotes greater lean mass accretion than does consumption of soy or carbohydrate in young, novice, male weightlifters. *Am. J. Clin. Nutr.* **2007**, *86*, 373–381. **[Google Scholar] [Green Version]**

52. Volek, J.S.; Volk, B.M.; Gomez, A.L.; Kunces, L.J.; Kupchak, B.R.; Freidenreich, D.J.; Aristizabal, J.C.; Saenz, C.; Dunn-Lewis, C.; Ballard, K.D.; et al. Whey protein supplementation during resistance training augments lean body mass. *J. Am. Coll. Nutr.* **2013**, *32*, 122–135. **[Google Scholar] [PubMed]**

53. Joy, J.M.; Lowery, R.P.; Wilson, J.M.; Purpura, M.; De Souza, E.O.; Wilson, S.M.; Kalman, D.S.; Dudeck, J.E.; Jäger, R. The effects of 8 weeks of whey or rice protein supplementation on body composition and exercise performance. *Nutr. J.* **2013**, *12*, 86. **[Google Scholar] [PubMed] [Green Version]**

54. Moon, J.M.; Ratliff, K.M.; Blumkaitis, J.C.; Harty, P.S.; Zabriskie, H.A.; Stecker, R.A.; Currier, B.S.; Jagim, A.R.; Jäger, R.; Purpura, M.; et al. Effects of daily 24-gram doses of rice or whey protein on resistance training adaptations in trained males. *J. Int. Soc. Sports Nutr.* **2020**, *17*, 60. **[Google Scholar] [PubMed]**

55. Moore, D.R. Maximizing Post-exercise Anabolism: The Case for Relative Protein Intakes. *Front. Nutr.* **2019**, *6*, 147. **[Google Scholar]**

56. Babault, N.; Paizis, C.; Deley, G.; Guerin-Deremaux, L.; Saniez, M.H.; Lefranc-Millot, C.; Allaert, F.A. Pea proteins oral supplementation promotes muscle thickness gains during resistance training: A double-blind, randomized, Placebo-controlled clinical trial vs. Whey protein. *J. Int. Soc. Sports Nutr.* **2015**, *12*, 3. **[Google Scholar] [Green Version]**

57. Reidy, P.T.; Borack, M.S.; Markofski, M.M.; Dickinson, J.M.; Deer, R.R.; Husaini, S.H.; Walker, D.K.; Igbinigie, S.; Robertson, S.M.; Cope, M.B.; et al. Protein Supplementation Has Minimal Effects on Muscle Adaptations during Resistance Exercise Training in Young Men: A Double-Blind Randomized Clinical Trial. *J. Nutr.* **2016**, *146*, 1660–1669. **[Google Scholar] [Green Version]**

58. Mobley, C.B.; Haun, C.T.; Roberson, P.A.; Mumford, P.W.; Romero, M.A.; Kephart, W.C.; Anderson, R.G.; Vann, C.G.; Osburn, S.C.; Pledge, C.D.; et al. Effects of Whey, Soy or Leucine Supplementation with 12 Weeks of Resistance Training on Strength, Body Composition, and Skeletal Muscle and Adipose Tissue Histological Attributes in College-Aged Males. *Nutrients* **2017**, *9*, 972. **[Google Scholar]**

59. Lynch, H.M.; Buman, M.P.; Dickinson, J.M.; Ransdell, L.B.; Johnston, C.S.; Wharton, C.M. No Significant Differences in Muscle Growth and Strength Development When Consuming Soy and Whey Protein Supplements Matched for Leucine Following a 12 Week Resistance Training Program in Men and Women: A Randomized Trial. *Int. J. Environ. Res. Public Health* **2020**, *17*, 3871. **[Google Scholar]**

60. Hevia-Larrain, V.; Gualano, B.; Longobardi, I.; Gil, S.; Fernandes, A.L.; Costa, L.A.R.; Pereira, R.M.R.; Artioli, G.G.; Phillips, S.M.; Roschel, H. High-Protein Plant-Based Diet Versus a Protein-Matched Omnivorous Diet to Support Resistance Training Adaptations: A Comparison Between Habitual Vegans and Omnivores. *Sports Med.* **2021**, 1–14. **[Google Scholar] [PubMed]**

61. Thomson, R.L.; Brinkworth, G.D.; Noakes, M.; Buckley, J.D. Muscle strength gains during resistance exercise training are attenuated with soy compared with dairy or usual protein intake in older adults: A randomized controlled trial. *Clin. Nutr.* **2016**, *35*, 27–33. **[Google Scholar]**

62. Kritikos, S.; Papanikolaou, K.; Draganidis, D.; Poulios, A.; Georgakouli, K.; Tsimeas, P.; Tzatzakis, T.; Batsilas, D.; Batrakoulis, A.; Deli, C.K.; et al. Effect of whey vs. soy protein supplementation on recovery kinetics following speed endurance training in competitive male soccer players: A randomized controlled trial. *J. Int. Soc. Sports Nutr.* **2021**, *18*, 23. **[Google Scholar] [PubMed]**

63. Xia, Z.; Cholewa, J.M.; Dardevet, D.; Huang, T.; Zhao, Y.; Shang, H.; Yang, Y.; Ding, X.; Zhang, C.; Wang, H.; et al. Effects of oat protein supplementation on skeletal muscle damage, inflammation and performance recovery following downhill running in untrained collegiate men. *Food Funct.* **2018**, *9*, 4720–4729. **[Google Scholar] [PubMed]**

64. Nieman, D.C.; Zwetsloot, K.A.; Simonson, A.J.; Hoyle, A.T.; Wang, X.; Nelson, H.K.; Lefranc-Millot, C.; Guerin-Deremaux, L. Effects of Whey and Pea Protein Supplementation on Post-Eccentric Exercise Muscle Damage: A Randomized Trial. *Nutrients* **2020**, *12*, 2382. **[Google Scholar]**

65. Saracino, P.G.; Saylor, H.E.; Hanna, B.R.; Hickner, R.C.; Kim, J.S.; Ormsbee, M.J. Effects of Pre-Sleep Whey vs. Plant-Based Protein Consumption on Muscle Recovery Following Damaging Morning Exercise. *Nutrients* **2020**, *12*, 2049. **[Google Scholar]**

66. Pasiakos, S.M.; Lieberman, H.R.; McLellan, T.M. Effects of protein supplements on muscle damage, soreness and recovery of muscle function and physical performance: A systematic review. *Sports Med.* **2014**, *44*, 655–670. **[Google Scholar] [PubMed]**

67. Doherty, T.J. Invited review: Aging and sarcopenia. *J. Appl. Physiol.* **2003**, *95*, 1717–1727. **[Google Scholar] [PubMed] [Green Version]**

68. Iannuzzi-Sucich, M.; Prestwood, K.M.; Kenny, A.M. Prevalence of sarcopenia and predictors of skeletal muscle mass in healthy, older men and women. *J. Gerontol. A Biol. Sci. Med. Sci.* **2002**, *57*, M772–M777. **[Google Scholar] [Green Version]**

69. Clark, B.C.; Manini, T.M. What is dynapenia? *Nutrition* **2012**, *28*, 495–503. **[Google Scholar] [Green Version]**

70. Phillips, S.M. Nutrient-rich meat proteins in offsetting age-related muscle loss. *Meat. Sci.* **2012**, *92*, 174–178. **[Google Scholar]**

71. Pannemans, D.L.; Wagenmakers, A.J.; Westerterp, K.R.; Schaafsma, G.; Halliday, D. Effect of protein source and quantity on protein metabolism in elderly women. *Am. J. Clin. Nutr.* **1998**, *68*, 1228–1235. **[Google Scholar] [PubMed] [Green Version]**

72. Giezenaar, C.; Chapman, I.; Luscombe-Marsh, N.; Feinle-Bisset, C.; Horowitz, M.; Soenen, S. Ageing Is Associated with Decreases in Appetite and Energy Intake--A Meta-Analysis in Healthy Adults. *Nutrients* **2016**, *8*, 28. **[Google Scholar] [Green Version]**

73. Moore, D.R.; Robinson, M.J.; Fry, J.L.; Tang, J.E.; Glover, E.I.; Wilkinson, S.B.; Prior, T.; Tarnopolsky, M.A.; Phillips, S.M. Ingested protein dose response of muscle and albumin protein synthesis after resistance exercise in young men. *Am. J. Clin. Nutr.* **2009**, *89*, 161–168. **[Google Scholar]**

74. Smith, G.I.; Atherton, P.; Reeds, D.N.; Mohammed, B.S.; Rankin, D.; Rennie, M.J.; Mittendorfer, B. Omega-3 polyunsaturated fatty acids augment the muscle protein anabolic response to hyperinsulinaemia-hyperaminoacidaemia in healthy young and middle-aged men and women. *Clin. Sci. (Lond)* **2011**, *121*, 267–278. **[Google Scholar] [Green Version]**

75. Smith, G.I.; Atherton, P.; Reeds, D.N.; Mohammed, B.S.; Rankin, D.; Rennie, M.J.; Mittendorfer, B. Dietary omega-3 fatty acid supplementation increases the rate of muscle protein synthesis in older adults: A randomized controlled trial. *Am. J. Clin. Nutr.* **2011**, *93*, 402–412. **[Google Scholar] [Green Version]**

76. Churchward-Venne, T.A.; Burd, N.A.; Mitchell, C.J.; West, D.W.; Philp, A.; Marcotte, G.R.; Baker, S.K.; Baar, K.; Phillips, S.M. Supplementation of a suboptimal protein dose with leucine or essential amino acids: Effects on myofibrillar protein synthesis at rest and following resistance exercise in men. *J. Physiol.* **2012**, *590*, 2751–2765. **[Google Scholar]**

77. Engelen, M.P.; Rutten, E.P.; De Castro, C.L.; Wouters, E.F.; Schols, A.M.; Deutz, N.E. Supplementation of soy protein with branched-chain amino acids alters protein metabolism in healthy elderly and even more in patients with chronic obstructive pulmonary disease. *Am. J. Clin. Nutr.* **2007**, *85*, 431–439. **[Google Scholar]** **[Green Version]**

78. Norton, L.E.; Wilson, G.J.; Layman, D.K.; Moulton, C.J.; Garlick, P.J. Leucine content of dietary proteins is a determinant of postprandial skeletal muscle protein synthesis in adult rats. *Nutr. Metab. (Lond)* **2012**, *9*, 67. **[Google Scholar]** **[PubMed]** **[Green Version]**

79. Paul, G.L. The rationale for consuming protein blends in sports nutrition. *J. Am. Coll. Nutr.* **2009**, *28 Suppl*, 464S–472S. **[Google Scholar]**

80. Reidy, P.T.; Walker, D.K.; Dickinson, J.M.; Gundermann, D.M.; Drummond, M.J.; Timmerman, K.L.; Fry, C.S.; Borack, M.S.; Cope, M.B.; Mukherjea, R.; et al. Protein blend ingestion following resistance exercise promotes human muscle protein synthesis. *J. Nutr.* **2013**, *143*, 410–416. **[Google Scholar]** **[PubMed]**

81. Kerksick, C.M.; Arent, S.; Schoenfeld, B.J.; Stout, J.R.; Campbell, B.; Wilborn, C.D.; Taylor, L.; Kalman, D.; Smith-Ryan, A.E.; Kreider, R.B.; et al. International society of sports nutrition position stand: Nutrient timing. *J. Int. Soc. Sports Nutr.* **2017**, *14*, 33. **[Google Scholar]** **[PubMed]**

82. Burd, N.A.; West, D.W.; Moore, D.R.; Atherton, P.J.; Staples, A.W.; Prior, T.; Tang, J.E.; Rennie, M.J.; Baker, S.K.; Phillips, S.M. Enhanced amino acid sensitivity of myofibrillar protein synthesis persists for up to 24 h after resistance exercise in young men. *J. Nutr.* **2011**, *141*, 568–573. **[Google Scholar]** **[PubMed]** **[Green Version]**

83. Pennings, B.; Koopman, R.; Beelen, M.; Senden, J.M.; Saris, W.H.; van Loon, L.J. Exercising before protein intake allows for greater use of dietary protein-derived amino acids for de novo muscle protein synthesis in both young and elderly men. *Am. J. Clin. Nutr.* **2011**, *93*, 322–331. **[Google Scholar]** **[PubMed]**

84. Stecker, R.A.; Moon, J.M.; Russo, T.J.; Ratliff, K.M.; Mumford, P.W.; Jäger, R.; Purpura, M.; Kerksick, C.M. Bacillus coagulans GBI-30, 6086 improves amino acid absorption from milk protein. *Nutr. Metab. (Lond)* **2020**, *17*, 93. **[Google Scholar]**

85. Jäger, R.; Zaragoza, J.; Purpura, M.; Iametti, S.; Marengo, M.; Tinsley, G.M.; Anzalone, A.J.; Oliver, J.M.; Fiore, W.; Biffi, A.; et al. Probiotic Administration Increases Amino Acid Absorption from Plant Protein: A Placebo-Controlled, Randomized, Double-Blind, Multicenter, Crossover Study. *Probiotics Antimicrob. Proteins* **2020**, *12*, 1330–1339. **[Google Scholar]** **[PubMed]**

# Chapter 4 NUTRITIONAL INTERVENTIONS TO ENHANCE SLEEP IN TEAM-SPORT ATHLETES: A NARRATIVE REVIEW

## 1. INTRODUCTION: AN OVERVIEW

High-performance team-sport athletes are required to train and compete to a high standard on a weekly basis. However, these athletes face the continual challenge of balancing the physiological, neuromuscular, and psychological stressors induced by training and competition [**1**]. Optimizing recovery to overcome these challenges and support performance is of utmost importance [**2**]. Sleep plays a crucial role in recovery and has restorative effects on physiological [**3**], perceptual [**3,4,5**], and immune [**6,7**] functions. Athletes, regardless of their sport, rate sleep as their most important recovery strategy [**8,9**]. A reduction in sleep quality has been associated with increased incidence of fatigue-related injury [**1**], reductions in the skeletal muscle remodeling [**10**], and disturbs cellular maintenance processes [**6,7**]. Despite evidence affirming the importance of restorative sleep [**11**], elite athletes appear to experience more sleep disturbances than the general population [**1,8**]. Behavioral and lifestyle strategies that promote sleep and sports performance will be welcomed by athletes and coaches.

Research examining athlete sleep indicates evening competition, travel, and training schedules can have a deleterious impact on sleep quality and quantity [**12**]. Up to ~50% of elite athletes experience sleep disturbances following late night competition or training sessions [**1,13**]. Night-time competition is widely associated with sleep issues and athletes can experience substantial disruptions (i.e., increased core temperature, muscle soreness, and delayed bedtime) to sleep quality and quantity compared with daytime competition [**12**]. Athletes also often face undesirable training schedules, including morning or late evening sessions, which can compromise an optimal recovery regime by reducing sleep quantity due to limited time in bed [**10,12,14**]. Athlete sleep quantity is also impacted by air travel, which can reduce sleep duration given a later sleep onset, delayed time in bed [**15**], and circadian rhythm misalignment [**12**]. A variety of interventions have been explored to negate the disturbances experienced by athletes, although not all have proven to be successful.

Evidence for the efficacy of interventions to improve sleep and related recovery outcomes in athletes is somewhat equivocal. Research investigating the effect of a sleep hygiene intervention in professional rugby league indicated sleep duration and efficiency increased immediately following the education seminars, but a follow-up one month later saw sleep behavior comparable to baseline levels [**16**]. Sleep hygiene and sleep extension interventions require athletes to change lifestyle behaviors (not always practical around training and competition schedules), which may yield poor compliance and limited effectiveness without regular follow-up [**16**]. Interventions that enhance athlete sleep and recovery regardless of situational changes (e.g., training times or travel demands) require further evaluation including both efficacy and practical means of implementation. Both sleep hygiene education and sleep extension interventions are effective short term, however long-term sustainability of their effects is questionable [**17**]. Furthermore, a recent survey study indicated female athletes may be resistant or less likely to implement sleep hygiene interventions [**18**]. Easily implemented techniques and strategies to improve sleep in the female athlete population are required.

It is well established that nutrition plays a vital role in performance and recovery; however, research investigating the role of selected foods, and macro- and micro-nutrients in the sleep–wake cycle is in its infancy. While the primary role of sports nutrition has been to support intensive training requirements and promote recovery [**19**], attention is shifting to the use of nutritional supplements for improving sleep [**10**]. The objective of this research was to examine dietary techniques that can improve sleep quality and duration, and how this knowledge can inform future nutritional therapies aimed at supporting sleep in athletes.

## 2. METHODS

A narrative review was performed from March to November 2020. The narrative review employed a semi-systematic methodology for article retrieval, incorporating explicit inclusion and exclusion criteria to ensure the relevance of the evaluated papers to athletes and sports contexts. Initial studies of interest were located through a search of six databases (PubMed, Scopus, CINAHL, EMBASE, SPORTDiscus, and Google Scholar) from inception up to November 2020. The following search terms were used: nutrition OR nutritional intervention AND sleep AND athletes OR athlete OR team-sport OR sportsman OR sportswoman. Another search was conducted using the following search terms: nutrition OR nutritional intervention AND sleep, to find interventions based on other populations.

Studies were included in the review if they were experimental, including randomized controlled trials, observation studies, case studies, and case reports conducted in elite or semi-elite athlete cohorts. Given the paucity of sleep nutrition research in the athlete population, we expanded our inclusion criteria to include studies that reported the outcomes of nutritional interventions to improve sleep in otherwise healthy adults. Studies were excluded if they included participants with concussions, included participants with other disorders unrelated to sleep, participants in shift work, described longitudinal dietary adjustment (e.g., low carbohydrate dieting), or an animal study. Reference lists of selected articles were also inspected to ensure all relevant literature was captured for review. The outcomes of nutritional intervention on sleep were detailed in four variables following existing recommendations [**20**]:

1. Total sleep time (TST, min)—total minutes of night-time sleep;
2. Sleep efficiency (SE, %)—the ratio of TST to time spent in bed;
3. Sleep onset latency (SOL, min)—the time between bedtime and sleep onset;
4. Wake after sleep onset (WASO, min)—the time awake after initial sleep onset but before the final awakening.

As this study was a review, ethical approval was not necessary. Narrative synthesis was employed to examine and analyze the similarities and differences between studies obtained through the two systematic searches and other pertinent secondary sources identified by the research team.

# 3. RESULTS

## 3.1. Included Studies and Characteristics

Evidence for the efficacy of nutritional interventions to improve sleep in human studies is limited, with even less research reporting their effectiveness in an athletic population. The results from the literature search for studies using athletic ($n = 4$) and both healthy ($n = 6$) and poor sleeping ($n = 10$) general population cohorts are displayed below in **Table 1.**

**Table 1. Characteristics of studies in athlete, and healthy and poor sleeping general population groups.**

| Study | Subjects Description | n | Age, y | Method of Sleep Assessment |
|---|---|---|---|---|
| **Athletes** | | | | |
| Killer, 2017 [**21**] | Trained male cyclists | 10 | 25.0 ± 5.8 | Wrist actigraphy |
| Daniel, 2019 [**22**] | State-level male basketball players | 8 | 18.0 ± 0.7 | Wrist actigraphy |
| Shamloo, 2019 [**23**] | Male athletes | 30 | 20.7 ± 3.7 | PSQI |
| MacInnis, 2020 [**24**] | Elite male and female track cyclists | 6 | 23 ± 6 | Wrist actigraphy |
| **General Population (Healthy)** | | | | |
| Afaghi, 2007 [**25**] | Healthy males | 12 | 18–35 | PSG |
| Afaghi, 2008 [**26**] | Health, non-obese males | 14 | 18–35 | PSG |
| Howatson, 2012 [**27**] | Healthy and physically active males and females | 20 | 26.6 ± 4.6 | Wrist actigraphy |
| Ong, 2017 [**28**] | Healthy males | 10 | 26.9 ± 5.3 | Wrist actigraphy |
| Bannai, 2012 [**29**] | Healthy males | 7 | 40.6 (30–61) | Subjective sleep questionnaires |
| Vlahoyiannis, 2018 [**30**] | Healthy males | 10 | 23.2 ± 1.8 | PSG |

| Study | Subjects Description | n | Age, y | Method of Sleep Assessment |
|---|---|---|---|---|
| General Population (Poor Sleepers) | | | | |
| Pigeon, 2010 [**31**] | Chronic insomnia, otherwise healthy | 15 | 71.6 ± 5.4 | Subjective sleep questionnaires |
| Lin, 2011 [**32**] | Poor sleepers, males and females | 24 | 20–55 | Wrist actigraphy and PSQI |
| Yamatsu, 2015 [**33**] | Poor sleepers, males and females | 16 | 36.8 ± 8.9 | One channel EEG |
| Byun, 2018 [**34**] | Poor sleepers, males and females | 30 | 49 ± 14 | PSG and PSQI |
| Simper, 2019 [**35**] | Poor sleepers, young male and female adults | 19 | 21.0 ± 1.0 | Wrist actigraphy |
| Ingawa, 2006 [**36**] | Poor sleepers, females | 15 | 31.1 (24–53) | Subjective sleep questionnaires |
| Yamadera, 2007 [**37**] | Poor sleepers, males and females | 11 | 40.5 ± 10.1 | PSG and subjective sleep questionnaires |
| Ito, 2014 [**38**] | Poor sleepers, males and females | 45 | 35 ± 8 | Subjective sleep questionnaires |
| Ito, 2014 [**38**] | Poor sleepers, males and females | 6 | 35 ± 8 | Wrist actigraphy |
| Yamatsu, 2016 [**39**] | Poor sleepers, males and females | 10 | 37.7 ± 11.5 | One channel EEG |

EEG: electroencephalogram, PSG: polysomnography, PSQI: Pittsburgh Sleep Quality Index, data presented as mean ± SD unless otherwise noted.

Athlete studies were in mixed sport disciplines, two in cycling [**21,22**] and another in basketball [**23**]. One study did not specify the discipline the athletes participated in [**24**]. Three athlete studies utilized wrist actigraphy and one the Pittsburgh Sleep Quality Index (PSQI). Healthy general population studies were predominantly in male participants ($n$ = 5), with one study utilizing a male and female population. Three studies used PSG to measure sleep following nutritional intervention, and two used wrist actigraphy. Poor sleeping general population studies implemented a mixture of sleep methods, from subjective sleep questionnaires to PSG. Study participants were classified as general population (poor sleepers) if they reported any of the following: subjective sleep problems; insomnia; diagnosed sleep pathology; and a PSQI score above the threshold for a 'sleep problem' (i.e., 5.0 or 6.0 depending on the specific study).

Details of the nutritional interventions, as well as the impact these interventions on sleep outcomes are outlined in **Table 2**. These outcomes are detailed below in the categories of carbohydrates, protein, tart-cherry juice, and other interventions.

**Table 2. Changes to sleep following carbohydrate, protein, tart cherry juice, and other nutritional interventions.**

| Study | Intervention Type | Timing | Days | TST (min) | SE (%) | SOL (min) | WASO (min) |
|---|---|---|---|---|---|---|---|
| **Carbohydrate** | | | | | | | |
| Afaghi, 2007 [25] | High GI dinner | 4 h pre-bed | 3 | ↑ 7.9 | ↑ 1.7 | ↓ 8.5* | ↑ 1.7 |
| Daniel, 2019 [24] | High GI dinner and evening snack | 4 h pre-bed | 1 | ↑ 26.5 | ↓ 1.2 | ↓ 12.5 | ↑ 9.0 |
| Afaghi, 2008 [26] | Very low carbohydrate diet (<1% total energy intake) | Over day | 4 | ↑ 22.7 | ↑ 3.3 | ↓ 5.4 * | ↓ 8.6 |
| Killer, 2017 [21] | High carbohydrate drinks | Pre-, during, and post-exercise | 9 | ↓ 19.0* | ↓ NR | ↔ NR | NR |
| Vlahoyiannis, 2018 [30] | High GI dinner | Post-exercise (~2 h pre-bed) | 1 | ↑ 62.4 * | ↑ 8.1 * | ↓ 18.9 * | ↓ 32.9 * |
| **Protein** | | | | | | | |
| Ong, 2017 [28] | Serving (20 g) of α-lactalbumin | 1 h pre-bed | 2 | ↑ 54.7 * | ↑ 7.0 * | ↓ 10.1 | ↓ 20.8 |
| MacInnis, 2020 [24] | Serving (40 g) of α-lactalbumin | 2 h pre-bed | 3 | ↔ NR | ↔ NR | ↔ NR | ↔ NR |
| **Tart Cherry Juice** | | | | | | | |
| Pigeon, 2010 [31] | Serving (240 mL) of tart Montmorency cherry juice | 8:00–10:00 and 1–2 h pre-bed | 14 | ↑ 29.3 ** | ↑ 3.7 * | ↓ 3.6 ** | ↓ 16.8 ** |
| Howatson, 2012 [27] | Serving (30 mL) of tart Montmorency cherry juice (with 200 mL water) | 30 min post-wake and 30 min pre-bed | 7 | ↑ 39.0 * | ↑ 2.7 | ↓ 9.1 | NR |

| Study | Intervention Type | Timing | Days | TST (min) | SE (%) | SOL (min) | WASO (min) |
|---|---|---|---|---|---|---|---|
| **Other** | | | | | | | |
| Lin, 2011 [**32**] | Two green kiwifruits | 1 h pre-bed | 28 | ↑ 54.8 ** | ↑ 2.0 ** | ↓ 13.9 ** | ↓ 6.1 ** |
| Yamatsu, 2015 [**33**] | GABA (100 mg) with AVLE (50 mg) | 30 min pre-bed | 14 | NR | NR | ↓ 4.3 | NR |
| Shamloo, 2019 [**23**] | Serving (100 mL) of beetroot juice | 2 h pre-exercise | 7 | NA | NA | NA | NA |
| Inagawa, 2006 [**30**] | Glycine (3 g) | 1 h pre-bed | 4 | NA | NA | NA | NA |
| Yamadera, 2007 [**37**] | Glycine (3 g) | 1 h pre-bed | 2 | ↔ NR | NA | ↓ NR ** | ↔ NR |
| Bannai, 2012 [**29**] | Glycine (3 g) | 30 min pre-bed | 3 | NA | NA | NA | NA |
| Ito, 2014 [**38**] | L-serine (3 g) | 30 min pre-bed | 4 | NA | NA | NA | NA |
| Ito, 2014 [**38**] | L-serine (3 g) | 30 min pre-bed | 2 | NA | NA | NA | NA |
| Yamatsu, 2016 [**39**] | GABA (100 mg) | 30 min pre-bed | 7 | NA | ↔ NR | ↓ 5.0 * | NA |
| Byun, 2018 [**34**] | GABA (300 mg) | 1 h pre-bed | 28 | ↑ 8.6 | ↑ 6.7 * | ↓ 7.7 ** | ↓ 19.6 * |
| Simper, 2019 [**35**] | Serving of "Night Time Recharge" sleep supplement | 1 h pre-bed | 7 | ↑ 0.37 | ↑ 5.9 | ↓ 10** | NR |

AVLE: *Apocynum venetum* leaf extract, GABA: γ-aminobutyric acid, GI: glycemic index, GL: glycemic load, NA: not applicable, NR: value not reported, SE: sleep efficiency, SOL: sleep onset latency, TST: total sleep time, ↑ increase, ↓ decrease, ↔ no change, * $p < 0.05$, ** $p < 0.01$.

## 3.2. Carbohydrates

The majority ($n$ = 3) of the identified carbohydrate nutritional intervention studies investigated the effect of high glycemic index (GI) carbohydrate consumption pre-sleep. Overall, high GI carbohydrate consumption resulted in increases in TST (7.9–62.4 min) and SE (0.4–8.1%), and consistent reductions in SOL (5.6–18.9 min). Afaghi and colleagues [**26**] also investigated the effect of a very low carbohydrate diet on sleep, showing an increase in TST (22.7 min) and SE (3.3%), and reduced SOL (5.6 min).

### 3.3. Protein

Two studies explored the effects of protein to improve sleep. Both studies used the whey protein isolate α-lactalbumin (dose range 20–40 g) [**24,28**]. In one study with healthy general populations, pre-sleep protein supplementation increased TST by 55 min, alongside a 7% increase in SE [**28**]. In the study by MacInnis et al. [**24**], α-lactalbumin had no effect on sleep variables in a small sample of cyclists ($n$ = 6).

### 3.4. Tart Cherry Juice

Interventions utilizing tart cherry juice resulted in a universal increase across studies in TST (range from 29–39 min). The studies also showed modest improvements in SE (2.7–3.7%), and slight reductions in SOL (3.6–9.1 min) and WASO (16.8 min). The tart cherry juice studies were all performed in general population cohorts (both healthy and poor sleepers).

### 3.5. Other Interventions

The combination of γ-aminobutyric acid (GABA; an amino acid produced by natural fermentation) and *Apocynum venetum* leaf extract treatment yielded a modest decrease in SOL of 4.3 min and shortening of deep non-REM sleep latency by 5.3 min [**33**]. Similar magnitude reductions in SOL were reported for 100 mg of GABA supplementation only [**39**], while supplementation with 300 mg of GABA induced reductions in SOL and WASO in concert with an increase in SE [**34**]. In comparison, the consumption of two kiwifruits 1 h before bedtime yielded a substantial increase in TST of 55 min, as well as a 2% increase in SE and decreased SOL (14 min) and WASO (6.1 min) [**32**]. In athletes, beetroot juice showed an improvement in subjective quality of sleep as measured by the PSQI [**23**]. In healthy adults, 3 g of glycine ingested an hour before bed decreased SOL and the onset latency of slow wave sleep [**37**]. Similarly, 3 g of glycine led to decreases in morning fatigue when ingested an hour before bed [**36**], and an improvement in cognitive function during periods of sleep restriction when ingested 30 min before bed [**29**]. In adults who were dissatisfied with sleep, 3 g of L-serine ingested 30 min before bed improved subjective sleep quality and sleep satisfaction; however, in a smaller sub-study, there were no improvements in actigraphy-measured sleep [**38**]. Finally, consuming a tart cherry-based sleep supplement powder reduced SOL (10 min) in poor sleeping young adults [**35**].

## 4. DISCUSSION

This study identified only four trials on nutritional therapies aimed at improving sleep quality and duration in an athletic group. Nonetheless, research conducted in various general population cohorts, encompassing individuals with diagnosed or self-reported sleep issues, demonstrates moderate evidence for the effectiveness of nutritional interventions in enhancing objective total sleep time (TST), objective sleep efficiency (SE), subjective sleep quality, and alleviating sleep-related complaints such as insomnia. Significantly more research is necessary in rigorously controlled dietary supplement trials to validate their efficacy and usefulness in enhancing sleep, recovery, and performance across the diverse environments that competitive athletes must navigate. The translation and execution of favorable experimental results will necessitate collaboration and management among athletes, coaches, and support personnel, particularly nutritionists and sports medicine professionals, who will offer tailored dietary recommendations.

## 4.1. Carbohydrate

Carbohydrates have historically been employed in sports to energize athletes participating in rigorous and extended physical activity [2,10].The conventional emphasis of carbohydrate supplementation often centers on replenishing muscle and liver glycogen stores between training sessions or competitions [40].Although the evidence regarding the quantity, type, and timing of carbohydrate consumption for recovery is well established, certain research have also investigated the role of carbohydrates in enhancing sleep quality.Most studies have focused on the effects of high and low glycemic index (GI) carbohydrate feeding [**22,30**]. Evidence from studies in athlete samples is limited and equivocal, with one study in Brazilian male basketballers reporting a non-significant increase in TST and decrease in SOL, but also reductions in SE and an increase in WASO [**22**]. However, studies in healthy populations are more definitive, with consistent reports of improvements in sleep following high GI carbohydrate feeding [**25,30**]. In a study of particular relevance to athletes, Vlahoyiannis and colleagues [**30**] provided healthy, physically active young males with either a high or low GI meal immediately following an evening bout of intermittent sprint exercise. While there were no effects of meal GI on sleep architecture (i.e., proportion of sleep time spent in different sleep stages), the high GI meal substantially improved TST, SE, SOL, and WASO. As such, high GI feeding may ameliorate the sleep disturbances experienced by athletes following evening training and competition.

The timing of a high GI meal may influence its subsequent impact on sleep. One study reported that SOL was longer and subjective sleepiness was lower when a high GI meal was ingested 1 h before bed rather than 4 h before bed [**25**]. The proposed mechanism for improvement in sleep following a high GI meal is an increase in the plasma ratio of tryptophan to large neutral amino acids (TRP/LNAA). Tryptophan is an essential amino acid and serves as a precursor to the synthesis of serotonin and melatonin [**41**], both important regulators of sleep. By increasing the TRP/LNAA, tryptophan can more readily cross the blood brain barrier, consequently leading to an increase in the synthesis of serotonin [**42**] and then downstream increases in secretion of melatonin [**25,30**]. Importantly, it appears that the TRP/LNAA peaks 2–4 h after ingestion of a high carbohydrate meal with minimal change in the first 1–2 h [**43**]. Therefore, high GI feeding should occur at least two hours before bedtime to maximize the potential impact on sleep.

In addition to manipulating glycemic load (which combines both the quality (GI) and the quantity of carbohydrates), studies have investigated the effects of restricting carbohydrate intake on sleep parameters [**26**]. Ingestion of a very low carbohydrate meal 4 h before bed increased the proportion of slow-wave sleep assessed by polysomnography (PSG), the gold standard of sleep assessment [**26**]. An increase in slow-wave sleep could be particularly beneficial to athletes as it is thought to play an important role in performance recovery [**44**] and assists in energy conservation and recuperation of the nervous system [**1,45**]. However, athletes also need to consider the impact of low carbohydrate feeding on muscle and liver glycogen restoration, and decisions on priorities for refueling versus sleep promotion will need to be made.

The impact of various evening carbohydrate meals on sleep remains ambiguous due to the variability in existing research results. Additional research focusing on the optimal timing, quantity, and source of carbohydrate consumption, along with its interaction with other macronutrients and micronutrients, is necessary within an athletic population to ascertain its effectiveness. Subsequent development of more definitive rules on carbohydrate consumption to enhance athlete sleep can occur.

## 4.2. Protein

Protein serves a crucial multifaceted purpose in an athlete's training and competition regimen by promoting muscle repair and rebuilding while bolstering immunological function. Whey protein supplementation after exercise and before sleep has been implemented to improve overall protein synthesis and muscle performance during overnight recovery. [**47**]. A specific whey protein which has recently been investigated as a nutritional pre-sleep intervention is α-lactalbumin [**42,48**]. α-Lactalbumin is reported to have the highest natural level of tryptophan in protein food sources [**48**]. Tryptophan is an essential amino acid and serves as a precursor to the synthesis of serotonin and melatonin, both of which are involved in the regulation of sleep [**41**].

The initial evidence demonstrating the potential effectiveness of α-lactalbumin on sleep was obtained from a series of studies conducted in stress-vulnerable participants with and without sleep complaints [**49,50**]. Although not directly investigating sleep parameters, sleep quality may have improved with a substantial reduction in sleepiness, and improved attention processes the morning following the intervention. In addition, these studies observed an increase in TRP/LNAA, which is essential for serotonin synthesis in the brain. Another study also reported decreases in depressive feelings under stress in stress-vulnerable participants consuming α-lactalbumin [**50**]. There are strong links between sleep and feelings of anxiety and depression, with women experiencing more insomnia complaints than males [**51**]. Supplementation with α-lactalbumin that can increase sleep quality and decrease depressive feelings may be beneficial during high-stress team-sport seasons, particularly for female athletes.

Ong and colleagues recently examined the effectiveness of an α-lactalbumin therapy (20 g, 1 hour before bedtime) in healthy male participants without known sleep disorders or impairments [28]. The quantity of sleep rose, with objective total sleep time (TST) rising by 13% as assessed by actigraphy and subjective TST increasing by 11% according to sleep diaries, in comparison to placebo. Additionally, objective sleep efficiency (SE) was 7% higher. In contrast, no differences were observed in any actigraphy-recorded sleep characteristics between α-lactalbumin and collagen peptide supplementation in a small group of cyclists [24]. Although preliminary evidence suggests that α-lactalbumin may enhance sleep, additional rigorously conducted research are necessary to validate its efficacy. Research on the chronic use of α-lactalbumin in an athletic population is necessary. To date, few investigations on nocturnal protein consumption have been conducted for periods beyond four weeks among the general population. Currently, there is no data supporting the efficacy of dietary therapies when applied chronically or in a field environment among athletic populations during training and competition.

## 4.3. Tart Cherry Juice

Tart cherries contain approximately 13 ng of melatonin per kg of cherry [**52**], which upon consumption can increase exogenous melatonin, which is critical for the sleep-wake cycle in humans [**53**]. The high antioxidant content of tart cherries purportedly reduces oxidative stress, in turn enhancing sleep in isolation and in conjunction with melatonin. The reported anti-inflammatory properties may influence the pro-inflammatory cytokines involved in sleep regulation and also the recovery process after exercise [**10,52**]. The majority of studies investigating tart cherry juice usage in an athletic population have examined its effect on aspects of recovery including muscle soreness [**54,55,56**]. While promoting recovery is beneficial to athletes, tart cherry juice has enhanced sleep indices as assessed by PSG and wrist actigraphy monitoring in healthy individuals without the presence of sleep problems [**31**], and individuals with sleep problems such as insomnia [**27**]. Other studies have demonstrated that tart cherry juice can increase TST and SE, regardless of the differences in participants (good sleepers compared to individuals with insomnia) [**27,57**]. Consumption of a liquid blend consisting of Montmorency tart cherries and apple juice improved sleep in older adults with chronic insomnia by decreasing WASO, and reducing their insomnia questionnaire score compared to baseline [**27**].

An authorized consensus group stated that tart cherry juice interventions for athletes are not recommended nor encouraged [60]. Additional research is required to evaluate the efficacy of tart cherry juice in athletic populations, particularly regarding its impact on sleep and physiological recovery.

## 4.4. Other Nutritional Strategies

There are a variety of other nutritional interventions that have been explored for their ability to improve sleep in poor sleepers, including kiwifruit and herbal supplements. Kiwifruits contain a range of nutrients that potentially augment sleep and recovery [**44**], including serotonin, a known sleep promoting hormone that helps regulate REM sleep [**61**]. Improved sleep was reported in poor sleepers who ingested two kiwifruits an hour before bed over a four-week intervention period [**32**]. Marked increases in wrist actigraphy monitored TST (16.9%) and SE (2.4%) were evident, while subjective sleep diary recordings showed a substantial decrease in WASO and SOL. The improved sleep quality may be attributable to high levels of folate in kiwifruit [**10,32**]. Folate deficiency has been linked to insomnia and restless leg syndrome, both of which cause large sleep disruptions and can hinder the restorative quality of sleep [**32,62**].

Akin to kiwifruit consumption, ingestion of GABA in different quantities has yielded improvements in the sleep quality of poor sleepers or those dissatisfied with sleep [**33,39**]. GABA is an inhibitory neurotransmitter that is often present in food, and its receptors in the central nervous system are often targeted by pharmacological agents such as benzodiazepines for treatment of several conditions including insomnia [**63**]. While benzodiazepines can improve sleep quality and quantity, they are also associated with substantial side-effects, including drowsiness, lethargy, fatigue, and, in extreme cases, impaired motor coordination and addiction [**63**], all of which would likely impair athletic performance. Importantly, studies in humans have reported no adverse effects of pre-sleep GABA ingestion on next-day sleepiness or fatigue, which suggests it may be useful in athletes to improve sleep.

Glycine is another inhibitory neurotransmitter that has been linked to improvements in subjective and objective sleep quality for poor sleepers [**36,37**], but also daytime fatigue and cognitive performance in healthy adults during simulated sleep restriction [**29**]. Similarly, ingestion of L-serine, a glycine precursor, reportedly leads to improvements in sleep satisfaction and subjective sleep quality in adults dissatisfied with their sleep [**38**]. While further evidence for the efficacy of glycine and L-serine in athlete populations is required, these results suggest both proteins may offer athletes dissatisfied with sleep issues, or facing situational sleep restriction, a means by which to improve their sleep.

Most studies included in this review have focused on the effects of single nutrients or ingredients. However, some recent studies have examined the effects of multi-nutrient supplements on sleep. In one study on the effects of a tart cherry powder-based supplement, there was a significant improvement in SOL and a tendency towards improvement in SE across seven days of supplementation in young adult poor sleepers [**35**]. However, chemical analysis undertaken as part of the study indicated the supplement contained no melatonin, despite being tart cherry based. Instead, the sleep improvement was likely due to the 3 g of tryptophan and 2 g of glycine, which is similar to the 3 g dose used in other studies that report sleep improvement [**29,36,37**], contained in the product. Another multi-nutrient sleep study determined both the most and least optimal combination of a variety of ingredients for sleep improvement [**64**]. Both combinations comprised a blend of components associated with enhanced sleep when utilized alone, including high glycemic index carbohydrates and tryptophan. The most effective combination resulted in a decrease in SOL among a cohort of healthy adults with adequate sleep. Significantly for athletes, the suboptimal combo drink resulted with elevated SOL compared to a placebo in the same cohort, underscoring the necessity to examine nutritional interactions that affect sleep.

## 5. TOWARDS THE FUTURE PATHS

There are numerous nutrients and foods that have demonstrated efficacy in isolation for enhancing sleep quality and quantity. As humans rarely consume single nutrients in isolation, and typically enjoy a variety of nutrients as part of mixed meals, it is important to clarify how the co-ingestion of food and supplements can help or hinder sleep. This information would not only be beneficial for athletes within the daily training environment, but also when traveling and crossing multiple time zones with national and international travel.

The growing interest in monitoring athlete sleep has led to an increase in commercial sleep technology (wearables such as Fitbit™ and Whoop™, nearables such as ResMed S+™, and smartphone applications). These consumer-based technologies have advantages in terms of low-cost and ease of use, however the reliability and validity of many of these devices remains to be established. Although caution needs to be taken when implementing these commercial sleep technology devices at present, the market for sleep monitoring technology is expanding rapidly. Ideally, this expansion will occur alongside research on the reliability and validity of these devices for use in applied settings.

With a plethora of supplements now available in different forms (powder, liquid, capsule), investigation is also required on the most effective form(s) of supplement to consume. For example, tart cherry is available as a liquid, powder, and in a capsule. Understanding the most effective dosage (for example g per kg body mass), timing (acute or chronic consumption), and the most effective supplement form (liquid, gel, powder, capsule), would enable practitioners to more accurately individualize and prescribe nutritional interventions and supplements to aid sleep. More work is needed to establish optimal nutrient dosing relative to body mass, rather than absolute dosing (fixed amount(s) of nutrients) used in the majority of existing studies.

## 6. PRACTICAL APPLICATIONS

The benefits of sleep for athletes are wellknown; nevertheless, in addition to the implementation of good sleep hygiene measures, such as developing a sleep pattern, avoiding electronic devices, and sleeping in a room that is cold, dark, and quiet, dietary treatments can be helpful in improving the quality and quantity of sleep.The following sleep enhancement strategies can be extrapolated from the studies that have been published up to this point, notwithstanding the fact that additional study is required to determine the precise timing and dosage of nutrition treatments to assist in improving sleep:

- Consume a diet rich in fiber, whole grains, fruits, and vegetables.
- Consume a high GI carbohydrate meal 2–4 h before bedtime.
- Incorporate tart cherry juice concentrate into an athlete's daily routine when sleep may be impaired (e.g., night competition), 1 × 30 mL upon waking and 1 × 30 mL before the evening meal.
- Consume 20–40 g of a protein source rich in tryptophan, such as α-lactalbumin enriched whey protein, 2 h before bedtime.
- Regular kiwifruit consumption an hour before bed.

- Glycine at a dosage of 3 g consumed before bed may enhance sleep quality and quantity.
- To identify if a nutritional intervention is enhancing the sleep of an individual athlete in an applied setting, we recommend:
- Using a reliable and valid device such as wrist actigraphy, and questionnaires that assess sleep quality (i.e., Pittsburgh Sleep Quality Index) [**65**] and quantify daytime sleepiness (Epworth Sleepiness Scale) [**66**].
- Considering alternative options available to monitor sleep depending on access to expertise, the simplicity of use, and reliability and validity of the method [**67**].
- In relation to nutritional interventions known to compromise sleep, we recommend that athletes avoid the following substances prior to sleep:
- Caffeine [**68**].
- Alcohol [**69**].
- Excess fluid ingestion [70].

A major challenge for athletes is to maintain high standard nutritional practices across the wide variety of settings they face: their personal home environment, the regular training facility, the home match venue, the away match venue, and during local, national, and international travel. Dieticians should work closely with and educate players, coaches, and team staff to ensure that both nutrition and sleep arrangements are given a high priority.

## 7. CONCISE SUMMARY

It would appear that certain nutritional interventions are an effective method for improving the quality and amount of sleep, provided that the appropriate dose, source, and time are supplied of the intervention. Given the low amount of studies that have been completed on this particular group of athletes, it is difficult to determine whether or not these nutritional interventions are helpful in the real world and whether or not they are effective in this context. It is necessary for future study to evaluate the capacity of these nutritional therapies to promote athlete sleep for both training and competition. This is because it is widely accepted that sleep is a crucial factor during training, travel, and competition.

## AT A GLANCE

Athletes frequently encounter sleep disturbances and inadequate sleep due to prolonged travel, the scheduling of training and competitions (e.g., early morning or evening), and muscular discomfort. Nutrition is essential for athletic performance and recovery, and several foods, beverages, and supplements are claimed to enhance both the quality and duration of sleep. This document reviews and discusses pertinent studies on nutrition, foods, supplements, and beverages that may enhance sleep quality and duration. Our narrative review employed a semi-systematic methodology for article retrieval, utilizing particular inclusion and exclusion criteria to ensure that the studied papers pertained to athletes and sports contexts. Six databases—PubMed, Scopus, CINAHL, EMBASE, SPORTDiscus, and Google Scholar—were queried for preliminary research of relevance from their start until November 2020. Due to the limited research on sleep nutrition in athletes, we broadened our inclusion criteria to encompass studies that documented the effects of dietary interventions on sleep in generally healthy individuals. The impact of carbohydrate consumption on sleep characteristics remains ambiguous, however foods with a high glycemic index seem to offer minor advantages. Tart cherry juice may increase sleep duration, herbal supplements can improve sleep quality, and kiwifruit and protein interventions have demonstrated efficacy in enhancing both sleep quality and duration. Nutritional therapies effectively enhance sleep quality and duration; however, additional research is necessary to ascertain the optimal dosage, source, and timing concerning training, travel, and competition needs.

## REFERENCES


1. Fullagar, H.H.; Duffield, R.; Skorski, S.; Coutts, A.J.; Julian, R.; Meyer, T. Sleep and Recovery in Team Sport: Current Sleep-Related Issues Facing Professional Team-Sport Athletes. *Int. J. Sport. Physiol. Perform.* **2015**, *10*, 950–957. [**Google Scholar**]
2. Heaton, L.E.; Davis, J.K.; Rawson, E.S.; Nuccio, R.P.; Witard, O.C.; Stein, K.W.; Baar, K.; Carter, J.M.; Baker, L.B. Selected in-season nutritional strategies to enhance recovery for team sport athletes: A practical overview. *Sport. Med.* **2017**, *47*, 2201–2218. [**Google Scholar**]
3. Skein, M.; Duffield, R.; Minett, G.M.; Snape, A.; Murphy, A. The Effect of Overnight Sleep Deprivation After Competitive Rugby League Matches on Postmatch Physiological and Perceptual Recovery. *Int. J. Sport. Physiol. Perform.* **2013**, *8*, 556–564. [**Google Scholar**]
4. Fullagar, H.H.K.; Skorski, S.; Duffield, R.; Julian, R.; Bartlett, J.; Meyer, T. Impaired sleep and recovery after night matches in elite football players. *J. Sport. Sci.* **2016**, *34*, 1333–1339. [**Google Scholar**]
5. Rae, D.E.; Chin, T.; Dikgomo, K.; Hill, L.; McKune, A.J.; Kohn, T.A.; Roden, L.C. One night of partial sleep deprivation impairs recovery from a single exercise training session. *Eur. J. Appl. Physiol.* **2017**, *117*, 699–712. [**Google Scholar**]
6. Majde, J.A.; Krueger, J.M. Links between the innate immune system and sleep. *J. Allergy Clin. Immunol.* **2005**, *116*, 1188–1198. [**Google Scholar**] [**PubMed**]
7. Swinbourne, R.R. Sleep, Recovery and Performance in Collision Sport Athletes. Ph.D. Thesis, Auckland University of Technology, Auckland, New Zealand, 2015. [**Google Scholar**]
8. Knufinke, M.; Nieuwenhuys, A.; Geurts, S.A.; Møst, E.I.; Maase, K.; Moen, M.H.; Coenen, A.M.; Kompier, M.A. Train hard, sleep well? Perceived training load, sleep quantity and sleep stage distribution in elite level athletes. *J. Sci. Med. Sport* **2018**, *21*, 427–432. [**Google Scholar**]
9. Venter, R.E. Perceptions of team athletes on the importance of recovery modalities. *Eur. J. Sport Sci.* **2011**, *14*, S69–S76. [**Google Scholar**]
10. Doherty, R.; Madigan, S.; Warrington, G.; Ellis, J. Sleep and Nutrition Interactions: Implications for Athletes. *Nutrients* **2019**, *11*, 822. [**Google Scholar**] [**Green Version**]
11. Tuomilehto, H.; Vuorinen, V.-P.; Penttilä, E.; Kivimäki, M.; Vuorenmaa, M.; Venojärvi, M.; Airaksinen, O.; Pihlajamäki, J. Sleep of professional athletes: Underexploited potential to improve health and performance. *J. Sport. Sci.* **2017**, *35*, 704–710. [**Google Scholar**] [**PubMed**]

12. Roberts, S.S.H.; Teo, W.-P.; Warmington, S.A. Effects of training and competition on the sleep of elite athletes: A systematic review and meta-analysis. *Br. J. Sport. Med.* **2019**, *53*, 513–522. **[Google Scholar] [Green Version]**

13. Lastella, M.; Roach, G.D.; Halson, S.L.; Sargent, C. Sleep/wake behaviours of elite athletes from individual and team sports. *Eur. J. Sport Sci.* **2015**, *15*, 94–100. **[Google Scholar] [Green Version]**

14. Halson, S.L. Sleep in Elite Athletes and Nutritional Interventions to Enhance Sleep. *Sport. Med.* **2014**, *44*, 13–23. **[Google Scholar] [PubMed] [Green Version]**

15. Fowler, P.M.; Knez, W.; Crowcroft, S.; Mendham, A.E.; Miller, J.; Sargent, C.; Halson, S.; Duffield, R. Greater Effect of East versus West Travel on Jet Lag, Sleep, and Team Sport Performance. *Med. Sci. Sport. Exerc.* **2017**, *49*, 2548–2561. **[Google Scholar]**

16. Caia, J.; Scott, T.J.; Halson, S.L.; Kelly, V.G. The influence of sleep hygiene education on sleep in professional rugby league athletes. *Sleep Health* **2018**, *4*, 364–368. **[Google Scholar] [PubMed]**

17. Vitale, K.C.; Owens, R.; Hopkins, S.R.; Malhotra, A. Sleep Hygiene for Optimizing Recovery in Athletes: Review and Recommendations. *Int. J. Sport Med.* **2019**, *40*, 535–543. **[Google Scholar] [PubMed]**

18. Miles, K.H.; Clark, B.; Fowler, P.M.; Miller, J.; Pumpa, K.L. Sleep practices implemented by team sport coaches and sports science support staff: A potential avenue to improve athlete sleep? *J. Sci. Med. Sport* **2019**, *22*, 748–752. **[Google Scholar]**

19. Leonarda, G.; Fedele, E.; Vitale, D.; Lucini, V.; Mirela, I.A.; Mirela, L. Healthy athlete's nutrition. *Med. Sport. J. Rom. Sport. Med. Soc.* **2018**, *14*, 2967–2985. **[Google Scholar]**

20. Reed, D.L.; Sacco, W.P. Measuring Sleep Efficiency: What Should the Denominator Be? *J. Clin. Sleep Med.* **2016**, *12*, 263–266. **[Google Scholar]**

21. Killer, S.C.; Svendsen, I.S.; Jeukendrup, A.E.; Gleeson, M. Evidence of disturbed sleep and mood state in well-trained athletes during short-term intensified training with and without a high carbohydrate nutritional intervention. *J. Sport. Sci.* **2017**, *35*, 1402–1410. **[Google Scholar] [Green Version]**

22. Daniel, N.V.; Zimberg, I.Z.; Estadella, D.; Garcia, M.C.; Padovani, R.C.; Juzwiak, C.R. Effect of the intake of high or low glycemic index high carbohydrate-meals on athletes' sleep quality in pre-game nights. *Anais Acad. Bras. Ciênc.* **2019**, *91*, e20180107. **[Google Scholar]**

23. Shamloo, S.; Irandoust, K.; Afif, A.H. The Effect of Beetroot Juice Supplementation on Physiological Fatigue and Quality of Sleep in Male Athletes. *Sleep Hypn. Int. J.* **2018**, *21*, 97–100. **[Google Scholar]**

24. MacInnis, M.J.; Dziedzic, C.E.; Wood, E.; Oikawa, S.Y.; Phillips, S.M. Presleep α-Lactalbumin Consumption Does Not Improve Sleep Quality or Time-Trial Performance in Cyclists. *Int. J. Sport Nutr. Exerc. Metab.* **2020**, *30*, 197–202. **[Google Scholar]**

25. Afaghi, A.; O'Connor, H.; Chow, C.M. High-glycemic-index carbohydrate meals shorten sleep onset. *Am. J. Clin. Nutr.* **2007**, *85*, 426–430. **[Google Scholar]**

26. Afaghi, A.; O'Connor, H.; Chow, C.M. Acute effects of the very low carbohydrate diet on sleep indices. *Nutr. Neurosci.* **2008**, *11*, 146–154. **[Google Scholar]**

27. Howatson, G.; Bell, P.G.; Tallent, J.; Middleton, B.; McHugh, M.P.; Ellis, J. Effect of tart cherry juice (Prunus cerasus) on melatonin levels and enhanced sleep quality. *Eur. J. Nutr.* **2012**, *51*, 909–916. **[Google Scholar] [PubMed]**

28. Ong, J.N.; Hackett, D.A.; Chow, C.-M. Sleep quality and duration following evening intake of alpha-lactalbumin: A pilot study. *Biol. Rhythm. Res.* **2017**, *48*, 507–517. **[Google Scholar]**

29. Bannai, M.; Kawai, N.; Ono, K.; Nakahara, K.; Murakami, N. The Effects of Glycine on Subjective Daytime Performance in Partially Sleep-Restricted Healthy Volunteers. *Front. Neurol.* **2012**, 3, 61. **[Google Scholar] [Green Version]**

30. Vlahoyiannis, A.; Aphamis, G.; Andreou, E.; Samoutis, G.; Sakkas, G.K.; Giannaki, C.D. Effects of High vs. Low Glycemic Index of Post-Exercise Meals on Sleep and Exercise Performance: A Randomized, Double-Blind, Counterbalanced Polysomnographic Study. *Nutrients* **2018**, *10*, 1795. **[Google Scholar]** **[Green Version]**

31. Pigeon, W.R.; Carr, M.; Gorman, C.; Perlis, M.L. Effects of a Tart Cherry Juice Beverage on the Sleep of Older Adults with Insomnia: A Pilot Study. *J. Med. Food* **2010**, *13*, 579–583. **[Google Scholar]** **[Green Version]**

32. Lin, H.-H.; Tsai, P.-S.; Fang, S.-C.; Liu, J.-F. Effect of kiwifruit consumption on sleep quality in adults with sleep problems. *Asia Pac. J. Clin. Nutr.* **2011**, *20*, 169–174. **[Google Scholar]**

33. Yamatsu, A.; Yamashita, Y.; Maru, I.; Yang, J.; Tatsuzaki, J.; Kim, M. The Improvement of Sleep by Oral Intake of GABA and Apocynum venetum Leaf Extract. *J. Nutr. Sci. Vitaminol.* **2015**, *61*, 182–187. **[Google Scholar]** **[PubMed]** **[Green Version]**

34. Byun, J.-I.; Shin, Y.Y.; Chung, S.-E.; Shin, W.C. Safety and Efficacy of Gamma-Aminobutyric Acid from Fermented Rice Germ in Patients with Insomnia Symptoms: A Randomized, Double-Blind Trial. *J. Clin. Neurol.* **2018**, *14*, 291–295. **[Google Scholar]**

35. Simper, T.; Gilmartin, M.; Allwood, D.; Taylor, L.; Chappell, A. The effects of a sleep/recovery supplement: 'Night Time Recharge' on sleep parameters in young adults. *Nutr. Health* **2019**, *25*, 265–274. **[Google Scholar]** **[PubMed]**

36. Inagawa, K.; Hiraoka, T.; Kohda, T.; Yamadera, W.; Takahashi, M. Subjective effects of glycine ingestion before bedtime on sleep quality. *Sleep Biol. Rhythm.* **2006**, *4*, 75–77. **[Google Scholar]**

37. Yamadera, W.; Inagawa, K.; Chiba, S.; Bannai, M.; Takahashi, M.; Nakayama, K. Glycine ingestion improves subjective sleep quality in human volunteers, correlating with polysomnographic changes. *Sleep Biol. Rhythm.* **2007**, *5*, 126–131. **[Google Scholar]**

38. Ito, Y.; Takahashi, S.; Shen, M.; Yamaguchi, K.; Satoh, M. Effects of L-serine ingestion on human sleep. *Springerplus* **2014**, *3*, 1–5. **[Google Scholar]** **[Green Version]**

39. Yamatsu, A.; Yamashita, Y.; Pandharipande, T.; Maru, I.; Kim, M. Effect of oral γ-aminobutyric acid (GABA) administration on sleep and its absorption in humans. *Food Sci. Biotechnol.* **2016**, *25*, 547–551. **[Google Scholar]**

40. Burke, L.M.; Hawley, J.A.; Wong, S.H.S.; Jeukendrup, A.E. Carbohydrates for training and competition. *J. Sport. Sci.* **2011**, *29*, S17–S27. **[Google Scholar]** **[PubMed]**

41. Heine, W.; Radke, M.; Wutzke, K.-D. The significance of tryptophan in human nutrition. *Amino Acids* **1995**, *9*, 91–205. **[Google Scholar]**

42. Layman, D.K.; Lönnerdal, B.; Fernstrom, J.D. Applications for α-lactalbumin in human nutrition. *Nutr. Rev.* **2018**, *76*, 444–460. **[Google Scholar]**

43. Wurtman, R.J.; Wurtman, J.J.; Regan, M.M.; McDermott, J.M.; Tsay, R.H.; Breu, J.J. Effects of normal meals rich in carbohydrates or proteins on plasma tryptophan and tyrosine ratios. *Am. J. Clin. Nutr.* **2003**, *77*, 128–132. **[Google Scholar]** **[PubMed]**

44. Halson, S.L. Sleep and the elite athlete. *Sport. Sci.* **2013**, *26*, 1–4. **[Google Scholar]**

45. Vyazovskiy, V.V.; Delogu, A. NREM and REM sleep: Complementary roles in recovery after wakefulness. *Neuroscientist* **2014**, *20*, 203–219. **[Google Scholar]**

46. Abbott, W.; Brett, A.; Cockburn, E.; Clifford, T. Presleep Casein Protein Ingestion: Acceleration of Functional Recovery in Professional Soccer Players. *Int. J. Sport. Physiol. Perform.* **2019**, *14*, 385–391. **[Google Scholar]** **[Green Version]**

47. West, D.W.D.; Sawan, S.A.; Mazzulla, M.; Williamson, E.; Moore, D.R. Whey Protein Supplementation Enhances Whole Body Protein Metabolism and Performance Recovery after Resistance Exercise: A Double-Blind Crossover Study. *Nutrients* **2017**, *9*, 735. **[Google Scholar]**

48. Rozé, J.-C.; Barbarot, S.; Butel, M.-J.; Kapel, N.; Waligora-Dupriet, A.-J.; De Montgolfier, I.; Leblanc, M.; Godon, N.; Soulaines, P.; Darmaun, D.; et al. An α-lactalbumin-enriched and symbiotic-supplemented v. a standard infant formula: A multicentre, double-blind, randomised trial. *Br. J. Nutr.* **2011**, *107*, 1616–1622. **[Google Scholar] [Green Version]**

49. Markus, C.R.; Jonkman, L.M.; Lammers, J.H.C.M.; Deutz, N.E.P.; Messer, M.H.; Rigtering, N. Evening intake of α-lactalbumin increases plasma tryptophan availability and improves morning alertness and brain measures of attention. *Am. J. Clin. Nutr.* **2005**, *81*, 1026–1033. **[Google Scholar]**

50. Markus, C.R.; Olivier, B.; Panhuysen, G.E.; Van Der Gugten, J.; Alles, M.S.; Tuiten, A.; Westenberg, H.G.; Fekkes, D.; Koppeschaar, H.F.; De Haan, E.E. The bovine protein α-lactalbumin increases the plasma ratio of tryptophan to the other large neutral amino acids, and in vulnerable subjects raises brain serotonin activity, reduces cortisol concentration, and improves mood under stress. *Am. J. Clin. Nutr.* **2000**, *71*, 1536–1544. **[Google Scholar] [PubMed] [Green Version]**

51. Schaal, K.; Tafflet, M.; Nassif, H.; Thibault, V.; Pichard, C.; Alcotte, M.; Guillet, T.; El Helou, N.; Berthelot, G.; Simon, S.; et al. Psychological Balance in High Level Athletes: Gender-Based Differences and Sport-Specific Patterns. *PLoS ONE* **2011**, *6*, e19007. **[Google Scholar] [PubMed] [Green Version]**

52. Burkhardt, S.; Tan, D.X.; Manchester, L.C.; Hardeland, R.; Reiter, R.J. Detection and quantification of the antioxidant melatonin in Montmorency and Balaton tart cherries (Prunus cerasus). *J. Agric. Food Chem.* **2001**, *49*, 4898–4902. **[Google Scholar]**

53. Hughes, R.J.; Sack, R.L.; Lewy, A.J. The Role of Melatonin and Circadian Phase in Age-related Sleep-maintenance Insomnia: Assessment in a Clinical Trial of Melatonin Replacement. *Sleep* **1998**, *21*, 52–68. **[Google Scholar] [PubMed] [Green Version]**

54. Bowtell, J.L.; Sumners, D.P.; Dyer, A.; Fox, P.; Mileva, K.N. Montmorency Cherry Juice Reduces Muscle Damage Caused by Intensive Strength Exercise. *Med. Sci. Sport. Exerc.* **2011**, *43*, 1544–1551. **[Google Scholar] [Green Version]**

55. Connolly, D.A.J.; McHugh, M.P.; Padilla-Zakour, O. Efficacy of a tart cherry juice blend in preventing the symptoms of muscle damage. *Br. J. Sport. Med.* **2006**, *40*, 679–683. **[Google Scholar] [PubMed]**

56. McCormick, R.; Peeling, P.; Binnie, M.; Dawson, B.; Sim, M. Effect of tart cherry juice on recovery and next day performance in well-trained Water Polo players. *J. Int. Soc. Sport. Nutr.* **2016**, *13*, 41. **[Google Scholar] [PubMed] [Green Version]**

57. Losso, J.N.; Finley, J.W.; Karki, N.; Liu, A.G.; Prudente, A.; Tipton, R.; Yu, Y.; Greenway, F.L. Pilot Study of the Tart Cherry Juice for the Treatment of Insomnia and Investigation of Mechanisms. *Am. J. Ther.* **2018**, *25*, e194–e201. **[Google Scholar] [PubMed]**

58. Howatson, G.; McHugh, M.P.; Hill, J.A.; Brouner, J.; Jewell, A.P.; Van Someren, K.A.; Shave, R.E.; Howatson, S.A. Influence of tart cherry juice on indices of recovery following marathon running. *Scand. J. Med. Sci. Sport.* **2009**, *20*, 843–852. **[Google Scholar]**

59. Gomez-Cabrera, M.-C.; Domenech, E.; Romagnoli, M.; Arduini, A.; Borras, C.; Pallardo, F.V.; Sastre, J.; Viña, J. Oral administration of vitamin C decreases muscle mitochondrial biogenesis and hampers training-induced adaptations in endurance performance. *Am. J. Clin. Nutr.* **2008**, *87*, 142–149. **[Google Scholar] [Green Version]**

60. Maughan, R.J.; Burke, L.M.; Dvorak, J.; Larson-Meyer, D.E.; Peeling, P.; Phillips, S.M.; Rawson, E.S.; Walsh, N.P.; Garthe, I.; Geyer, H.; et al. IOC Consensus Statement: Dietary Supplements and the High-Performance Athlete. *Int. J. Sport Nutr. Exerc. Metab.* **2018**, *28*, 104–125. **[Google Scholar] [Green Version]**

61. Monti, J.M. Serotonin control of sleep-wake behavior. *Sleep Med. Rev.* **2011**, *15*, 269–281. **[Google Scholar]**

62. Kelly, G.S. Folates: Supplemental forms and therapeutic applications. *Altern. Med. Rev. A J. Clin. Ther.* **1998**, *3*, 208–220. **[Google Scholar]**

63. Griffen, C.E.; Kaye, A.M.; Rivera Bueno, F.; Kaye, A.D. Benzodiazepine pharmacology and central nervous system-mediated effects. *Oschner J.* **2013**, *13*, 214–223. **[Google Scholar]**

64. Halson, S.L.; Shaw, G.; Versey, N.; Miller, D.J.; Sargent, C.; Roach, G.D.; Nyman, L.; Carter, J.M.; Baar, K. Optimisation and Validation of a Nutritional Intervention to Enhance Sleep Quality and Quantity. *Nutrients* **2020**, *12*, 2579. **[Google Scholar]**

65. Buysse, D.J.; Reynolds, C.F.; Monk, T.H.; Berman, S.R.; Kupfer, D.J. The Pittsburgh sleep quality index: A new instrument for psychiatric practice and research. *Psychiatry Res.* **1989**, *28*, 193–213. **[Google Scholar]**

66. Johns, M.W. A new method for measuring daytime sleepiness: The Epworth sleepiness scale. *Sleep* **1991**, *14*, 540–545. **[Google Scholar]** **[Green Version]**

67. Halson, S.L. Sleep monitoring in athletes: Motivation, methods, miscalculations and why it matters. *Sport. Med.* **2019**, *49*, 1487–1497. **[Google Scholar]** **[PubMed]**

68. Dunican, I.C.; Higgins, C.C.; Jones, M.J.; Clarke, M.W.; Murray, K.; Dawson, B.; Caldwell, J.A.; Halson, S.L.; Eastwood, P.R. Caffeine use in a Super Rugby game and its relationship to post-game sleep. *Eur. J. Sport Sci.* **2018**, *18*, 513–523. **[Google Scholar]** **[PubMed]**

69. Thakkar, M.M.; Sharma, R.; Sahota, P. Alcohol disrupts sleep homeostasis. *Alcohol* **2015**, *49*, 299–310. **[Google Scholar]** **[Green Version]**

70. Geoghegan, P.; O'Donovan, M.T.; Lawlor, B.A. Investigation of the effects of alcohol on sleep using actigraphy. *Alcohol Alcohol.* **2012**, *47*, 538–544. **[Google Scholar]** **[Green Version]**

# 5 Chapter NUTRITION FOR ELDERLY ATHLETES

## 1. INTRODUCTION: AN OVERVIEW

Nutrition and physical activity are the primary modifiable determinants of health and well-being in contemporary society. These two components are frequently examined and regarded as distinct entities, despite their actual interrelation in multiple aspects. Physical activity (PA) can alter the nutrient spectrum utilized by human metabolism; insufficient PA results in the accumulation of ectopic fat in the liver, muscle, and possibly other organs [1,2]; malnutrition impairs both physical and cognitive performance; excessive feeding causes the expansion of fat deposits, thereby increasing body inertia and compromising physical fitness [3]. This review aims to enhance knowledge of the relationship between nutrition and physical activity/performance for readers from both backgrounds.

The subject of diet and physical activity is especially pertinent in relation to aging, as aging is typically linked to widespread inflammation and an increased disease burden [4]. Substantial data indicates that consistent physical activity and enhanced diet can mitigate disease load [5,6,7]. Consequently, the World Health Organization (WHO) has initiated efforts to promote physical activity across all age groups, and numerous governments have formulated national programs aimed at alleviating age-related morbidity. Nevertheless, older individuals generally become increasingly sedentary with advancing age, making it often difficult to include them in consistent physical activity.

In this regard, masters athletes can provide valuable information. These individuals train for and participate in athletic competitions beyond the conventional retirement age for sports. Numerous individuals adhere to stringent training protocols, frequently spanning decades or encompassing their entire adult existence. In addition to their inherent motivation for physical activity, individuals are compelled by the aspiration to excel in sports and to preserve their health. The scientific literature has historically overlooked this subject, with a notable rise in papers concerning various facets of masters sports occurring just in the last decade (Figure 1).

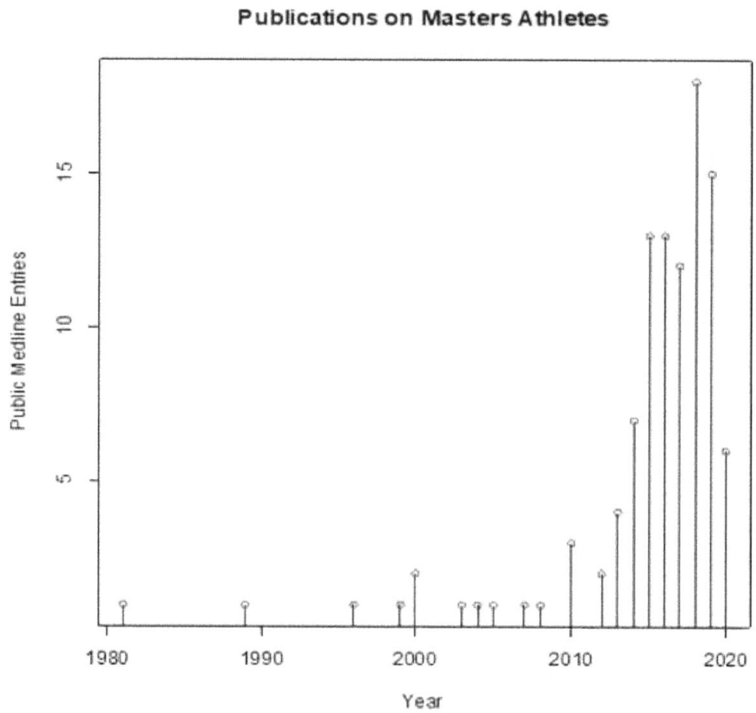


**Figure 1. Publications on masters athletes, plotted against year of publication. Date are the result of a literature research on public Medline on 1 October 2021, using the following search terms: ((master athlete (Title/Abstract)) OR (masters athlete (Title/Abstract)) OR (veteran athlete (Title/Abstract)).**

Naturally, a plethora of questions arise with regard to the nutritional support for these aging athletes. Thus, as with any athlete, also the masters athletes wish to reduce their body fat, in order to optimize athletic performance. But what are the energetic requirements, given that resting metabolic rate (RMR) typically dwindles with age? How can the requirements for the intake of protein, vitamins and other micronutrients be met when the total intake is reduced for the sake of body composition? Which nutrients are physiologically opportune for optimized performance, and which ones should be recommended to facilitate recovery and prevention of injury? The field of nutritional support for athletes has traditionally focused on young elite athletes, and there is no clear answer to these and other questions pertinent to the topic. Hence, the present paper attempts to collate the relevant information in order to (a) provide recommendations where evidence is available, and to (b) flag the most important open question for future research.

## 2. PHYSIOLOGICAL CHANGES IN OLDER ATHLETES

### 2.1. Oxygen Delivery and Utilization Systems

The exercising skeletal muscles rely on continuous oxygen supply that is precisely matched to the metabolic requirements of the exercise intensity. If, at any intensity, the oxygen supply becomes limited, anaerobic metabolism compensates for the lacking oxygen, indicated by increasing lactate concentration **[9,10]**. Oxygen has to be transported from the ambient air to the oxygen-respiring mitochondria of the working muscles. This is involving a series of steps, namely oxygen diffusion (driven by the existing pressure gradient) from the alveoli into the pulmonary capillary blood, the oxygenated blood (oxygen is primarily bound to hemoglobin) is pumped by the heart to the skeletal muscles, where oxygen is converted to adenosine triphosphate (ATP), providing energy to power the working muscles (**Figure 2**). Oxygen delivery ($DO_2$) to the muscles is determined by the cardiac output (heart rate x stroke volume, Q), the hemoglobin concentration (Hb) and the level of its saturation ($SaO_2$), according to the equation:

$$DO_2 = Q \times Hb \times SaO_2 \times K$$

K indicates the Hüfner coefficient for hemoglobin-oxygen binding capacity which is 1.33 mL/g.

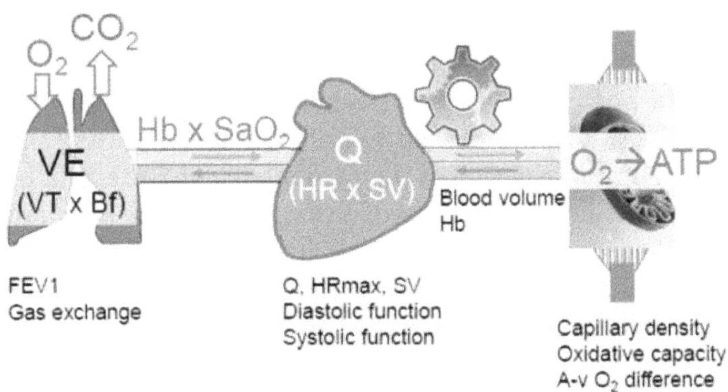


**Figure 2. The lung-heart-muscle axis involved in oxygen delivery and utilization. Main cardiorespiratory parameters specifying organ function at rest and during exercise: minute ventilation (VE), cardiac output (Q), and oxygen extraction in the skeletal muscle. Parameters listed below the organs represent those which are primarily affected by the aging process. Oxygen, $O_2$; carbon dioxide, $CO_2$; tidal volume, VT; breathing frequency, Bf; hemoglobin concentration, Hb; arterial oxygen saturation, $SaO_2$; heart rate, HR; adenosine triphosphate, ATP.**

The extraction of oxygen utilized by the mitochondria is represented by the arterio-venous oxygen difference (a-v $O_2$ difference). As the need for oxygen is increasing with increasing exercise intensity, minute ventilation, cardiac output, muscle perfusion and oxygen extraction all have to increase. According to the Fick principle for individual aerobic capacity, the highest achievable rate of oxygen uptake ($VO_2max$) equals Q × a-v $O_2$ extraction. All organs involved in oxygen transport and utilization may contribute to $VO_2max$ decline in the aging athlete.

### 2.1.1. The Pulmonary System

Although data on the breathing reserve (BR; maximal voluntary ventilation related to minute ventilation during maximal exercise) do not indicate a considerable ventilatory limitation of $VO_2max$ in healthy older individuals [**11**], it can become a limiting factor in some highly trained aged athletes [**12**]. In addition, diffusion capacity of the lung is predictive of marathon performance, and it decreases markedly with age, an effect from which masters athletes are not exempt [**13**]. Probably as a consequence of this, exercise-induced hypoxemia is more prevalent in highly fit older individuals compared to the healthy general population and fatiguing work of the respiratory muscles may provoke vasoconstriction in the leg muscles and compromise Q [**14**]. Thus, $VO_2max$ restriction by the pulmonary system depends on the level of fitness (the higher the more likely) and the age-related degree of decrease in respiratory function along with structural changes, i.e., declining respiratory muscle strength and endurance, enhanced rigidity of the chest wall, loss of elastic recoil, reduction of the alveolar surface area and the number of capillaries perfusing the lung [**11,15,16**]. A low BR, reduced forced expiratory volume in one second (FEV1) and exercise-induced hypoxemia are potential markers for pulmonary limitations of $VO_2max$ in the older athlete [**17**] (**Figure 2**).

### 2.1.2. The Cardiovascular System

It is obvious that a precise interplay between pulmonary ventilation, $DO_2$ and the extraction of oxygen by the muscle tissue is a prerequisite for properly matching oxygen need and demand. The contribution of the cardiovascular system, in particular Qmax, is considered as the main determinant of $VO_2max$ in young people when including large skeletal muscle groups, e.g., leg cycling, running or cross-country skiing [**18,19**]. The demand of oxygen by these working muscles increases tremendously (about 10 to 20-fold, depending on the individual fitness) from rest to maximal work [**10**]. Consequently, a large amount of oxygenated blood has to be transported to muscles driven by the pumping heart. Thus, a 72% contribution of Qmax to $VO_2max$ changes has been demonstrated in sedentary young and older subjects of both sexes, and the Qmax increased to 81–89% in trained young and older subjects of both sexes [**18**]. The age-related decrease in cardiovascular function (particularly decline of Q which is HR x SV) will considerably affect $VO_2max$. HRmax decreases according to the formula (208 (beats per min)—0.7 × age) in healthy sedentary and trained subjects, probably due to the decrease in intrinsic heart rate [**20**]. In addition, lower SV associated with reduced left ventricular (LV) compliance (diminished diastolic function) was shown in healthy sedentary people but seems to be preserved in masters athletes [**21**]. Impaired ability to modulate sympathetic vasoconstrictor activity (functional sympatholysis) and a reduced exercise hyperemia are also characteristics of aging. Again, regular PA was shown to offset these impairments [**22**].

### 2.1.3. Skeletal Muscle and Mitochondria

Capillarization of skeletal muscles and muscle oxidative capacity decrease likewise with aging at least in rather sedentary subjects [**23,24**]. However, long-term engaging in endurance sports can largely prevent the reduction in muscle capillarization and muscle oxidative enzymatic activity with aging, e.g., in 65- to 75-year-old athletes

[25]. The oxidative capacity of skeletal muscles is not considered as an important limitation of $VO_2max$ because it exceeds the amount of oxygen consumed during whole body exercise [26]. Thus, benefits of regular training on adaptations in the skeletal muscle rather promote improved submaximal exercise performance than $VO_2max$. Such adaptations include increases in capillary supply and mitochondrial key enzyme activities favoring a higher rate of fat oxidation and a concomitant reduction in the glycolytic flux, as well as a tighter control of the acid-base status [10]. Consequently, the anaerobic threshold (submaximal endurance performance) declines at a slower rate with aging (especially in trained individuals) than $VO_2max$ [27,28]. A noteworthy observation is the inverse relationship between mechanical efficiency and $VO_2max$ (shown in elite cyclers), which was attributed to variations in the amount of efficient type I and less efficient type II fibers of working muscles [29].

## 2.2. Body Composition and Metabolism

Although aging is generally associated with a loss of lean muscle mass, exercise can modulate such losses. According to population-based studies, the prevalence of sarcopenia in healthy adults aged 60 years and older is about 10% for men and 10% for women, respectively [30]. Intriguingly, in a cross-sectional study including 156 female and male masters athletes aged between 40–79 years, no individual was categorized as sarcopenic, i.e., below normal levels of muscle mass and muscle strength or performance, according to the definition of the European Working Group for Sarcopenia in Older People [31,32]. Data from cross-sectional studies indicate that lean muscle mass and muscle strength did not decline with age in individuals aged 40–81 years who trained 4 to 5 times per week [33]. These data could indicate that declines in physical function may not be related to age alone but are rather confounded by muscle disuse and decreased levels of PA in the elderly general population [34]. On the other hand, two previous cross-sectional studies based on an anthropometric assessment of lower limb muscle volume [35] in male 115 track and field masters [36] and in 54 male master weight lifters [37] indicated a volume reduction of approximately 6% per age decade. This figure has been confirmed by a recent longitudinal study in 71 track-and-field master athletes with a mean follow-up of 4.2 years that found a reduction in calf muscle cross section, as assessed with computed tomography, by 0.6% per year in men, but no significant change in women [38]. Moreover, a recent cross-sectional study in 256 track and field masters aged 35–91 years in which whole body skeletal muscle mass was assessed via bio-electrical impedance indicates a reduction by 3.2% and 2.8% per decade in women in men, respectively [39], which was equalized by a commensurate increase in fat mass. On the other hand, older athletes of 68 years showed 17% lower body fat percentage and 12% greater leg lean mass, respectively [40]. In the general population, fat-free mass is expected to decrease the 6th decade of life onwards by approximately 2% per decade in men but not in women, while both men and women gain fat mass by 7.5% per decade [41]. Thus, whilst masters athletes likely experience muscle wasting and adipose tissue accumulation, their body composition may still be better preserved than in the non-athletic counterparts.

The question arises, which factors may trigger the age-related adipose tissue accumulation. Lifelong training increased the proportion of type I muscle fibres with a concomitant decrease of carbohydrate oxidation independent of intensity level in older athletes compared to younger man [**42**]. While fat oxidation capacity was similar in both groups, older athletes compensated with a higher exercise metabolic efficiency [**42**]. While sports and recreational activity decreased to a higher extent in men than in women over a course of ~10 years, activity levels as well as baseline age were inversely related to changes in fat mass in women only [**41**]. Low RMR may predispose to future weight gain. As PA contributes considerably to total energy expenditure, the question is whether regular exercise can curb age-related reductions in RMR. Although it is difficult to disentangle changes in metabolic rate from alterations of body composition with aging, evidence suggests that RMR is lower in older men and women, even after adjusting for differences in body composition, waist-to-hip ratio and smoking status [**43,44**]. A paper, based on the cohort of 256 track and field masters athletes mentioned above, has found that the effect of age on RMR is mostly attributable to changes in body composition [**45**]. While fat-free mass is a main determinant of RMR, other factors that are unrelated to differences in body composition can also explain differences in RMR of young and older individuals. Although the decline of RMR also occurs in highly physically active individuals, it is associated with reductions of exercise volume and energy intake that occur with age. However, these age-related adaptations are blunted in individuals who maintain these two components at a similar level as young physically active men [**46**]. Also, a higher aerobic capacity is related to a higher RMR in older athletes [**47**]. In a sample of 65 healthy women ranging from 21–72 years, those individuals who were regularly performing endurance exercise were spared from an age-related decline in RMR assessed by indirect calorimetry compared to their sedentary counterparts [**48**]. This metabolic difference may in part explain lower body weight and fat mass in active, older individuals.

In summary, the reduction in metabolic rate, coupled with concurrent decreases and increases in lean mass and fat mass in the elderly, can only partially be attributed to the aging process itself. Instead, these impacts appear to be complicated by reduced physical activity levels and insufficient calorie consumption in this demographic. Despite older athletes exhibiting superior body composition compared to their less active peers of the same age, they still experience age-related declines and changes in body composition and metabolism, which can be partially mitigated by enhanced exercise metabolic efficiency.

## 2.3. Effects of Aging on the Endocrine System and Metabolic Pathways

The aging process is associated with many endocrine modifications, as well as adjustments in practically all biological systems, encompassing body composition, functional performance, and bone mass. The impacts of aging are frequently complicated by additional factors, including chronic diseases and alterations in eating patterns, with malnutrition typically occurring simultaneously during the aging process. This section does not aim to provide a comprehensive overview of endocrine changes; rather, it addresses the significant hormonal shifts associated with aging that relate to appetite regulation, glucose homeostasis, and energy expenditure, as well as the modulatory function of physical activity.

### 2.3.1. Thyroid Hormones

The important role of thyroid hormones in determining energy expenditure and basal metabolic rate has long been recognized [**49**]. With aging, there is a general increase of the incidence of thyroid diseases [**50**]. Apart from this increase and according to several population studies, aging is associated with subclinical hypothyroidism, i.e., increased levels of thyroid-stimulating hormone (TSH) with free thyroxine (FT4) levels remaining in the normal range [**51,52**]. Some authors even ascribe a beneficial adaptation of physiological aging to these reduced TSH levels in the elderly by preventing excessive catabolism [**53**]. While the free triiodothyronine resistance index was negatively associated with aging in males, TSH levels were positively associated with age in females [**54**]. These results underline a possible sex-specific effect of alterations of thyroid hormones with aging.

Although endocrine effects have to be separated from alterations of body composition and PA behavior with aging, RMR is lower in older individuals, potentially even after adjusting for differences in body composition [**43**]. The age-related decline of RMR, however, cannot fully be ascribed to alterations of body composition or differences in thyroid hormone status [**55**].

### 2.3.2. Hypothalamic Growth Hormone-Insulin-Like Growth Factor-I Axis

This axis includes the secretion of growth hormone (GH; somatotropin) from the somatotropes of the pituitary gland into the circulation, and the successive stimulation of insulin-like growth factor-1 (IGF-1). This endocrine system drives anabolic effects on protein synthesis and growth and hence plays an important role in maintaining muscle mass. In elderly individuals, GH secretion, together with IGF-1 levels decrease starting with the third decade [**56**]. There is also a reduction in GH releasing hormone (GHRH)-induced GH secretion, likely reflecting changes of neurotransmitter control and reduced hypothalamic GHRH synthesis related to the aging brain [**57**]. Regular physical exercise is thought to modulate activity of the GH-IGF-1 axis throughout the lifespan, potentially preserving muscle mass in the elderly. With regard to that, GH responses to a cycling sprint, resistance or endurance exercise bout were compared in young and middle- aged men. While resting GH concentration and objective parameters of exertion were not different between groups, GH response to exercise was greater in the young compared to their older counterparts [**58**]. When investigating the effect of a 12-week resistance training program on GH and testosterone secretion in young (23 years) and older (63 years) individuals, the authors found that, regardless of age, this training modality elicits GH and testosterone secretion. Response and magnitude, however, was different between the two groups [**59**]. Mechano growth factor (MGF), a splice variant of the IGF-1 gene, is supposed to be an important local factor promoting satellite cell proliferation in muscle. Although short-term (5-week) resistance exercise failed to increase expression of MGF in elderly as compared to young individuals [60], longer-term training of 12-weeks was still able to upregulate expression of this factor in the elderly [61]. Exercise training can stimulate the GH-IGF-1 axis as well as MGF in the elderly, albeit somewhat less so in older as compared to younger individuals. This may reflect an age-related desensitization to mechanical loading. It has to be noted that short study duration, differences in training motivation or the inability to achieve a sufficient absolute exercise intensity in the elderly as well as a sex-bias towards male study participants may bias these findings.

### 2.3.3. Hormones Regulating Appetite and Food Intake

Above the age of 65 years, there seems to be a decrease in appetite and food intake, which predisposes to undernutrition. A negative energy balance has implications for chronic disease progression and mortality rate [62]. Hormones mediating the anorexic effect of aging include cholecystokinin (CCK), leptin, and ghrelin. CCK is a gastrointestinal peptide hormone produced by enteroendocrine cells of the duodenum that mediate satiating effects by binding to receptors in the central nervous system. Aging is associated with increased CCK concentrations as well as a greater sensitivity to the satiety-inducing effect of this hormone [63]. In line with that, whey protein ingestion resulted in greater plasma concentrations of CCK and gastric inhibitory peptide in older compared to younger individuals [64]. In addition, the increased activity of the anorexigenic hormone leptin, an adipokine derived from adipose tissue in humans as well as the reduced activity of the orexigenic hormone ghrelin, a gastrointestinal molecule derived from the stomach, seem to further reduce hunger and thereby hamper energy intake in the elderly [65,66]. Obesity is another factor that can dysregulate the endocrine role of leptin secretion from adipocytes, so that hyperleptinemia due to high fat mass fails to negatively regulate food intake, a state termed leptin resistance [67]. A recent study showed that higher fitness levels in older individuals were associated with lower leptin levels and inflammation, regardless of adiposity, suggesting a protective effect of physical fitness towards development of leptin resistance [68]. Nevertheless, the modulatory role of PA on hormones governing appetite and food intake in the elderly remains understudied. In general, individuals with higher levels of PA experience blunted satiety and amplified hunger compared to those being less physically active, likely in order to compensate for the increased PA induced energy expenditure [69]. It seems, however, that chronic exercise can affect perceptions of hunger and energy intake independent of body composition and sex. Individuals being physically active may be more sensitive to regulating energy balance by improved adjustments of energy intake and density of food [70]. The paucity of data on this subject in older athletes of both sexes, however, does not allow definitive conclusions with regard to this age group.

### 2.3.4. Insulin, Glucose and Metabolic Pathways Mediating Glucose Homeostasis

Insulin is the most important hormone mediating control of glucose homeostasis, i.e., cellular uptake, utilisation and endogenous production. Aging is associated with deteriorating glucose homeostasis [**71**]. It has been suggested that, starting from the fourth decade, fasting plasma glucose increases by about 0.055 mmol/L per decade, alongside with a gradual rise of glucose concentrations obtained after 120 min of a 75 g oral glucose tolerance test [**72**]. Further to that, aging is a risk factor for brain insulin resistance, i.e., impaired sensitivity of central nervous pathways to insulin [**73**]. Interestingly, high insulin action in the brain influences long-term weight management and is associated with a favorable body fat distribution [**74**]. In general, insulin is secreted in a pulsatile manner. During the basal as well as insulin-stimulated state, both amplitude and number of pulses are reduced with aging [**75**]. This goes hand in hand with decreased effectiveness in reducing hepatic glucose output and increased liver insulin clearance [**76**]. Glucagon concentrations, in turn, do not seem to be affected by age [**77**]. However, the rise in hepatic glucose production after glucagon stimulation, i.e., hepatic sensitivity to glucagon, is increased in elderly individuals compared to their younger counterparts [**78**].

Seminal studies from the lab of John Holloszy and colleagues point towards the importance of physical training for maintaining glucose tolerance. The researchers studied older lean and overweight untrained as well as trained individuals compared to young untrained and trained individuals. They found that oral glucose tolerance, defined as the area under the glucose curve, was twofold poorer in the untrained older individuals as compared to the other groups. Also, the insulin response to glucose was higher in the untrained groups as compared to the older and younger trained groups [**79**]. These results are suggestive of reduced glucose tolerance and insulin sensitivity with aging and a counter regulatory role of lifelong exercise training.

A similar, more recent study used the glucose clamp technique to assess insulin sensitivity in younger (age range 24–47 years) and older (age range 60–75 years) athletes as well as younger and older normal-weight and obese individuals. Insulin sensitivity was highest and similar in young and older athletes, followed by normal weight individuals and lowest in obese young and old individuals [**80**]. This study underlines the fact that body composition and physical inactivity, but not age per se are related to the development of insulin resistance. As glucose disposal decreases over the lifespan, several factors contributing to reduced insulin action have to be considered. These include a rise in total body fat, in particular visceral fat, and reductions of caloric intake, PA and consequent decrements in lean mass or certain drugs and age-related diseases.

In this context, it is important to also scrutinize cellular mechanisms responsible for age-induced reductions in insulin-stimulated glucose uptake. In brief, upon binding to its receptor, insulin stimulates autophosphorylation of the insulin receptor, tyrosine phosphorylation of the insulin receptor substrate-1 (IRS-1) and association with phosphoinositide 3-kinase (PI3K) and subsequent phosphorylation of Akt2 at serine 473 and threonine 308 sites and AS160 phosphorylation, which finally promotes glucose transporter type 4 (GLUT4) translocation to the plasma membrane to stimulate glucose uptake [**81**]. Aging can selectively affect elements of this signalling cascade.

For instance, Akt phosphorylation by insulin was ~40% lower in healthy, lean, elderly individuals compared to young body mass index (BMI)-, fat mass- and habitual PA-matched volunteers [**82**]. This was in line with a 25% reduction in insulin-stimulated rates of muscle glucose uptake. Another study found that AS160 phosphorylation under insulin-stimulated conditions was reduced, together with ~30% lower whole-body insulin sensitivity, in aged compared to young individuals [**83**]. Participation in an exercise training program of either strength or endurance exercise improved whole-body insulin sensitivity and abrogated impairments in AS160 phosphorylation in these individuals. Different factors have been discussed that could contribute to this reduction in insulin action in elderly individuals. Among these, a reduction in oxidative capacity [**84**], impaired mitochondrial metabolic flexibility during insulin stimulation [**82**], oxidative stress [**85**] or dysfunctional regulation of mitochondrial dynamics [**86**] may contribute to alterations of mitochondria with aging. These changes in turn promote increased deposition of ectopic lipids within the myocyte as intramyocellular lipids (IMCL). This site of lipid deposition has repeatedly been shown to be particularly detrimental to insulin action [**87**]. Compared to younger volunteers, IMCL content, assessed by $^{1}$H magnetic resonance spectroscopy, was 70% higher in elderly individuals [**82**]. Decrements in mitochondrial activity together with excess caloric intake promote lipid synthesis and storage and yield bioactive diacylglycerols, which are known to accumulate within the plasma membrane, where they recruit novel protein kinase C isoforms that facilitate inhibitory phosphorylation of IRS1 [**81**]. Ceramides, another important class of bioactive lipids, may inhibit Akt phosphorylation [**81**]. These intracellular processes impair the insulin signalling pathway and eventually contribute to impaired insulin-stimulated cellular glucose uptake.

In summary, aging is associated with deteriorating glucose homeostasis. While insulin secretion is diminished over the lifespan, glucagon action is only marginally affected. Besides decrements in hormones mediating control of glucose homeostasis, decreased PA, together with reduced mitochondrial function will promote ectopic lipid deposition in muscle, which further impairs insulin signalling and glucose uptake.

## 2.4. Bone and Bone Metabolism

Bone is a hard tissue that derives its tensile stiffness from the organic extracellular matrix and its stiffness in shear and compression from an inorganic calcium-phosphate compound (so-called bone apatite). Whilst the majority of the organic matrix consists of type 1 collagen (>90%), there are also other collagens as well as other protein constituents, such as proteoglycans, carboxylated osteocalcin, osteopontin and TGF-β (Transforming growth factor beta (TGF-β)). The role of these latter constituents is only just evolving and seems to be primarily related to endocrine and regulatory functions, rather than serving mechanical purposes. Four different types of cells govern biological activity in bone. Ostoeblasts lay down bone protein onto existing bone surfaces, and they also initiate mineralization. When such bone formation drifts cease, osteocytes either become dormant as bone lining cells, or they transform into osteocytes that are fully covered by bone matrix and thus remote to the bone's surface.

However, osteocytes still communicate via gap junctions with other osteocytes and lining cells, which allows trafficking of electrolytes and small organic compounds. Osteocytes are also thought to sense mechanical strains, to transfer that information into biological signals that help to adapt bone to its mechanical purposes, and also to initiate the repair of bone microdamage through the process of bone remodeling [**88,89**]. Osteoclasts, finally, trans-differentiate from peripheral blood mononuclear cells and have capacity to dissolve the inorganic matrix through acidification, and subsequently also the protein phase in order to resorb bone tissue.

The four types of bone cells work in co-operation with each other. Thus, the activity of osteoclasts is under the control of osteoblasts through receptor activator of NFKB ligand (RANKL), as well as under the control of osteocytes by sclerostin [**90**]. In addition, TGF-β from the bone matrix stimulates activation of osteoblasts [**91**]. The reciprocal control of osteoblastic activity by osteoclasts is less well established, but may involve compounds such as ephrinB2 and other factors [**92**]. These cell-cell interactions seem fundamental for the bone remodeling process [**93**]. Herein, osteoclastic bone resorption precedes osteoblastic bone formation, a process that is often triggered by material microdamage [**94**], thus helping to repair damaged bone. Modeling, on the other hand, serves the purpose of 'shaping' bones through formation and resorption that occurs on opposing surfaces of the bone, thus resulting in bone 'drifts' [**95**]. Thus, remodeling and modeling are two diverse processes. Whilst modeling is the main contributor to bone turn-over at young age, the bone turn-over after closure of the growth plate is mostly due to remodeling. With regards to aging, it is also noteworthy that bone turn-over is typically greater in young than in older people [**96**]. This is partly due to a slowing of the remodeling process, i.e., the entire cycle from activation of osteoclasts until closure of the resorption cavity, which takes approximately 90 days in young people but 120 days in old people [**93**]. In addition, it has been demonstrated that the ability to respond to bone microdamage becomes blunted with increasing age [**97**].

It is important to understand that the largest forces that bones experience emerge from regional muscle forces and impact loading, rather than from body weight per se. As a result, muscle mass and bone mass are well-adapted to each other [**98**]. This mutual relationship between muscle and bone is largely driven through the bone's response to local tissue strains [**99**]. Thus, the mechanostat theory proposes that bone counteracts excessive deformations with enhanced bone formation, whereas sub-threshold deformations are answered by streamlining the bone's structure [**100**]. In addition, evidence suggests also an independent effect of strain rate on bone accrual. There are also several signaling pathways that interact with muscle and bone. For example, bone morphogenetic protein 1 (BMP1) has been shown to positively affect muscle growth in mice [**101**]. TGF-β, which initially had been known for its stimulating role for osteoblasts, has now been recognized to negatively affect calcium handling within skeletal muscle, and to thereby hamper muscles electro-mechanical coupling [**102**]. Moreover, undercarboxylated osteocalcin from the bone enhances insulin production, cognitive functioning and muscular fuel utilization [**103**]. Thus, there are several compounds from bone's non-collagen protein phase that unfold important systemic actions on skeletal muscle and athletic performance.

In addition to the mechanical determinants, bone is also under control of several endocrine systems. Both sex hormones have important effects, with the estrogens and androgens being more effective on the endocortical and periosteal surfaces, respectively **[104]**. From an evolutionary perspective, estrogens may serve the role of 'packing' bone minerals that are not mechanically required **[98]**, so that sufficient calcium depots are available when breastfeeding taps on the calcium resources **[105]**. In this regard, the complete withdrawal of estrogen after menopause is a catastrophic event for the female skeleton, leading to bone loss and an incidence rate for vertebral and femoral fractures of 1% per year, respectively **[106]**. In female endurance athletes, the so-called female athlete triad may occur, where underfeeding is associated with amenorrhea, low bone mineral density and fractures, even at young age **[107]**. In addition to sex steroids, there are also other hormones impinging on bone, such as parathyroid hormone, the D-hormone and insulin-like growth factors.

Bones are responsive to exercise **[108]**, which is primarily thought to be through mechanical effects. Rapid running and jumping elicits larger strains and strain rates than static exercises **[109]**, and power athletes have stronger leg bones than endurance athletes **[110,111,112]**. The largest effects have been observed for the humerus, the structure of which can be twice as strong in tennis and baseball players in the active as compared in the passive arm **[113,114]**. Side-to-side differences in the legs of jumpers are much smaller than in the arm **[115]**, which could be due to the fact that jumpers load both legs substantially during run-ups, whereas tennis players place only small loads on their passive arms.

With advancing age, bone mass is lost in the general population, a phenomenon that is much more pronounced in the spine and in the upper extremity than in the legs **[116]**. Bone benefits acquired through exercise at young age can still persist several decades after cessation of exercise training **[117]**. Conversely, when taking up an exercise activity during adulthood, i.e., after fusion of the growth plates, then it is still possible to moderately enhance bone mass and bone strength in the loaded bones, as demonstrated by observations in masters tennis players achieved in adulthood **[118]**. As to another question, namely what happens to masters athletes if exercise is continued across the life span, results from cross-sectional studies suggest that the bone benefits attained at young age **[119]** persist into old age, although they may fade away with advancing age **[120]**. A recent longitudinal study in 71 track and field masters with 4-year follow-up, however, demonstrates that tibia bone mass and strength can be preserved, or even increased in male power athletes, whilst male endurance athletes and female track-and-field masters lose tibia epiphyseal bone mass at a rate of approximately 5% per decade **[38]**. It has to be considered, however, that some of the female masters athletes in that study were aged between 50 and 60 years, i.e., within the perimenopausal decade, and that this study could not discern between the effects of aging and of menopause. It therefore seems fair to conclude that engagement in track and field events such as sprint running and jumping has potential to maintain or increase bone health into old age.

# 3. PERFORMANCE AND TRAINABILITY OF OLDER ATHLETES

## 3.1. Performance Decline in the Aging Athlete

Declines in cardiovascular fitness and physical performance are the main features of aging human beings [**121,122**]. The decline starts in the third to fourth decade and depends on genetic and life-style characteristics, in particular on PA through life-span. High cardiorespiratory fitness (CRF: aerobic capacity, $VO_2max$) and regular PA are associated with longevity even when adjusted for relevant confounders [**122,123**]. Differences of the slope in performance decline between aging athletes and their sedentary peers are still a matter of debate, but absolute performance levels remain considerably high in masters athletes of both sexes at all ages [**28**]. Whereas most studies primarily focused on age-dependent changes in running and swimming performance [**124,125**], only a few have considered a broader range of sports [**126**]. Data derived from mean winning performance times in track and field events of 10,000 participants in Senior Olympic Games demonstrate a slow decline from the age of 50 to 75 years which became dramatically steeper after the age of 75 [**126**]. Those findings have been expanded by a recent study suggesting an additional steepening of the endurance performance (in track and field events) in very old masters athletes aged 80+ [**127**]. Whereas no differences in performance decline in sprint versus endurance events were found for men, sprint performance declined more steeply than that of endurance in women [**128**]. However, when accounting for kinetic energy contributions to the metabolic costs, sprint and distance running world records depicted remarkably similar age trends [**129**]. A similar decline was shown in mountain runners from 50 to 70+ years; this decline was, however, slightly more pronounced in females compared to males [**28**]. Although the performance decline in this study seemed to be slightly steeper in masters athletes than in sedentary persons of the general population, it is important to note that endurance performance remained about 3.5 times higher in older athletes [**28**]. A recent review confirmed, based on current data from masters athletes, that most of the physiological mechanisms determining $VO_2max$ (i.e., pulmonary and cardiovascular function, blood oxygen transport capacity, skeletal muscle capillary density and oxidative capacity) are profoundly modulated by regular PA during the entire life-span [**9**]. In contrast to cardiovascular and skeletal muscle adaptations to PA and exercise training, pulmonary adaptations seem to play a rather minor role for the maintenance of performance in the aging athletes [**9,10**]. In summary, all these findings indicate that endurance performance (i.e., $VO_2max$) inevitably declines when getting older but can be favorably modified by regular PA and especially by exercise training at all ages in both sexes (**Figure 3**).

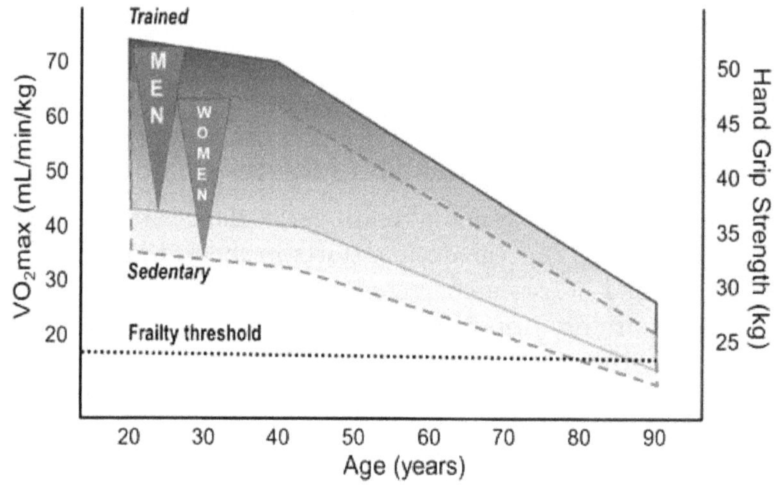


**Figure 3. Schematic presentation of the age-related performance decline, i.e., in aerobic capacity ($VO_2$max) and maximal grip strength, for both sexes, depending on physical training status, ranging from well-trained to sedentary. The figure is based on the meta-analysis from Fitzgerald et al. (1997) [130], with contributions from Burtscher et al. (2008) [28], Booth et al. (2010) [131], Landi et al. (2017) [132], and (defining frailty threshold as $VO_2$max of 18 mL/min/kg) Carr et al. (2006) [133].**

## 3.2. Sex Differences in Performance, Decline Rates, and Training Effects

### 3.2.1. Aerobic Fitness

Upper limits of $VO_2$max values can exceed 90 mL/min/kg in young male elite athletes [**134**] compared to about 35 to 37 mL/min/kg in the general population aged 35–45 years [**135**]. Above the third age decade, $VO_2$max values decline by approximately 10% per decade but this decline may be considerably modulated by training [**9,10**]. Extraordinarily high aerobic capacity has been reported in lifelong physically active very old individuals of both sexes. For instance, $VO_2$max values of 38 (±1) vs. 21 (±1) mL/min/kg were shown for 81-year-old male endurance athletes ($n$ = 9) vs. age-matched healthy untrained persons [**136**]. Even more impressive, a $VO_2$max of 42.3 mL/min/kg has been recently reported in a 83-year old female masters runner [**137**]. On top, a 101-yr old athlete improved his $VO_2$max following 2 years of specific training (to 103 years of age) from 31 to 35 mL/min/kg [**138**]. Baker and Tang compared the aging-related rates in performance decline of masters records of both sexes [**126**]. The age of males/females when performance had declined to 50% of the maximum performance at 30–35 years were 90/84 years for walking, 87/84 years for swimming, 78/72 years for jumping, and 74/60 years for weight lifting [**126**]. The larger sex differences in weight lifting compared to walking or swimming might be attributable to differences between lower and upper body performance (composition). While 12% sex difference was reported for running, swimming and cycling [**139,140**], the sex difference was 17% in cross country skiing (skating technique), again indicating different lower and upper body performance between sexes [**135**]. The relative (to body mass) $VO_2max$ differs by about 10% between male and female athletes, which is primarily explained by the higher percentage of body fat and lower hemoglobin levels in women [**135,141**]. Although this indicates similar overall effectiveness of the oxygen delivery and utilization systems in men and women, specific differences in cardiac and skeletal muscle adaptations exist. With regard to cardiac adaptation to regular exercise training, greater LV end-diastolic cavity sizes and LV mass are observed in trained versus untrained individuals, which is more pronounced in male athletes [**142**]. Sex differences in LV mass cannot completely be explained by the lower body size of the female athletes, but may at least partly result in the larger blood pressure increase at peak exercise in men [**143**]. Performance in sprint cycling (200 m) was effectively halved (from the maximum performance at 30–35 years) at an age of 80 years in males compared to an age of 59 years in female masters athletes [**126**]. Regular exercise training of masters athletes can prevent the shrinking of type I muscle fibers [**144**], and minimize loss of type II fibers, and it may also prevent fiber type grouping [**145**] following denervation-reinnervation cycles with aging in both sexes. Notably, females seem to develop a slower muscle fiber phenotype due to progressive slowing of discharge rates [**146**], likely explaining the relatively large sex difference in the decline of sprint cycling performance [**126**] (see below).

### 3.2.2. Muscular Strength and Power

Muscular strength and power significantly contribute to physical fitness and play an independent function in preventing numerous chronic illnesses and premature mortality [147]. The aging process leads to a reduction in muscle mass and strength of around 1% annually, commencing in the fourth decade of life [148]. Peak instantaneous power diminishes by roughly 7% every decade, as evaluated through vertical leap tests in endurance runners, sprinters, and the general population, with comparable findings noted in ergometric lower extremity power assessments [36,144,149,150]. Muscle wastage varies considerably across individuals due to inherent variances in the aging process, although it can be substantially influenced by physical activity levels and exercise training. The primary characteristics linked to aging are muscle architecture and fiber type composition, tendon qualities, and vascular regulation of contracting muscle. In athletes, the decline in power-lifting performance is more significant and accelerates more swiftly than that of endurance performance; specifically, both men's and women's power-lifting performance begins to diminish by 3% year in the fourth decade and by 1% annually afterward [152]. The immediate and significant effects of resistance training on muscle mass, strength, and power are well-documented in both young and elderly adults, similar to endurance training's impact on cardiovascular fitness. Consequently, elevated muscle strength and power in aged athletes is unsurprising, primarily attributed to hypertrophy of the remaining fibers, while the reduction in fiber quantity is unpreventable through lifelong physical activity. The extent of disparities in physical strength across sexes is extensively documented and may mostly be attributed to variations in muscle size among equally trained men and women, suggesting comparable muscle quality traits for both genders. males possess greater overall muscle mass and power compared to women, and the absolute increases in muscle mass after resistance training are likewise more pronounced in males; however, the relative changes in strength and muscle hypertrophy are comparable across both sexes [155]. A cross-sectional study encompassing a broad age spectrum of men and women shown that females exhibit superior preservation of eccentric peak torque and an enhanced ability to store and utilize elastic energy with aging compared to males [156]. Eccentric actions in hypertrophy-focused resistance training appear to be marginally more effective than concentric actions; nonetheless, both modalities should be incorporated. Skeletal muscles in males are often stronger and more powerful than those in females; yet, male muscles may be more susceptible to fatigue. Muscular strength and power significantly contribute to physical fitness and play an independent function in preventing numerous chronic illnesses and premature mortality [147]. The aging process leads to a reduction in muscle mass and strength of around 1% annually, commencing in the fourth decade of life [148]. Peak instantaneous power diminishes by roughly 7% every decade, as evaluated through vertical leap tests in endurance runners, sprinters, and the general population, with comparable findings noted in ergometric lower extremity power assessments [36,144,149,150]. Muscle wastage varies considerably across individuals due to inherent variances in the aging process, although it can be substantially influenced by physical activity levels and exercise training. The primary characteristics linked to aging are muscle architecture and fiber type composition, tendon qualities, and vascular regulation of contracting muscle. In athletes, the decline in power-lifting performance is more significant and accelerates more swiftly than that of endurance performance; specifically, both men's and women's power-lifting performance begins to diminish by 3% year in the fourth decade and by 1% annually afterward [152]. The immediate and significant effects of resistance training on muscle mass, strength, and power are well-documented in both young and elderly adults, similar to endurance training's impact on cardiovascular fitness. Consequently, elevated muscle strength and power in aged athletes is unsurprising, primarily attributed to hypertrophy of the remaining fibers, while the reduction in fiber quantity is unpreventable through lifelong physical activity. The extent of disparities in physical strength across sexes is extensively documented and may mostly be attributed to variations in muscle size among equally trained men and women, suggesting comparable muscle quality traits for both genders. males possess greater overall muscle mass and power compared to women, and the absolute increases in muscle mass after resistance training are likewise more pronounced in males; however, the relative changes in strength and muscle hypertrophy are comparable across both sexes [155]. A cross-sectional study encompassing a broad age spectrum of men and women shown that females exhibit superior preservation of eccentric peak torque and an enhanced ability to store and utilize elastic energy with aging compared to males [156]. Eccentric actions in hypertrophy-focused resistance training appear to be marginally more effective than concentric actions; nonetheless, both modalities should be incorporated. Skeletal muscles in males are often stronger and more powerful than those in females; yet, male muscles may be more susceptible to fatigue. The observed sex differences are mainly attributed to variations in contractile processes; however, other factors such as muscle perfusion and voluntary activation also play a role (Figure 4) [158].The observed sex differences are mainly attributed to variations in contractile processe Muscular strength and power significantly contribute to physical fitness and play an independent function in preventing numerous chronic illnesses and premature mortality [147]. The aging process leads to a reduction in muscle mass and strength of around 1% annually, commencing in the fourth decade of life [148]. Peak instantaneous power diminishes by roughly 7% every decade, as evaluated through vertical leap tests in endurance runners, sprinters, and the general population, with comparable findings noted in ergometric lower extremity power assessments [36,144,149,150]. Muscle wastage varies considerably across individuals due to inherent variances in the aging process, although it can be substantially influenced by physical activity levels and exercise training. The primary characteristics linked to aging are muscle architecture and fiber type composition, tendon qualities, and vascular regulation of contracting muscle. In athletes, the decline in power-lifting performance is more significant and accelerates more swiftly than that of endurance performance; specifically, both men's and women's power-lifting performance begins to diminish by 3% year in the fourth decade and by 1% annually afterward [152]. The immediate and significant effects of resistance training on muscle mass, strength, and power are well-documented in both young and elderly adults, similar to endurance training's impact on cardiovascular fitness. Consequently, elevated muscle strength and power in aged athletes is unsurprising, primarily attributed to hypertrophy of the remaining fibers, while the reduction in fiber quantity is unpreventable through lifelong physical activity. The extent of disparities in physical strength across sexes is extensively documented and may mostly be attributed to variations in muscle size among equally trained men and women, suggesting comparable muscle quality traits for both genders. males possess greater overall muscle mass and power compared to women, and the absolute increases in muscle mass after resistance training are likewise more pronounced in males; however, the relative changes in strength and muscle hypertrophy are comparable across both sexes [155]. A cross-sectional study encompassing a broad age spectrum of men and women shown that females exhibit superior preservation of eccentric peak torque and an enhanced ability to store and utilize elastic energy with aging compared to males [156]. Eccentric actions in hypertrophy-focused resistance training appear to be marginally more effective than concentric actions; nonetheless, both modalities should be incorporated. Skeletal muscles in males are often stronger and more powerful than those in females; yet, male muscles may be more susceptible to fatigue. The observed sex differences are mainly attributed to variations in contractile processes; however, other factors such as muscle perfusion and voluntary activation also play a role (Figure 4) [158].s; however, other factors such as muscle perfusion and voluntary activation also play a role (Figure 4) [158].

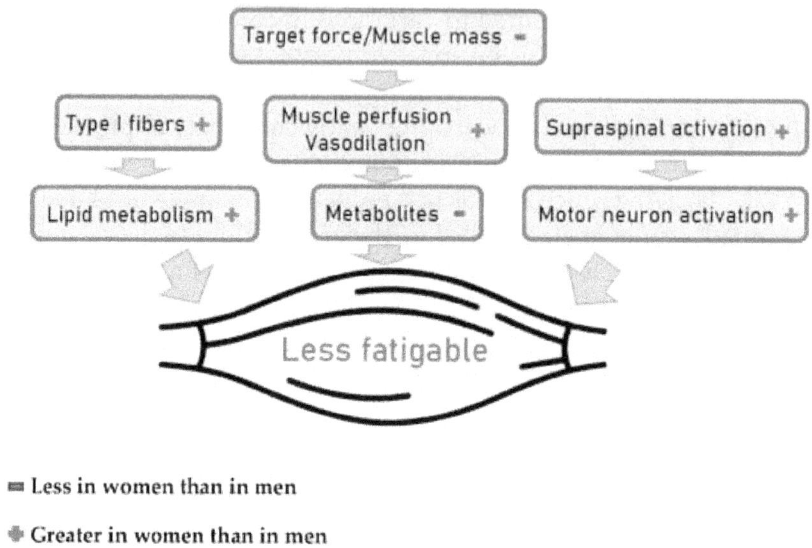


**Figure 4. Mechanisms potentially contributing to the less fatigability of skeletal muscles in females. Modified according to Hunter [158].**

### 3.2.3. Mitochondria

Mitochondria are extremely adaptable organelles that respond dynamically to environmental stimuli, including dietary conditions and physical activity. The increase in mitochondrial mass, facilitated by mitochondrial biogenesis, is governed by several molecules, including the co-transcriptional factor peroxisome-proliferator-activated receptor γ co-activator-1α (PGC-1α). Conversely, mitochondrial mass may be diminished through mitophagy, a mechanism that facilitates the removal of faulty mitochondria and hence enhances mitochondrial quality control. The quantity of mitochondria is additionally governed by mitochondrial dynamics (i.e., fusion and fission) [160], which do not necessarily alter mitochondrial mass. Physical activity enhances mitochondrial biogenesis, turnover, and respiration, while mitochondrial quality correlates positively with physical performance. AMP-activated protein kinase (AMPK) modulates PGC-1α [165] and mitochondrial quality control [166], thereby serving as a crucial regulator of mitochondrial biogenesis by PA. Mitochondrial functions, including ATP synthesis, are impaired in senior age [167]. Aging is correlated with oxidative stress, inflammation, and compromised mitochondrial biogenesis. The latter is partially mediated by diminished AMPK activity with advancing age, an impact that can be significantly mitigated in skeletal muscle by exercise. Although sex dimorphisms of mitochondria have been described, they are still a matter of debate and the functional consequences are not well understood. In aged rat brain a higher mitochondrial mass has been reported in males, while females had more efficient mitochondria with a better redox balance, which was in line with reduced levels of uncoupling proteins (UCP4 and UCP5) that are implicated in oxidative stress reduction [**165**]. This sexual mitochondrial dimorphism may be associated with higher life span and protection from some age-related neurological diseases [**171**]. Similarly, more efficient mitochondria in female rats have been described in the liver [172,173], cardiac muscle [174] and skeletal muscle [175]. A review of sex-related differences in mitochondria by Ventura-Clapier and colleagues [176] provides an overview on several further rodent studies in which mitochondria of female in most tissues appear to be more efficient and less affected by oxidative stress as compared to males [176]. On the other hand, the transcription of mitochondrial biogenesis-related factors has been reported to be tissue-specifically different in mice; with no differences in the liver but higher levels of related RNAs in brain and kidney of male as compared to female mice [177]. In humans, mitochondrial biogenesis could be higher in blood of females than in blood of men [178]. Conversely, ATP production rates in skeletal muscles have been observed to be lower in women than in men in another study [179].

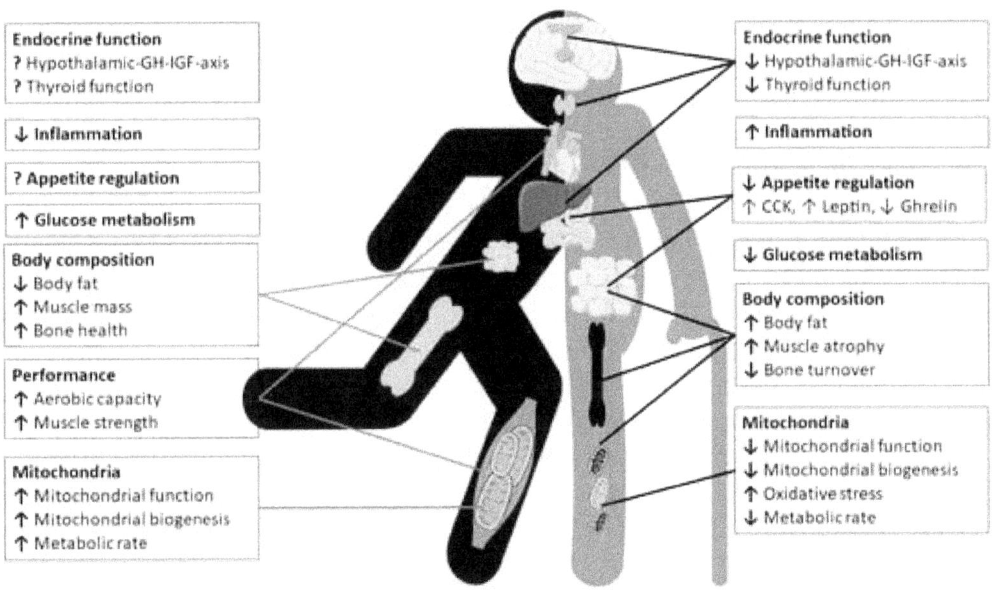


**Figure 5. Pleiotropic effects of physical exercise and nutrition on healthy aging. The right side depicts effects of aging on endocrine function, appetite regulation, glucose metabolism, body composition and mitochondria. The left side illustrates how physical exercise can potentially mitigate effects of aging on the human body of masters athletes. ↑, positive change; ↓, negative change; ?, unknown effect. Cholecystokinine, CCK; growth hormone, GH; insulin-like growth factor, IGF.**

In conclusion, mitochondrial sexual dimorphism seems to differ among cell types, tissues, species, and is influenced by age, health, and physical fitness levels. Comprehensive research is necessary to elucidate sex-related differences in mitochondrial ATP production, reactive oxygen species (ROS) generation, oxidative stress, mitochondrial biogenesis, and their functional implications. The significance of mitochondrial integrity and efficiency for human health is well recognized, and mitochondrial quality and biogenesis can be improved, for instance, by PA, in both genders. Figure 5 illustrates the pleiotropic effects of physical activity and nutrition on the physiology of master's athletes.

## 4. NUTRITIONAL CONSIDERATIONS FOR MASTERS ATHLETES

Masters athletes are often considered as a role model for successful aging and their physical capacities provide useful insight into strategies for healthy aging [**183**]. Although training is the primary stimulus for exercise-induced adaptations, nutrition can have a major impact on the physiological adaptations that result from exercise training and competition. However, nutrition for the older athletes needs to consider the physiological and diet-related challenges associated with aging and exercise (e.g., changing gut function and nutrient requirements with age) that affect training capacity or nutrient absorption. The most important challenges that masters athletes may face to stay competitive is, first, the maintenance of energy balance, including the risk of low energy availability and, second, anabolic resistance, where the synthetic response to muscle contraction and/or protein ingestion is blunted. For example, a protein-energy deficit can quickly lead to a loss of muscle mass, strength and function together with a transient depression of immune function so that exercise performance is compromised [**184**]. Furthermore, changes in body composition and hormones in the andropausal/menopausal transition can influence both muscle and bone. The aging muscle is a significant predictor for falls and fractures. Immobilization of a limb due to injury results in a sudden and dramatic muscle wasting and bone loss in conjunction with an inflammatory response, both of which may have detrimental metabolic and functional consequences. This section therefore highlights nutritional aspects that may support health and physical performance for older athletes. Key nutrition-related concerns include the need for adequate energy and protein intake for preventing low bone and muscle mass and a higher demand for specific nutrients (e.g., vitamin D and probiotics) that may reduce the inflammatory burden in masters athletes. In older adults, gut microbiota composition may represent a marker of health status and probably a predictor of functional decline. With this review, we highlight important research findings on the association between exercise, nutrition and the microbiota, which represents a rapidly developing field in sports nutrition.

### 4.1. Dietary Protein and Energy Requirements

It is well known that a balanced diet that provides enough energy to allow physical exercise is of utmost importance to stay healthy, and this is a yet more crucial factor for athletes with specific dietary needs. In sports nutrition, energy availability is defined as the energy available to promote good health once the energy cost of exercise is deducted from energy intake, relative to an athlete's fat-free mass. Low energy availability (<30 kcal/kg of lean body mass/day) is associated with a number of disorders seen in both female and male athletes, including reduced metabolic rate, hormonal changes (e.g., satiety hormones, reproductive hormones, GH and IGF-1), poor bone health and impairments of muscle protein synthesis, immune health and performance [**185,186**]. Females may have special or different needs due to differences in body size and nutritional status (e.g., energy availability or iron status) as well as due to fluctuations in sex steroid hormones, for example via menopause [**187**]. Furthermore, physiological changes associated with aging per se such as a gradual decrease in lean body mass and subsequently in RMR, loss of appetite, changes in the composition and function of the gut microbiota but also diminished salivary secretion may increase the risk of inadequate energy intake and might require modification of the master athletes' diet [**188**]. Although regular PA may lower the risk of inadequate energy intake and has the potential to maintain muscle mass and RMR with aging [**46,48**], recent findings including athletic populations suggest that masters athletes are still at risk of nutritional deficit [**189**]. In this study in master triathletes, post-exercise energy and protein intakes relative to body mass were significantly lower than the recommended dietary allowance (RDA) for younger athletes, with -40% for energy (22.7 kJ/kg), and -25% for protein (19.6 g), which may affect post-exercise recovery. Furthermore, dietary analysis revealed that female masters athletes in particular consumed significantly less carbohydrates (0.7 g/kg) post-exercise than recommended (1.0 to 1.2 g/kg).

### 4.1.1. Optimizing Post-Exercise Recovery

Carbohydrates provide key substrates for the muscle and central nervous system during rest and exercise. It is still unclear if the recommended carbohydrate intake of 1.2 g/kg/h [**190**] is sufficient for this, or if a surplus could enhance post-exercise muscle glycogen resynthesis and whether female athletes or older individuals are affected differently. Until now, there is no evidence that post-exercise carbohydrate fuelling recommendations differ between ages and sexes. Thus, it is likely that carbohydrate loading strategies act in the same way in masters athletes, provided that they consume at least 8.0 g/kg body mass/day for daily fuel needs and recovery [**190**], additionally 30 to 70 g carbohydrates per hour of exercise—depending on exercise intensity and duration—for immune system recovery after intense exercise boots [**191**].

Proteins are essential nutrients for recovery from exercise. Post-exercise protein ingestion stimulates muscle protein synthesis (MPS), and the balance between synthesis and breakdown of muscle proteins determines recovery and adaptation to the exercise stimulus. Thus, sufficient provision of amino acids is critical to build muscle mass and strength with exercise training, as well as enhancing other adaptations [**192**]. In particular resistance exercise augments the ability of muscle to respond to protein intake. The optimal daily dietary protein intake depends on many factors, including age, sex, body size, habitual energy and nutrient intake as well as habitual exercise and PA. Moreover, acute dietary factors such as the quality of protein, defined by the spectrum of amino acids contained, the amount of protein ingested and the timing of protein ingestion and also the intake of other nutrients can influence the response of muscle to protein intake [**193**]. It is clear that the essential amino acids are critical for optimal stimulation of MPS, but also as signals to stimulate the process. The essential amino acid leucine is of particular interest as it is a powerful signal for stimulation of the mammalian target of rapamycin (mTORC) 1 pathway, which is responsible for the initiation of protein translation and is thus often used as a proxy measure for MPS [**194**]. The recommended protein intake for professional athletes is between 20–25 g of high-quality protein consumed after exercise [**195**], preferably through the ingestion of whole foods [**196**], which are rich in dietary protein, vitamins, minerals, and other macronutrients (e.g., whole milk or eggs). Recent data suggest that this amount may be suboptimal and insufficient for older people [**197**]. Thus, dietary protein recommendations for older adults should be increased (i.e., ≥30 g/meal or ≥1.2 g/kg body mass/day), which contain higher amounts of leucine (i.e., 78.5 mg/kg body mass/day) than current recommendations [**198**], and also considered on a meal-by-meal (every 3–4 h) basis [**199,200**]. Experts even suggested higher protein intakes for masters athletes (35–40 g/meal) to meet a daily target of ~1.5–1.6 g/kg body mass/day to optimize lean mass gains during resistance training [**201**]. Protein intakes in female masters athletes with energy intakes less than 1800 kcal/day are likely to be too low. To preserve lean tissue during periods of energy restriction, protein requirements are greater (i.e., 1.6–2.4 g/kg body mass/day) than during periods of energy balance [**202**]. Vegetarian athletes can increase the muscle anabolic potential by blending animal and plant protein sources [**203**], and vegan athletes should combine various plant-based proteins in a 50/50 ratio to provide a more balanced amino acid profile (e.g., maize/soybean, rice/soybean, rice/pea) or by fortifying plant-based proteins with leucine (3 g/meal) [**204,205**].

#### 4.1.2. Mastering Anabolic Resistance

At old age, the stimulating effects of exercise on MPS become blunted, which is referred to as anabolic resistance [**206**]. It was also recently demonstrated that masters triathletes aged >50 years display lower MPS rates following a bout of downhill running than younger triathletes, suggesting slower acute recovery with aging [**207**]. However, the latter study was not designed to address the impact of chronic exercise training on muscle anabolism with aging. The only study to date to investigate MPS in masters athletes compared to untrained older individuals reported that endurance-trained masters athletes, with an average of ~50 years of continuous training, do not display an elevated capacity to upregulate intramuscular signalling and integrated myofibrillar protein synthesis in response to unaccustomed resistance exercise training [**208**]. This is somewhat surprising, since masters athletes typically display superior physiological function and indices of muscle morphology compared with healthy untrained older individuals (see above, [**209**]). Obviously, lifelong exercise is the best approach to achieve whole-body health, but even starting later on in life will help delay age-related muscle weakness and physical disability.

There is a great interest how modifiable factors, such as diet and PA, can modulate the rate of age-related muscle loss. Stable isotope approaches revealed that the older muscle displays a reduced responsiveness to anabolic properties of amino acid feeding [**210,211**]. Older women in particular exhibit a blunted MPS response to feeding [**206**]. This anabolic resistance is now widely believed to be a key factor responsible for age-related muscle loss [**212**]. However, performing exercise in close temporal proximity to protein ingestion, and increasing the amount of protein ingested per meal (see above) can—at least to some extent—overcome anabolic resistance [**213,214**]. In support of this, cross sectional data show that senior athletes who consume protein modestly above the RDA experience higher muscle strength and quality than those consuming the RDA [**215**]. Moreover, supplementing with a daily dose of ~3.5 g omega-3 fatty acids has been shown to stimulate MPS and may improve muscle mass and function in healthy older adults [**216,217**].

## 4.2. Bone Health and Injury Recovery

In addition to its mechanical susceptibility, bone is also a nutritionally modulated tissue and nutritional inadequacies are a risk factor for low bone mass in athletic individuals [**218**]. What is less clear is the influence of feeding practices on the bone response to intense exercise and training, and the current knowledge is well covered in the recent review by Sale et al. [**219**]. Evidence suggests that an energy availability >30 kcal/kg of lean body mass/day minimize negative effects on the bone and an energy availability of 45 kcal/kg of lean body mass/day is optimal to support bone health in the athlete [**220**]. This requirement is particular important to prevent the female athlete triad and to thereby prevent fatigue fractures [**107**]. Apart from energy availability, low carbohydrate availability negatively affects the bone, while consuming carbohydrate before, during or after exercise attenuates bone resorption to intense exercise and training in the athlete [**221**]. Masters athletes require protein intakes higher than the RDA (between 1.2 and 1.6 up to 2.2 g/kg body mass/day) through its support for muscle mass and function [**201**], but also via the increase in circulating hormones and growth factors, such as IGF-1, which have an anabolic effect on bone [**222**]. Nevertheless, it seems unlikely that a diet high in animal protein (~2 g/kg) is harmful for bone health, provided that dietary calcium intake is adequate [**223**]. Findings even indicate beneficial effects of animal protein sources on bone strength in older adults with exercise training [**224**]. In addition, diets high in animal protein appear to protect against bone loss during periods of weight loss [**225**]. Fermented dairy products, in particular, exert beneficial effects on bone growth and mineralization, attenuation of bone loss, and reduce fracture risk [**226**]. Perhaps more attention should be paid to increasing fruit and vegetable intake in older athletes, because of their potassium alkali salts that the body metabolizes to bicarbonate [**227,228**], rather than reducing animal protein sources. An important direct or indirect mediator of bone and skeletal health is vitamin D. Vitamin D is mainly obtained through sunlight ultraviolet-B exposure (UVB) of the skin, with a small amount typically coming from the diet. It is now clear that vitamin D has important roles beyond its well-known effects on calcium and bone homeostasis. Vitamin D deficiency and insufficiency are common in athletes [**229**] and associated with a greater risk of low bone mass and bone injuries, such as fatigue fractures [**230**], which appeared to be protected by calcium (2000 mg/day) and vitamin D (800 IU/day) supplementation [**231**]. Higher doses with at least 1500–2000 IU/day vitamin D are required in athletes with insufficient status (circulating 25(OH) D < 40 nmol/L) [**232**].

### 4.2.1. Muscle Disuse Atrophy

Skeletal muscle injuries account for over 40% of all sports-related injuries, with a two times higher risk in male than female athletes [**233**]. Fatigue fractures are the most common bone injuries in athletes (0.7% to 20% of all injuries), especially in women with reduced energy availability [**218**], and often occur during periods of high-volume and high-intensity training that are characterized by excessive and rapid increases in training and competition load [**234**]. Fatigue fractures emerge from prolonged mechanical overuse, so that bone's capacity to repair microdamage through the remodelling process is overwhelmed by the emergence of new bone microdamage sites, which ultimately results in bone material fatigue [**94**]. Thus, the factors that predispose to fatigue fractures include the intensity, frequency and duration of loading exercises, as well as short recovery periods between loading cycles [**235**]. Based on the current epidemiological evidence, the masters athlete's age, per se, does not increase the prevalence and risk of injury within competition [**236**], although little is known about injuries during training, including the incidence of fatigue fractures. It is rather that inadequate energy intake and/or deficits in muscle strength, flexibility or aerobic fitness increases the risk of sustained sports injuries.

Muscle disuse due to prolonged best rest (e.g., hospitalization, recovery from surgery), limb immobilization or reduced PA due to illness result in rapid muscle atrophy (~0.5% of muscle mass per day of immobilization) and deconditioning of muscle tissue [**237,238**]. Furthermore, short-term (5 days) muscle disuse has been demonstrated to lower post-absorptive and post-prandial MPS rates and to induce anabolic resistance to protein ingestion in healthy young adults [**239**]. Thus, muscle disuse represents a unique metabolic and nutritional challenge for the young but even more so for the masters athlete as energy and macronutrient requirements are altered considerably. Although robust data on the consequences of these changing metabolic demands and the efficacy of nutritional interventions in injured athletes are still lacking, models of muscle disuse (i.e., bed-rest, step reduction) have revealed insights into the likelihood for deleterious metabolic adaptations that occur during a short-term reduction in PA with increased sedentary behavior [**2,240,241**]. A recent study in young adults with a habitually active lifestyle (>10,000 steps/day) provided direct evidence of a number of unfavourable adaptations to body composition with loss of lean mass (~0.3 kg) and accretion of abdominal and liver fat, with development of whole-body insulin resistance, after 2 weeks of physical inactivity (>80% step reduction) [**2**]. Older adults with lower baseline lean mass and slower rate of recovery following physical inactivity may be even more prone to these acute periods of muscle disuse when compared to young people [**2,241**].

### 4.2.2. Nutrition for Injury Recovery

While sports nutrition has typically focused on augmenting performance and adaptations, far less attention has been given to nutrition for the injured athlete. Injury, per se, results in significant stress response and increases energy expenditure by 15% to 50%, depending on the type and severity of the injury. During the first stage following an injury, an inflammatory response is initiated accompanied by an increase in catabolic hormones (i.e., cortisol and catecholamines) and a decrease in anabolic hormones (i.e., GH, testosterone), resulting in a catabolic environment that can lead to a sudden and large loss of lean body mass [**242**].

Nutritional strategies have been proposed to help improve recovery from exercise-induced injuries involving immobilization and/or reduced activity [**243,244,245,246,247**]. One of the key considerations during the injury is to ensure that sufficient energy is consumed to prevent excessive muscle disuse atrophy and to support repair, without significantly increasing body fat. Hence, identifying energy needs during injury via indirect calorimetry or estimated using predictive equations is an important first step to maintain the caloric balance. Thereby, total daily energy expenditure can be calculated as: resting metabolic rate x stress factor (bone fracture, minor surgery = 1.2) × activity coefficient (sedentary = 1.2, lightly active = 1.4) [**245**]. Especially in the older athlete, where the muscle could develop anabolic resistance, it is crucial to ensure a higher protein intake for repair. The recommendation is 1.6–2.5 g/kg body mass, evenly spread across the day, every 3–4 h around a rehabilitation session, and before sleep, in amounts of 20–35 g, which contain high amounts of leucine (2.5–3 g), and additionally casein prior to sleep [**246,248,249**]. Other nutrients, such as creatine monohydrate (10 g/day for 2 weeks), fish oil-derived omega-3 fatty acids (4 g/day), and ß-hydroxy-ß-methylbutyrate (3 g/day) have been proposed as beneficial for the treatment of injury [**248**]. However, although dietary-supplement strategies may be useful if caloric intake and appetite is reduced, nutritional considerations to promote injury recovery should be explored in a food first approach, rather than a reliance on supplements [**243**].

## 4.3. Immune Function and Risk of Infection

Age-related declines of both the innate as well as the adaptive immune system contribute to the increased susceptibility of older individuals to acute and chronic infections, autoimmune diseases, and systemic inflammatory diseases. While a lack of PA, decreased muscle mass, and poor nutritional status facilitate immunosenescence (namely, a decline of naïve T cells and the CD4/CD8 T-cell ratio, an increase in memory/effector T-cells and senescent/exhausted T-cells) and inflammaging (characterized by elevated levels of IL-6, TNF-α, and IL-1β), moderate exercise training positively affects the composition of the T cell compartment, the function of various leukocyte subpopulations, and counteracts hallmarks of immunosenescence [**250**]. Thus, maintaining regular PA throughout life helps to maintain function of the immune system during aging, which could play a role in preventing infection. A recent study in masters cyclists aged 55 to 80 years found that compared with inactive older adults, the cyclists showed reduced evidence of a decline in thymic output and inflammaging [**251**]. Masters cyclists showed higher serum levels of the thymo-protective cytokine IL-7 and lower IL-6, which promotes thymic atrophy. In addition, maintaining high levels of aerobic fitness during aging may help prevent the accumulation of senescent T-cells [**252**]. While moderate exercise reduces the risk of illness [**253**], prolonged intense exercise is associated with a transient depression of immune function and can lead to immune impairment in athletes associated with an increased susceptibility to infections (mainly of the upper respiratory tract) [**254**]. There has been much interest in how dietary strategies can improve immunity in athletes. So far, there is limited evidence that the dietary practices of athletes such as low energy or carbohydrate availability suppress immunity. Athletes are recommended to follow a balanced diet to avoid a nutrient deficiencies required for proper immune function [**255**]. A metabolomics approach offered by Nieman and Mitmesser [**191**] highlights the potential impact of high carbohydrate-polyphenol food sources to counter post-exercise inflammation and to enhance oxidative and anti-viral capacity, with reduced upper respiratory illness (URI) rates [**256**]. Another intervention by which the immunomodulatory effects of high-intensity training might be countered is by manipulating dietary protein intake. For example, a reduced incidence of URI was observed in elite cyclists undertaking 2 weeks of high-intensity exercise training while consuming a high protein diet (3 g/kg body mass/day) [**257**]. The authors concluded that it is possible that immune surveillance might be maintained during heavy training by consuming a high protein diet. The new theoretical perspective offered by Walsh et al. [**258**] sharpens the focus on tolerogenic nutritional supplements (e.g., probiotics, vitamin C and vitamin D) shown to reduce the burden of infection in athletes at a non-damaging level. In the present section, we focus on vitamin D and probiotics, with a particular interest in the gut microbiota because of the close relationship between the microbiome and the immune system.

### 4.3.1. Anti-Inflammatory Vitamin D

There has been increasing interest in the benefits of supplementing vitamin D during the winter months as studies demonstrate vitamin D insufficiency (25(OH)D < 50 nmol/L) in more than half of all athletes living at northerly latitudes [**259**]. It is important to avoid vitamin D deficiency (25(OH)D < 30 nmol/L) in order to maintain immunity and prevent URI, particularly in settings where profound vitamin D deficiency is common [**260**]. URI tend to be more prevalent in female endurance athletes when engaging in similarly high training loads than their male counterparts (~11 h/week of moderate-vigorous activity) [**261,262**]. Evidence supports an optimal circulating 25(OH)D of 75 nmol/L to prevent URI in athletes and military personnel and, furthermore, to enhance immune function and to induce anti-inflammatory actions through the induction of regulatory T cells and the inhibition of pro-inflammatory cytokine production [**263**]. Reducing inflammation is a key mechanism that can improve age-related skeletal muscle changes through either direct catabolic effects or indirect mechanisms (e.g., higher GH and IGF-1 concentrations, less anorexia) [**264**]. A recent study in sarcopenic older adults participating in a 12-week controlled resistance training program found a significant beneficial effect of daily supplementation with whey protein (22 g), essential amino acids (including 4 g leucine), and vitamin D (100 IU) compared to placebo, with a gain of 1.7 kg in fat free mass, significant decreases in C-reactive protein concentrations, and significant increases in IGF-I concentrations, accompanied by a reduced risk of malnutrition [**265**]. Although the authors were not able to assess the effects of vitamin D supplementation separately from essential amino acid supplementation, this study suggests that whey protein, essential amino acid and vitamin D supplementation, together with resistance training, can reduce inflammatory markers and improve anabolic markers in sarcopenic elderly. Interestingly, long-term supplementation with calcium-vitamin D fortified milk may negate these benefits because of the concomitant gains in fat mass [**266**]. Despite the decline in vitamin D production with aging, vitamin D sufficiency can be achieved in older athletes by regular sunlight exposure in the summer and daily 1000 IU vitamin D3 supplementation in the winter months [**267**].

### 4.3.2. Gut Microbiota and Probiotics

A healthy, resilient gut microbiota is characterized by its high richness and biodiversity [268]. The intestinal microbiota significantly contributes to several metabolic activities advantageous to the host, including vitamin synthesis and short-chain fatty acid (SCFA) generation, as well as the maturation of the mucosal immune system [269]. Conversely, it has been linked to chronic inflammation due to the dysfunction of the mucosal barrier, hence facilitating the onset of inflammatory, autoimmune, and metabolic illnesses [270]. Reduced bacterial diversity has been noted with advancing age, and growing evidence indicates that the gut microbiota correlates with health condition in the elderly [271]. Diet, especially protein consumption, and physical activity can alter the composition, variety, and metabolic capability of the gut microbiota, potentially serving as an effective method to improve gut and systemic immune function. Exercise-induced alterations in the microbiota, such as enhanced butyrate-regulating bacterial taxa and increased short-chain fatty acid (SCFA) production capacity, are reportedly more pronounced in lean adults compared to their obese counterparts and are predominantly reversed upon cessation of exercise training, indicating a correlation among microbial diversity, body composition, and physical function. Cardiorespiratory fitness (VO2max) has been found to connect with gut microbial diversity and fecal butyrate, a short-chain fatty acid linked to gut health, in healthy young people [275], and with intestinal Bacteroides in healthy elderly women [276]. Consequently, VO2max appears to be an effective indicator of gut microbial diversity and metabolic function in healthy individuals. Recent studies from the American Gut Project indicate that persistent exercise training aids older persons by preserving the integrity of the gut microbiota (microbial composition and function) affected by aging [277]. Recent data demonstrated that masters athletes can be seen as a model of healthy aging also from the perspective of the microbiota [**278**]. Compared to community-dwelling older adults, senior orienteering athletes displayed a more homogeneous composition of gut microbiota, with higher levels of *F. prausnitzii* that is associated with positive health benefits, such as good gastrointestinal health, as well as psychological well-being that is most likely due to changes in the gut–brain axis [**279**]. Conversely, a substantial proportion of endurance athletes report gastrointestinal problems (e.g., abdominal discomfort, diarrhoea) during long-distance runs or competitive events and these symptoms may be related to gut ischaemia-associated leakage of bacterial endotoxins into the circulation [**280**]. Excessive exercise, but also other factors, such as drugs or illness, may be linked with dysbiosis of the gut microbiome, promoting inflammation and a catabolic state that can negatively influence muscle mass and function, particularly during aging [**281**].

Probiotics are live microorganisms that are thought to confer immunomodulation properties on both local and systemic immunity. Probiotics have been found to modify the population of the gut microflora and have been shown to increase some aspects of mucosal and systemic immunity in healthy humans such as altered cytokine production, increased natural killer cell cytotoxic activity, increased secretory immunoglobulin A (IgA) levels, and enhanced resistance to infections [**282**]. On the other hand, probiotics exert important anti-inflammatory 'tolerogenic' effects that may reduce the infection risk of athletes at a harmless level [**258**] and there is now some evidence from a number of studies in support of this [**283,284,285,286,287**].The proposed mechanism behind the protective effects of probiotics against infections in athletes may be attributable to modulation of the gut microbiota (enhanced intestinal barrier function and protection from pathogens) the mucosal immune system (enhanced bioactive metabolite production, such as SCFA and neurotransmitters) and lung macrophage and T lymphocyte functions [**288,289**]. Data from our own study indicate that some of these effects appeared to be connected with alterations in tryptophan metabolism [**287**]. Daily supplementation with a multi-species probiotics ($1 \times 10^{10}$ colony-forming units (CFUs) during 12 weeks of winter training limited exercise-induced drops in tryptophan levels and reduced the incidence of URI. Trained young athletes who developed URI demonstrated higher degradation rates of tryptophan compared to those without URI. A previous study undertaken by well-trained cyclists reported sex differences with probiotic supplementation ($1 \times 10^9$ CFUs of *L. fermentum* PCC®) for 11 weeks with a significant reduction in lower respiratory illness symptoms (duration and severity) in males, but with some evidence of an increase in symptoms in females, while the effects of probiotic supplementation on URI were unclear in males and females [**290**]. Although anti-inflammatory effects of probiotics exist in young athletes, these results cannot be directly extrapolated to masters athletes due to changes in the immune system that occur with ageing. The influence of probiotics on immune function and infection risk in the elderly has been studied only sporadically. The most comprehensive study so far in free-living elderly aged >65 years demonstrated a clear association between probiotic ($3 \times 10^7$ CFUs of *L. delbrueckii* ssp. *bulgaricus* 8481) consumption for 6 months and enhanced systemic immunity in older people [**291**]. Clinical benefits by probiotics are reported from respiratory infection studies where in one study the rate of common cold infections was decreased by dietary intake of yoghurt fermented with *L. delbrueckii* ssp. *bulgaricus* OLL1073R-1 [**292**] and in another study the duration but not the incidence of episodes decreased with *L. casei* DN-114001 [**293**]. Theoretically, combining probiotics with omega-3 fatty acids may offer a promising nutritional strategy to counteract metabolic challenges associated with aging via the gut microbiota, especially relevant for older people that suffer from anabolic resistance, systemic inflammation, and mood disorders (through the gut–brain axis) [279,294,295]. However, more research is required to understand the connection between exercise, nutrition and the gut microbiota in the elderly population in general and in master athletes in particular.

## 5. CONCISE SUMMARY

In summary, physiological and diet-related challenges that occur with the aging process can be positively influenced by chronic exercise training and appropriate nutrition. Even though limited evidence exists on nutritional requirements for masters athletes, based on the analysis of current nutrition guidelines for young athletes and older non-athletic populations, recommendations can be suggested for older athletes (**Figure 6**). Particular attention should be given to proper energy and protein intake for preventing low bone and muscle mass and optimizing post-exercise recovery. Furthermore, a higher demand for specific nutrients (e.g., vitamin D, probiotics omega-3 fatty acids) should be considered in older athletes to improve both mucosal and systemic immunity, enhance resistance towards inflammatory and metabolic diseases (including infections), and, last but not least, to preserve psychological well-being, which itself can help boost the masters athletes' immune system.

Despite our recommended nutritional guidelines for senior athletes, numerous inquiries regarding the nutritional needs of masters athletes remain unresolved. What are the training and dietary practices of senior athletes, and what is their knowledge and application of nutrition? What is the significance of nutrition in reducing fracture risk and facilitating the healing process post-fracture? Moreover, additional research is necessary to elucidate the immunological advantages of tolerogenic foods in older athletes. Research on the effects of exercise adaptations on gut microbiota and the influence of nutritional variables, such as caloric restriction or increased protein intake, in older athletes is sparse. Consequently, further longitudinal research should investigate the optimal diet and specific nutrients conducive to the athletic lifespan, thereby enhancing support for masters athletes.

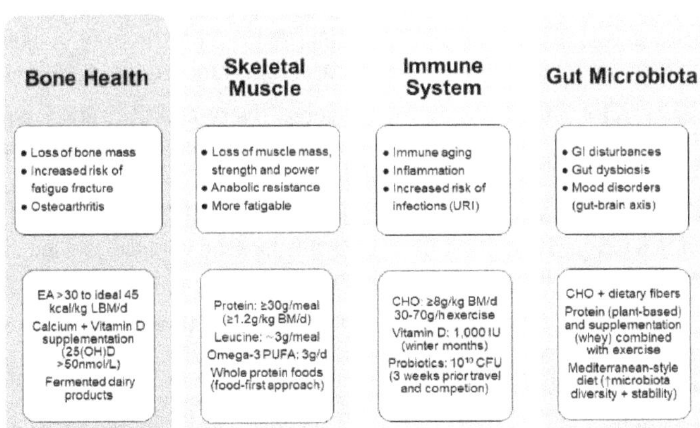


**Figure 6. Overview of physiological and diet-related challenges associated with aging and nutritional strategies to assist masters athletes to stay healthy, optimize adaptation and post-exercise recovery. Body mass, BM; colony-forming units, CFU; carbohydrates, CHO; energy availability, EA; gastrointestinal, GI; international units, IU; lean body mass, LBM; polyunsaturated fatty acids, PUFA; upper respiratory illness, URI.**

## REFERENCES


1. Breen, L.; Stokes, K.A.; Churchward-Venne, T.A.; Moore, D.R.; Baker, S.K.; Smith, K.; Atherton, P.J.; Phillips, S.M. Two weeks of reduced activity decreases leg lean mass and induces "anabolic resistance" of myofibrillar protein synthesis in healthy elderly. *J. Clin. Endocrinol. Metab.* **2013**, *98*, 2604–2612. **[Google Scholar] [PubMed] [Green Version]**

2. Bowden Davies, K.A.; Sprung, V.S.; Norman, J.A.; Thompson, A.; Mitchell, K.L.; Halford, J.C.G.; Harrold, J.A.; Wilding, J.P.H.; Kemp, G.J.; Cuthbertson, D.J. Short-term decreased physical activity with increased sedentary behaviour causes metabolic derangements and altered body composition: Effects in individuals with and without a first-degree relative with type 2 diabetes. *Diabetologia* **2018**, *61*, 1282–1294. **[Google Scholar] [PubMed] [Green Version]**

3. Yamada, Y.; Buehring, B.; Krueger, D.; Anderson, R.M.; Schoeller, D.A.; Binkley, N. Electrical Properties Assessed by Bioelectrical Impedance Spectroscopy as Biomarkers of Age-related Loss of Skeletal Muscle Quantity and Quality. *J. Gerontol. Ser. A Biol. Sci. Med. Sci.* **2017**, *72*, 1180–1186. **[Google Scholar] [PubMed] [Green Version]**

4. Furman, D.; Campisi, J.; Verdin, E.; Carrera-Bastos, P.; Targ, S.; Franceschi, C.; Ferrucci, L.; Gilroy, D.W.; Fasano, A.; Miller, G.W.; et al. Chronic inflammation in the etiology of disease across the life span. *Nat. Med.* **2019**, *25*, 1822–1832. **[Google Scholar]**

5. Pedersen, B.K.; Saltin, B. Exercise as medicine-evidence for prescribing exercise as therapy in 26 different chronic diseases. *Scand J. Med. Sci. Sports* **2015**, *25* (Suppl. 3), 1–72. **[Google Scholar] [PubMed] [Green Version]**

6. Booth, F.W.; Roberts, C.K.; Thyfault, J.P.; Ruegsegger, G.N.; Toedebusch, R.G. Role of Inactivity in Chronic Diseases: Evolutionary Insight and Pathophysiological Mechanisms. *Physiol. Rev.* **2017**, *97*, 1351–1402. **[Google Scholar] [PubMed]**

7. Health effects of dietary risks in 195 countries, 1990-2017: A systematic analysis for the Global Burden of Disease Study 2017. *Lancet* **2019**, *393*, 1958–1972. **[Green Version]**

8. World Health Organization. *Physical Activity for Health. Report to the Director-General. WHO Executive Board, 142nd Session*; World Health Organization: Geneva, Switzerland, 2018. **[Google Scholar]**

9. Valenzuela, P.L.; Maffiuletti, N.A.; Joyner, M.J.; Lucia, A.; Lepers, R. Lifelong Endurance Exercise as a Countermeasure Against Age-Related [Formula: See text] Decline: Physiological Overview and Insights from Masters Athletes. *Sports Med.* **2020**, *50*, 703–716. **[Google Scholar]**

10. Burtscher, M. Exercise limitations by the oxygen delivery and utilization systems in aging and disease: Coordinated adaptation and deadaptation of the lung-heart muscle axis-a mini-review. *Gerontology* **2013**, *59*, 289–296. **[Google Scholar]**

11. Habedank, D.; Reindl, I.; Vietzke, G.; Bauer, U.; Sperfeld, A.; Gläser, S.; Wernecke, K.D.; Kleber, F.X. Ventilatory efficiency and exercise tolerance in 101 healthy volunteers. *Eur. J. Appl. Physiol. Occup. Physiol.* **1998**, *77*, 421–426. **[Google Scholar] [PubMed]**

12. McClaran, S.R.; Babcock, M.A.; Pegelow, D.F.; Reddan, W.G.; Dempsey, J.A. Longitudinal effects of aging on lung function at rest and exercise in healthy active fit elderly adults. *J. Appl. Physiol.* **1995**, *78*, 1957–1968. **[Google Scholar]**

13. Lavin, K.M.; Straub, A.M.; Uhranowsky, K.A.; Smoliga, J.M.; Zavorsky, G.S. Alveolar-membrane diffusing capacity limits performance in Boston marathon qualifiers. *PLoS ONE* **2012**, *7*, e44513. **[Google Scholar] [PubMed] [Green Version]**

14. Amann, M. Pulmonary system limitations to endurance exercise performance in humans. *Exp. Physiol.* **2012**, *97*, 311–318. **[Google Scholar] [Green Version]**

15. Taylor, B.J.; Johnson, B.D. The pulmonary circulation and exercise responses in the elderly. *Semin. Respir. Crit. Care Med.* **2010**, *31*, 528–538. **[Google Scholar] [Green Version]**

16. Burtscher, M.; Schocke, M.; Koch, R. Ventilation-limited exercise capacity in a 59-year-old athlete. *Respir. Physiol. Neurobiol.* **2011**, *175*, 181–184. **[Google Scholar]**

17. Degens, H.; Maden-Wilkinson, T.M.; Ireland, A.; Korhonen, M.T.; Suominen, H.; Heinonen, A.; Radak, Z.; McPhee, J.S.; Rittweger, J. Relationship between ventilatory function and age in master athletes and a sedentary reference population. *Age* **2013**, *35*, 1007–1015. **[Google Scholar] [Green Version]**

18. Ogawa, T.; Spina, R.J.; Martin, W.H.; Kohrt, W.M.; Schechtman, K.B.; Holloszy, J.O.; Ehsani, A.A. Effects of aging, sex, and physical training on cardiovascular responses to exercise. *Circulation* **1992**, *86*, 494–503. **[Google Scholar] [Green Version]**

19. Di Prampero, P.E. Factors limiting maximal performance in humans. *Eur. J. Appl. Physiol.* **2003**, *90*, 420–429. **[Google Scholar] [PubMed]**

20. Tanaka, H.; Monahan, K.D.; Seals, D.R. Age-predicted maximal heart rate revisited. *J. Am. Coll. Cardiol.* **2001**, *37*, 153–156. **[Google Scholar] [Green Version]**

21. Arbab-Zadeh, A.; Dijk, E.; Prasad, A.; Fu, Q.; Torres, P.; Zhang, R.; Thomas, J.D.; Palmer, D.; Levine, B.D. Effect of aging and physical activity on left ventricular compliance. *Circulation* **2004**, *110*, 1799–1805. **[Google Scholar] [PubMed] [Green Version]**

22. Mortensen, S.P.; Nyberg, M.; Gliemann, L.; Thaning, P.; Saltin, B.; Hellsten, Y. Exercise training modulates functional sympatholysis and α-adrenergic vasoconstrictor responsiveness in hypertensive and normotensive individuals. *J. Physiol.* **2014**, *592*, 3063–3073. **[Google Scholar] [PubMed]**

23. Groen, B.B.; Hamer, H.M.; Snijders, T.; van Kranenburg, J.; Frijns, D.; Vink, H.; van Loon, L.J. Skeletal muscle capillary density and microvascular function are compromised with aging and type 2 diabetes. *J. Appl. Physiol.* **2014**, *116*, 998–1005. **[Google Scholar] [PubMed] [Green Version]**

24. Bori, Z.; Zhao, Z.; Koltai, E.; Fatouros, I.G.; Jamurtas, A.Z.; Douroudos, I.I.; Terzis, G.; Chatzinikolaou, A.; Sovatzidis, A.; Draganidis, D.; et al. The effects of aging, physical training, and a single bout of exercise on mitochondrial protein expression in human skeletal muscle. *Exp. Gerontol.* **2012**, *47*, 417–424. **[Google Scholar] [Green Version]**

25. Iversen, N.; Krustrup, P.; Rasmussen, H.N.; Rasmussen, U.F.; Saltin, B.; Pilegaard, H. Mitochondrial biogenesis and angiogenesis in skeletal muscle of the elderly. *Exp. Gerontol.* **2011**, *46*, 670–678. **[Google Scholar] [Green Version]**

26. Saltin, B. Hemodynamic adaptations to exercise. *Am. J. Cardiol.* **1985**, *55*, 42D–47D. **[Google Scholar]**

27. Stathokostas, L.; Jacob-Johnson, S.; Petrella, R.J.; Paterson, D.H. Longitudinal changes in aerobic power in older men and women. *J. Appl. Physiol.* **2004**, *97*, 781–789. **[Google Scholar] [PubMed]**

28. Burtscher, M.; Forster, H.; Burtscher, J. Superior endurance performance in aging mountain runners. *Gerontology* **2008**, *54*, 268–271. **[Google Scholar]**

29. Lucía, A.; Hoyos, J.; Pérez, M.; Santalla, A.; Chicharro, J.L. Inverse relationship between VO2max and economy/efficiency in world-class cyclists. *Med. Sci. Sports Exerc.* **2002**, *34*, 2079–2084. **[Google Scholar]**

30. Shafiee, G.; Keshtkar, A.; Soltani, A.; Ahadi, Z.; Larijani, B.; Heshmat, R. Prevalence of sarcopenia in the world: A systematic review and meta- analysis of general population studies. *J. Diabetes Metab. Disord.* **2017**, *16*, 21. **[Google Scholar] [PubMed] [Green Version]**

31. Cruz-Jentoft, A.J.; Baeyens, J.P.; Bauer, J.M.; Boirie, Y.; Cederholm, T.; Landi, F.; Martin, F.C.; Michel, J.-P.; Rolland, Y.; Schneider, S.M.; et al. Sarcopenia: European consensus on definition and diagnosis: Report of the European Working Group on Sarcopenia in Older People. *Age Ageing* **2010**, *39*, 412–423. **[Google Scholar] [PubMed] [Green Version]**

32. Fien, S.; Climstein, M.; Quilter, C.; Buckley, G.; Henwood, T.; Grigg, J.; Keogh, J.W.L. Anthropometric, physical function and general health markers of Masters athletes: A cross-sectional study. *PeerJ* **2017**, *5*, e3768. **[Google Scholar] [Green Version]**

33. Wroblewski, A.P.; Amati, F.; Smiley, M.A.; Goodpaster, B.; Wright, V. Chronic exercise preserves lean muscle mass in masters athletes. *Phys. Sportsmed* **2011**, *39*, 172–178. **[Google Scholar]** **[PubMed]** **[Green Version]**

34. Milanović, Z.; Pantelić, S.; Trajković, N.; Sporiš, G.; Kostić, R.; James, N. Age-related decrease in physical activity and functional fitness among elderly men and women. *Clin. Interv. Aging* **2013**, *8*, 549–556. **[Google Scholar]** **[PubMed]** **[Green Version]**

35. Jones, P.R.; Pearson, J. Anthropometric determination of leg fat and muscle plus bone volumes in young male and female adults. *J. Physiol.* **1969**, *204*, 63p–66p. **[Google Scholar]**

36. Grassi, B.; Cerretelli, P.; Narici, M.V.; Marconi, C. Peak anaerobic power in master athletes. *Eur. J. Appl. Physiol. Occup. Physiol.* **1991**, *62*, 394–399. **[Google Scholar]** **[PubMed]**

37. Pearson, S.J.; Young, A.; Macaluso, A.; Devito, G.; Nimmo, M.A.; Cobbold, M.; Harridge, S.D. Muscle function in elite master weightlifters. *Med. Sci. Sports Exerc.* **2002**, *34*, 1199–1206. **[Google Scholar]**

38. Ireland, A.; Mittag, U.; Degens, H.; Felsenberg, D.; Ferretti, J.L.; Heinonen, A.; Koltai, E.; Korhonen, M.T.; McPhee, J.S.; Mekjavic, I.; et al. Greater maintenance of bone mineral content in male than female athletes and in sprinting and jumping than endurance athletes: A longitudinal study of bone strength in elite masters athletes. *Arch. Osteoporos.* **2020**, *15*, 87. **[Google Scholar]**

39. Alvero Cruz, J.R.; Brikis, M.; Chilibeck, P.; Frings-Meuthen, P.; Vico Guzmán, J.; Mittag, U.; Michely, S.; Mulder, E.; Tanaka, H.; Tank, J.; et al. Age-Related Decline in Vertical Jumping Performance in Masters Track and Field Athletes: Concomitant Influence of Body Composition. *Front. Physiol.* **2021**, in press. **[Google Scholar]**

40. Piasecki, J.; Ireland, A.; Piasecki, M.; Deere, K.; Hannam, K.; Tobias, J.; McPhee, J.S. Comparison of Muscle Function, Bone Mineral Density and Body Composition of Early Starting and Later Starting Older Masters Athletes. *Front. Physiol.* **2019**, *10*, 1050. **[Google Scholar]**

41. Hughes, V.A.; Frontera, W.R.; Roubenoff, R.; Evans, W.J.; Singh, M.A.F. Longitudinal changes in body composition in older men and women: Role of body weight change and physical activity. *Am. J. Clin. Nutr.* **2002**, *76*, 473–481. **[Google Scholar]**

42. Dubé, J.J.; Broskey, N.T.; Despines, A.A.; Stefanovic-Racic, M.; Toledo, F.G.S.; Goodpaster, B.H.; Amati, F. Muscle Characteristics and Substrate Energetics in Lifelong Endurance Athletes. *Med. Sci. Sports Exerc.* **2016**, *48*, 472–480. **[Google Scholar]** **[PubMed]** **[Green Version]**

43. Piers, L.S.; Soares, M.J.; McCormack, L.M.; O'Dea, K. Is there evidence for an age-related reduction in metabolic rate? *J. Appl. Physiol.* **1998**, *85*, 2196–2204. **[Google Scholar]**

44. Krems, C.; Lührmann, P.M.; Straßburg, A.; Hartmann, B.; Neuhäuser-Berthold, M. Lower resting metabolic rate in the elderly may not be entirely due to changes in body composition. *Eur. J. Clin. Nutr.* **2005**, *59*, 255–262. **[Google Scholar]** **[PubMed]**

45. Frings-Meuthen, P.; Henkel, S.; Boschmann, M.; Chilibeck, P.D.; Alvero Cruz, J.R.; Hoffmann, F.; Möstl, S.; Mittag, U.; Mulder, E.; Rittweger, N.; et al. Resting Energy Expenditure of Master Athletes: Accuracy of Predictive Equations and Primary Determinants. *Front. Physiol.* **2021**, *12*, 641455. **[Google Scholar]** **[PubMed]**

46. Van Pelt, R.E.; Dinneno, F.A.; Seals, D.R.; Jones, P.P. Age-related decline in RMR in physically active men: Relation to exercise volume and energy intake. *Am. J. Physiol. Endocrinol. Metab.* **2001**, *281*, E633–E639. **[Google Scholar]**

47. Sullo, A.; Cardinale, P.; Brizzi, G.; Fabbri, B.; Maffulli, N. Resting metabolic rate and post-prandial thermogenesis by level of aerobic power in older athletes. *Clin. Exp. Pharmacol. Physiol.* **2004**, *31*, 202–206. **[Google Scholar]** **[PubMed]**

48. Van Pelt, R.E.; Jones, P.P.; Davy, K.P.; DeSouza, C.A.; Tanaka, H.; Davy, B.M.; Seals, D.R. Regular Exercise and the Age-Related Decline in Resting Metabolic Rate in Women*. *J. Clin. Endocrinol. Metab.* **1997**, *82*, 3208–3212. **[Google Scholar]**

49. Kim, B. Thyroid hormone as a determinant of energy expenditure and the basal metabolic rate. *Thyroid Off. J. Am. Thyroid Assoc.* **2008**, *18*, 141–144. **[Google Scholar]**

50. Cooper, D.S.; Biondi, B. Subclinical thyroid disease. *Lancet* **2012**, *379*, 1142–1154. **[Google Scholar]**

51. Bremner, A.P.; Feddema, P.; Leedman, P.J.; Brown, S.J.; Beilby, J.P.; Lim, E.M.; Wilson, S.G.; O'Leary, P.C.; Walsh, J.P. Age-related changes in thyroid function: A longitudinal study of a community-based cohort. *J. Clin. Endocrinol. Metab.* **2012**, *97*, 1554–1562. **[Google Scholar] [Green Version]**

52. Waring, A.C.; Arnold, A.M.; Newman, A.B.; Bùzková, P.; Hirsch, C.; Cappola, A.R. Longitudinal changes in thyroid function in the oldest old and survival: The cardiovascular health study all-stars study. *J. Clin. Endocrinol. Metab.* **2012**, *97*, 3944–3950. **[Google Scholar] [PubMed] [Green Version]**

53. Mariotti, S.; Barbesino, G.; Caturegli, P.; Bartalena, L.; Sansoni, P.; Fagnoni, F.; Monti, D.; Fagiolo, U.; Franceschi, C.; Pinchera, A. Complex alteration of thyroid function in healthy centenarians. *J. Clin. Endocrinol. Metab.* **1993**, *77*, 1130–1134. **[Google Scholar]**

54. Suzuki, S.; Nishio, S.-I.; Takeda, T.; Komatsu, M. Gender-specific regulation of response to thyroid hormone in aging. *Thyroid Res.* **2012**, *5*, 1. **[Google Scholar] [Green Version]**

55. Meunier, N.; Beattie, J.H.; Ciarapica, D.; O'Connor, J.M.; Andriollo-Sanchez, M.; Taras, A.; Coudray, C.; Polito, A. Basal metabolic rate and thyroid hormones of late-middle-aged and older human subjects: The ZENITH study. *Eur. J. Clin. Nutr.* **2005**, *59* (Suppl. 2), S53–S57. **[Google Scholar] [PubMed] [Green Version]**

56. Le Roith, D.; Butler, A.A. Insulin-like growth factors in pediatric health and disease. *J. Clin. Endocrinol. Metab.* **1999**, *84*, 4355–4361. **[Google Scholar]**

57. Ghigo, E.; Arvat, E.; Gianotti, L.; Lanfranco, F.; Broglio, F.; Aimaretti, G.; Maccario, M.; Camanni, F. Hypothalamic growth hormone-insulin-like growth factor-I axis across the human life span. *J. Pediatric Endocrinol. Metab.* **2000**, *13* (Suppl. 6), 1493–1502. **[Google Scholar]**

58. Gilbert, K.L.; Stokes, K.A.; Hall, G.M.; Thompson, D. Growth hormone responses to 3 different exercise bouts in 18- to 25- and 40- to 50-year-old men. *Appl. Physiol. Nutr. Metab.* **2008**, 33, 706–712. **[Google Scholar]**

59. Craig, B.W.; Brown, R.; Everhart, J. Effects of progressive resistance training on growth hormone and testosterone levels in young and elderly subjects. *Mech. Ageing Dev.* **1989**, *49*, 159–169. **[Google Scholar]**

60. Hameed, M.; Orrell, R.W.; Cobbold, M.; Goldspink, G.; Harridge, S.D. Expression of IGF-I splice variants in young and old human skeletal muscle after high resistance exercise. *J. Physiol.* **2003**, *547*, 247–254. **[Google Scholar]**

61. Hameed, M.; Lange, K.H.; Andersen, J.L.; Schjerling, P.; Kjaer, M.; Harridge, S.D.; Goldspink, G. The effect of recombinant human growth hormone and resistance training on IGF-I mRNA expression in the muscles of elderly men. *J. Physiol.* **2004**, *555*, 231–240. **[Google Scholar] [PubMed] [Green Version]**

62. Cruz-Jentoft, A.J.; Kiesswetter, E.; Drey, M.; Sieber, C.C. Nutrition, frailty, and sarcopenia. *Aging Clin. Exp. Res.* **2017**, *29*, 43–48. **[Google Scholar]**

63. MacIntosh, C.G.; Andrews, J.M.; Jones, K.L.; Wishart, J.M.; Morris, H.A.; Jansen, J.B.; Morley, J.E.; Horowitz, M.; Chapman, I.M. Effects of age on concentrations of plasma cholecystokinin, glucagon-like peptide 1, and peptide YY and their relation to appetite and pyloric motility. *Am. J. Clin. Nutr.* **1999**, *69*, 999–1006. **[Google Scholar]**

64. Giezenaar, C.; Hutchison, A.T.; Luscombe-Marsh, N.D.; Chapman, I.; Horowitz, M.; Soenen, S. Effect of Age on Blood Glucose and Plasma Insulin, Glucagon, Ghrelin, CCK, GIP, and GLP-1 Responses to Whey Protein Ingestion. *Nutrients* **2017**, *10*, 2. **[Google Scholar] [Green Version]**

65. Chapman, I.M. Endocrinology of anorexia of ageing. *Best Pract. Res. Clin. Endocrinol. Metab.* **2004**, *18*, 437–452. **[Google Scholar]**

66. Johnson, K.O.; Shannon, O.M.; Matu, J.; Holliday, A.; Ispoglou, T.; Deighton, K. Differences in circulating appetite-related hormone concentrations between younger and older adults: A systematic review and meta-analysis. *Aging Clin. Exp. Res.* **2020**, *32*, 1233–1244. **[Google Scholar]** **[Green Version]**

67. Zhang, Y.; Scarpace, P.J. The role of leptin in leptin resistance and obesity. *Physiol. Behav.* **2006**, *88*, 249–256. **[Google Scholar]**

68. Nicholson, E.; Allison, D.J.; Bullock, A.; Heisz, J.J. Examining the obesity paradox: A moderating effect of fitness on adipose endocrine function in older adults. *Mech. Ageing Dev.* **2020**, *193*, 111406. **[Google Scholar]** **[PubMed]**

69. Gregersen, N.T.; Møller, B.K.; Raben, A.; Kristensen, S.T.; Holm, L.; Flint, A.; Astrup, A. Determinants of appetite ratings: The role of age, gender, BMI, physical activity, smoking habits, and diet/weight concern. *Food Nutr. Res.* **2011**, 55. **[Google Scholar]** **[Green Version]**

70. Dorling, J.; Broom, D.R.; Burns, S.F.; Clayton, D.J.; Deighton, K.; James, L.J.; King, J.A.; Miyashita, M.; Thackray, A.E.; Batterham, R.L.; et al. Acute and Chronic Effects of Exercise on Appetite, Energy Intake, and Appetite-Related Hormones: The Modulating Effect of Adiposity, Sex, and Habitual Physical Activity. *Nutrients* **2018**, *10*, 1140. **[Google Scholar]** **[PubMed]** **[Green Version]**

71. Reaven, G.M.; Chen, N.; Hollenbeck, C.; Chen, Y.D. Effect of age on glucose tolerance and glucose uptake in healthy individuals. *J. Am. Geriatr. Soc.* **1989**, *37*, 735–740. **[Google Scholar]** **[PubMed]**

72. Van den Beld, A.W.; Kaufman, J.M.; Zillikens, M.C.; Lamberts, S.W.J.; Egan, J.M.; van der Lely, A.J. The physiology of endocrine systems with ageing. *Lancet Diabetes Endocrinol.* **2018**, *6*, 647–658. **[Google Scholar]** **[Green Version]**

73. Kullmann, S.; Heni, M.; Hallschmid, M.; Fritsche, A.; Preissl, H.; Häring, H.U. Brain Insulin Resistance at the Crossroads of Metabolic and Cognitive Disorders in Humans. *Physiol. Rev.* **2016**, *96*, 1169–1209. **[Google Scholar]** **[PubMed]** **[Green Version]**

74. Kullmann, S.; Valenta, V.; Wagner, R.; Tschritter, O.; Machann, J.; Häring, H.-U.; Preissl, H.; Fritsche, A.; Heni, M. Brain insulin sensitivity is linked to adiposity and body fat distribution. *Nat. Commun.* **2020**, *11*, 1841. **[Google Scholar]** **[Green Version]**

75. Meneilly, G.S.; Veldhuis, J.D.; Elahi, D. Disruption of the pulsatile and entropic modes of insulin release during an unvarying glucose stimulus in elderly individuals. *J. Clin. Endocrinol. Metab.* **1999**, *84*, 1938–1943. **[Google Scholar]**

76. Basu, R.; Dalla Man, C.; Campioni, M.; Basu, A.; Klee, G.; Toffolo, G.; Cobelli, C.; Rizza, R.A. Effects of age and sex on postprandial glucose metabolism: Differences in glucose turnover, insulin secretion, insulin action, and hepatic insulin extraction. *Diabetes* **2006**, *55*, 2001–2014. **[Google Scholar]** **[PubMed]** **[Green Version]**

77. Elahi, D.; Muller, D.C.; Tzankoff, S.P.; Andres, R.; Tobin, J.D. Effect of age and obesity on fasting levels of glucose, insulin, glucagon, and growth hormone in man. *J. Gerontol.* **1982**, *37*, 385–391. **[Google Scholar]**

78. Simonson, D.C.; DeFronzo, R.A. Glucagon physiology and aging: Evidence for enhanced hepatic sensitivity. *Diabetologia* **1983**, *25*, 1–7. **[Google Scholar]** **[PubMed]** **[Green Version]**

79. Seals, D.R.; Hagberg, J.M.; Allen, W.K.; Hurley, B.F.; Dalsky, G.P.; Ehsani, A.A.; Holloszy, J.O. Glucose tolerance in young and older athletes and sedentary men. *J. Appl. Physiol. Respir. Environ. Exerc. Physiol.* **1984**, *56*, 1521–1525. **[Google Scholar]**

80. Amati, F.; Dubé, J.J.; Coen, P.M.; Stefanovic-Racic, M.; Toledo, F.G.S.; Goodpaster, B.H. Physical inactivity and obesity underlie the insulin resistance of aging. *Diabetes Care* **2009**, *32*, 1547–1549. **[Google Scholar]** **[Green Version]**

81. Roden, M.; Shulman, G.I. The integrative biology of type 2 diabetes. *Nature* **2019**, *576*, 51–60. **[Google Scholar] [PubMed] [Green Version]**

82. Petersen, K.F.; Morino, K.; Alves, T.C.; Kibbey, R.G.; Dufour, S.; Sono, S.; Yoo, P.S.; Cline, G.W.; Shulman, G.I. Effect of aging on muscle mitochondrial substrate utilization in humans. *Proc. Natl. Acad. Sci. USA* **2015**, *112*, 11330–11334. **[Google Scholar] [Green Version]**

83. Consitt, L.A.; Van Meter, J.; Newton, C.A.; Collier, D.N.; Dar, M.S.; Wojtaszewski, J.F.; Treebak, J.T.; Tanner, C.J.; Houmard, J.A. Impairments in site-specific AS160 phosphorylation and effects of exercise training. *Diabetes* **2013**, *62*, 3437–3447. **[Google Scholar] [Green Version]**

84. Conley, K.E.; Jubrias, S.A.; Esselman, P.C. Oxidative capacity and ageing in human muscle. *J. Physiol.* **2000**, *526 Pt 1*, 203–210. **[Google Scholar]**

85. Gianni, P.; Jan, K.J.; Douglas, M.J.; Stuart, P.M.; Tarnopolsky, M.A. Oxidative stress and the mitochondrial theory of aging in human skeletal muscle. *Exp. Gerontol.* **2004**, *39*, 1391–1400. **[Google Scholar]**

86. Sharma, A.; Smith, H.J.; Yao, P.; Mair, W.B. Causal roles of mitochondrial dynamics in longevity and healthy aging. *Embo. Rep.* **2019**, *20*, e48395. **[Google Scholar]**

87. Krssak, M.; Falk Petersen, K.; Dresner, A.; DiPietro, L.; Vogel, S.M.; Rothman, D.L.; Roden, M.; Shulman, G.I. Intramyocellular lipid concentrations are correlated with insulin sensitivity in humans: A 1H NMR spectroscopy study. *Diabetologia* **1999**, *42*, 113–116. **[Google Scholar] [PubMed] [Green Version]**

88. Henriksen, K.; Neutzsky-Wulff, A.V.; Bonewald, L.F.; Karsdal, M.A. Local communication on and within bone controls bone remodeling. *Bone* **2009**, *44*, 1026–1033. **[Google Scholar] [PubMed]**

89. Bonewald, L.F. The amazing osteocyte. *J. Bone Miner. Res. Off. J. Am. Soc. Bone Miner. Res.* **2011**, *26*, 229–238. **[Google Scholar] [PubMed]**

90. Robling, A.G.; Niziolek, P.J.; Baldridge, L.A.; Condon, K.W.; Allen, M.R.; Alam, I.; Mantila, S.M.; Gluhak-Heinrich, J.; Bellido, T.M.; Harris, S.E.; et al. Mechanical stimulation of bone in vivo reduces osteocyte expression of Sost/sclerostin. *J. Biol. Chem.* **2008**, *283*, 5866–5875. **[Google Scholar] [Green Version]**

91. Mundy, G.R. The effects of TGF-beta on bone. *Ciba Found. Symp.* **1991**, *157*, 137–143, discussion 143–151. **[Google Scholar]**

92. Matsuo, K.; Irie, N. Osteoclast-osteoblast communication. *Arch. Biochem. Biophys.* **2008**, *473*, 201–209. **[Google Scholar] [PubMed]**

93. Ott, S.M. Chapter 19-Histomorphometric Analysis of Bone Remodeling. In *Principles of Bone Biology*, 2nd ed.; Bilezikian, J.P., Raisz, L.G., Rodan, G.A., Eds.; Academic Press: San Diego, CA, USA, 2002; p. 303. **[Google Scholar]**

94. Burr, D.B.; Martin, R.B.; Schaffler, M.B.; Radin, E.L. Bone remodeling in response to in vivo fatigue microdamage. *J. Biomech* **1985**, *18*, 189–200. **[Google Scholar]**

95. Frost, H.M. Skeletal structural adaptations to mechanical usage (SATMU): 1. Redefining Wolff's law: The bone modeling problem. *Anat. Rec.* **1990**, *226*, 403–413. **[Google Scholar] [PubMed]**

96. Buehlmeier, J.; Frings-Meuthen, P.; Mohorko, N.; Lau, P.; Mazzucco, S.; Ferretti, J.L.; Biolo, G.; Pisot, R.; Simunic, B.; Rittweger, J. Markers of bone metabolism during 14 days of bed rest in young and older men. *J. Musculoskelet. Neuronal. Interact.* **2017**, *17*, 399–408. **[Google Scholar] [PubMed]**

97. Diab, T.; Condon, K.W.; Burr, D.B.; Vashishth, D. Age-related change in the damage morphology of human cortical bone and its role in bone fragility. *Bone* **2006**, *38*, 427–431. **[Google Scholar]**

98. Schiessl, H.; Frost, H.M.; Jee, W.S. Estrogen and bone-muscle strength and mass relationships. *Bone* **1998**, *22*, 1–6. **[Google Scholar]**

99. Rubin, C.T.; Lanyon, L.E. Kappa Delta Award paper. Osteoregulatory nature of mechanical stimuli: Function as a determinant for adaptive remodeling in bone. *J. Orthop. Res. Off. Publ. Orthop. Res. Soc.* **1987**, *5*, 300–310. **[Google Scholar]**

100. Frost, H.M. Bone "mass" and the "mechanostat": A proposal. *Anat. Rec.* **1987**, *219*, 1–9. **[Google Scholar]**

101. Sartori, R.; Schirwis, E.; Blaauw, B.; Bortolanza, S.; Zhao, J.; Enzo, E.; Stantzou, A.; Mouisel, E.; Toniolo, L.; Ferry, A.; et al. BMP signaling controls muscle mass. *Nat. Genet.* **2013**, *45*, 1309–1318. **[Google Scholar]**

102. Regan, J.N.; Trivedi, T.; Guise, T.A.; Waning, D.L. The Role of TGFβ in Bone-Muscle Crosstalk. *Curr. Osteoporos. Rep.* **2017**, *15*, 18–23. **[Google Scholar]**

103. Lee, N.K.; Sowa, H.; Hinoi, E.; Ferron, M.; Ahn, J.D.; Confavreux, C.; Dacquin, R.; Mee, P.J.; McKee, M.D.; Jung, D.Y.; et al. Endocrine regulation of energy metabolism by the skeleton. *Cell* **2007**, *130*, 456–469. **[Google Scholar] [PubMed] [Green Version]**

104. Vanderschueren, D.; Venken, K.; Ophoff, J.; Bouillon, R.; Boonen, S. Clinical Review: Sex steroids and the periosteum—Reconsidering the roles of androgens and estrogens in periosteal expansion. *J. Clin. Endocrinol. Metab.* **2006**, *91*, 378–382. **[Google Scholar] [Green Version]**

105. Prentice, A. Calcium intakes and bone densities of lactating women and breast-fed infants in The Gambia. *Adv. Exp. Med. Biol.* **1994**, *352*, 243–255. **[Google Scholar] [PubMed]**

106. Cauley, J.A. Estrogen and bone health in men and women. *Steroids* **2015**, *99*, 11–15. **[Google Scholar]**

107. Nattiv, A.; Loucks, A.B.; Manore, M.M.; Sanborn, C.F.; Sundgot-Borgen, J.; Warren, M.P. American College of Sports Medicine position stand. The female athlete triad. *Med. Sci. Sports Exerc.* **2007**, *39*, 1867–1882. **[Google Scholar] [PubMed]**

108. Khan, K. *Physical Activity and Bone Health*; Human Kinetics: Champaign, IL, USA, 2001. **[Google Scholar]**

109. Milgrom, C.; Finestone, A.; Simkin, A.; Ekenman, I.; Mendelson, S.; Millgram, M.; Nyska, M.; Larsson, E.; Burr, D. In-vivo strain measurements to evaluate the strengthening potential of exercises on the tibial bone. *J. Bone Jt. Surg. Br. Vol.* **2000**, *82*, 591–594. **[Google Scholar]**

110. Nikander, R.; Sievänen, H.; Heinonen, A.; Kannus, P. Femoral neck structure in adult female athletes subjected to different loading modalities. *J. Bone Miner. Res. Off. J. Am. Soc. Bone Miner. Res.* **2005**, *20*, 520–528. **[Google Scholar]**

111. Nichols, J.F.; Palmer, J.E.; Levy, S.S. Low bone mineral density in highly trained male master cyclists. *Osteoporos. Int.* **2003**, *14*, 644–649. **[Google Scholar]**

112. Wilks, D.C.; Gilliver, S.F.; Rittweger, J. Forearm and tibial bone measures of distance- and sprint-trained master cyclists. *Med. Sci. Sports Exerc.* **2009**, *41*, 566–573. **[Google Scholar]**

113. Ireland, A.; Maden-Wilkinson, T.; McPhee, J.; Cooke, K.; Narici, M.; Degens, H.; Rittweger, J. Upper limb muscle-bone asymmetries and bone adaptation in elite youth tennis players. *Med. Sci. Sports Exerc.* **2013**, *45*, 1749–1758. **[Google Scholar] [Green Version]**

114. Warden, S.J. Extreme skeletal adaptation to mechanical loading. *J. Orthop Sports Phys.* **2010**, *40*, 188. **[Google Scholar] [Green Version]**

115. Ireland, A.; Korhonen, M.; Heinonen, A.; Suominen, H.; Baur, C.; Stevens, S.; Degens, H.; Rittweger, J. Side-to-side differences in bone strength in master jumpers and sprinters. *J. Musculoskelet. Neuronal. Interact.* **2011**, *11*, 298–305. **[Google Scholar]**

116. Riggs, B.L.; Melton, L.J.; Robb, R.A.; Camp, J.J.; Atkinson, E.J.; McDaniel, L.; Amin, S.; Rouleau, P.A.; Khosla, S. A population-based assessment of rates of bone loss at multiple skeletal sites: Evidence for substantial trabecular bone loss in young adult women and men. *J. Bone Miner. Res. Off. J. Am. Soc. Bone Miner. Res.* **2008**, *23*, 205–214. **[Google Scholar] [PubMed]**

117. Warden, S.J.; Mantila Roosa, S.M.; Kersh, M.E.; Hurd, A.L.; Fleisig, G.S.; Pandy, M.G.; Fuchs, R.K. Physical activity when young provides lifelong benefits to cortical bone size and strength in men. *Proc. Natl. Acad. Sci. USA* **2014**, *111*, 5337–5342. **[Google Scholar] [PubMed] [Green Version]**

118. Ireland, A.; Maden-Wilkinson, T.; Ganse, B.; Degens, H.; Rittweger, J. Effects of age and starting age upon side asymmetry in the arms of veteran tennis players: A cross-sectional study. *Osteoporos. Int.* **2014**, *25*, 1389–1400. **[Google Scholar] [Green Version]**

119. Wilks, D.C.; Winwood, K.; Gilliver, S.F.; Kwiet, A.; Chatfield, M.; Michaelis, I.; Sun, L.W.; Ferretti, J.L.; Sargeant, A.J.; Felsenberg, D.; et al. Bone mass and geometry of the tibia and the radius of master sprinters, middle and long distance runners, race-walkers and sedentary control participants: A pQCT study. *Bone* **2009**, *45*, 91–97. **[Google Scholar] [PubMed]**

120. Wilks, D.C.; Winwood, K.; Gilliver, S.F.; Kwiet, A.; Sun, L.W.; Gutwasser, C.; Ferretti, J.L.; Sargeant, A.J.; Felsenberg, D.; Rittweger, J. Age-dependency in bone mass and geometry: A pQCT study on male and female master sprinters, middle and long distance runners, race-walkers and sedentary people. *J. Musculoskelet. Neuronal Interact.* **2009**, *9*, 236–246. **[Google Scholar] [PubMed]**

121. Strasser, B.; Burtscher, M. Survival of the fittest: VO. *Front. BioSci.* **2018**, *23*, 1505–1516. **[Google Scholar]**

122. Burtscher, J.; Burtscher, M. Run for your life: Tweaking the weekly physical activity volume for longevity. *Br. J. Sports Med.* **2019**. **[Google Scholar] [PubMed]**

123. Kodama, S.; Saito, K.; Tanaka, S.; Maki, M.; Yachi, Y.; Asumi, M.; Sugawara, A.; Totsuka, K.; Shimano, H.; Ohashi, Y.; et al. Cardiorespiratory fitness as a quantitative predictor of all-cause mortality and cardiovascular events in healthy men and women: A meta-analysis. *JAMA* **2009**, *301*, 2024–2035. **[Google Scholar] [PubMed] [Green Version]**

124. Tanaka, H.; Seals, D.R. Invited Review: Dynamic exercise performance in Masters athletes: Insight into the effects of primary human aging on physiological functional capacity. *J. Appl. Physiol.* **2003**, *95*, 2152–2162. **[Google Scholar]**

125. Tanaka, H.; Seals, D.R. Endurance exercise performance in Masters athletes: Age-associated changes and underlying physiological mechanisms. *J. Physiol.* **2008**, *586*, 55–63. **[Google Scholar] [PubMed]**

126. Baker, A.B.; Tang, Y.Q. Aging performance for masters records in athletics, swimming, rowing, cycling, triathlon, and weightlifting. *Exp. Aging Res.* **2010**, *36*, 453–477. **[Google Scholar] [PubMed]**

127. Ganse, B.; Drey, M.; Hildebrand, F.; Knobe, M.; Degens, H. Performance Declines Are Accelerated in the Oldest-Old Track and Field Athletes 80 to 94 Years of Age. *Rejuvenation Res.* **2020**. **[Google Scholar]**

128. Wright, V.J.; Perricelli, B.C. Age-related rates of decline in performance among elite senior athletes. *Am. J. Sports Med.* **2008**, *36*, 443–450. **[Google Scholar] [PubMed]**

129. Rittweger, J.; Di Prampero, P.E.; Maffulli, N.; Narici, M.V. Sprint and endurance power and ageing: An analysis of master athletic world records. *Proc. Biol. Sci.* **2009**, *276*, 683–689. **[Google Scholar] [Green Version]**

130. Fitzgerald, M.D.; Tanaka, H.; Tran, Z.V.; Seals, D.R. Age-related declines in maximal aerobic capacity in regularly exercising vs. sedentary women: A meta-analysis. *J. Appl. Physiol.* **1997**, *83*, 160–165. **[Google Scholar] [PubMed]**

131. Booth, F.W.; Zwetsloot, K.A. Basic concepts about genes, inactivity and aging. *Scand. J. Med. Sci. Sports* **2010**, *20*, 1–4. **[Google Scholar] [Green Version]**

132. Landi, F.; Calvani, R.; Tosato, M.; Martone, A.M.; Fusco, D.; Sisto, A.; Ortolani, E.; Savera, G.; Salini, S.; Marzetti, E. Age-Related Variations of Muscle Mass, Strength, and Physical Performance in Community-Dwellers: Results From the Milan EXPO Survey. *J. Am. Med. Dir. Assoc.* **2017**, *18*, 88.e17–88.e24. **[Google Scholar]**

133. Carr, D.B.; Flood, K.; Steger-May, K.; Schechtman, K.B.; Binder, E.F. Characteristics of frail older adult drivers. *J. Am. Geriatr. Soc.* **2006**, *54*, 1125–1129. **[Google Scholar] [PubMed]**

134. Burtscher, M.; Nachbauer, W.; Wilber, R. The upper limit of aerobic power in humans. *Eur. J. Appl. Physiol.* **2011**, *111*, 2625–2628. **[Google Scholar] [PubMed]**

135. Sandbakk, Ø.; Ettema, G.; Holmberg, H.C. Gender differences in endurance performance by elite cross-country skiers are influenced by the contribution from poling. *Scand. J. Med. Sci. Sports* **2014**, *24*, 28–33. **[Google Scholar] [PubMed]**

136. Trappe, S.; Hayes, E.; Galpin, A.; Kaminsky, L.; Jemiolo, B.; Fink, W.; Trappe, T.; Jansson, A.; Gustafsson, T.; Tesch, P. New records in aerobic power among octogenarian lifelong endurance athletes. *J. Appl. Physiol.* **2013**, *114*, 3–10. **[Google Scholar] [PubMed] [Green Version]**

137. Cattagni, T.; Gremeaux, V.; Lepers, R. The Physiological Characteristics of an 83-Year-Old Champion Female Master Runner. *Int. J. Sports Physiol. Perform.* **2019**, 1–5. **[Google Scholar]**

138. Billat, V.; Dhonneur, G.; Mille-Hamard, L.; Le Moyec, L.; Momken, I.; Launay, T.; Koralsztein, J.P.; Besse, S. Case Studies in Physiology: Maximal oxygen consumption and performance in a centenarian cyclist. *J. Appl. Physiol.* **2017**, *122*, 430–434. **[Google Scholar]**

139. Seiler, S.; De Koning, J.J.; Foster, C. The fall and rise of the gender difference in elite anaerobic performance 1952–2006. *Med. Sci. Sports Exerc.* **2007**, *39*, 534–540. **[Google Scholar]**

140. Coast, J.R.; Blevins, J.S.; Wilson, B.A. Do gender differences in running performance disappear with distance? *Can. J. Appl. Physiol.* **2004**, *29*, 139–145. **[Google Scholar]**

141. Calbet, J.A.; Joyner, M.J. Disparity in regional and systemic circulatory capacities: Do they affect the regulation of the circulation? *Acta Physiol.* **2010**, *199*, 393–406. **[Google Scholar]**

142. Yilmaz, D.C.; Buyukakilli, B.; Gurgul, S.; Rencuzogullari, I. Adaptation of heart to training: A comparative study using echocardiography & impedance cardiography in male & female athletes. *Indian J. Med. Res.* **2013**, *137*, 1111–1120. **[Google Scholar]**

143. Karjalainen, J.; Mäntysaari, M.; Viitasalo, M.; Kujala, U. Left ventricular mass, geometry, and filling in endurance athletes: Association with exercise blood pressure. *J. Appl. Physiol.* **1997**, *82*, 531–537. **[Google Scholar]**

144. Korhonen, M.T.; Cristea, A.; Alén, M.; Häkkinen, K.; Sipilä, S.; Mero, A.; Viitasalo, J.T.; Larsson, L.; Suominen, H. Aging, muscle fiber type, and contractile function in sprint-trained athletes. *J. Appl. Physiol.* **2006**, *101*, 906–917. **[Google Scholar]**

145. Messa, G.A.M.; Piasecki, M.; Rittweger, J.; McPhee, J.S.; Koltai, E.; Radak, Z.; Simunic, B.; Heinonen, A.; Suominen, H.; Korhonen, M.T.; et al. Absence of an aging-related increase in fiber type grouping in athletes and non-athletes. *Scand. J. Med. Sci. Sports* **2020**, *30*, 2057–2069. **[Google Scholar] [PubMed]**

146. Piasecki, J.; Inns, T.B.; Bass, J.J.; Scott, R.; Stashuk, D.W.; Phillips, B.E.; Atherton, P.J.; Piasecki, M. Influence of sex on the age-related adaptations of neuromuscular function and motor unit properties in elite masters athletes. *J. Physiol.* **2020**. **[Google Scholar]**

147. Strasser, B.; Volaklis, K.; Fuchs, D.; Burtscher, M. Role of Dietary Protein and Muscular Fitness on Longevity and Aging. *Aging Dis.* **2018**, *9*, 119–132. **[Google Scholar] [Green Version]**

148. Goodpaster, B.H.; Park, S.W.; Harris, T.B.; Kritchevsky, S.B.; Nevitt, M.; Schwartz, A.V.; Simonsick, E.M.; Tylavsky, F.A.; Visser, M.; Newman, A.B. The loss of skeletal muscle strength, mass, and quality in older adults: The health, aging and body composition study. *J. Gerontol. A Biol. Sci. Med. Sci.* **2006**, *61*, 1059–1064. **[Google Scholar] [PubMed]**

149. Michaelis, I.; Kwiet, A.; Gast, U.; Boshof, A.; Antvorskov, T.; Jung, T.; Rittweger, J.; Felsenberg, D. Decline of specific peak jumping power with age in master runners. *J. Musculoskelet Neuronal. Interact.* **2008**, *8*, 64–70. **[Google Scholar]**

150. Runge, M.; Rittweger, J.; Russo, C.R.; Schiessl, H.; Felsenberg, D. Is muscle power output a key factor in the age-related decline in physical performance? A comparison of muscle cross section, chair-rising test and jumping power. *Clin. Physiol. Funct. Imaging* **2004**, *24*, 335–340. **[Google Scholar] [PubMed]**

151. Lexell, J. Human aging, muscle mass, and fiber type composition. *J. Gerontol. A Biol Sci. Med. Sci.* **1995**, *50*, 11–16. **[Google Scholar]**

152. Galloway, M.T.; Kadoko, R.; Jokl, P. Effect of aging on male and female master athletes' performance in strength versus endurance activities. *Am. J. Orthop* **2002**, *31*, 93–98. **[Google Scholar] [PubMed]**

153. Faulkner, J.A.; Davis, C.S.; Mendias, C.L.; Brooks, S.V. The aging of elite male athletes: Age-related changes in performance and skeletal muscle structure and function. *Clin. J. Sport Med.* **2008**, *18*, 501–507. **[Google Scholar] [PubMed]**

154. Bishop, P.; Cureton, K.; Collins, M. Sex difference in muscular strength in equally-trained men and women. *Ergonomics* **1987**, *30*, 675–687. **[Google Scholar]**

155. Cureton, K.J.; Collins, M.A.; Hill, D.W.; McElhannon, F.M. Muscle hypertrophy in men and women. *Med. Sci. Sports Exerc.* **1988**, *20*, 338–344. **[Google Scholar] [PubMed]**

156. Lindle, R.S.; Metter, E.J.; Lynch, N.A.; Fleg, J.L.; Fozard, J.L.; Tobin, J.; Roy, T.A.; Hurley, B.F. Age and gender comparisons of muscle strength in 654 women and men aged 20–93 yr. *J. Appl. Physiol.* **1997**, *83*, 1581–1587. **[Google Scholar] [Green Version]**

157. Schoenfeld, B.J.; Ogborn, D.I.; Vigotsky, A.D.; Franchi, M.V.; Krieger, J.W. Hypertrophic Effects of Concentric vs. Eccentric Muscle Actions: A Systematic Review and Meta-analysis. *J. Strength Cond Res.* **2017**, *31*, 2599–2608. **[Google Scholar] [PubMed]**

158. Hunter, S.K. The Relevance of Sex Differences in Performance Fatigability. *Med. Sci. Sports Exerc.* **2016**, *48*, 2247–2256. **[Google Scholar] [PubMed] [Green Version]**

159. Popov, L.-D. Mitochondrial biogenesis: An update. *J. Cell Mol. Med.* **2020**, *24*, 4892–4899. **[Google Scholar] [PubMed] [Green Version]**

160. Schrepfer, E.; Scorrano, L. Mitofusins, from Mitochondria to Metabolism. *Mol. Cell* **2016**, *61*, 683–694. **[Google Scholar] [Green Version]**

161. Hood, D.A.; Memme, J.M.; Oliveira, A.N.; Triolo, M. Maintenance of Skeletal Muscle Mitochondria in Health, Exercise, and Aging. *Annu. Rev. Physiol.* **2019**, *81*, 19–41. **[Google Scholar]**

162. Granata, C.; Oliveira, R.S.; Little, J.P.; Renner, K.; Bishop, D.J. Mitochondrial adaptations to high-volume exercise training are rapidly reversed after a reduction in training volume in human skeletal muscle. *FASEB J.* **2016**, *30*, 3413–3423. **[Google Scholar] [Green Version]**

163. Jacobs, R.A.; Rasmussen, P.; Siebenmann, C.; Díaz, V.; Gassmann, M.; Pesta, D.; Gnaiger, E.; Nordsborg, N.B.; Robach, P.; Lundby, C. Determinants of time trial performance and maximal incremental exercise in highly trained endurance athletes. *J. Appl. Physiol.* **2011**, *111*, 1422–1430. **[Google Scholar] [Green Version]**

164. Jacobs, R.A.; Lundby, C. Mitochondria express enhanced quality as well as quantity in association with aerobic fitness across recreationally active individuals up to elite athletes. *J. Appl. Physiol.* **2013**, *114*, 344–350. **[Google Scholar] [Green Version]**

165. Jornayvaz, F.R.; Shulman, G.I. Regulation of mitochondrial biogenesis. *Essays Biochem.* **2010**, *47*, 69–84. **[Google Scholar] [PubMed] [Green Version]**

166. Radak, Z.; Torma, F.; Berkes, I.; Goto, S.; Mimura, T.; Posa, A.; Balogh, L.; Boldogh, I.; Suzuki, K.; Higuchi, M.; et al. Exercise effects on physiological function during aging. *Free Radic. Biol. Med.* **2019**, *132*, 33–41. **[Google Scholar] [Green Version]**

167. Petersen, K.F.; Befroy, D.; Dufour, S.; Dziura, J.; Ariyan, C.; Rothman, D.L.; DiPietro, L.; Cline, G.W.; Shulman, G.I. Mitochondrial dysfunction in the elderly: Possible role in insulin resistance. *Science* **2003**, *300*, 1140–1142. **[Google Scholar]** **[Green Version]**

168. Campisi, J.; Kapahi, P.; Lithgow, G.J.; Melov, S.; Newman, J.C.; Verdin, E. From discoveries in ageing research to therapeutics for healthy ageing. *Nature* **2019**, *571*, 183–192. **[Google Scholar]** **[Green Version]**

169. Reznick, R.M.; Zong, H.; Li, J.; Morino, K.; Moore, I.K.; Hannah, J.Y.; Liu, Z.-X.; Dong, J.; Mustard, K.J.; Hawley, S.A. Aging-associated reductions in AMP-activated protein kinase activity and mitochondrial biogenesis. *Cell Metab.* **2007**, *5*, 151–156. **[Google Scholar]** **[PubMed]** **[Green Version]**

170. Vainshtein, A.; Hood, D.A. The regulation of autophagy during exercise in skeletal muscle. *J. Appl. Physiol.* **2016**, *120*, 664–673. **[Google Scholar]** **[Green Version]**

171. Guevara, R.; Santandreu, F.M.; Valle, A.; Gianotti, M.; Oliver, J.; Roca, P. Sex-dependent differences in aged rat brain mitochondrial function and oxidative stress. *Free Radic. Biol. Med.* **2009**, *46*, 169–175. **[Google Scholar]**

172. Valle, A.; Guevara, R.; Garcia-Palmer, F.J.; Roca, P.; Oliver, J. Sexual dimorphism in liver mitochondrial oxidative capacity is conserved under caloric restriction conditions. *Am. J. Physiol. Cell Physiol.* **2007**, *293*, C1302–C1308. **[Google Scholar]**

173. Justo, R.; Boada, J.; Frontera, M.; Oliver, J.; Bermúdez, J.; Gianotti, M. Gender dimorphism in rat liver mitochondrial oxidative metabolism and biogenesis. *Am. J. Physiol. Cell Physiol.* **2005**, *289*, C372–C378. **[Google Scholar]** **[PubMed]** **[Green Version]**

174. Colom, B.; Oliver, J.; Roca, P.; Garcia-Palmer, F.J. Caloric restriction and gender modulate cardiac muscle mitochondrial $H_2O_2$ production and oxidative damage. *Cardiovasc Res.* **2007**, *74*, 456–465. **[Google Scholar]** **[PubMed]** **[Green Version]**

175. Colom, B.; Alcolea, M.; Valle, A.; Oliver, J.; Roca, P.; García-Palmer, F. Skeletal muscle of female rats exhibit higher mitochondrial mass and oxidative-phosphorylative capacities compared to males. *Cell. Physiol. Biochem.* **2007**, *19*, 205–212. **[Google Scholar]**

176. Ventura-Clapier, R.; Moulin, M.; Piquereau, J.; Lemaire, C.; Mericskay, M.; Veksler, V.; Garnier, A. Mitochondria: A central target for sex differences in pathologies. *Clin. Sci.* **2017**, *131*, 803–822. **[Google Scholar]**

177. Zawada, I.; Masternak, M.M.; List, E.O.; Stout, M.B.; Berryman, D.E.; Lewinski, A.; Kopchick, J.J.; Bartke, A.; Karbownik-Lewinska, M.; Gesing, A. Gene expression of key regulators of mitochondrial biogenesis is sex dependent in mice with growth hormone receptor deletion in liver. *Aging* **2015**, *7*, 195. **[Google Scholar]** **[PubMed]** **[Green Version]**

178. Van Leeuwen, N.; Beekman, M.; Deelen, J.; van den Akker, E.B.; de Craen, A.J.; Slagboom, P.E.; t Hart, L.M. Low mitochondrial DNA content associates with familial longevity: The Leiden Longevity Study. *Age* **2014**, *36*, 9629. **[Google Scholar]** **[PubMed]** **[Green Version]**

179. Karakelides, H.; Irving, B.A.; Short, K.R.; O'Brien, P.; Nair, K.S. Age, obesity, and sex effects on insulin sensitivity and skeletal muscle mitochondrial function. *Diabetes* **2010**, *59*, 89–97. **[Google Scholar]** **[PubMed]** **[Green Version]**

180. Howald, H.; Hoppeler, H.; Claassen, H.; Mathieu, O.; Straub, R. Influences of endurance training on the ultrastructural composition of the different muscle fiber types in humans. *Pflügers Arch.* **1985**, *403*, 369–376. **[Google Scholar]**

181. Howald, H.; Boesch, C.; Kreis, R.; Matter, S.; Billeter, R.; Essen-Gustavsson, B.; Hoppeler, H. Content of intramyocellular lipids derived by electron microscopy, biochemical assays, and 1H-MR spectroscopy. *J. Appl. Physiol.* **2002**, *92*, 2264–2272. **[Google Scholar]** **[Green Version]**

182. Tarnopolsky, M.A.; Rennie, C.D.; Robertshaw, H.A.; Fedak-Tarnopolsky, S.N.; Devries, M.C.; Hamadeh, M.J. Influence of endurance exercise training and sex on intramyocellular lipid and mitochondrial ultrastructure, substrate use, and mitochondrial enzyme activity. *Am. J. Physiol. Regul. Integr. Comp. Physiol.* **2007**, *292*, R1271–R1278. **[Google Scholar] [Green Version]**

183. Tanaka, H.; Tarumi, T.; Rittweger, J. Aging and Physiological Lessons from Master Athletes. *Compr. Physiol.* **2019**, *10*, 261–296. **[Google Scholar]**

184. Sloane, P.D.; Marzetti, E.; Landi, F.; Zimmerman, S. Understanding and Addressing Muscle Strength, Mass, and Function in Older Persons. *J. Am. Med. Dir. Assoc.* **2019**, *20*, 1–4. **[Google Scholar]**

185. Melin, A.K.; Heikura, I.A.; Tenforde, A.; Mountjoy, M. Energy Availability in Athletics: Health, Performance, and Physique. *Int J. Sport Nutr. Exerc. Metab.* **2019**, *29*, 152–164. **[Google Scholar]**

186. Mountjoy, M.; Sundgot-Borgen, J.K.; Burke, L.M.; Ackerman, K.E.; Blauwet, C.; Constantini, N.; Lebrun, C.; Lundy, B.; Melin, A.K.; Meyer, N.L.; et al. IOC consensus statement on relative energy deficiency in sport (RED-S): 2018 update. *Br. J. Sports Med.* **2018**, *52*, 687–697. **[Google Scholar] [Green Version]**

187. Tarnopolsky, M.A. Sex differences in exercise metabolism and the role of 17-beta estradiol. *Med. Sci. Sports Exerc.* **2008**, *40*, 648–654. **[Google Scholar]**

188. Cox, N.J.; Ibrahim, K.; Sayer, A.A.; Robinson, S.M.; Roberts, H.C. Assessment and Treatment of the Anorexia of Aging: A Systematic Review. *Nutrients* **2019**, *11*, 144. **[Google Scholar] [PubMed] [Green Version]**

189. Doering, T.M.; Reaburn, P.R.; Cox, G.R.; Jenkins, D.G. Comparison of Postexercise Nutrition Knowledge and Postexercise Carbohydrate and Protein Intake Between Australian Masters and Younger Triathletes. *Int. J. Sport Nutr. Exerc. Metab.* **2016**, *26*, 338–346. **[Google Scholar] [PubMed]**

190. Burke, L.M.; Hawley, J.A.; Wong, S.H.; Jeukendrup, A.E. Carbohydrates for training and competition. *J. Sports Sci.* **2011**, *29* (Suppl. 1), S17–S27. **[Google Scholar] [PubMed]**

191. Nieman, D.C.; Mitmesser, S.H. Potential Impact of Nutrition on Immune System Recovery from Heavy Exertion: A Metabolomics Perspective. *Nutrients* **2017**, *9*, 513. **[Google Scholar] [Green Version]**

192. Tipton, K.D. Efficacy and consequences of very-high-protein diets for athletes and exercisers. *Proc. Nutr Soc.* **2011**, *70*, 205–214. **[Google Scholar] [Green Version]**

193. Trommelen, J.; Betz, M.W.; van Loon, L.J.C. The Muscle Protein Synthetic Response to Meal Ingestion Following Resistance-Type Exercise. *Sports Med.* **2019**, *49*, 185–197. **[Google Scholar] [Green Version]**

194. Drummond, M.J.; Dreyer, H.C.; Fry, C.S.; Glynn, E.L.; Rasmussen, B.B. Nutritional and contractile regulation of human skeletal muscle protein synthesis and mTORC1 signaling. *J. Appl. Physiol.* **2009**, *106*, 1374–1384. **[Google Scholar] [Green Version]**

195. Witard, O.C.; Jackman, S.R.; Breen, L.; Smith, K.; Selby, A.; Tipton, K.D. Myofibrillar muscle protein synthesis rates subsequent to a meal in response to increasing doses of whey protein at rest and after resistance exercise. *Am. J. Clin. Nutr.* **2014**, *99*, 86–95. **[Google Scholar] [Green Version]**

196. Burd, N.A.; Beals, J.W.; Martinez, I.G.; Salvador, A.F.; Skinner, S.K. Food-First Approach to Enhance the Regulation of Post-exercise Skeletal Muscle Protein Synthesis and Remodeling. *Sports Med.* **2019**, *49*, 59–68. **[Google Scholar] [Green Version]**

197. Holwerda, A.M.; Paulussen, K.J.M.; Overkamp, M.; Goessens, J.P.B.; Kramer, I.F.; Wodzig, W.K.W.H.; Verdijk, L.B.; van Loon, L.J.C. Dose-Dependent Increases in Whole-Body Net Protein Balance and Dietary Protein-Derived Amino Acid Incorporation into Myofibrillar Protein During Recovery from Resistance Exercise in Older Men. *J. Nutr.* **2019**, *149*, 221–230. **[Google Scholar] [PubMed]**

198. Szwiega, S.; Pencharz, P.B.; Rafii, M.; Lebarron, M.; Chang, J.; Ball, R.O.; Kong, D.; Xu, L.; Elango, R.; Courtney-Martin, G. Dietary leucine requirement of older men and women is higher than current recommendations. *Am. J. Clin. Nutr.* **2020.** **[Google Scholar]**

199. Bauer, J.; Biolo, G.; Cederholm, T.; Cesari, M.; Cruz-Jentoft, A.J.; Morley, J.E.; Phillips, S.; Sieber, C.; Stehle, P.; Teta, D.; et al. Evidence-based recommendations for optimal dietary protein intake in older people: A position paper from the PROT-AGE Study Group. *J. Am. Med. Dir. Assoc.* **2013**, *14*, 542–559. **[Google Scholar]** **[PubMed]**

200. Loenneke, J.P.; Loprinzi, P.D.; Murphy, C.H.; Phillips, S.M. Per meal dose and frequency of protein consumption is associated with lean mass and muscle performance. *Clin. Nutr.* **2016**, *35*, 1506–1511. **[Google Scholar]** **[PubMed]**

201. Morton, R.W.; Murphy, K.T.; McKellar, S.R.; Schoenfeld, B.J.; Henselmans, M.; Helms, E.; Aragon, A.A.; Devries, M.C.; Banfield, L.; Krieger, J.W.; et al. A systematic review, meta-analysis and meta-regression of the effect of protein supplementation on resistance training-induced gains in muscle mass and strength in healthy adults. *Br. J. Sports Med.* **2018**, *52*, 376–384. **[Google Scholar]**

202. Hector, A.J.; Phillips, S.M. Protein Recommendations for Weight Loss in Elite Athletes: A Focus on Body Composition and Performance. *Int. J. Sport. Nutr. Exerc. Metab.* **2018**, *28*, 170–177. **[Google Scholar]** **[PubMed]** **[Green Version]**

203. Deane, C.S.; Bass, J.J.; Crossland, H.; Phillips, B.E.; Atherton, P.J. Animal, Plant, Collagen and Blended Dietary Proteins: Effects on Musculoskeletal Outcomes. *Nutrients* **2020**, *12*, 2670. **[Google Scholar]** **[PubMed]**

204. Van Vliet, S.; Burd, N.A.; Van Loon, L.J. The Skeletal Muscle Anabolic Response to Plant- versus Animal-Based Protein Consumption. *J. Nutr.* **2015**, *145*, 1981–1991. **[Google Scholar]** **[Green Version]**

205. Gorissen, S.H.M.; Witard, O.C. Characterising the muscle anabolic potential of dairy, meat and plant-based protein sources in older adults. *Proc. Nutr. Soc.* **2018**, *77*, 20–31. **[Google Scholar]**

206. Smith, G.I.; Atherton, P.; Villareal, D.T.; Frimel, T.N.; Rankin, D.; Rennie, M.J.; Mittendorfer, B. Differences in muscle protein synthesis and anabolic signaling in the postabsorptive state and in response to food in 65-80 year old men and women. *PLoS ONE* **2008**, *3*, e1875. **[Google Scholar]** **[Green Version]**

207. Doering, T.M.; Jenkins, D.G.; Reaburn, P.R.; Borges, N.R.; Hohmann, E.; Phillips, S.M. Lower Integrated Muscle Protein Synthesis in Masters Compared with Younger Athletes. *Med. Sci. Sports Exerc.* **2016**, *48*, 1613–1618. **[Google Scholar]** **[PubMed]**

208. McKendry, J.; Shad, B.J.; Smeuninx, B.; Oikawa, S.Y.; Wallis, G.; Greig, C.; Phillips, S.M.; Breen, L. Comparable Rates of Integrated Myofibrillar Protein Synthesis Between Endurance-Trained Master Athletes and Untrained Older Individuals. *Front. Physiol.* **2019**, *10*, 1084. **[Google Scholar]** **[PubMed]**

209. McKendry, J.; Joanisse, S.; Baig, S.; Liu, B.; Parise, G.; Greig, C.A.; Breen, L. Superior Aerobic Capacity and Indices of Skeletal Muscle Morphology in Chronically Trained Master Endurance Athletes Compared With Untrained Older Adults. *J. Gerontol. A Biol. Sci. Med. Sci.* **2020**, *75*, 1079–1088. **[Google Scholar]** **[PubMed]**

210. Burd, N.A.; Gorissen, S.H.; van Loon, L.J. Anabolic resistance of muscle protein synthesis with aging. *Exerc. Sport Sci. Rev.* **2013**, *41*, 169–173. **[Google Scholar]**

211. Wall, B.T.; Gorissen, S.H.; Pennings, B.; Koopman, R.; Groen, B.B.; Verdijk, L.B.; van Loon, L.J. Aging Is Accompanied by a Blunted Muscle Protein Synthetic Response to Protein Ingestion. *PLoS ONE* **2015**, *10*, e0140903. **[Google Scholar]** **[PubMed]**

212. Wilkinson, D.J.; Piasecki, M.; Atherton, P.J. The age-related loss of skeletal muscle mass and function: Measurement and physiology of muscle fibre atrophy and muscle fibre loss in humans. *Ageing Res. Rev.* **2018**, *47*, 123–132. **[Google Scholar]** **[PubMed]**

213. Cermak, N.M.; Res, P.T.; de Groot, L.C.; Saris, W.H.; van Loon, L.J. Protein supplementation augments the adaptive response of skeletal muscle to resistance-type exercise training: A meta-analysis. *Am. J. Clin. Nutr.* **2012**, *96*, 1454–1464. **[Google Scholar] [Green Version]**

214. Yang, Y.; Breen, L.; Burd, N.A.; Hector, A.J.; Churchward-Venne, T.A.; Josse, A.R.; Tarnopolsky, M.A.; Phillips, S.M. Resistance exercise enhances myofibrillar protein synthesis with graded intakes of whey protein in older men. *Br. J. Nutr.* **2012**, *108*, 1780–1788. **[Google Scholar] [PubMed] [Green Version]**

215. Di Girolamo, F.G.; Situlin, R.; Fiotti, N.; Tence, M.; De Colle, P.; Mearelli, F.; Minetto, M.A.; Ghigo, E.; Pagani, M.; Lucini, D.; et al. Higher protein intake is associated with improved muscle strength in elite senior athletes. *Nutrition* **2017**, *42*, 82–86. **[Google Scholar] [PubMed]**

216. Smith, G.I.; Atherton, P.; Reeds, D.N.; Mohammed, B.S.; Rankin, D.; Rennie, M.J.; Mittendorfer, B. Dietary omega-3 fatty acid supplementation increases the rate of muscle protein synthesis in older adults: A randomized controlled trial. *Am. J. Clin. Nutr.* **2011**, *93*, 402–412. **[Google Scholar] [PubMed] [Green Version]**

217. Smith, G.I.; Julliand, S.; Reeds, D.N.; Sinacore, D.R.; Klein, S.; Mittendorfer, B. Fish oil-derived n-3 PUFA therapy increases muscle mass and function in healthy older adults. *Am. J. Clin. Nutr.* **2015**, *102*, 115–122. **[Google Scholar] [Green Version]**

218. Papageorgiou, M.; Dolan, E.; Elliott-Sale, K.J.; Sale, C. Reduced energy availability: Implications for bone health in physically active populations. *Eur. J. Nutr.* **2018**, *57*, 847–859. **[Google Scholar] [PubMed]**

219. Sale, C.; Elliott-Sale, K.J. Nutrition and Athlete Bone Health. *Sports Med.* **2019**, *49*, 139–151. **[Google Scholar] [PubMed] [Green Version]**

220. Ihle, R.; Loucks, A.B. Dose-response relationships between energy availability and bone turnover in young exercising women. *J. Bone Min. Res.* **2004**, *19*, 1231–1240. **[Google Scholar]**

221. Hammond, K.M.; Sale, C.; Fraser, W.; Tang, J.; Shepherd, S.O.; Strauss, J.A.; Close, G.L.; Cocks, M.; Louis, J.; Pugh, J.; et al. Post-exercise carbohydrate and energy availability induce independent effects on skeletal muscle cell signalling and bone turnover: Implications for training adaptation. *J. Physiol.* **2019**, *597*, 4779–4796. **[Google Scholar]**

222. Locatelli, V.; Bianchi, V.E. Effect of GH/IGF-1 on Bone Metabolism and Osteoporsosis. *Int. J. Endocrinol.* **2014**, *2014*, 235060. **[Google Scholar] [Green Version]**

223. Kerstetter, J.E.; Kenny, A.M.; Insogna, K.L. Dietary protein and skeletal health: A review of recent human research. *Curr. Opin. Lipidol.* **2011**, *22*, 16–20. **[Google Scholar]**

224. Holm, L.; Olesen, J.L.; Matsumoto, K.; Doi, T.; Mizuno, M.; Alsted, T.J.; Mackey, A.L.; Schwarz, P.; Kjaer, M. Protein-containing nutrient supplementation following strength training enhances the effect on muscle mass, strength, and bone formation in postmenopausal women. *J. Appl. Physiol.* **2008**, *105*, 274–281. **[Google Scholar]**

225. Bowen, J.; Noakes, M.; Clifton, P.M. A high dairy protein, high-calcium diet minimizes bone turnover in overweight adults during weight loss. *J. Nutr.* **2004**, *134*, 568–573. **[Google Scholar]**

226. Geiker, N.R.W.; Mølgaard, C.; Iuliano, S.; Rizzoli, R.; Manios, Y.; Van Loon, L.J.C.; Lecerf, J.M.; Moschonis, G.; Reginster, J.Y.; Givens, I.; et al. Impact of whole dairy matrix on musculoskeletal health and aging-current knowledge and research gaps. *Osteoporos Int.* **2020**, *31*, 601–615. **[Google Scholar] [Green Version]**

227. Frassetto, L.; Morris, R.C.; Sellmeyer, D.E.; Todd, K.; Sebastian, A. Diet, evolution and aging—The pathophysiologic effects of the post-agricultural inversion of the potassium-to-sodium and base-to-chloride ratios in the human diet. *Eur. J. Nutr.* **2001**, *40*, 200–213. **[Google Scholar]**

228. New, S.A.; Robins, S.P.; Campbell, M.K.; Martin, J.C.; Garton, M.J.; Bolton-Smith, C.; Grubb, D.A.; Lee, S.J.; Reid, D.M. Dietary influences on bone mass and bone metabolism: Further evidence of a

positive link between fruit and vegetable consumption and bone health? *Am. J. Clin. Nutr.* **2000**, *71*, 142–151. **[Google Scholar] [PubMed] [Green Version]**

229. Close, G.L.; Russell, J.; Cobley, J.N.; Owens, D.J.; Wilson, G.; Gregson, W.; Fraser, W.D.; Morton, J.P. Assessment of vitamin D concentration in non-supplemented professional athletes and healthy adults during the winter months in the UK: Implications for skeletal muscle function. *J. Sports Sci.* **2013**, *31*, 344–353. **[Google Scholar]**
230. Ruohola, J.P.; Laaksi, I.; Ylikomi, T.; Haataja, R.; Mattila, V.M.; Sahi, T.; Tuohimaa, P.; Pihlajamäki, H. Association between serum 25(OH)D concentrations and bone stress fractures in Finnish young men. *J. Bone Min. Res.* **2006**, *21*, 1483–1488. **[Google Scholar]**
231. Lappe, J.; Cullen, D.; Haynatzki, G.; Recker, R.; Ahlf, R.; Thompson, K. Calcium and vitamin d supplementation decreases incidence of stress fractures in female navy recruits. *J. Bone Min. Res.* **2008**, *23*, 741–749. **[Google Scholar] [PubMed]**
232. Larson-Meyer, D.E.; Willis, K.S. Vitamin D and athletes. *Curr. Sports Med. Rep.* **2010**, *9*, 220–226. **[Google Scholar] [Green Version]**
233. Edouard, P.; Branco, P.; Alonso, J.M. Muscle injury is the principal injury type and hamstring muscle injury is the first injury diagnosis during top-level international athletics championships between 2007 and 2015. *Br. J. Sports Med.* **2016**, *50*, 619–630. **[Google Scholar] [PubMed]**
234. Fredericson, M.; Jennings, F.; Beaulieu, C.; Matheson, G.O. Stress fractures in athletes. *Top. Magn. Reson. Imaging* **2006**, *17*, 309–325. **[Google Scholar] [PubMed]**
235. Soligard, T.; Schwellnus, M.; Alonso, J.M.; Bahr, R.; Clarsen, B.; Dijkstra, H.P.; Gabbett, T.; Gleeson, M.; Hägglund, M.; Hutchinson, M.R.; et al. How much is too much? (Part 1) International Olympic Committee consensus statement on load in sport and risk of injury. *Br. J. Sports Med.* **2016**, *50*, 1030–1041. **[Google Scholar] [Green Version]**
236. Ganse, B.; Degens, H.; Drey, M.; Korhonen, M.T.; McPhee, J.; Müller, K.; Johannes, B.W.; Rittweger, J. Impact of age, performance and athletic event on injury rates in master athletics-first results from an ongoing prospective study. *J. Musculoskelet Neuronal. Interact.* **2014**, *14*, 148–154. **[Google Scholar]**
237. Wall, B.T.; Dirks, M.L.; Snijders, T.; Senden, J.M.; Dolmans, J.; van Loon, L.J. Substantial skeletal muscle loss occurs during only 5 days of disuse. *Acta Physiol.* **2014**, *210*, 600–611. **[Google Scholar]**
238. LeBlanc, A.D.; Schneider, V.S.; Evans, H.J.; Pientok, C.; Rowe, R.; Spector, E. Regional changes in muscle mass following 17 weeks of bed rest. *J. Appl. Physiol.* **1992**, *73*, 2172–2178. **[Google Scholar] [PubMed]**
239. Wall, B.T.; Dirks, M.L.; Snijders, T.; Stephens, F.B.; Senden, J.M.; Verscheijden, M.L.; van Loon, L.J. Short-term muscle disuse atrophy is not associated with increased intramuscular lipid deposition or a decline in the maximal activity of key mitochondrial enzymes in young and older males. *Exp. Gerontol.* **2015**, *61*, 76–83. **[Google Scholar] [PubMed]**
240. Rudrappa, S.S.; Wilkinson, D.J.; Greenhaff, P.L.; Smith, K.; Idris, I.; Atherton, P.J. Human Skeletal Muscle Disuse Atrophy: Effects on Muscle Protein Synthesis, Breakdown, and Insulin Resistance-A Qualitative Review. *Front. Physiol.* **2016**, *7*, 361. **[Google Scholar]**
241. Bowden Davies, K.A.; Pickles, S.; Sprung, V.S.; Kemp, G.J.; Alam, U.; Moore, D.R.; Tahrani, A.A.; Cuthbertson, D.J. Reduced physical activity in young and older adults: Metabolic and musculoskeletal implications. *Adv. Endocrinol. Metab.* **2019**, 10. **[Google Scholar]**
242. Demling, R.H. Nutrition, anabolism, and the wound healing process: An overview. *Eplasty* **2009**, *9*, e9. **[Google Scholar] [PubMed]**
243. Close, G.L.; Sale, C.; Baar, K.; Bermon, S. Nutrition for the Prevention and Treatment of Injuries in Track and Field Athletes. *Int. J. Sport Nutr. Exerc. Metab.* **2019**, *29*, 189–197. **[Google Scholar] [Green Version]**

244. Papadopoulou, S.K. Rehabilitation Nutrition for Injury Recovery of Athletes: The Role of Macronutrient Intake. *Nutrients* **2020**, *12*, 2449. **[Google Scholar]** **[PubMed]**

245. Smith-Ryan, A.E.; Hirsch, K.R.; Saylor, H.E.; Gould, L.M.; Blue, M.N.M. Nutritional Considerations and Strategies to Facilitate Injury Recovery and Rehabilitation. *J. Athl. Train.* **2020**, *55*, 918–930. **[Google Scholar]** **[PubMed]**

246. Tipton, K.D. Nutritional Support for Exercise-Induced Injuries. *Sports Med.* **2015**, *45* (Suppl. 1), S93–S104. **[Google Scholar]** **[PubMed]** **[Green Version]**

247. Wall, B.T.; Van Loon, L.J. Nutritional strategies to attenuate muscle disuse atrophy. *Nutr. Rev.* **2013**, *71*, 195–208. **[Google Scholar]**

248. Wall, B.T.; Morton, J.P.; van Loon, L.J. Strategies to maintain skeletal muscle mass in the injured athlete: Nutritional considerations and exercise mimetics. *Eur. J. Sport Sci.* **2015**, *15*, 53–62. **[Google Scholar]**

249. Trommelen, J.; Van Loon, L.J. Pre-Sleep Protein Ingestion to Improve the Skeletal Muscle Adaptive Response to Exercise Training. *Nutrients* **2016**, *8*, 763. **[Google Scholar]** **[Green Version]**

250. Weyh, C.; Krüger, K.; Strasser, B. Physical Activity and Diet Shape the Immune System during Aging. *Nutrients* **2020**, *12*, 622. **[Google Scholar]** **[Green Version]**

251. Duggal, N.A.; Pollock, R.D.; Lazarus, N.R.; Harridge, S.; Lord, J.M. Major features of immunesenescence, including reduced thymic output, are ameliorated by high levels of physical activity in adulthood. *Aging Cell* **2018**, 17. **[Google Scholar]** **[Green Version]**

252. Minuzzi, L.G.; Rama, L.; Chupel, M.U.; Rosado, F.; Dos Santos, J.V.; Simpson, R.; Martinho, A.; Paiva, A.; Teixeira, A.M. Effects of lifelong training on senescence and mobilization of T lymphocytes in response to acute exercise. *Exerc. Immunol. Rev.* **2018**, *24*, 72–84. **[Google Scholar]**

253. Nieman, D.C.; Henson, D.A.; Austin, M.D.; Sha, W. Upper respiratory tract infection is reduced in physically fit and active adults. *Br. J. Sports Med.* **2011**, *45*, 987–992. **[Google Scholar]**

254. Simpson, R.J.; Campbell, J.P.; Gleeson, M.; Krüger, K.; Nieman, D.C.; Pyne, D.B.; Turner, J.E.; Walsh, N.P. Can exercise affect immune function to increase susceptibility to infection? *Exerc. Immunol. Rev.* **2020**, *26*, 8–22. **[Google Scholar]** **[PubMed]**

255. Passos, B.N.; Lima, M.C.; Sierra, A.P.R.; Oliveira, R.A.; Maciel, J.F.S.; Manoel, R.; Rogante, J.I.; Pesquero, J.B.; Cury-Boaventura, M.F. Association of Daily Dietary Intake and Inflammation Induced by Marathon Race. *Mediat. Inflamm.* **2019**, *2019*, 1537274. **[Google Scholar]** **[PubMed]** **[Green Version]**

256. Nieman, D.C.; Henson, D.A.; Gross, S.J.; Jenkins, D.P.; Davis, J.M.; Murphy, E.A.; Carmichael, M.D.; Dumke, C.L.; Utter, A.C.; McAnulty, S.R.; et al. Quercetin reduces illness but not immune perturbations after intensive exercise. *Med. Sci. Sports Exerc.* **2007**, *39*, 1561–1569. **[Google Scholar]** **[Green Version]**

257. Witard, O.C.; Turner, J.E.; Jackman, S.R.; Kies, A.K.; Jeukendrup, A.E.; Bosch, J.A.; Tipton, K.D. High dietary protein restores overreaching induced impairments in leukocyte trafficking and reduces the incidence of upper respiratory tract infection in elite cyclists. *Brain Behav. Immun.* **2014**, *39*, 211–219. **[Google Scholar]** **[Green Version]**

258. Walsh, N.P. Recommendations to maintain immune health in athletes. *Eur. J. Sport Sci.* **2018**, *18*, 820–831. **[Google Scholar]** **[Green Version]**

259. Farrokhyar, F.; Tabasinejad, R.; Dao, D.; Peterson, D.; Ayeni, O.R.; Hadioonzadeh, R.; Bhandari, M. Prevalence of vitamin D inadequacy in athletes: A systematic-review and meta-analysis. *Sports Med.* **2015**, *45*, 365–378. **[Google Scholar]**

260. Martineau, A.R.; Jolliffe, D.A.; Greenberg, L.; Aloia, J.F.; Bergman, P.; Dubnov-Raz, G.; Esposito, S.; Ganmaa, D.; Ginde, A.A.; Goodall, E.C.; et al. Vitamin D supplementation to prevent acute respiratory infections: Individual participant data meta-analysis. *Health Technol. Assess.* **2019**, *23*, 1–44. **[Google Scholar]** **[PubMed]**

261. He, C.S.; Handzlik, M.; Fraser, W.D.; Muhamad, A.; Preston, H.; Richardson, A.; Gleeson, M. Influence of vitamin D status on respiratory infection incidence and immune function during 4 months of winter training in endurance sport athletes. *Exerc. Immunol. Rev.* **2013**, *19*, 86–101. **[Google Scholar] [PubMed]**

262. He, C.S.; Bishop, N.C.; Handzlik, M.K.; Muhamad, A.S.; Gleeson, M. Sex differences in upper respiratory symptoms prevalence and oral-respiratory mucosal immunity in endurance athletes. *Exerc. Immunol. Rev.* **2014**, *20*, 8–22. **[Google Scholar] [PubMed]**

263. He, C.S.; Aw Yong, X.H.; Walsh, N.P.; Gleeson, M. Is there an optimal vitamin D status for immunity in athletes and military personnel? *Exerc. Immunol. Rev.* **2016**, *22*, 42–64. **[Google Scholar] [PubMed]**

264. Roubenoff, R. Catabolism of aging: Is it an inflammatory process? *Curr. Opin. Clin. Nutr. Metab. Care* **2003**, *6*, 295–299. **[Google Scholar]**

265. Rondanelli, M.; Klersy, C.; Terracol, G.; Talluri, J.; Maugeri, R.; Guido, D.; Faliva, M.A.; Solerte, B.S.; Fioravanti, M.; Lukaski, H.; et al. Whey protein, amino acids, and vitamin D supplementation with physical activity increases fat-free mass and strength, functionality, and quality of life and decreases inflammation in sarcopenic elderly. *Am. J. Clin. Nutr.* **2016**, *103*, 830–840. **[Google Scholar]**

266. Peake, J.; Nosaka, K.; Suzuki, K. Characterization of inflammatory responses to eccentric exercise in humans. *Exerc. Immunol. Rev.* **2005**, *11*, 64–85. **[Google Scholar]**

267. Logan, V.F.; Gray, A.R.; Peddie, M.C.; Harper, M.J.; Houghton, L.A. Long-term vitamin D3 supplementation is more effective than vitamin D2 in maintaining serum 25-hydroxyvitamin D status over the winter months. *Br. J. Nutr.* **2013**, *109*, 1082–1088. **[Google Scholar] [PubMed] [Green Version]**

268. Heiman, M.L.; Greenway, F.L. A healthy gastrointestinal microbiome is dependent on dietary diversity. *Mol. Metab.* **2016**, *5*, 317–320. **[Google Scholar] [PubMed]**

269. Rowland, I.; Gibson, G.; Heinken, A.; Scott, K.; Swann, J.; Thiele, I.; Tuohy, K. Gut microbiota functions: Metabolism of nutrients and other food components. *Eur. J. Nutr.* **2018**, *57*, 1–24. **[Google Scholar] [PubMed] [Green Version]**

270. Tilg, H.; Zmora, N.; Adolph, T.E.; Elinav, E. The intestinal microbiota fuelling metabolic inflammation. *Nat. Rev. Immunol.* **2020**, *20*, 40–54. **[Google Scholar] [PubMed]**

271. Stavropoulou, E.; Bezirtzoglou, E. Human microbiota in aging and infection: A review. *Crit. Rev. Food Sci. Nutr.* **2019**, *59*, 537–545. **[Google Scholar]**

272. Rinninella, E.; Cintoni, M.; Raoul, P.; Lopetuso, L.R.; Scaldaferri, F.; Pulcini, G.; Miggiano, G.A.D.; Gasbarrini, A.; Mele, M.C. Food Components and Dietary Habits: Keys for a Healthy Gut Microbiota Composition. *Nutrients* **2019**, *11*, 2393. **[Google Scholar] [Green Version]**

273. Clarke, S.F.; Murphy, E.F.; O'Sullivan, O.; Lucey, A.J.; Humphreys, M.; Hogan, A.; Hayes, P.; O'Reilly, M.; Jeffery, I.B.; Wood-Martin, R.; et al. Exercise and associated dietary extremes impact on gut microbial diversity. *Gut* **2014**, *63*, 1913–1920. **[Google Scholar] [PubMed] [Green Version]**

274. Allen, J.M.; Mailing, L.J.; Cohrs, J.; Salmonson, C.; Fryer, J.D.; Nehra, V.; Hale, V.L.; Kashyap, P.; White, B.A.; Woods, J.A. Exercise training-induced modification of the gut microbiota persists after microbiota colonization and attenuates the response to chemically-induced colitis in gnotobiotic mice. *Gut Microbes* **2018**, *9*, 115–130. **[Google Scholar] [Green Version]**

275. Estaki, M.; Pither, J.; Baumeister, P.; Little, J.P.; Gill, S.K.; Ghosh, S.; Ahmadi-Vand, Z.; Marsden, K.R.; Gibson, D.L. Cardiorespiratory fitness as a predictor of intestinal microbial diversity and distinct metagenomic functions. *Microbiome* **2016**, *4*, 42. **[Google Scholar] [Green Version]**

276. Morita, E.; Yokoyama, H.; Imai, D.; Takeda, R.; Ota, A.; Kawai, E.; Hisada, T.; Emoto, M.; Suzuki, Y.; Okazaki, K. Aerobic Exercise Training with Brisk Walking Increases Intestinal Bacteroides in Healthy Elderly Women. *Nutrients* **2019**, *11*, 868. **[Google Scholar] [Green Version]**

277. Zhu, Q.; Jiang, S.; Du, G. Effects of exercise frequency on the gut microbiota in elderly individuals. *Microbiologyopen* **2020**, *9*, e1053. **[Google Scholar]**

278. Fart, F.; Rajan, S.K.; Wall, R.; Rangel, I.; Ganda-Mall, J.P.; Tingö, L.; Brummer, R.J.; Repsilber, D.; Schoultz, I.; Lindqvist, C.M. Differences in Gut Microbiome Composition between Senior Orienteering Athletes and Community-Dwelling Older Adults. *Nutrients* **2020**, *12*, 2610. **[Google Scholar]**

279. Bear, T.L.K.; Dalziel, J.E.; Coad, J.; Roy, N.C.; Butts, C.A.; Gopal, P.K. The Role of the Gut Microbiota in Dietary Interventions for Depression and Anxiety. *Adv. Nutr.* **2020**, *11*, 890–907. **[Google Scholar] [PubMed] [Green Version]**

280. Jeukendrup, A.E.; Vet-Joop, K.; Sturk, A.; Stegen, J.H.; Senden, J.; Saris, W.H.; Wagenmakers, A.J. Relationship between gastro-intestinal complaints and endotoxaemia, cytokine release and the acute-phase reaction during and after a long-distance triathlon in highly trained men. *Clin. Sci.* **2000**, *98*, 47–55. **[Google Scholar] [Green Version]**

281. Ticinesi, A.; Lauretani, F.; Tana, C.; Nouvenne, A.; Ridolo, E.; Meschi, T. Exercise and immune system as modulators of intestinal microbiome: Implications for the gut-muscle axis hypothesis. *Exerc. Immunol. Rev.* **2019**, *25*, 84–95. **[Google Scholar] [PubMed]**

282. Wu, D.; Lewis, E.D.; Pae, M.; Meydani, S.N. Nutritional Modulation of Immune Function: Analysis of Evidence, Mechanisms, and Clinical Relevance. *Front. Immunol.* **2018**, *9*, 3160. **[Google Scholar]**

283. Cox, A.J.; Pyne, D.B.; Saunders, P.U.; Fricker, P.A. Oral administration of the probiotic Lactobacillus fermentum VRI-003 and mucosal immunity in endurance athletes. *Br. J. Sports Med.* **2010**, *44*, 222–226. **[Google Scholar] [Green Version]**

284. Gleeson, M.; Bishop, N.C.; Oliveira, M.; Tauler, P. Daily probiotic's (Lactobacillus casei Shirota) reduction of infection incidence in athletes. *Int. J. Sport Nutr. Exerc. Metab.* **2011**, *21*, 55–64. **[Google Scholar] [PubMed]**

285. West, N.P.; Horn, P.L.; Pyne, D.B.; Gebski, V.J.; Lahtinen, S.J.; Fricker, P.A.; Cripps, A.W. Probiotic supplementation for respiratory and gastrointestinal illness symptoms in healthy physically active individuals. *Clin. Nutr.* **2014**, *33*, 581–587. **[Google Scholar] [PubMed] [Green Version]**

286. Michalickova, D.; Minic, R.; Dikic, N.; Andjelkovic, M.; Kostic-Vucicevic, M.; Stojmenovic, T.; Nikolic, I.; Djordjevic, B. Lactobacillus helveticus Lafti L10 supplementation reduces respiratory infection duration in a cohort of elite athletes: A randomized, double-blind, placebo-controlled trial. *Appl. Physiol. Nutr. Metab.* **2016**, *41*, 782–789. **[Google Scholar] [PubMed] [Green Version]**

287. Strasser, B.; Geiger, D.; Schauer, M.; Gostner, J.M.; Gatterer, H.; Burtscher, M.; Fuchs, D. Probiotic Supplements Beneficially Affect Tryptophan-Kynurenine Metabolism and Reduce the Incidence of Upper Respiratory Tract Infections in Trained Athletes: A Randomized, Double-Blinded, Placebo-Controlled Trial. *Nutrients* **2016**, *8*, 752. **[Google Scholar] [Green Version]**

288. Pyne, D.B.; West, N.P.; Cox, A.J.; Cripps, A.W. Probiotics supplementation for athletes-clinical and physiological effects. *Eur. J. Sport Sci.* **2015**, *15*, 63–72. **[Google Scholar]**

289. Colbey, C.; Cox, A.J.; Pyne, D.B.; Zhang, P.; Cripps, A.W.; West, N.P. Upper Respiratory Symptoms, Gut Health and Mucosal Immunity in Athletes. *Sports Med.* **2018**, *48*, 65–77. **[Google Scholar] [Green Version]**

290. West, N.P.; Pyne, D.B.; Cripps, A.W.; Hopkins, W.G.; Eskesen, D.C.; Jairath, A.; Christophersen, C.T.; Conlon, M.A.; Fricker, P.A. Lactobacillus fermentum (PCC®) supplementation and gastrointestinal and respiratory-tract illness symptoms: A randomised control trial in athletes. *Nutr. J.* **2011**, *10*, 30. **[Google Scholar] [Green Version]**

291. Moro-García, M.A.; Alonso-Arias, R.; Baltadjieva, M.; Fernández Benítez, C.; Fernández Barrial, M.A.; Díaz Ruisánchez, E.; Alonso Santos, R.; Alvarez Sánchez, M.; Saavedra Miján, J.; López-Larrea, C. Oral supplementation with Lactobacillus delbrueckii subsp. bulgaricus 8481 enhances systemic immunity in elderly subjects. *Age* **2013**, *35*, 1311–1326. **[Google Scholar]**

292. Makino, S.; Ikegami, S.; Kume, A.; Horiuchi, H.; Sasaki, H.; Orii, N. Reducing the risk of infection in the elderly by dietary intake of yoghurt fermented with Lactobacillus delbrueckii ssp. bulgaricus OLL1073R-1. *Br. J. Nutr.* **2010**, *104*, 998–1006. **[Google Scholar]** **[Green Version]**

293. Guillemard, E.; Tanguy, J.; Flavigny, A.; de la Motte, S.; Schrezenmeir, J. Effects of consumption of a fermented dairy product containing the probiotic Lactobacillus casei DN-114 001 on common respiratory and gastrointestinal infections in shift workers in a randomized controlled trial. *J. Am. Coll. Nutr.* **2010**, *29*, 455–468. **[Google Scholar]** **[PubMed]**

294. Lalia, A.Z.; Dasari, S.; Robinson, M.M.; Abid, H.; Morse, D.M.; Klaus, K.A.; Lanza, I.R. Influence of omega-3 fatty acids on skeletal muscle protein metabolism and mitochondrial bioenergetics in older adults. *Aging* **2017**, *9*, 1096–1129. **[Google Scholar]** **[Green Version]**

295. Costantini, L.; Molinari, R.; Farinon, B.; Merendino, N. Impact of Omega-3 Fatty Acids on the Gut Microbiota. *Int. J. Mol. Sci.* **2017**, *18*, 2645. **[Google Scholar]** **[Green Version]**

# 6 Chapter

# RETURN SKINFOLDS, ALL IS PARDONED: A NARRATIVE REVIEW OF THE EFFICACY OF COMMON BODY COMPOSITION METHODS IN APPLIED SPORTS PRACTICE

## 1. INTRODUCTION: AN OVERVIEW

The evaluation of body composition is standard procedure in numerous sports organizations. Although total body mass (BM) evaluations may be significant in certain contexts, such as weight-classified sports, a comprehensive analysis of body composition, particularly lean mass (LM) and fat mass (FM), provides greater insight for athletes and their coaches. The assessment of fat mass (FM), commonly expressed as the body fat percentage (BF%), is significantly pertinent in various sports, as excess fat mass may be regarded as 'dead weight' when the body counteracts gravitational forces during activities like jumping and running. Although optimizing and evaluating body composition is crucial in elite sports, there is no universally recognized measurement technique. Practitioners frequently choose methods that align with their daily routines rather than possessing a comprehensive understanding of the methodologies and their limitations.

Historically, academics have endeavored to investigate and precisely quantify human anthropometry through various methodologies, from initial cadaver studies to contemporary imaging technologies like dual-energy X-ray absorptiometry (DXA). In anthropometry, the body is frequently categorized into divisions based on conceptual rather than physical distinctions. The two-compartment model is the most straightforward, dividing the body into fat mass (FM) and fat-free mass (FFM), based on the assumption that if one component is measured, the other may be inferred. The three-compartment model comprises bone mineral content (BMC), fat mass (FM), and fat-free mass (FFM), which encompasses all non-mineral tissues, including organs. In contrast, the four-compartment model further include total body water (TBW) [1]. Figure 1 illustrates a graphic representation of the compartment model.

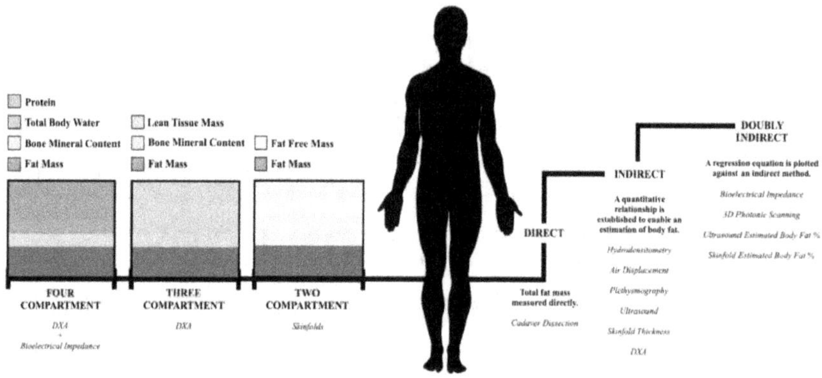


**Figure 1. The 2-, 3- and 4-compartmental models of human body composition (left hand side), alongside the validation hierarchy (right hand side).**

Whilst various methods were developed to measure specific body tissues, cadaveric dissection is the only 'direct' method and therefore less invasive, more practical 'indirect' methods have been developed (**Figure 1**). Indirect methods include hydro-densitometry, which whilst accurate, has limited application in the elite sporting environment, as discussed below. Certain methods are deemed 'doubly indirect' and use predictive regression equations to quantify body composition based on an indirect technique, e.g., skinfold thickness measures with subsequent prediction equations. All of these methods may be deemed 'suitable practice' in specific situations and given there is no gold-standard body composition methodology in free-living individuals, it is crucial that athletes and coaches are fully aware of the various methodologies available and their limitations. Therefore, the aims of this current review are to (1) provide an overview of common methodologies used within sport to measure body composition; (2) compare the efficacy of what is widely believed to be the most valid (DXA) and most practical (skinfold thickness) measurement techniques within applied sports practice; and (3) provide a framework to help select the most appropriate body composition method in applied sports practice.

## 2. MEASUREMENT METHODOLOGIES THAT CAN BE USED IN APPLIED SPORT FOR THE ASSESSMENT OF BODY COMPOSITION

Over the centuries, numerous techniques have been developed and utilised in an attempt to gain a greater understanding of the evaluation of body composition. However, the validity, accuracy, precision and reliability when employing some of these measures can be questionable, with methods often selected based on factors such as expense, safety, portability, invasiveness and requisite expertise for operation, rather than the most suitable for the required assessment. Whilst it is not possible to review every method of assessing body composition, this section will highlight those that have been used in the applied sport environment and critically evaluate their efficacy. Specifically, hydro-densitometry, air displacement plethysmography (ADP), bioelectrical impedance analysis and spectroscopy (BIA and BIS), ultrasound (US), three-dimensional (3D) scanning, DXA and skinfold thickness will be discussed. An overview of these techniques is provided in **Table 1.**

**Table 1. An overview of the different methodologies for assessing body composition in sport. The authors of the current paper met to rate each technique on a number of key consideration based upon the current balance of evidence within the scientific literature.**

| Method of Assessment | Evidence of Reliability | Speed of Measurement | Affordability of the Unit | Ease of Standardisation | Suitability for Sport |
|---|---|---|---|---|---|
| Hydro-Denitrometry (Two-Compartmental Doubly Indirect) | *** | ** | ** | ** | Inappropriate – lack of specialised equipment available and uncomfortable for the athlete |
| Air Displacement Plethysmography (Two-Compartmental Doubly Indirect) | *** | *** | *** | *** | May not be suitable to measure in-season changes to body composition and inappropriate for athletes at extremes of the BMI |
| Bioelectrical Impedance Spectroscopy (Multi-Compartmental Doubly Indirect) | *** | ***** | *** | ** | Useful to detect changes over time but not to measure LBM/ FM and many standardisation factors to consider |
| Ultrasound A-Mode (Single-Compartmental (Doubly) Indirect) | ** | **** | **** | **** | Time and cost effective with good potential application in sport but needs further research |
| 3D Photonic Scanning (Single-Compartmental (Doubly) Indirect) | Data lacking | ***** | *** | Data lacking | Given the lack of data in athletic populations, this method requires further study before being utilized in sport |
| Dual-Energy X-ray Absorptiometry (DXA) (Three-Compartmental Indirect) | ***** | **** | * | ** | Best when segment specific LM changes, or bone density measures are required i.e. following injury or suspected low energy availability. Use heavily dependent on access and available finance with many standardisation factors to consider |
| Skinfold Thickness (Two-Compartmental (Doubly) Indirect) | **** | **** | ***** | ***** | Time and cost effective method to assess FM and track change over time |

Classifications range between 1 * (low) and 5 ***** (high) star ratings. It should be noted that star ratings are based on ideal conditions/equipment, for example taken by an accredited, suitably trained practitioner with the best available equipment. * Low, ** Low-Medium, *** Medium, **** Medium-High, ***** High.

## 2.1. Hydro-Densitometry—Two Compartmental, Indirect

The indirect method of underwater weighing, termed hydro-densitometry, dates back to ~300 BC and uses assumed densities [**2**] and prediction formulae for determination of two-compartmental FFM and FM [**2,3**]. Historically, measures of body density established via underwater weighing have represented the 'criterion' for both accurate and reliable measurement of body composition and as a means for other methods to be validated against [**4**]. Employing the 'Archimedes principle' of measuring body volume, this technique is based upon the understanding that when an object is submerged underwater, the measurement of the 'buoyant force' is deemed to be equal to the weight of the water that it displaces [**5**]. When carried out by a qualified technician, the method can be accurate and reliable. However, limitations include (1) assumption of specific tissue densities, which may differ in elite athletic populations; (2) residual lung volume can be a source of error, given an individual must exhale all of their air whilst remaining static for a stable value; (3) some individuals may become claustrophobic whilst underwater or not be comfortable in water; (4) the equipment is now uncommon and costly, whilst needing to be maintained, sterilised and cleaned regularly; (5) the technique cannot measure distribution of FFM or FM; (6) air can be contained within an individual's swimsuit, skin, head, and/or body hair or internally such as in their digestive tract, all of which can be included in false estimations [**6**]; (7) air temperature, barometric pressure, nitrogen analyser and force sensor calibrations all contain sources of error, which could contribute to the overall measurement error [**7**]; and (8) is time consuming and potentially uncomfortable. Despite the fact that hydro-densitometry has long been considered a criterion assessment of body composition, the emergence of accurate surrogate techniques are now seen as more suitable alternates in applied sport [**8**] and in laboratory-based sport science research [**9,10,11**].

## 2.2. Air Displacement Plethysmography—Two Compartmental, Indirect

Air displacement plethysmography (ADP) is an alternative to hydrostatic weighing and has more practicality in applied sport, where instead of water, air is utilised to measure body density. Some consider ADP to overcome several of the aforementioned limitations of hydro-densitometry [**6**]. Machines such as the BOD POD (COSMED, Rome, ITA), use Poisson's Law to calculate air displacement and thus volumetric calculation. Isothermal air is then measured via inbuilt systems or generated via a prediction formula and combined to calculate a corrected body volume and body composition via numerous predictive equations [**12**]. Correlations of body density to assess validity when compared to hydro-densitometry have been found to be high [**4,13,14**]. Additionally, ADP has a high level of reliability (CV = 1.7 ± 1.1%) [**4**]. Despite these benefits, ADP is (1) insufficiently sensitive to detect in-competition changes in elite athletic body composition [**15**]; (2) sensitive to clothing, body hair, air movement, moisture, pressure and temperature changes [**12,21,22,23**]; and (3) expensive to purchase for those in the applied sports setting. When compared with hydro-densitometry, ADP overestimates BF% by 'at least 1.28%' [**6**]. When estimating adiposity in comparison to DXA, which will be covered later in this review, ADP diverges at the extremes of the BMI spectrum [**24**], which may be a cause for concern when used with certain athletic populations. Additionally, much like the use of hydro-densitometry, ADP is considered to be limited by its lack of ability to differentiate FM distribution, which may be of interest to practitioners. As such, this technique is not commonly used in applied sports practice and is primarily utilised in laboratory-based sport science research.

## 2.3. Bioelectrical Impedance Analysis and Spectroscopy—Multi-Compartmental, Doubly Indirect

Bioelectrical impedance methods are commonly used within general populations for assessment of body composition due to the speed of procedure, minimal expertise required to administer the test, portability and cost in comparison to other approaches. Indeed, it is not uncommon to see such units in gymnasiums and sports clubs. The methods of bioelectrical impedance are categorised by the number of frequencies used for analysis [**25**]. Techniques which are single frequency are commonly referred to as bioelectrical impedance analysis (BIA) devices (i.e., hand to hand), while multiple frequency methods are described as bioelectrical impedance spectroscopy (BIS) devices (i.e., hand and foot contact) [**25**]. BIS methods are considered superior to BIA methods as the calculation of body fluid volumes are based on Cole modelling and mixture theories as opposed to the simple regression equations used by BIA (for a more in-depth review see [**25**]). Despite this, the majority of previous research using bioelectrical impedance cites BIA methods. For both techniques, the currents are generated and measured using electrodes or metal contacts, which send a small voltage through the body to indirectly assess TBW volume. Based on the resistance to current flow observed within the body, FFM has more water and is less resistant than FM, which contains less water and is therefore more resistant. Bioelectrical impedance was previously validated for measuring TBW volume and may also distinguish between intracellular and extracellular fluid compartments [**26,27**]. Nevertheless, this method has several limitations including (1) outputs that can be affected by temperature and hydration status [**28**]; (2) sensitivity to conductive surface of electrodes and electrode placement [**29**]; (3) makes assumptions on the composition of the body in formula and calculations, irrespective of population group [**30**]; and (4) the limbs contribute a large proportion to whole-body impedance, despite the relatively low contribution to overall BM [**31**].

Within athletic populations, there are a limited amount of studies that have assessed the validation of bioelectrical impedance methods to measure FM and FFM, with conflicting findings when compared to DXA. Some investigations reported an underestimation of FM and overestimation of FFM [**32,33,34,35,36**], with others that reported overestimations of FM [37]. There is also large variability between devices [38], alongside large differences in the equations used to estimate body composition, making comparisons highly complex [25]. However, using bioelectrical impedance as a way of assessing change (provided methods are standardised) may be a useful tool [38] and is re-emerging in an applied sport context.

## 2.4. Ultrasound—Multi-Compartmental, Indirect (or Doubly Indirect If Prediction Equations Used)

A relatively new method in the measurement of body composition is ultrasound (US). This method measures uncompressed subcutaneous adipose tissue thickness through US imaging [39] by transmitting a high-frequency beam through the skin at a chosen surface anthropometry site(s) via a handheld transducer head. Once the beam meets an interface (such as subcutaneous fat or muscle tissues) an image is partially echoed back to the transducer, whereby specific types of tissues transmit differing acoustic impedance (i.e., FM content increases the time required for sound reflections off BMC to return to the probe [40]). An image can then be produced from the echo reflected back to the transducer, allowing the integrated software to produce an estimation of the thickness of the tissue (for a more in-depth review see [39]). The use of US can be an accurate measure of subcutaneous adipose tissue; however, it can be altered by (1) the chosen US frequency; (2) pressure and orientation of the probe causing measurement error; (3) the technician's ability to choose the representative sites for measurements. Furthermore, US can be expensive and impractical within the applied setting, even with improved portability. One reported advantage of US is that intra-abdominal fat can be assessed more reliably than anthropometric measures [41], although, whilst this is useful to assess metabolic risk factors for cardiovascular disease, it is not routinely required in applied sport.

With regards to the application of US in applied sport, it is considered a reliable [42] and accurate measure [39] of subcutaneous adipose tissue thickness, but is limited by the plasticity of fat tissue and uneven tissue borders. More recently, Gomes et al. [43] reported US provides similar results for FM in comparison to skinfold and DXA across a range of athletes. However, the aforementioned study used a high-resolution B-mode US unit, which can be time-consuming (>20 min) and requires costly medical devices (>£11,000) along with expensive analysis software (>£1000) [44], that limits the application of such a method in an applied setting. Within an applied context, one of the more widely used methods is A-mode US devices which are commercially available at a considerably lower cost (such as the BodyMetrix® (Intelmetrix, Brentwood, CA, USA) device (<£2000)). However, research on the validity of such devices is at best equivocal, with poor agreeability reported in comparison with DXA in both non-athletic [45,46,47] and athletic young adults [48], and when compared to BOD POD in NCAA Division I athletes [44]. Moreover, Peréz-Chirinos Buxadé and colleagues [49] reported that the A-mode US devices produced significantly lower skinfold thickness scores in comparison with skinfold caliper measures performed by The International Society for the Advancement of Kinanthropometry (ISAK) qualified technicians. In terms of the reliability of A-mode devices, mixed results have been reported, from excellent [**44,50**], to acceptable [**51**] and also poor [**49**]. However, it is important to note there are a range of devices available and results may be specific to the device assessed. It should also be noted that the US method involves converting uncompressed subcutaneous adipose tissue thickness into a percentage body fat using regression equations, which adds another layer of inaccuracy that is discussed in more detail in **Section 3.2**. One advantage of the US device is that it has better inter-rater reliability than skinfolds in novice (non ISAK trained) practitioners [**52**]. Whilst the use of portable US may prove an exciting avenue for assessment of body composition in the future, this requires further development and research to assess the accuracy and reliability of available devices; however, it could be an effective tool to produce repeatable data when there is no access to suitably trained skinfold practitioners (see **Section 2.7**).

## 2.5. 3D Photonic Scanning—One Compatmental, Doubly Indirect

The use of 3D scanners, a form of digital anthropometry, originates from the assessment of human body shape for garment manufacture [**53**]. Three-dimensional scanners are now used for a variety of purposes, including assessment of body composition. Briefly, data with a 3D scanner involves the use of visible and infrared light to create an avatar of the human body, with the subject required to stand still in a particular posture whilst wearing minimal clothing. The reflection of the light off the body allows for a series of points to be captured with triangulation [**54**]. These points are connected to create a 3D mesh, with the use of landmarks to calculate circumferences, volumes, lengths and surface areas (for a more in-depth explanation of data acquisition and processing, see [**55**]). In comparison to DXA and computerised tomography (CT) scans, 3D scanners do not require ionising radiation or principal component analysis, the outcome can be used to create a pseudo-DXA scan [**55**]. The use of 3D scanners is time efficient (a scan takes approx. 10 s), which provides advantages over other time-consuming methods. Theoretically, this method could be employed on a regular basis within athletic populations for frequent assessments of body composition, providing visualisations for retrospective comparisons. Conversely, the cost of using 3D scanners and the operative expertise required may make it a prohibitive method in most applied settings.

The first published data on the use of 3D scanners to assess the body composition of athletes were by Schranz et al. [**56**], who compared elite Australian rowers to age-matched non-athletic controls. They observed elite rowers had greater segmental volumes and cross-sectional areas, variables which cannot be measured with a one compartment method. Therefore, the authors suggested for talent identification purposes, 3D scanning may be implemented in the testing of potential athletes, with the same research group subsequently observing that 3D methods are better than 1D methods for predicting junior rowing performance [**57**]. Evidence exists for the accuracy and reliability of 3D scanning when estimating body composition [**56,58,59,60**], although there are differences between commercially available scanners, which is partly due to the differences in the algorithms used [60]. Indeed, the development and refinement of the most valid algorithm and post-processing technique are still required [61]. Nonetheless, not all data support the validity of 3D scanning [62,63]. Cabre et al. [63] observed high typical errors and significant under and over predicting of BF%, FM and FFM using 3D scans compared to a four component model (combined DXA, ADP and BIS) in a non-athletic population. However, the authors observed no significant differences between 3D and DXA measures. Conversely, Tinsley et al. [60] observed high limits of agreement (LoA) for BF% (7–9.5%) and FM/FFM (5.3–7.2 kg) when compared to a four component model. As these LoA are in excess of expected changes from typical dietary and exercise interventions, longitudinal data that compare 3D scanning to other methods of body composition assessment during interventions aimed to alter body composition are required. In summary, given the expense and lack of athlete-specific validation data, this technique is uncommon in applied sport and is mainly suitable for laboratory-based research.

## 2.6. Dual-Energy X-ray Absorptiometry—Three Compartmental, Indirect

Whilst DXA was first developed for the measurement of bone mineral density (BMD), it has been extensively utilised in athletic populations for the assessment of body composition [11,64,65,66]. Indeed, DXA is now considered by many in the field as the 'criterion standard' of body composition assessment, despite being used in clinical settings for the diagnosis of bone related disorders such as osteoporosis. DXA operates by passing both high and low energy x-ray photons in either a pencil or fan-based beam, through differing body regions. The energy of these beams is attenuated by the density and volume of differing tissues, with soft tissues such as FM and LM allowing greater passage of photons when compared with denser tissues such as bone. The system software then produces an image in a rectilinear fashion and measurements of cross-sectional areas are completed with quantification of FM, LM and BMC in a two-dimensional image, calculated from the coefficient of two differing peaks in order to generate an R-value. For an further in depth description of the technical aspects of DXA measurement in differing systems, readers are directed to a recent review by Bazzocchi and colleagues [67]. Although DXA can be a reliable measure of body composition [68,69], utilisation of this method is not without its limitations, inclusive of legal and ethical constraints and technical considerations that will be discussed in more detail in subsequent sections. The major strength of DXA is the ability to measure BMC, which is growing in importance in due to the increasing awareness of low energy availability and the consequences of this on bone mineral content [70]. Furthermore, DXA provides limb-specific estimations of FM and FFM which can be useful when tracking injured athletes and the magnitude of fat loss in weight-making athletes [9,10].

## 2.7. Skinfold Thickness—Two Compartmental, Indirect (or Doubly Indirect If Prediction Equations Used)

Skinfold thickness assessment involves the use of a caliper to measure a double fold of gripped skin, over a range of differing sites to establish an overall measurement of subcutaneous adiposity [**71**]. This method is an inexpensive technique, requiring minimal equipment (calibrated calipers and anthropometric tape measure), allowing assessment to be conducted in a number of different field-based settings making it a popular method for estimating FM [**71,72**]. Detailed methodology of specific protocols are outlined in a number of texts [**73,74**]. The number of anatomical sites measured and equations used to predict both body density and FM using this technique varies significantly, which can create discrepancies in the data collected. As a consequence, ISAK was founded in 1986 to provide training courses and accreditation worldwide, setting professional standards for using skinfold thickness to assess body composition, with the eight site method now considered by many as best practice in applied sport settings. Although traditionally the most popular and suitable method for field testing, this doubly indirect method was previously deemed unsuitable for the assessment of FFM and estimation of BF% [**30**]. The limitations and practical application of this technique will be covered in more detail in **Section 3**.

# 3. PRACTICAL CONSIDERATIONS WHEN USING DXA AND SKINFOLDS AS MEASURES OF BODY COMPOSITION IN APPLIED SPORT PRACTICE

Although traditionally skinfold thickness measurement has been the most popular method of body composition assessment in applied settings, DXA assessment has become increasingly more common in recent years [**68**], most likely due to a greater availability of machines and a belief that this is now the criterion standard. Despite these methods being used extensively in applied practice, both techniques produce outcomes based on a number of assumptions and require a high degree of standardisation for both accurate and reliable assessment, which is often ignored or not considered in applied sport settings. The following sections will serve to draw attention to these considerations, in the context of an applied sport setting, whilst providing a framework for best practice should these methods be considered and utilised.

## 3.1. DXA

The following practical considerations when using DXA to assess body composition are important to generate valid and reproducible data: (1) machine and software types, (2) legal and ethical considerations and (3) technical standardisation.

### 3.1.1. Machine and Software Types

As highlighted earlier, DXA was originally developed to measure BMD within the general population and therefore quantifies FM and LM as a secondary measure. DXA scanning assesses the composition of photographic pixels, directly distinguishing bone (usually 40–45% of pixels) from other soft tissues (FM and LM). The remaining pixels are used to calculate the remaining soft tissue using a FM:LM ratio [**75**]. Where no bone is present, the ratio of the attenuation of the two beams is linearly proportional to fat within the soft tissue, with this relationship used to estimate FM and LM, respectively [**76**]. There are also variations between manufacturers, such as energy levels emitted, pixel size, beam path, software algorithms and scanning frequencies [**67**].

A further consideration often not considered are both inter-machine and inter-manufacturer variability, causing issues with athletes who are required to travel and may be scanned at different locations. Additionally, even when the same model of DXA machine is used, results may vary significantly between hardware and software version. For example, **Table 2** shows data collected on elite female soccer players assessed on units produced by the same DXA manufacturer, yet with different models. These measurements were made within weeks of each other and despite players reporting with the same total BM, there was an 18% increase in FM and a 4% decrease in LM. Furthermore, the algorithm used within differing software packages can be modified with numerous iterations available for scan analysis, all of which may produce conflicting values. Within the published literature it is not common for authors to report which algorithm they have used for analysis, rather, only the make and model of machinery used. Furthermore, the software on DXA scanning systems often only allow allocation of athletes to a single racial classification, thereby not allowing further options for individuals who may be of multi-ethnic backgrounds. Such issues do not detract from the use of DXA; however, they must be taken into consideration when comparing athletes who may have been scanned at differing sites and even at the same site if the software on the machine has been updated.

**Table 2. Example of the differences observed in practice using real-world data derived from English Premier League and Women's Super League soccer players. This includes using different DXA scanners made by the same company, on the same individuals, alongside an example of the effect of different predictive equations on collected skinfold data.**

| **Real World DXA Data** | | | | | |
|---|---|---|---|---|---|
| Participant & DXA Characteristics | Multi-ethnic backgrounds, Females, Soccer Players ($n$ = 5), Age: 25 ± 5 years, Height: 167.5 ± 4.0 cm | | | | |
| | SCAN 1: QDR Series Discovery A, Hologic Inc., Bedford, MA, Software Version 12.4, Weight: 64.0 ± 7.7 kg | | | | |
| | SCAN 2: QDR Series Horizon A, Hologic Inc., Bedford, MA, Software Version 13.6.0.2, Weight: 64.0 ± 6.8 kg | | | | |
| **Scan Details** | **Fat Mass (kg)** | **Lean Mass (kg)** | **BMC (kg)** | **Body Mass (kg)** | **Body Fat (%)** |
| SCAN 1 | 12.1 ± 2.1 | 50.0 ± 6.1 | 2.9 ± 0.2 | 65.0 ± 7.9 | 18.6 ± 1.7 |
| SCAN 2 | 14.2 ± 2.0 | 48.0 ± 5.1 | 2.8 ± 0.2 | 63.0 ± 10.0 | 21.9 ± 1.6 |

| | Δ Fat Mass (%) | Δ Lean Mass (%) | Δ BMC (%) | Δ Body Mass (%) | Δ Body Fat (%) |
|---|---|---|---|---|---|
| SCAN 1 vs. SCAN 2 | 18.0 | -4.0 | -2.2 | -3.3 | 18.0 |
| **Real World Skinfold Data** | | | | | |
| Participant Characteristics | ATHLETE 1: Caucasian, Male, Soccer Player, Age: 26 years, Height: 180.0 cm, Weight: 79.4 kg, Bicep, 4.0 mm; Tricep, 4.2 mm; Chest, 4.4 mm; Axilla, 5.2 mm; Subscapular, 7.6 mm; Abdominal, 7.4 mm; Supraspinale, 4.6 mm; Iliac Crest, 9.0 mm; Thigh, 4.6 mm; Calf, 4.0 mm. | | | | |
| | ATHLETE 2: Caucasian, Male, Rugby Player, Age: 27 years, Height: 195.5 cm, Weight: 133.7 kg, Bicep, 6.2 mm; Tricep, 8.0 mm; Chest, 14.4 mm; Axilla, 18.4 mm; Subscapular, 25.2 mm; Abdominal, 29.8 mm; Supraspinale, 27.2 mm; Iliac Crest, 31.2 mm; Thigh, 12.5 mm; Calf, 13.4 mm. | | | | |
| **Equation Used** | **Designed For** | **Sites Used** | **Calculation** | **Body Fat (%)** | |
| | | | | **Athlete 1** | **Athlete 2** |
| Durnin & Womersley (1974) [**16**] & Siri (1961) [**17**] | Age Specific Male Population | Biceps, Triceps, Subscapular, Suoprailiac | Body Density = 1.1631 - (0.0632 × Log ΣSF)Body Fat Percentage: ((495/body density) - 450) | 8.2% | 23.1% |
| Jackson & Pollock (1978) [**18**] & Siri (1961) [**17**] | General Male Population | Chest, Abdominal, Thigh | Body Density = 1.10938 - (0.0008267 × ΣSF) + (0.0000016 × $\Sigma SF^2$) - (0.0002574 × age)Body Fat Percentage = ((495/body density) - 450) | 4.3% | 16.6% |
| Jackson & Pollock (1978) [**18**]& Siri (1961) [**17**] | General Male Population | Chest, Axilla, Triceps, Subscapular, Abdominal, Suprailiac, Thigh | Body Density = 1.112 - (0.00043499 × ΣSF) + (0.00000055 × $\Sigma SF^2$) - (0.00028826 × age)Body Fat Percentage = ((495/body density) - 450) | 5.4% | 19.4% |

| | | | | | |
|---|---|---|---|---|---|
| Withers et al., (1987) [19]& Siri (1961) [17] | Athletic Male Population | Biceps, Triceps, Subscapular, Suprailiac, Abdominal, Thigh, Calf | Body Density = 1.0988 - (0.0004 × ΣSF)Body Fat Percentage = ((495/body density) - 450) | 7.3% | 22.2% |
| Reilly et al., (2009) [20] | Athletic Male Soccer Population | Thigh, Abdominal, Triceps, Calf | Body Fat Percentage = 5.174 + (0.124 × Thigh) + (0.147 × Abdominal) + (0.196 × Triceps) + (0.130 × Calf) | 8.2% | 14.4% |

Dual-energy X-ray absorptiometry (DXA); bone mineral content (BMC); skinfolds (SF).

### 3.1.2. Legal and Ethical Considerations

DXA exposes athletes to low radiation doses (ranging between 0.1 and 75 μSy dependent upon manufacturer, model and scan mode used). Considering this in perspective, the effective dose of two of the most widely used commercially available DXA systems (Hologic Discovery A system and GE-Lunar iDXA), which are relatively similar in radiation exposure (4–5 μSy), is less than the average natural daily background radiation experienced (5–8 μSy per day) in the United Kingdom [**67,75,77,78**]. However, due to radiation exposure, there are still legal and ethical constraints surrounding the dose of radiation emitted during DXA scanning (for both athlete and operator), which despite being relatively minimal when compared to other radiographic devices, is a factor that requires consideration. For example, in the United Kingdom, scanning for research purposes requires either ethical approval at a national level (a local ethics committee is not sufficient) or a referral from a qualified medical practitioner. Moreover, whist radiation is low, there is currently considerable debate as to the maximum times per annum this technique can be utilised and it is therefore not suitable if teams wish to assess body composition regularly throughout the season, i.e., monthly. Furthermore, it would also be inappropriate to scan females who may be pregnant.

### 3.1.3. Technical Standardisation Requirements

Despite DXA scanner hardware/software limitations and the legal/ethical considerations, whole-body DXA measurements can be a reliable measure of body composition in athletic populations when standardised protocols are used [**79**], with technical error of measurements of ~0.1% for total mass, ~0.4% for total LM, ~1.9% for total FM and ~0.7% for total BMC [**69**]. Whilst measurements should always be taken from the whole body within the limits of the bed, this can be problematic with athletes such as rugby players, who may be both wider and taller than the bed. Taller athletes cannot always fit within the ~195 cm limit of the scanning area [**80**], which can significantly alter the outcome results. An example of this is indicated in **Table 3**, where a 201 cm tall athlete was placed on the DXA scanner on the same day in a number of positions including head off/feet on, head on/feet off and head and feet on, but with knees bent to 90 degrees. These varying positions altered FM by over 3 kg and total body mass by 7 kg, with BF% ranging from 13.8% to 16.6% (**Table 3**). Indeed, DXA may fail to accurately assess athletes who are often considered within the 'extremes' of physiology, such as tall and extremely muscular athletes. Specifically, historical data have shown issues with those who have a chest depth >25 cm [**81**] and particularly lean athletes, where negative fat values were found for the torso [**82**]. Given that many sports teams often set arbitrary non-discriminatory BF% targets for athletes (often 15% with sanctions in place when this is not achieved), positioning can lead to errors and thus major consequences for the athlete. To date, there is no approved standardisation procedure for tall athletes (in our experience most teams opt for head off feet on) and we would suggest that, as a minimum, this needs to be considered and reproduced for each scan, whilst future studies should establish best practice for such situations.

**Table 3. An example of failure to fit different athletic body types within the confinements of the DXA bed and how this affects results: (a) head on, feet off; (b) head off, feet on; (c) head on, feet on with 90° bend of the knee.**

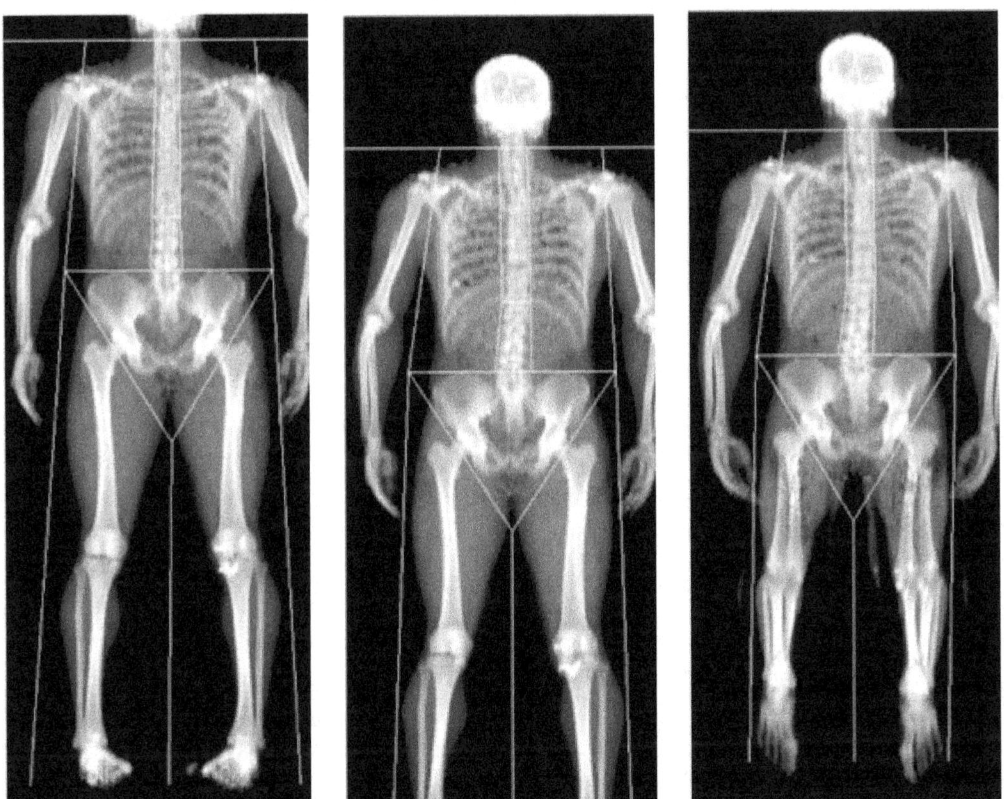

**Head Off/Feet On (A)** **Head On/Feet Off (B)** **Head On/Legs On - 90° Bend (C)**

Characteristics - Caucasian, Male, Age: 35 years, Height: 201.0 cm, Weight: 103.5 kg
DXA - QDR Series Horizon, Hologic Inc., Bedford, MA, USA

| Scan | Fat Mass (kg) | Lean Mass (kg) | BMC (kg) | Body Mass (kg) | Body Fat (%) |
|---|---|---|---|---|---|
| Head Off/Feet On | 13.3 | 79.3 | 4.0 | 96.5 | 13.8 |
| Head On/Feet Off | 16.6 | 79.4 | 4.1 | 103.0 | 16.6 |
| Head On/Legs On | 14.2 | 79.1 | 4.2 | 97.6 | 14.6 |

All measurements collected one after the other by one of the research team. dual-energy X-ray absorptiometry (DXA); bone mineral content (BMC).

**Table 4** summarises a number of emerging technical considerations that must be accounted for and/or controlled to generate reliable DXA body composition data. It is important that athletes have fasted overnight when being scanned, which can be challenging when assessing large squads of individuals [**79**]. Given that a typical DXA scan can take 10–15 min per individual, when testing an entire sporting squad in one day it is possible that some athletes may need to be fasted until the late afternoon, which is often not feasible. Given that it is unusual for a sports team to own their own DXA unit, assessment can involve visiting a local University, which poses challenges when ensuring pre-scanning standardisation procedures. Indeed, studies have suggested that eating a meal can lead to as much as a 2.6% increase in FM [**83**]. Another key consideration is the effect of muscle glycogen on the reliability of DXA body composition measures. It is now common practice for athletes to periodise carbohydrate intake, commencing some training sessions with low and often competing with high muscle glycogen, utilising the 'fuel for the work required' concept [**84,85,86,87**]. Glycogen depletion significantly affects DXA results, with a 2.5% increase in LM when glycogen super compensated [**83**]. Conversely, this could have major implications for athletes who may feel they have lost LM, when in reality they may simply have depleted glycogen stores due to training. Similarly, creatine loading can have major effects on the reliability of the data obtained [**88**]. Other factors to consider include time of day, hydration status and previous exercise activity [**83,89**]. Careful planning is required for the use of DXA to give the best possibility of reproducible data, which from an applied perspective is often difficult to control on a regular basis. Perhaps the strongest example of the effects of diet and exercise on DXA data veracity is in a series of case studies from our research group, summarised in **Table 4.** These reports involved professional combat sport athletes 'making weight' for competition utilising acute weight loss (AWL) strategies, inclusive of the manipulation of carbohydrate intake and hydration status. Post AWL, LM and FM was reduced by 17.5% and 10.4% respectively, across a 4 day period of intense energy and water restriction. These values rebounded by 25.4% and 40.6%, respectively following a two week period of rehydration, refuelling and recovery, inclusive of total cessation of training activity [**9**]. In addition, when assessing another weight making athlete one day prior and following weigh in, LM and FM were both reduced by 4.0% and 5.8%, followed by a 10.0% and 4.6% rebound [**10**]. These values are physiologically impossible and highlight the effects that acute changes in nutrition and exercise status can have on DXA body composition data, further illustrating the importance of pre scan standardisation to enhance reproducibility of the outcome data. It is crucial coaches are aware of these limitations and create conditions where such controls can be implemented. Indeed, if it is not possible to implement such controls, it would seem unethical to subject an athlete to a radiation dose, albeit a very low concentration, if the data produced have limited validity and could result in inaccurate practical outcomes. It could therefore be argued that if it is not necessary to assess BMC and/or limb-specific measurements of FM and FFM, then skinfold thickness measures may provide a suitable and more reliable alternate in free-living conditions. Where using DXA as a technique to measure body composition, it is imperative to ensure standardised, best practice protocols are followed **[69]** and all information considered within the Committee on Medical Aspects of Radiation in the Environment's (COMARE) report considered **[90]**.

**Table 4. A summary of differences in DXA scan results over the course of a habitual day [83]; following creatine supplementation [88]; exercise activity [89]; glycogen storage [88]; rapid weight loss and gain [9,10]; dual-energy X-ray absorptiometry (DXA); bone mineral content (BMC).**

<table>
<tr><td>[83]</td><td colspan="6">Characteristics - Race Unknown, Males, Age: 28 ± 6 years, Height: 178.0 ± 6.0 cm, Weight: 75.0 ± 9.0 kg, DXA: Lunar Prodigy, GE Healthcare, Madison, WI, USA</td></tr>
<tr><td>[89]</td><td colspan="6">Characteristics - Race Unknown, Males, Age: 30 ± 6 years, Height: 178.6 ± 6.0 cm, Weight: 80.6 ± 10.2 kg, DXA: Lunar Prodigy, GE Healthcare, Madison, WI, USA</td></tr>
<tr><td>[88]</td><td colspan="6">Characteristics - Race Unknown, Males, Age: 31 ± 6 years, Height: 182.7 ± 7.2 cm, Weight: 78.2 ± 8.8 kg, DXA: Lunar Prodigy, GE Healthcare, Madison, WI, USA</td></tr>
<tr><td>[9]</td><td colspan="6">Characteristics - Caucasian, Male, Age: 22 years, Height: 180.0 cm, Weight: 75.8 kg, DXA: QDR Series Horizon, Hologic Inc., Bedford, MA, USA</td></tr>
<tr><td>[10]</td><td colspan="6">Characteristics - Caucasian, Male, Age: 19 years, Height: 166.0 cm, Weight: 72.5 kg, DXA: QDR Series Horizon, Hologic Inc., Bedford, MA, USA</td></tr>
<tr><th>Effect of:</th><th>Δ Fat Mass (%)</th><th>Δ Lean Mass (%)</th><th>Δ BMC (%)</th><th>Δ Body Mass (%)</th><th>Δ Body Fat (%)</th><th>Reference</th></tr>
<tr><td colspan="7">Experimental Research Derived Data</td></tr>
<tr><td>No Intervention (Immediate Retest)</td><td>-0.4</td><td>0.0</td><td>0.3</td><td>0.0</td><td>0.1</td><td>[83]</td></tr>
<tr><td>Habitual Day (Am To Pm, ~12H)</td><td>-1.7</td><td>0.8</td><td>0.3</td><td>0.4</td><td>0.3</td><td>[83]</td></tr>
<tr><td>Habitual Day (Am To Am, ~24H)</td><td>-0.6</td><td>-0.2</td><td>-0.2</td><td>-0.2</td><td>0.1</td><td>[83]</td></tr>
<tr><td>Meal Consumption</td><td>2.6</td><td>1.5</td><td>0.4</td><td>1.5</td><td>-0.2</td><td>[83]</td></tr>
</table>

| | | | | | | |
|---|---|---|---|---|---|---|
| Exercise Activity | 0.2 | 0.4 | 0.0 | 0.4 | -0.3 | [**89**] |
| Creatine Loading | 0.4 | 1.1 | 0.0 | 1.3 | 3.3 | [**88**] |
| Glycogen Depletion | -0.2 | -1.1 | 0.0 | -1.3 | -2.0 | [**88**] |
| Glycogen Loading | 0.5 | 1.8 | 0.0 | 2.3 | 4.5 | [**88**] |
| Glycogen & Creatine Loading | 0.6 | 2.5 | 0.0 | 3.0 | 5.2 | [**88**] |
| **Case Study Derived Data** | | | | | | |
| Rapid Weight Depletion (Time Course: 4D) | -10.4 | -17.5 | -3.1 | -12.7 | 3.8 | [**9**] |
| Rapid Weight Depletion (Time Course: 1D) | -5.8 | -4.0 | -0.8 | -2.8 | 0.0 | [**10**] |
| Rapid Weight Regain (Time Course: 1D) | 4.6 | 10.0 | 0.0 | 4.5 | 5.5 | [**10**] |
| Rapid Weight Regain (Time Course: 14D) | 40.6 | 25.4 | -2.1 | 26.3 | 10.9 | [**9**] |

## 3.2. Skinfold Thickness Assessment

Despite the aforementioned simplicity of skinfold measurement, which makes this method popular within applied settings, there are a number of technical limitations that must be considered when employing this technique. Initially, there is an assumption of constant skin thickness and compressibility in the double fold between differing intra and inter individual measurement sites. This is also affected by the grip of the practitioner and the applied pressure of the caliper, and an athlete's age, sex and skin temperature. However, skinfold assessment has also been shown to be the least affected method by everyday activities, ingestion of a meal and changes in hydration status [**79,91**]. To that end, the experience of the anthropometrist is crucial in obtaining accurate skinfold data. From our own experiences and previous reports, as little as a 1 cm difference in the assessed measurement site can have significant effects on the outcome data [**92**]. Even with ISAK-accredited practitioners, it is not uncommon to see large discrepancies in assessment outcomes, particularly in larger athletes, which can create issues when multiple testers perform the measurements across groups of individuals.

A key issue when utilising skinfold thickness in the applied setting is the desire for FM measurements to be reported as a BF%, which adds another layer of complexity and turns an indirect method into doubly indirect. Doubly-indirect methods incorporate regression equations by plotting results against a criterion standard to create an estimate of composition. The conundrum with these regression equations is there are currently over one hundred such formulae for the estimation of BF% from skinfold thickness measurements alone [**73**], and these equations have not yet been validated when tracking regular changes in body composition [93]. These formulae are also established across varying populations, using numerous protocols, with deviations in sites measured and often have intra-practitioner and criterion variability and reliability issues. This can be characterised by the use of different equations on the same set of individual data producing resounding differences (as highlighted in **Table 2**), where data on a Caucasian male soccer player resulted in ranges between 4 and 8% body fat dependent upon the equation used. Therefore, the conversion of skinfold thickness into a BF% should be discouraged with data presented as a sum of the 8 skinfold sites providing a more accurate and reliable outcome of body composition assessment [20,94,95]. Indeed, the sum of skinfold thicknesses has a high degree of agreement with whole-body measures from DXA [96]. However, there are some considerations with this approach. Firstly, it is not possible to further estimate FFM, which is often useful information for those in the field. The second problem is that many coaches are not familiar with being given data as a 'sum of mm' and often still request relativiseddata. This is compounded by limited normative data of 8 skinfold measures in athletes and thus coaches can be somewhat confused when presented with such information. We therefore present a set of normative data taken from applied practitioners working in the field, which we believe can help to address this problem (**Table 5**). Finally, even in ISAK-accredited practitioners, it is not uncommon to see sum of 4, 7 or 8 sites reported. This can cause confusion and make it difficult to compare data. If the field is to move away from percentage values then it is important that a widely accepted methodology is adopted, which we would suggest is the standard ISAK sum of 8 sites as presented in **Table 4**.

**Table 5. Overview of Σ8 skinfold ranges (mm) in a variety of sports (data compiled from personal communications with peers working in elite performance). Lower, middle and upper ranges suggested are based upon typical values measured in elite sport although it must be stressed that attributing performance to skinfold measures is difficult to establish.**

| | Males | | | Females | | |
|---|---|---|---|---|---|---|
| | Lower | Middle | Upper | Lower | Middle | Upper |
| Combat Athletes | 35–40 | 40–55 | 55–65 | 45–50 | 50–65 | 65–75 |
| Cricket Batsmen | 45–55 | 55–65 | 65–70 | 90–100 | 100–120 | 120–140 |
| Cricket Bowlers | 40–50 | 50–60 | 60–70 | 75–80 | 80–100 | 100–120 |
| Distance Running | 30–40 | 40–45 | 45–55 | 40–55 | 55–70 | 70–85 |
| Field Hockey | 35–40 | 40–55 | 55–65 | 50–65 | 65–80 | 80–90 |
| Football | 40–45 | 45–55 | 55–65 | 60–65 | 65–75 | 75–85 |
| Road Cycling | 30–35 | 35–40 | 40–50 | – | – | – |
| Rowing Lightweight | 30–35 | 35–45 | 45–55 | 40–45 | 45–50 | 50–55 |
| Rowing Openweight | 35–45 | 45–60 | 60–70 | 55–65 | 65–80 | 80–95 |
| Rugby Backs | 40–45 | 45–60 | 60–75 | 55–60 | 60–70 | 70–80 |
| Rugby Forwards | 40–55 | 55–70 | 70–90 | 65–70 | 70–80 | 80–95 |

| | Males | | | Females | | |
|---|---|---|---|---|---|---|
| | Lower | Middle | Upper | Lower | Middle | Upper |
| Rugby 7s | 45–50 | 50–65 | 65–75 | – | – | – |
| Swimming | 40–45 | 45–55 | 55–65 | 55–70 | 70–80 | 80–95 |
| Tennis | 40–45 | 45–55 | 55–65 | 50–55 | 55–65 | 65–75 |

## 4. CONCISE SUMMARY

Although body composition measurement is a standard procedure in applied sports contexts, the methodologies employed for this evaluation seem to lack uniformity. Each method examined in this analysis possesses distinct advantages and disadvantages, and may occasionally be regarded as 'best practice' in particular athletic contexts and for specific inquiries. Figure 2 illustrates a schematic representation of the relevant factors to consider when selecting the optimal approach for analyzing body composition. We recommend that when BMC requires evaluation or when limb-specific measurements of FM and FFM are essential, DXA is the preferred assessment technology, provided that pre-scan circumstances can be regulated as previously stated. Nonetheless, considering the straightforwardness of the skinfold approach, the rapidity of its implementation and evaluation, the frequency of its use, and the little costs involved with the procedure. For the purpose of monitoring variations in body fat over time, one could contend that skinfold measurements, when expressed as a cumulative millimeter value rather than a relative percentage, may offer the most effective answer. Considering that skinfold assessments are the least influenced by uncontrollable factors in athletes (such as dietary intake, hydration levels, and daily activity), it may be appropriate to reinstate their use in applied sports practice, stating, 'Welcome back, skinfolds; all is forgiven.'

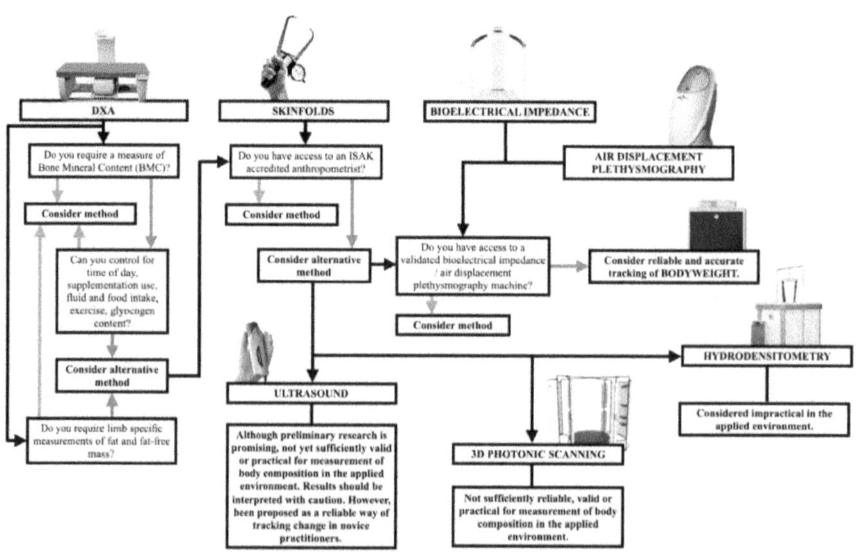


**Figure 2. A proposed body composition method decision-making tree. Evidence base and applicability of all methods should be considered within the specific context in which**

**they are being applied, be conducted by a suitably accredited/trained individual with all risks managed and should deliberate all points made throughout the current article prior to application of the chosen method. Green arrows indicate yes as the answer, red arrows indicate no as the answer, and black arrows indicate the potential flow of questioning when considering different methods of anthropometrical assessment.**

## AT A GLANCE

Although the evaluation of body composition is standard in sports, there is significant contention on the most effective instruments, with the selected method being determined by convenience rather than a comprehension of the technique and its constraints. The objective of this paper was threefold: (1) Present an overview of prevalent methodologies employed in sports to assess body composition, specifically hydro-densitometry, air displacement plethysmography, bioelectrical impedance analysis and spectroscopy, ultrasound, three-dimensional scanning, dual-energy X-ray absorptiometry (DXA), and skinfold thickness; (2) evaluate the effectiveness of what are commonly regarded as the most accurate (DXA) and practical (skinfold thickness) assessment tools; and (3) offer a framework for selecting the most suitable assessment in applied sports practice, incorporating insights from the authors' experiences in elite sports. Historically, skinfold thickness has been the predominant method for assessing body composition; nevertheless, the utilization of DXA has surged in recent years, with a widely accepted assumption that it represents the criteria standard. DXA is the preferred method for assessing bone mineral content and for obtaining limb-specific estimations of fat and fat-free mass. However, it is essential to consider the logistical constraints necessary for generating reliable data, such as regulating food intake, prior exercise, and hydration status. Nevertheless, in light of the necessity for simplicity and after evaluating the evidence from all assessment techniques, skinfold measurements seem to be the least influenced by daily variability, resulting in the conclusion, 'return to skinfolds, everything is forgiven.'

## REFERENCES

1. Behnke, A.R.; Wilmore, J.H. *Evaluation and Regulation of Body Build and Composition*; International Research Monograph Series in Physical Education; Prentice-Hall: Englewood Cliffs, NJ, USA, 1974. **[Google Scholar]**
2. Siri, W.E. Body Composition from Fluid Spaces and Density: Analysis of Methods. *Nutr. Burbank Los Angel. Cty. Calif.* **1993**, *9*, 480–491. **[Google Scholar]**
3. Brožek, J.; Grande, F.; Anderson, J.T.; Keys, A. Densitometric analysis of body composition: Revision of some quantitative Assumptions. *Ann. N. Y. Acad. Sci.* **2006**, *110*, 113–140. **[Google Scholar]**
4. McCrory, M.A.; Gomez, T.D.; Bernauer, E.M.; Molé, P.A. Evaluation of a New Air Displacement Plethysmograph for Measuring Human Body Composition. *Med. Sci. Sports Exerc.* **1995**, *27*, 1686–1691. **[Google Scholar]** **[PubMed]** **[Green Version]**
5. Stewart, D.M. The Role of Tension in Muscle Growth A2. In *Regulation of Organ and Tissue Growth*; Academic Press: Cambridge, MA, USA, 1972; pp. 77–100. **[Google Scholar]**

6. Gibby, J.T.; Njeru, D.K.; Cvetko, S.T.; Heiny, E.L.; Creer, A.R.; Gibby, W.A. Whole-Body Computed Tomography–Based Body Mass and Body Fat Quantification: A Comparison to Hydrostatic Weighing and Air Displacement Plethysmography. *J. Comput. Assist. Tomogr.* **2017**, *41*, 302–308. **[Google Scholar]**

7. Biaggi, R.R.; Vollman, M.W.; Nies, M.A.; Brener, C.E.; Flakoll, P.J.; Levenhagen, D.K.; Sun, M.; Karabulut, Z.; Chen, K.Y. Comparison of Air-Displacement Plethysmography with Hydrostatic Weighing and Bioelectrical Impedance Analysis for the Assessment of Body Composition in Healthy Adults. *Am. J. Clin. Nutr.* **1999**, *69*, 898–903. **[Google Scholar] [PubMed] [Green Version]**

8. Schubert, M.M.; Seay, R.F.; Spain, K.K.; Clarke, H.E.; Taylor, J.K. Reliability and Validity of Various Laboratory Methods of Body Composition Assessment in Young Adults. *Clin. Physiol. Funct. Imaging* **2019**, *39*, 150–159. **[Google Scholar]**

9. Kasper, A.M.; Crighton, B.; Langan-Evans, C.; Riley, P.; Sharma, A.; Close, G.L.; Morton, J.P. Case Study: Extreme Weight Making Causes Relative Energy Deficiency, Dehydration, and Acute Kidney Injury in a Male Mixed Martial Arts Athlete. *Int. J. Sport Nutr. Exerc. Metab.* **2019**, *29*, 331–338. **[Google Scholar] [Green Version]**

10. Langan-Evans, C.; Germaine, M.; Artukovic, M.; Oxborough, D.L.; Areta, J.L.; Close, G.L.; Morton, J.P. The Psychological and Physiological Consequences of Low Energy Availability in a Male Combat Sport Athlete. *Med. Sci. Sports Exerc.* **2020. [Google Scholar]**

11. Milsom, J.; Naughton, R.; O'Boyle, A.; Iqbal, Z.; Morgans, R.; Drust, B.; Morton, J.P. Body Composition Assessment of English Premier League Soccer Players: A Comparative DXA Analysis of First Team, U21 and U18 Squads. *J. Sports Sci.* **2015**, *33*, 1799–1806. **[Google Scholar]**

12. Higgins, P.B.; Fields, D.A.; Hunter, G.R.; Gower, B.A. Effect of Scalp and Facial Hair on Air Displacement Plethysmography Estimates of Percentage of Body Fat. *Obesity* **2001**, *9*, 326–330. **[Google Scholar] [PubMed] [Green Version]**

13. Wagner, D.R.; Heyward, V.H.; Gibson, A.L. Validation of Air Displacement Plethysmography for Assessing Body Composition. *Med. Sci. Sports Exerc.* **2000**, *32*, 1339–1344. **[Google Scholar]**

14. Levenhagen, D.K.; Borel, M.J.; Welch, D.C.; Piasecki, J.H.; Piasecki, D.P.; Chen, K.Y.; Flakoll, P.J. A Comparison of Air Displacement Plethysmography with Three Other Techniques to Determine Body Fat in Healthy Adults. *J. Parenter. Enter. Nutr.* **1999**, *23*, 293–299. **[Google Scholar]**

15. Eston, R.; Reilly, T. *Kinanthropometry and Exercise Physiology Laboratory Manual: Volume One: Anthropometry and Volume Two*; Exercise Physiology: Ottawa, ON, Canada, 2003. **[Google Scholar]**

16. Durnin, J.V.G.A.; Womersley, J. Body fat assessed from total body density and its estimation from skinfold thickness: Measurements on 481 men and women aged from 16 to 72 years. *Br. J. Nutr.* **1974**, *32*, 77–97. **[Google Scholar] [Green Version]**

17. Siri, W.E. Body composition from fluid spaces and density: Analysis of methods. In *Techniques for Measuring Body Compositions*; Brozek, J., Henschel, A., Eds.; National Academy of Sciences: Washington, DC, USA, 1961; pp. 223–244. **[Google Scholar]**

18. Jackson, A.S.; Pollock, M.L. Generalized equations for predicting body density of men. *Br. J. Nutr.* **1978**, *40*, 497–504. **[Google Scholar] [PubMed] [Green Version]**

19. Withers, R.T.; Craig, N.P.; Bourdon, P.C.; Norton, K. Relative body fat and anthropometric prediction of body density of male athletes. *Eur. J. Appl. Physiol. Occup. Physiol.* **1987**, *56*, 191–200. **[Google Scholar]**

20. Reilly, T.; George, K.; Marfell-Jones, M.; Scott, M.; Sutton, L.; Wallace, J. How Well Do Skinfold Equations Predict Percent Body Fat in Elite Soccer Players? *Int. J. Sports Med.* **2009**, *30*, 607–613. **[Google Scholar] [PubMed]**

21. Fields, D.A.; Higgins, P.B.; Hunter, G.R. Assessment of Body Composition by Air-Displacement Plethysmography: Influence of Body Temperature and Moisture. *Dyn. Med.* **2004**, *3*, 3. **[Google Scholar] [Green Version]**

22. Fields, D.; Hunter, G.; Goran, M. Validation of the BOD POD with Hydrostatic Weighing: Influence of Body Clothingin. *Int. J. Obes.* **2000**, *24*, 200–205. **[Google Scholar] [PubMed] [Green Version]**

23. Peeters, M.W.; Claessens, A.L. Effect of Different Swim Caps on the Assessment of Body Volume and Percentage Body Fat by Air Displacement Plethysmography. *J. Sports Sci.* **2011**, *29*, 191–196. **[Google Scholar]**

24. Lowry, D.W.; Tomiyama, A.J. Air Displacement Plethysmography versus Dual-Energy X-ray Absorptiometry in Underweight, Normal-Weight, and Overweight/Obese Individuals. *PLoS ONE* **2015**, *10*, e0115086. **[Google Scholar] [Green Version]**

25. Moon, J.R. Body Composition in Athletes and Sports Nutrition: An Examination of the Bioimpedance Analysis Technique. *Eur. J. Clin. Nutr.* **2013**, *67*, S54–S59. **[Google Scholar] [Green Version]**

26. Matias, C.N.; Santos, D.A.; Júdice, P.B.; Magalhães, J.P.; Minderico, C.S.; Fields, D.A.; Lukaski, H.C.; Sardinha, L.B.; Silva, A.M. Estimation of Total Body Water and Extracellular Water with Bioimpedance in Athletes: A Need for Athlete-Specific Prediction Models. *Clin. Nutr.* **2016**, *35*, 468–474. **[Google Scholar]**

27. Moon, J.R.; Stout, J.R.; Smith, A.E.; Tobkin, S.E.; Lockwood, C.M.; Kendall, K.L.; Graef, J.L.; Fukuda, D.H.; Costa, P.B.; Stock, M.S.; et al. Reproducibility and Validity of Bioimpedance Spectroscopy for Tracking Changes in Total Body Water: Implications for Repeated Measurements. *Br. J. Nutr.* **2010**, *104*, 1384–1394. **[Google Scholar] [PubMed] [Green Version]**

28. Koulmann, N.; Jimenez, C.; Regal, D.; Bolliet, P.; Launay, J.-C.; Savourey, G.; Melin, B. Use of Bioelectrical Impedance Analysis to Estimate Body Fluid Compartments after Acute Variations of the Body Hydration Level. *Med. Sci. Sports Exerc.* **2000**, *32*, 857–864. **[Google Scholar]**

29. Baumgartner, R.N.; Chumle, C.; Roche, A.F. Bioelectric Impedance for Body Composition. *Exerc. Sport Sci. Rev.* **1990**, *18*, 193–224. **[Google Scholar] [PubMed]**

30. Ackland, T.R.; Lohman, T.G.; Sundgot-Borgen, J.; Maughan, R.J.; Meyer, N.L.; Stewart, A.D.; Müller, W. Current Status of Body Composition Assessment in Sport: Review and Position Statement on Behalf of the Ad Hoc Research Working Group on Body Composition Health and Performance, Under the Auspices of the I.O.C. Medical Commission. *Sports Med.* **2012**, *42*, 227–249. **[Google Scholar] [PubMed]**

31. Coppini, L.Z.; Waitzberg, D.L.; Campos, A.C.L. Limitations and Validation of Bioelectrical Impedance Analysis in Morbidly Obese Patients. *Curr. Opin. Clin. Nutr. Metab. Care* **2005**, *8*, 329–332. **[Google Scholar]**

32. Syed-Abdul, M.M.; Soni, D.S.; Barnes, J.T.; Wagganer, J.D. Comparative Analysis of BIA, IBC, and DXA for Determining Body Fat in American Football Players. *J. Sports Med. Phys. Fitness* **2021**. **[Google Scholar]**

33. Svantesson, U.; Zander, M.; Klingberg, S.; Slinde, F. Body Composition in Male Elite Athletes, Comparison of Bioelectrical Impedance Spectroscopy with Dual Energy X-ray Absorptiometry. *J. Negat. Results Biomed.* **2008**, *7*, 1. **[Google Scholar] [PubMed] [Green Version]**

34. Pichard, C.; Kyle, U.G.; Gremion, G.; Gerbase, M.; Slosman, D.O. Body Composition by X-ray Absorptiometry and Bioelectrical Impedance in Female Runners. *Med. Sci. Sports Exerc.* **1997**, *29*, 1527–1534. **[Google Scholar]**

35. Hartmann Nunes, R.F.; de Souza Bezerra, E.; Orssatto, L.B.; Moreno, Y.M.; Loturco, I.; Duffield, R.; Silva, D.A.; Guglielmo, L.G. Assessing Body Composition in Rugby Players: Agreement between Different Methods and Association with Physical Performance. *J. Sports Med. Phys. Fitness* **2020**, *60*. **[Google Scholar]**

36. Esco, M.R.; Olson, M.S.; Williford, H.N.; Lizana, S.N.; Russell, A.R. The Accuracy of Hand-to-Hand Bioelectrical Impedance Analysis in Predicting Body Composition in College-Age Female Athletes. *J. Strength Cond. Res.* **2011**, *25*, 1040–1045. **[Google Scholar] [PubMed]**

37. Houtkooper, L.B.; Mullins, V.A.; Going, S.B.; Brown, C.H.; Lohman, T.G. Body Composition Profiles of Elite American Heptathletes. *Int. J. Sport Nutr. Exerc. Metab.* **2001**, *11*, 162–173. **[Google Scholar]** **[Green Version]**

38. Carrion, B.M.; Wells, A.; Mayhew, J.L.; Koch, A.J. Concordance Among Bioelectrical Impedance Analysis Measures of Percent Body Fat in Athletic Young Adults. *Int. J. Exerc. Sci.* **2019**, *12*, 324–331. **[Google Scholar]**

39. Müller, W.; Horn, M.; Fürhapter-Rieger, A.; Kainz, P.; Kröpfl, J.M.; Maughan, R.J.; Ahammer, H. Body Composition in Sport: A Comparison of a Novel Ultrasound Imaging Technique to Measure Subcutaneous Fat Tissue Compared with Skinfold Measurement. *Br. J. Sports Med.* **2013**, *47*, 1028–1035. **[Google Scholar]**

40. Wagner, D.R. Ultrasound as a Tool to Assess Body Fat. *J. Obes.* **2013**, *2013*, 1–9. **[Google Scholar]** **[PubMed]**

41. Stolk, R.P.; Meijer, R.; Mali, W.P.; Grobbee, D.E.; van der Graaf, Y.; on behalf of the Secondary Manifestations of Arterial Disease (SMART) Study Group. Ultrasound Measurements of Intraabdominal Fat Estimate the Metabolic Syndrome Better than Do Measurements of Waist Circumference. *Am. J. Clin. Nutr.* **2003**, *77*, 857–860. **[Google Scholar]** **[Green Version]**

42. Müller, W.; Horn, M.; Fürhapter-Rieger, A.; Kainz, P.; Kröpfl, J.M.; Ackland, T.R.; Lohman, T.G.; Maughan, R.J.; Meyer, N.L.; Sundgot-Borgen, J.; et al. Body Composition in Sport: Interobserver Reliability of a Novel Ultrasound Measure of Subcutaneous Fat Tissue. *Br. J. Sports Med.* **2013**, *47*, 1036–1043. **[Google Scholar]** **[PubMed]**

43. Gomes, A.C.; Landers, G.J.; Binnie, M.J.; Goods, P.S.R.; Fulton, S.K.; Ackland, T.R. Body Composition Assessment in Athletes: Comparison of a Novel Ultrasound Technique to Traditional Skinfold Measures and Criterion DXA Measure. *J. Sci. Med. Sport* **2020**, *23*, 1006–1010. **[Google Scholar]**

44. Wagner, D.R.; Cain, D.L.; Clark, N.W. Validity and Reliability of A-Mode Ultrasound for Body Composition Assessment of NCAA Division I Athletes. *PLoS ONE* **2016**, *11*, e0153146. **[Google Scholar]** **[PubMed]**

45. Baranauskas, M.N.; Johnson, K.E.; Juvancic-Heltzel, J.A.; Kappler, R.M.; Richardson, L.; Jamieson, S.; Otterstetter, R. Seven-Site versus Three-Site Method of Body Composition Using BodyMetrix Ultrasound Compared to Dual-Energy X-ray Absorptiometry. *Clin. Physiol. Funct. Imaging* **2017**, *37*, 317–321. **[Google Scholar]**

46. Johnson, K.E.; Miller, B.; Gibson, A.L.; McLain, T.A.; Juvancic-Heltzel, J.A.; Kappler, R.M.; Otterstetter, R. A Comparison of Dual-Energy X-ray Absorptiometry, Air Displacement Plethysmography and A-Mode Ultrasound to Assess Body Composition in College-Age Adults. *Clin. Physiol. Funct. Imaging* **2017**, *37*, 646–654. **[Google Scholar]**

47. Loenneke, J.P.; Barnes, J.T.; Wagganer, J.D.; Wilson, J.M.; Lowery, R.P.; Green, C.E.; Pujol, T.J. Validity and Reliability of an Ultrasound System for Estimating Adipose Tissue. *Clin. Physiol. Funct. Imaging* **2014**, *34*, 159–162. **[Google Scholar]**

48. Loenneke, J.P.; Barnes, J.T.; Wagganer, J.D.; Pujol, T.J. Validity of a Portable Computer-Based Ultrasound System for Estimating Adipose Tissue in Female Gymnasts. *Clin. Physiol. Funct. Imaging* **2014**, *34*, 410–412. **[Google Scholar]**

49. Pérez-Chirinos Buxadé, C.; Solà-Perez, T.; Castizo-Olier, J.; Carrasco-Marginet, M.; Roy, A.; Marfell-Jones, M.; Irurtia, A. Assessing Subcutaneous Adipose Tissue by Simple and Portable Field Instruments: Skinfolds versus A-Mode Ultrasound Measurements. *PLoS ONE* **2018**, *13*, e0205226. **[Google Scholar]** **[PubMed]**

50. Kopinski, S.; Engel, T.; Cassel, M.; Fröhlich, K.; Mayer, F.; Carlsohn, A. Ultrasound Applied to Subcutaneous Fat Tissue Measurements in International Elite Canoeists. *Int. J. Sports Med.* **2015**, *36*, 1134–1141. **[Google Scholar]** **[PubMed]**

51. Ribeiro, G.; de Aguiar, R.A.; Penteado, R.; Lisbôa, F.D.; Raimundo, J.A.G.; Loch, T.; Meira, Â.; Turnes, T.; Caputo, F. A-Mode Ultrasound Reliability in Fat and Muscle Thickness Measurement. *J. Strength Cond. Res.* **2020**. **[Google Scholar] [PubMed]**

52. Wagner, D.R.; Teramoto, M. Interrater Reliability of Novice Examiners Using A-Mode Ultrasound and Skinfolds to Measure Subcutaneous Body Fat. *PLoS ONE* **2020**, *15*, e0244019. **[Google Scholar] [PubMed]**

53. Stewart, A.D. Kinanthropometry and Body Composition: A Natural Home for Three-Dimensional Photonic Scanning. *J. Sports Sci.* **2010**, *28*, 455–457. **[Google Scholar]**

54. Eder, M.; Brockmann, G.; Zimmermann, A.; Papadopoulos, M.A.; Schwenzer-Zimmerer, K.; Zeilhofer, H.F.; Sader, R.; Papadopulos, N.A.; Kovacs, L. Evaluation of Precision and Accuracy Assessment of Different 3-D Surface Imaging Systems for Biomedical Purposes. *J. Digit. Imaging* **2013**, *26*, 163–172. **[Google Scholar] [PubMed] [Green Version]**

55. Heymsfield, S.B.; Bourgeois, B.; Ng, B.K.; Sommer, M.J.; Li, X.; Shepherd, J.A. Digital Anthropometry: A Critical Review. *Eur. J. Clin. Nutr.* **2018**, *72*, 680–687. **[Google Scholar]**

56. Schranz, N.; Tomkinson, G.; Olds, T.; Daniell, N. Three-Dimensional Anthropometric Analysis: Differences between Elite Australian Rowers and the General Population. *J. Sports Sci.* **2010**, *28*, 459–469. **[Google Scholar]**

57. Schranz, N.; Tomkinson, G.; Olds, T.; Petkov, J.; Hahn, A.G. Is Three-Dimensional Anthropometric Analysis as Good as Traditional Anthropometric Analysis in Predicting Junior Rowing Performance? *J. Sports Sci.* **2012**, *30*, 1241–1248. **[Google Scholar]**

58. Medina-Inojosa, J.; Somers, V.K.; Ngwa, T.; Hinshaw, L.; Lopez-Jimenez, F. Reliability of a 3D Body Scanner for Anthropometric Measurements of Central Obesity. *Obes. Open Access* **2016**, *2*. **[Google Scholar]**

59. Adler, C.; Steinbrecher, A.; Jaeschke, L.; Mähler, A.; Boschmann, M.; Jeran, S.; Pischon, T. Validity and Reliability of Total Body Volume and Relative Body Fat Mass from a 3-Dimensional Photonic Body Surface Scanner. *PLoS ONE* **2017**, *12*, e0180201. **[Google Scholar] [PubMed] [Green Version]**

60. Tinsley, G.M.; Moore, M.L.; Benavides, M.L.; Dellinger, J.R.; Adamson, B.T. 3-Dimensional Optical Scanning for Body Composition Assessment: A 4-Component Model Comparison of Four Commercially Available Scanners. *Clin. Nutr.* **2020**, *39*, 3160–3167. **[Google Scholar]**

61. Chiu, C.-Y.; Pease, D.L.; Fawkner, S.; Dunn, M.; Sanders, R.H. Comparison of Automated Post-Processing Techniques for Measurement of Body Surface Area from 3D Photonic Scans. *Comput. Methods Biomech. Biomed. Eng. Imaging Vis.* **2019**, *7*, 227–234. **[Google Scholar]**

62. Harbin, M.M.; Kasak, A.; Ostrem, J.D.; Dengel, D.R. Validation of a Three-Dimensional Body Scanner for Body Composition Measures. *Eur. J. Clin. Nutr.* **2018**, *72*, 1191–1194. **[Google Scholar]**

63. Cabre, H.E.; Blue, M.N.M.; Hirsch, K.R.; Brewer, G.J.; Gould, L.M.; Nelson, A.G.; Smith-Ryan, A.E. Validity of a Three-Dimensional Body Scanner: Comparison Against a 4-Compartment Model and Dual Energy X-ray Absorptiometry. *Appl. Physiol. Nutr. Metab.* **2020**. **[Google Scholar] [PubMed]**

64. Deutz, R.C.; Benardot, D.; Martin, D.E.; Cody, M.M. Relationship between Energy Deficits and Body Composition in Elite Female Gymnasts and Runners. *Med. Sci. Sports Exerc.* **2000**, *32*, 659–668. **[Google Scholar] [PubMed]**

65. Bilsborough, J.C.; Kempton, T.; Greenway, K.; Cordy, J.; Coutts, A.J. Longitudinal Changes and Seasonal Variation in Body Composition in Professional Australian Football Players. *Int. J. Sports Physiol. Perform.* **2017**, *12*, 10–17. **[Google Scholar]**

66. Bartlett, J.D.; Hatfield, M.; Parker, B.B.; Roberts, L.A.; Minahan, C.; Morton, J.P.; Thornton, H.R. DXA-Derived Estimates of Energy Balance and Its Relationship with Changes in Body Composition across a Season in Team Sport Athletes. *Eur. J. Sport Sci.* **2020**, *20*, 859–867. **[Google Scholar] [PubMed]**

67. Bazzocchi, A.; Ponti, F.; Albisinni, U.; Battista, G.; Guglielmi, G. DXA: Technical Aspects and Application. *Eur. J. Radiol.* **2016**, *85*, 1481–1492. **[Google Scholar]**

68. Nana, A.; Slater, G.J.; Stewart, A.D.; Burke, L.M. Methodology Review: Using Dual-Energy X-ray Absorptiometry (DXA) for the Assessment of Body Composition in Athletes and Active People. *Int. J. Sport Nutr. Exerc. Metab.* **2015**, *25*, 198–215. **[Google Scholar]**

69. Nana, A.; Slater, G.J.; Hopkins, W.G.; Halson, S.L.; Martin, D.T.; West, N.P.; Burke, L.M. Importance of Standardized DXA Protocol for Assessing Physique Changes in Athletes. *Int. J. Sport Nutr. Exerc. Metab.* **2016**, *26*, 259–267. **[Google Scholar]** **[PubMed]**

70. Sale, C.; Elliott-Sale, K.J. Nutrition and Athlete Bone Health. *Sports Med.* **2019**, *49* (Suppl. S2), 139–151. **[Google Scholar]** **[Green Version]**

71. Martin, A.D.; Ross, W.D.; Drinkwater, D.T.; Clarys, J.P. Prediction of Body Fat by Skinfold Caliper: Assumptions and Cadaver Evidence. *Int. J. Obes.* **1985**, *9* (Suppl. S1), 31–39. **[Google Scholar]**

72. Meyer, N.L.; Sundgot-Borgen, J.; Lohman, T.G.; Ackland, T.R.; Stewart, A.D.; Maughan, R.J.; Smith, S.; Müller, W. Body Composition for Health and Performance: A Survey of Body Composition Assessment Practice Carried out by the Ad Hoc Research Working Group on Body Composition, Health and Performance under the Auspices of the IOC Medical Commission. *Br. J. Sports Med.* **2013**, *47*, 1044–1053. **[Google Scholar]** **[PubMed]**

73. Lohman, T.G.; Roche, A.F. (Eds.) *Anthropometric Standardization Reference Manual*; Human Kinetics Books: Champaign, IL, USA, 1988. **[Google Scholar]**

74. Stewart, A.; Sutton, L. (Eds.) *Body Composition in Sport, Exercise, and Health*; Routledge: London, UK, 2012. **[Google Scholar]**

75. Toombs, R.J.; Ducher, G.; Shepherd, J.A.; De Souza, M.J. The Impact of Recent Technological Advances on the Trueness and Precision of DXA to Assess Body Composition. *Obesity* **2012**, *20*, 30–39. **[Google Scholar]** **[PubMed]**

76. Laskey, M.A. Dual-Energy X-ray Absorptiometry and Body Composition. *Nutrition* **1996**, *12*, 45–51. **[Google Scholar]**

77. Hawkinson, J.; Timins, J.; Angelo, D.; Shaw, M.; Takata, R.; Harshaw, F. Technical White Paper: Bone Densitometry. *J. Am. Coll. Radiol.* **2007**, *4*, 320–327. **[Google Scholar]** **[PubMed]**

78. Boudousq, V.; Goulart, D.M.; Dinten, J.M.; de Kerleau, C.C.; Thomas, E.; Mares, O.; Kotzki, P.O. Image Resolution and Magnification Using a Cone Beam Densitometer: Optimizing Data Acquisition for Hip Morphometric Analysis. *Osteoporos. Int.* **2005**, *16*, 813–822. **[Google Scholar]**

79. Kerr, A.; Slater, G.J.; Byrne, N. Impact of Food and Fluid Intake on Technical and Biological Measurement Error in Body Composition Assessment Methods in Athletes. *Br. J. Nutr.* **2017**, *117*, 591–601. **[Google Scholar]** **[PubMed]**

80. Nana, A.; Slater, G.J.; Hopkins, W.G.; Burke, L.M. Techniques for Undertaking Dual-Energy X-ray Absorptiometry Whole-Body Scans to Estimate Body Composition in Tall and/or Broad Subjects. *Int. J. Sport Nutr. Exerc. Metab.* **2012**, *22*, 313–322. **[Google Scholar]**

81. Jebb, S.A.; Goldberg, G.R.; Elia, M. DXA Measurements of Fat and Bone Mineral Density in Relation to Depth and Adiposity. In *Human Body Composition*; Ellis, K.J., Eastman, J.D., Eds.; Springer: Boston, MA, USA, 1993; pp. 115–119. **[Google Scholar]**

82. Stewart, A.D.; Hannan, W.J. Prediction of Fat and Fat-Free Mass in Male Athletes Using Dual X-ray Absorptiometry as the Reference Method. *J. Sports Sci.* **2000**, *18*, 263–274. **[Google Scholar]** **[PubMed]**

83. Nana, A.; Slater, G.J.; Hopkins, W.G.; Burke, L.M. Effects of Daily Activities on Dual-Energy X-ray Absorptiometry Measurements of Body Composition in Active People. *Med. Sci. Sports Exerc.* **2012**, *44*, 180–189. **[Google Scholar]** **[Green Version]**

84. Morehen, J.C.; Bradley, W.J.; Clarke, J.; Twist, C.; Hambly, C.; Speakman, J.R.; Morton, J.P.; Close, G.L. The Assessment of Total Energy Expenditure During a 14-Day In-Season Period of Professional Rugby League Players Using the Doubly Labelled Water Method. *Int. J. Sport Nutr. Exerc. Metab.* **2016**, *26*, 464–472. **[Google Scholar] [Green Version]**

85. Anderson, L.; Orme, P.; Naughton, R.J.; Close, G.L.; Milsom, J.; Rydings, D.; O'Boyle, A.; Di Michele, R.; Louis, J.; Hambly, C.; et al. Energy Intake and Expenditure of Professional Soccer Players of the English Premier League: Evidence of Carbohydrate Periodization. *Int. J. Sport Nutr. Exerc. Metab.* **2017**, *27*, 228–238. **[Google Scholar]**

86. Impey, S.G.; Hearris, M.A.; Hammond, K.M.; Bartlett, J.D.; Louis, J.; Close, G.L.; Morton, J.P. Fuel for the Work Required: A Theoretical Framework for Carbohydrate Periodization and the Glycogen Threshold Hypothesis. *Sports Med.* **2018**, *48*, 1031–1048. **[Google Scholar] [Green Version]**

87. Maughan, R.J.; Depiesse, F.; Geyer, H. The Use of Dietary Supplements by Athletes. *J. Sports Sci.* **2007**, *25* (Suppl. S1), S103–S113. **[Google Scholar]**

88. Bone, J.L.; Ross, M.L.; Tomcik, K.A.; Jeacocke, N.A.; Hopkins, W.G.; Burke, L.M. Manipulation of Muscle Creatine and Glycogen Changes Dual X-ray Absorptiometry Estimates of Body Composition. *Med. Sci. Sports Exerc.* **2017**, *49*, 1029–1035. **[Google Scholar] [PubMed] [Green Version]**

89. Nana, A.; Slater, G.J.; Hopkins, W.G.; Burke, L.M. Effects of Exercise Sessions on DXA Measurements of Body Composition in Active People. *Med. Sci. Sports Exerc.* **2013**, *45*, 178–185. **[Google Scholar] [PubMed] [Green Version]**

90. Martin, C.; de Vocht, F.; Kadhim, M.; Currell, K.; Brooke-Wavell, K.; Dunn, M.; Smith, F.; Kemp, R.; Chell, I. Medical Radiation Dose Issues Associated with Dual-Energy X-ray Absorptiometry (DXA) Scans for Sports Performance Assessments and Other Non-Medical Practices. 18th Report. 2019. Available online: **https://assets.publishing.service.gov.uk/government/uploads/system/uploads/attachment_data/file/817530/Committee_on_Medical_Aspects_of_Radiation_in_the_Environment_COMARE_18th_report.pdf** (accessed on 22 February 2021).

91. Norton, K.; Olds, T.; Dolman, J. Kinanthropometry VI: Proceedings of the sixth scientific conference of the International Society for the Advancement of Kinanthropometry. *Adelaide, 13–16 October 1998.* Available online: **https://trove.nla.gov.au/nbdid/22043824** (accessed on 22 February 2021).

92. Hume, P.; Marfell-Jones, M. The Importance of Accurate Site Location for Skinfold Measurement. *J. Sports Sci.* **2008**, *26*, 1333–1340. **[Google Scholar] [PubMed]**

93. Silva, A.M.; Fields, D.A.; Quitério, A.L.; Sardinha, L.B. Are Skinfold-Based Models Accurate and Suitable for Assessing Changes in Body Composition in Highly Trained Athletes? *J. Strength Cond. Res.* **2009**, *23*, 1688–1696. **[Google Scholar] [PubMed]**

94. Johnston, F.E. Relationships between Body Composition and Anthropometry. *Hum. Biol.* **1982**, *54*, 221–245. **[Google Scholar]**

95. Kerr, D.; Stewart, A. Body Composition in Sport. *Appl. Anat. Biomech. Sports Ed. Ackland TR Elliott BC Bloom. J.* **2009**, *2*, 67–81. **[Google Scholar]**

96. Doran, D.; Mc Geever, S.; Collins, K.; Quinn, C.; McElhone, R.; Scott, M. The Validity of Commonly Used Adipose Tissue Body Composition Equations Relative to Dual Energy X-ray Absorptiometry (DXA) in Gaelic Games Players. *Int. J. Sports Med.* **2013**, *35*, 95–100. **[Google Scholar]**

# 8 Chapter

# MECHANISMS AND EFFECTIVENESS OF CREATINE SUPPLEMENTATION, PHYSICAL EXERCISE, AND OXIDATIVE STRESS MARKERS

## 1. INTRODUCTION: AN OVERVIEW

Many athletes have utilized ergogenic aids to maintain fitness, improve recovery, and physiological adaptations in long-term exercise programs. Therefore, the effects of ergogenic aids have always attracted a lot of attention, and many researchers have tried to combine exercise programs and ergogenic aids to enhance the benefits of exercise [**1,2**].

One of the favorite ergogenic supplements among athletes (at all levels) is creatine. Studies have shown that creatine supplementation combined with resistance training had a higher effectiveness in training and increased muscle strength and lean mass [**1,2**]. As a popular creatine supplement in the sports and fitness industry, it is believed that creatine supplementation helps maintain high-energy phosphate stores during exercise. Moreover, specific mechanisms of creatine supplementation have been identified in improving athletic performance [**3,4**]; there are ambiguities about its effects on oxidative stress and its mechanism of action. The antioxidant effects of creatine may be due to various functional mechanisms, such as indirect mechanisms involved in the cell membrane stabilization and improvement of cellular energy capacity [**5**] and its direct antioxidant properties [**6**]. Oxidative stress reduces strength and performance [**7**]; mechanically, reactive oxygen species (ROS) can speed up skeletal muscle fatigue by reducing calcium sensitivity [**8**] and can decrease maximal calcium-activated force [**9**]. ROS are free radical molecules that can oxidatively alter cellular compounds such as lipids, proteins, and DNA, and damage cells [**10**]. They are also associated with several diseases such as cancer, cardiovascular disease, Parkinson's, Alzheimer's, etc. [**11**]. Increased ROS production due to certain diseases or exercise can exceed the capacity of the antioxidant system, which can lead to oxidative stress and dysfunction. However, its predominant impact on the human health and function is still controversial [12].

One of the common physiological conditions associated with the enhancement of oxidative stress is exercise [13,14]. Exercise can have positive and negative effects on oxidative stress [15]. High-intensity exercise can lead to a temporary imbalance between the active oxygen/nitrogen species production and removal, which can lead to oxidative stress. Although exercise-induced ROS is required for the production of natural force in the muscles, high levels of ROS appear to cause contractile dysfunction [16]. Exercise-induced ROS production is important for exercise-induced mitochondrial biogenesis [17], because ROS are used as signaling molecules to activate redox-sensitive signaling pathways [16]. Evidence suggests that exercise intensity and duration are associated with oxidative stress in humans, and has been confirmed by several studies [18,19]. Intense exercise or exercise in untrained people is associated with a greater increase in oxidative stress compared to moderate and regular aerobic exercise [20]. In addition, long-term regular training may improve some antioxidant defense mechanisms, and thus may limit mitochondrial oxidative damage [21,22].

Using antioxidant supplements along with physical activity can reduce the harmful effects of oxidative stress caused by exercise, increase the antioxidant defense system associated with exercise and increase the positive effects of physical activity. Creatine is one of the most popular supplements for athletes; it can act as a cellular energy buffer, increase creatine phosphate (CrP) and adenosine triphosphate (ATP) regeneration [23]; additionally, creatine compounds can have different effects. It seems that creatine has significant antioxidant effects. In general, the purpose of this study was to investigate the available information on the effects of endurance, resistance, and combination exercise along with the creatine supplementation on oxidative stress and their mechanism of action. Therefore, the present study tried to summarize the available information and research on the effects of creatine supplement consumption and physical exercise on oxidative stress and how it works, together with the mechanisms of action.

## 2. MATERIALS AND METHODS

A search was conducted in the MEDLINE, PubMed, Scopus, Directory of Open Access Journals, and Science Direct databases, guided by the research objective. The keywords employed were physical activity, creatine supplementation, and oxidative stress. We concentrated on English papers published between 2008 and 2020. Figure 1 illustrates that initially, 341 publications were examined. Following the elimination of duplicates and articles irrelevant to the research aims via multiple stages, 8 papers were chosen for comprehensive analysis of their findings. Following the selection of papers and the examination of their conclusions regarding physical activity and creatine supplementation, data was gathered with an emphasis on the research objectives (Figure 1).

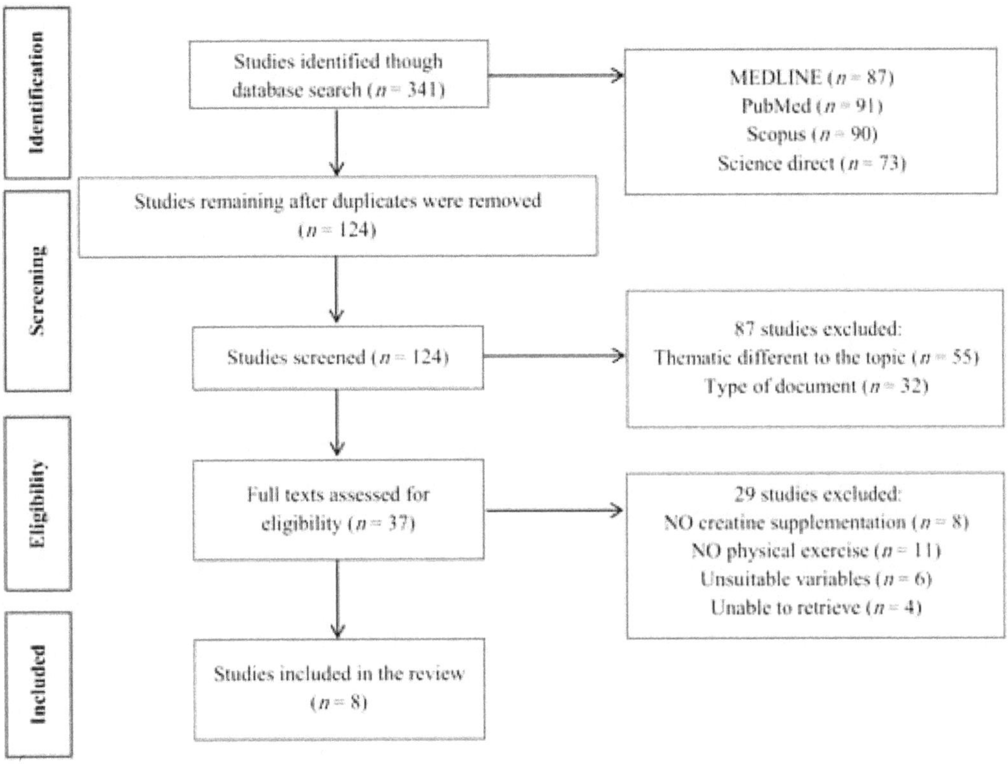


**Figure 1. Flowchart of the study selection.**

## 3. OXIDATIVE STRESS

Oxidative stress is an enclosed physiological pathway regulated by the antioxidant mechanisms. Improper regulation of oxidative stress is correlated with several recurrent pathological or physiological conditions [**14**]. Oxidative stress can be defined as an imbalance between the generation of harmful free radicals and their removal by the antioxidant defense system. Highly reactive unstable free radicals are composed of many compounds. However, the most common are ROS (superoxide, hydroxile, alcoxile, peroxile, hydrogen peroxide) and reactive nitrogen species (RNS) (nitric oxide, nitrogen dioxide, peroxinitrile); collectively called reactive oxygen and nitrogen species (RONS) [**24**]. Free radicals are very reactive atoms or molecules that have one or more unpaired electrons in their outer shell and can be formed by the interaction of oxygen with specific molecules [**25**]. These radicals are produced by the loss or acceptance of an electron in cells, therefore behaving as the oxidants or reductants [**26**]. The endogenous sources of RONS consist of: nicotinamide adenine dinucleotide phosphate (NADPH) oxidase, myeloperoxidase (MPO), lipoxygenase, and angiotensin II [**27**]. External sources of RONS are air pollution, tobacco, alcohol, drugs, industrial solvents, etc., which are metabolized to free radicals in the body [**28**].

NADPH oxidase is a common source of the superoxide anion ($O_2^-$) formed by the reduction of one electron of the molecular oxygen by electrons supplied by the NADPH during cellular respiration. Most $O_2^-$ is catalyzed by superoxide dismutase (SOD) to hydrogen peroxide ($H_2O_2$) [**29**]. $H_2O_2$ is not a free radical because it has no unpaired electrons, but via the Fenton or Haber-Weiss reaction, it is able to form very reactive hydroxyl radicals ($OH^-$). Hydroxyl radicals are highly reactive and react especially with phospholipids in cell membranes and proteins [**30**].

Too much RONS can cause irreversible damage to the biological molecules, proteins, carbohydrates, lipids, RNA and DNA, leading to the spread of many pathological problems and oxidative tissue damage [**31**]. Antioxidant systems suitable with enzymatic (e.g., SOD, catalase (CAT) and glutathione peroxidase (GPX)) and non-enzymatic (e.g., uric acid, bilirubin, vitamin E, vitamin C, glutathione (GSH), ascorbic acid, and α-tocopherol) processes, both act to reduce the oxidation potential of RONS through direct and indirect mechanisms. Direct antioxidants activate redox reactions and trap and inactivate RONS in a process that is sacrificed and must be regenerated [**32**]. On the other hand, indirect antioxidants may or may not be redox-active and apply their antioxidant effects via the up-regulation of cytoprotective proteins [**32**].

The ROS involve many physiological functions. The intracellular concentration of ROS increases transiently in response to a stimulus such as cytokines, growth factors, or other hormones; this pattern is common in many physiological conditions, where the release of ROS is quickly controlled by the antioxidant regulatory mechanisms. If stable or unbalanced, increased oxidative stress may suppress antioxidant capabilities, and the ROS can cause damage [**14**]. The ROS release is involved in major cellular signaling pathways and allows the transmission of extracellular stimuli and changes in cell physiology by modulating the transcription of some genes or by post-transcriptional modulation. To date, "redox-responsive" signaling pathways have been implicated in important functions such as nitric oxide (NO) generation, vascular tone regulation and neurotransmission, cell adhesion, immune responses, and hypoxia and apoptosis [**11,33**].

## 4. CREATINE AND OXIDATIVE STRESS

Creatine is a metabolite of three amino acids (arginine, glycine, and methionine) that are synthesized by the cooperation of various organs, including the liver, pancreas, and kidneys [**34**]. Beef is a rich source of arginine, glycine and methionine. In contrast, all plant-based foods contain small amounts of glycine and methionine, and most plant foods (except soy, peanuts, and other nuts) also contain small amounts of arginine [**35**]. The beginning of creatine synthesis is by arginine; the guanidino group from arginine to glycine is transferred by glycine amidinotransferase, and produces guanidinoacetate and ornithine (**Figure 2**). It seems that the arginine-glycine aminotransferase is fundamentally expressed in the kidney tubules, pancreas, and a little in the liver and other organs. Thus, guanidineacetate is produced by renal components. The guanidinoacetate released by the kidneys is methylated by guanidinoacetate N-methyltransferase, which is mainly found in the liver, pancreas, and to a very small extent in the kidneys, and produces creatine [**36**].

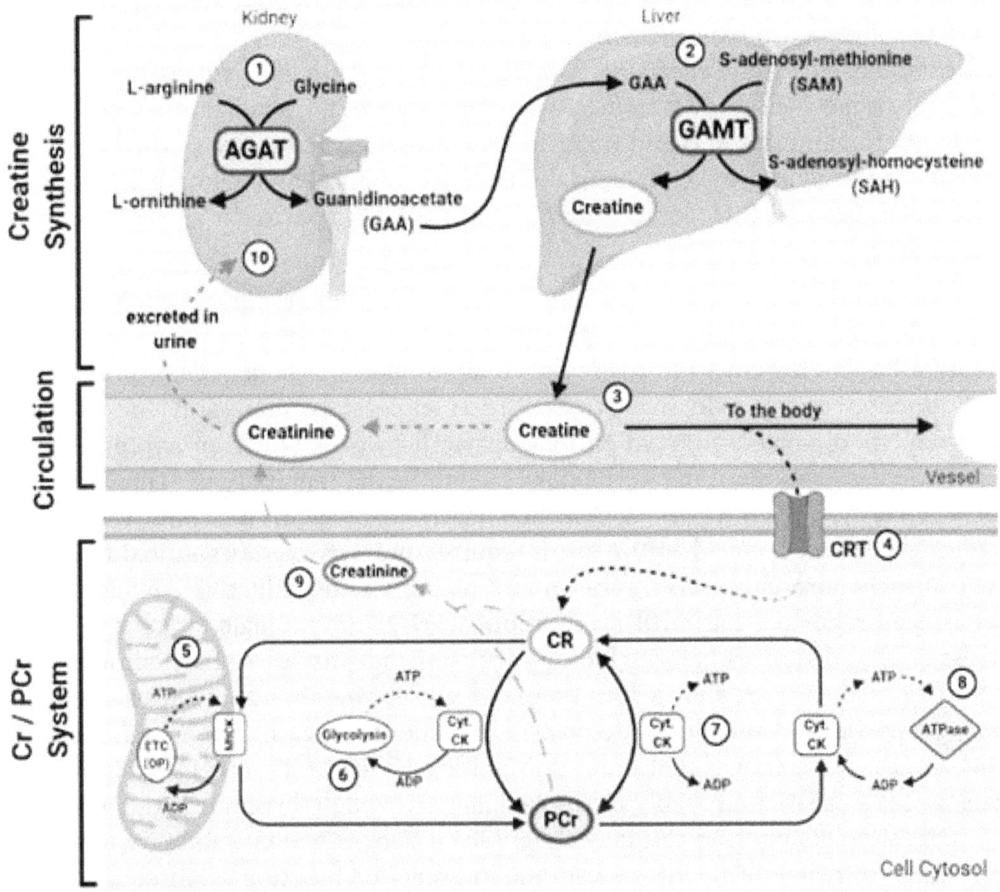


**Figure 2. Physiological structure of creatine. Adopted from Clarke et al. [41]. L-arginine: glycine amidinotransferase (AGAT); anidinoacetate N-methyltransferase (GAMT); phosphocreatine (PCr); cytosolic creatine kinase (Cyt. CK); electron transport chain (ETC); adenosine diphosphate (ADP); mitochondrial creatine kinase (mtCK); and adenosine triphosphate (ATP).**

Creatine synthesis is primarily regulated as follows: (1) changes in the renal arginine expression: glycine aminotransferase in rats and humans; and (2) the availability of substrates. Dietary creatine intake and circulating growth hormone (GH) levels are major factors influencing new creatine synthesis [**36**]. Creatine supplements and GHs do not affect the hepatic activity of guanidinoacetate N-methyltransferase in animals. Thus, a creatine supplement helps to store arginine, glycine, and methionine for use through other vital metabolic pathways such as protein synthesis, NO, and glutathione. This is of great nutritional and physiological importance [**34,37**].

Studies have shown that creatine supplementation can have antioxidant properties. The first evidence of creatine-like antioxidant activity was reported by Matthews et al. [**13**]. They stated that creatine supplementation could protect rats against nitropropionic acid intoxication (an animal model of Huntington's disease). Moreover,

Hosamani et al. showed a reduction in mitochondrial oxidative damage induced by rotenone and neurotoxicty in Drosophila melanogaster when supplemented with creatine [**38**]. The exact mechanism of action of creatine antioxidant is not known. However, it has been shown to increase the activity of antioxidant enzymes and the capability to eliminate ROS and RONS [**6,13,39**]. Furthermore, 90% of the body's total creatine is stored in the skeletal muscle, and mitochondria are an important source of ROS, which includes $H_2O_2$ and $O_2^-$, and possibly $OH^-$ and peroxynitrite in the skeletal muscle [**40**].

Creatine protects two different and important cellular targets, mitochondrial deoxyribonucleic acid (mtDNA) and RNA against oxidative damage. In addition, creatine has been shown to cause other related effects that help the cell to survive and function under oxidative stress. Creatine possibly maintains mitochondrial integrity via organelle-directed antioxidant activity [**42**], which promotes adequate mitochondrialogenesis, and provides a significant amount of thiol contents intracellularly, preventing the RNA from oxidative damage in situations where robust messenger ribonucleic acid (mRNA) use is required and thus exerts its antioxidant effects [**42**]. Mitochondria and mtDNA are important targets for oxidative damage. Indeed, it has been reported that mtDNA mutations work as an etiologic factor in oxidative stress-related disorders [**43**], including cardiovascular disease, inherited or acquired neurological disorders, and various types of tumors. Mitochondrial antioxidants have been proposed as a valuable tool to protect mitochondria against pathological changes [**44**]. Studies have shown that creatine significantly protects mtDNA from oxidative damage [**42**]. Creatine probably prevents damage through direct antioxidant activity. Thus, its supplementation can play a significant role in genome stability, which can normalize mitochondrial mutagenesis and intercept its functional consequences such as reduced oxygen consumption, mitochondrial membrane potential, ATP content, and cell survival [**45,46**].

Furthermore, RNA molecules interfere with all stages of gene expression and several other biological activities. RNA damage can also affect the balance between protein breakdown and synthesis and the repair and regeneration processes in the skeletal muscle that ultimately determine muscle mass [**46**]. RNA damage can be related to exposure to xenobiotics [**46**]. The protective effect of creatine against doxorubicin activity, which causes RNA damage, can be attributed in part to the production of CrP sources that increase ATP regeneration. Creatine's protective activity against radicals also points to its role as an antioxidant [**47**]. Creatine also increases the expression of myogenic transcriptional regulators (MRFs) and IGF-1 mRNAs [**48,49**] and increases CrP sources [**50**]. In the case of non-muscle tissue, empirical reports suggested that creatine mightplay a significant role in the differentiation and function of the central nervous system (CNS) neurons. For example, creatine can act as an exocytosis transmitter by nerve cells [**51**] and adjust gamma-aminobutyric acid (GABA) receptors (inhibitory [**52**] or stimulant [**53**]). It is worth noting that the GABA receptor activity plays a main role in the neuronal differentiation [**46**]. A study by Young et al. showed that mitochondrial reductase and cytoplasm (peroxiredoxin-4, a type 2 peroxiredoxin 2 and thioredoxin-dependent peroxide reductase) were increased in the creatine-treated cells [**54**]. Incremental regulation of these enzymes may also effectively help several protective effects. Studies have shown that creatine helps cells function and survive under oxidative stress, especially in the differentiation of myoblasts [**46**].

In addition, the antioxidant properties of creatine may be related to the presence of arginine in its molecule. Arginine is a substrate of the NO synthase family and can enhance NO generation (a free radical that modulates metabolism, contraction, and glucose uptake into the skeletal muscle) [**55**]. Other amino acids such as glycine and methionine may be particularly sensitive to the oxidation of free radicals due to the presence of sulfhydryl groups (**Figure 3**) [**56**].

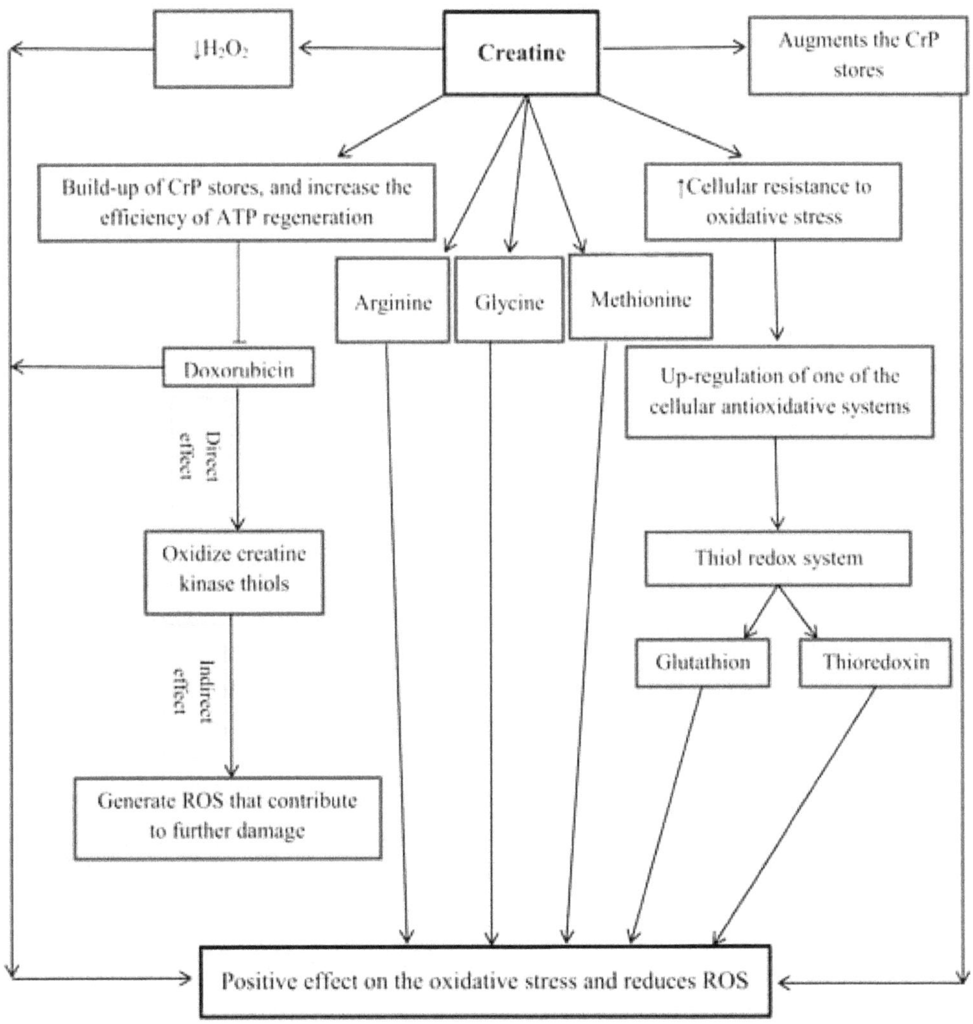


**Figure 3. The effect of creatine on oxidative stress. Hydrogen peroxide ($H_2O_2$); creatine phosphate (CrP); adenosine triphosphate (ATP); and reactive oxygen species (ROS).**

## 5. THE IMPACT OF PHYSICAL EXERCISE ON OXIDATIVE STRESS

Physical workouts are typically categorized into two primary types: endurance exercises and resistance exercises. Endurance or extreme aerobic exercise is known to induce reactive oxygen species and overproduce active nitrogen species due to heightened metabolism, resulting in oxidative stress and associated damage. [**57**]. Aerobic exercise is estimated to increase $O_2^-$ 1–3-fold during muscle contraction [**58**]. However, mitochondria account for only a small fraction of $O_2^-$ production during aerobic exercise [**58,59**]. In fact, mitochondrial-derived $O_2^-$ formation in the skeletal muscle decreases during the exercise relative to the rest. This is because contractile activity changes the redox state in the muscles to a more oxidative state and reduces the NADH/NAD ratio in the mitochondria. Decrease in the NADH/NAD ratio is related to decreased release of I-dependent $O_2^-$ [**58**]. During the endurance exercise, ATP is broken down into adenosine diphosphate (ADP) to release energy and support continuous muscle contraction. In some situations, adenosine monophosphate (AMP) is formed, and by a biochemical process involving xanthine oxidase (XO) it can be broken down into hypoxanthine, xanthine, and uric acid. The XO, using molecular oxygen, stimulates the formation of $O_2^-$ and thus exacerbates oxidative stress [**60**]. In addition, special precautions should be taken for exercise in people with conditions such as asthma; asthma can cause significant ROS and oxidative stress, therefore it can jeopardize the benefits of exercise [**61**].

Although a period of intense aerobic training may cause oxidative damage to muscle fibers, regular aerobic exercise helps increase the cells' ability to reduce ROS over-accumulation [**62**]. Regular moderate-intensity exercise has been shown to increase the activity of endogenous antioxidant enzymes such as SOD, GPX, and CAT [**63**]. The body's protection facing chronic low-to-moderate ROS exposure occurs via exercise through elementary conditioning relevant to the redox consisting of repair systems acting as the oxidative damage [**62,64**]. This adaptation through moderate-intensity exercise also includes an increase in the myocellular antioxidant capacity, which helps reduce the ROS levels [**65**]. In addition, increasing the ROS formation in the active skeletal muscle by modulating muscle contraction plays an essential role in the adaptation to exercise [**62,63**]. For example, endurance running is considered important for survival in human development because it can stimulate exercise-related contractile responses through metabolic and redox challenges [**62,66**]. However, current lifestyles caused reduced physical activity and inhibits human adaptation capacity in redox metabolism and homeostasis [**62**]. Basic evidence has shown that at least 30 min of exercise (moderate intensity) each day is essential to maintain good health and decrease the potential risks of disease [**65**].

Accordingly, Zarrindast et al. stated that moderate-intensity aerobic training for eight weeks on the land and water reduces oxidative stress and improves antioxidant status [**67**]. Moreover, Done et al. concluded that regular aerobic exercise increases resistance to oxidative stress [**68**]. Estébanez et al. showed that aerobic exercise does not cause significant changes in the oxidative stress biomarkers among the elderly

[69]. In addition, Leelarungrayub et al. reported that moderate-intensity aerobic dance for six weeks could reduce malondialdehyde (MDA) and increase total antioxidant capacity (TAC) among inactive women [70]. In general, moderate to intermittent ROS production during a short period of aerobic training program can activate signaling pathways that lead to cellular adaptation and protection against subsequent stresses. In contrast, moderate levels of ROS production over a long period of time (e.g., several hours) or high levels generated during high-intensity short-term training can lead to tissue and structural damage [69].

Despite the need for less oxygen during resistance activities compared to aerobic exercise, the generation of free radicals during the resistance exercise is significant and results from the XO pathway, respiratory burst of neutrophils, catecholamine autoxidation, local muscle ischemia and conversion of weak superoxide to powerful hydroxyl radical with lactate which causes oxidative stress [71,72]. In the case of skeletal muscle, it has been shown that increased ROS formation may impair cellular redox status and lead to the attack of macrophages and other phagocytes, culminating in tissue damage and impaired muscle function [19,73]. Evidence suggests that oxidative damage to biomolecules in cells during acute myeloid leukemia leads to a continuous enhancement in ROS levels and a reduction in the antioxidant cellular defense [74]. Skeletal muscle and myogenic cells are equipped with antioxidants. The antioxidant system inactivates excess ROS/RNS, causing myogenic regeneration and affecting inflammatory reactions, thus stimulating angiogenesis and reducing fibrosis [75]. The oxidative stress-responsive muscle cells include: nuclear factor kappa B (NF-κB), activator protein 1 (AP-1), Nrf2, and peroxisome proliferator-activated receptor gamma coactivator-1 alpha (PGC-1α) [76]. The main role of ROS in the skeletal muscle has been confirmed, both in physiological processes and in fatigue and muscle wasting, aging, and excessive exercise [73]. Skeletal muscle is the biggest tissue in the human body; this system, like other systems, requires the severe regulation of redox homeostasis, such as energy requirements, calcium signaling, and glucose uptake [76]. Skeletal muscle consumes large amounts of molecular oxygen and can produce large amounts of ROS [77].

Resistance training increases the activity of antioxidant enzymes if performed regularly for a long time [78,79]. In this regard, da Silva et al. stated that six months of resistance training can improve people's response to oxidative stress and this mechanism maybe help better performance and health. Their results showed an increase in the CAT activity and no change in the SOD activity [80]. Furthermore, Vezzoli et al. concluded that 12 weeks of moderate-intensity resistance training can minimize the generation of ROS and oxidative stress. They stated that moderate-intensity resistance training can overcome anabolic resistance and maximize protein synthesis in older adults [81]. In the case of acute resistance exercise, Motameni et al. showed that three types of resistance exercise (hypertrophy, strength, and power) did not worsen oxidative stress in women who practiced resistance exercise. They did not observe a significant change in $H_2O_2$ and MDA levels due to the resistance training [82]. In contrast, they reported that plasma MDA levels had increased after three sets of resistance exercises in untrained men [**83**]. Based on the evidence, variations of training intensity and volume, or both (high volume-low intensity or low volume-high intensity training) likely have a positive influence on the elevation of GSH concentration [**84**].

No research has been conducted as of yet on the effects of order of exercise (first strength or endurance exercises) with concurrent exercises on oxidative stress, and it is not clear how they affect it; the need for research in this field is felt. However, in research on the benefits of strength–endurance or endurance–strength training, the results showed that endurance–strength training increases aerobic capacity more than strength–endurance, and the strength–endurance training further increases strength, power and muscle hypertrophy than the endurance–strength training [**85**]. The order of exercise in the concurrent training depends on the purpose of the training and the needs of the sport. In addition, the phosphatidylinositol 3-kinase (PI3K)–protein kinase B (AKT)–mammalian target of rapamycin (mTOR) signaling pathways are disrupted when resistance training is performed after glycogen depletion during endurance training [**86,87**].

Ammar et al. stated in their study that aerobic, anaerobic, and combined training can alter antioxidant status in response to the elevated lipid peroxidation. They stated that under the aerobic and anaerobic conditions, a faster response occurs after training, with higher levels of MDA occurring 5 min after the aerobic training, as well as higher levels of SOD and GPX occurring during anaerobic training (immediately and 5 min after training) and aerobic training (20 min after training). They concluded that the response to oxidative stress depends on the intensity and duration of activity [**88**]. Mitochondria, in addition to producing ATP during aerobic exercise, appear to be the main intracellular source of pro-oxidants. The mitochondrial electron transfer chain consists of several redox centers, which possibly lead to electron leakage to oxygen and its reduction to $O_2^-$. This is engaged in the dissemination of reactions related to the oxidative chain, which is a progenitor of other ROS [**89**]. Findings have shown that pro-oxidants of aerobic exercise are much higher than those of anaerobic exercise, and it has been suggested that the response to oxidative stress depends on the type of exercise (such as intensity and duration) [**12**]. Parker et al. stated that aerobic exercise produces a much higher pro-oxidant status than anaerobic exercise [**90,91**]. They also stated that increasing the intensity of exercise creates more endogenous antioxidant defenses. These results maybe reflect an enhancement in ROS generation, which stimulates the release of plasma antioxidants and subsequently inhibits ROS with high-intensity exercise [**14,64**]. High-intensity exercises maybe create redox-related health adaptations by readjusting endogenous antioxidant defenses [**62**]. A study by Azizbeigi et al. concluded that the endurance, resistance, and concurrent training (endurance + resistance) reduced oxidative stress (MDA) and increased the enzymatic and non-enzymatic antioxidant capacity (SOD, erythrocyte GPx) in untrained men. TAC levels rose considerably solely in the endurance training and concurrent groups. They indicated that it remains ambiguous whether the enhancement in enzyme activity in the concurrent group was from adaptive responses to endurance or resistance training, and it is uncertain which had a more significant impact [92].

## 6. MECHANISM OF THE IMPACT OF CREATINE SUPPLEMENTATION IN CONJUNCTION WITH PHYSICAL ACTIVITY ON OXIDATIVE STRESS

As mentioned, acute and chronic exercises have various effects on oxidative stress. Findings have shown that regular exercise stimulates the endogenous antioxidant system and protects the body against the dangers of oxidative stress. PGC-1α plays a pivotal role in regulating the expression of subunits cytochrome C and cytochrome oxidase in response to a period of treadmill training and long-term training; which indicating that exercise-induced changes in the oxidation capacity are regulated by PGC-1α [**88**]. Increased expression of PGC-1α is associated with increased expression of nuclear respiratory factor-1 (Nrf-1) and Nrf-2 [**70**]. In addition to regulating mitochondrial biogenesis, PGC-1α can regulate the expression of endogenous antioxidants in skeletal muscle [**90,91**]. Nrf-2 is a redox-sensing transcription factor, a major regulator of antioxidants as well as other protective factors responsible for strengthening the antioxidant defense system [**82,93**]. Additionally, PGC-1α in cell culture can regulate mRNA expression of uncoupling proteins 2 and 3 [**94**]; this indicates that PGC-1α can increase binding capacity while reducing ROS production in mitochondria [**91**]. During exercise, several other stimuli are activated that help increase the PGC-1α response; these include increasing cytosolic calcium concentrations, decreasing high-energy phosphate levels and activating AMP-activated protein kinase (AMPK), stimulating the adrenergic system that synthesizes cyclic adenosine monophosphate (c-AMP), and activating protein kinase A and other kinases, including mitogen activated protein kinase (MAPK) [**90**]. PGC-1α expression appears to be upregulated by ROS. Studies have shown the role of PGC-1α in the increasing of ROS, eliminating enzymes due to elevations in ROS [**70**]. In skeletal muscle, physical activity upregulates peroxisome proliferator-activated receptors γ (PPARγ)-controlled genes to augment mitochondrial biogenesis, aerobic respiration, and other physical activity-triggered affairs; it has been shown that PPARγ is a coactivator of PGC-1α [**71**]. A set of adaptations in the body enables PPARγ to regulate antioxidant defense. Evidence confirms that PPARγ is involved in the direct transcriptional regulation of several major endogenous antioxidants [**72,73,74**]. Unlike chronic physical activity, acute exercise can increase the generation of free radicals and cause oxidative damage to cells. Intensity and duration of physical activity, nutrition, and training status are the main factors influencing oxidative stress caused by physical activity [**95**]. In addition, aging, dehydration, hypoxia, and gender have many effects on oxidative stress caused by physical activity [**96,97,98**].

It is clear that enhanced demand for ATP used during exercise enhances ROS levels. Oxidative phosphorylation (OXPHOS) is the main source of ATP production in cells. Changes in the process of increasing ROS production lead to oxidative damage [**23**]. Endogenous antioxidants could not completely prevent oxidative damage under the physiological and pathological conditions in this case (exercise at altitude). These conditions may disturb the endogenous antioxidant balance and increase oxidative stress. In this case, the use of antioxidant supplements such as creatine can have positive effects on the antioxidant system. Few studies have been performed on the effects of short-term and long-term creatine supplementation along with physical exercise on oxidative stress (**Table 1**). In this regard, Stefani et al. [**99**] noted that creatine supplement consumption combined with resistance exercise could reduce oxidative stress (reduced lipoperoxidation in plasma, heart and liver, and gastrocnemius). Moreover, supplementation had positive effects on the SOD activity in all groups. Creatine supplement consumptions possibly have a synergistic effect with resistance training in modulating SOD activity in the heart [**99**]. In conditions of progressive chronic stress and in resistance training, the supplementation seems to exert a synergistic effect due to the compatibility of resistance training with creatine, which includes the enzymatic compatibility of cellular signaling with SOD in heart tissue. This mechanism happens by the activation of the NADPH oxidase system, which modulates the expression of antioxidant enzymes in a short time through angiotensin II and inflammatory mediators [**11,100**]. Additionally, the results of Araujo et al. revealed that creatine consumption acts in an additive manner to exercise to raise the antioxidant enzymes in rat livers [**101**]. Their results showed an increase in glutathione peroxidase (GSH-GPx) activity in the training and training + creatine groups compared to the control group. Regular exercise activates transcription factors (NF-κB and Nrf2), which are responsible for stimulating various genes including mitochondrial GSH-GPx [**102,103**]. The results of Silva et al. showed that the increase in thiobarbituric acid reactive substance (TBARS) is independent of creatine supplementation [**23**]. Actually, about 2–5% of the oxygen involved in OXPHOS during physical activity is changed to potentially detrimental oxygen formatives named ROS [**104**]. Creatine increases intracellular CrP which acts as a cellular energy buffer, thus reducing the OXPHOS dependence on the high-intensity, short-term exercise (**Figure 3**) [**23**]. Creatine supplementation may be more effective in short-term training than in long-term training, by reducing intracellular calcium accumulation and limiting ROS formation and reducing oxidative damage [**23**]. Rahimi stated that consuming 20 g of creatine per day for seven days reduces MDA and 8-hydroxy-2′-deoxyguanosine (8-OHdG) after resistance training. He stated that a resistance exercise using the flat pyramid loading pattern system increases oxidative DNA damage and lipid peroxidation in athletes. Additionally, the antioxidant effects of creatine may be related to its compounds (arginine, glycine and methionine) [**40**]. Deminice and Jordao concluded that creatine supplement consumption reduces the oxidative stress markers induced by a moderate aerobic exercise [**105**]. They stated that acute aerobic exercise increases TBARS and total lipid hydroperoxide, and that creatine supplementation can have positive effects on these variables. Mitochondrial protection is very important because this process is required to maintain mitochondrial activity and mitochondriogenesis [**106**]. As mentioned, creatine has direct antioxidant activity through normalizing mitochondrial mutagenesis, prevents its functional outcomes, and perhaps plays the main role in the stability of mitochondrial activity. Additionally, creatine can prevent mtDNA damage and protect mitochondria by reducing extracellular $H_2O_2$ levels [**45,46**]. Young et al. reported the capacity of creatine exposure to promote the thiol redox system, of which the GSH and thioredoxin pathways are important components (indirect antioxidant effect) [54]. In addition, studies have shown other indirect antioxidant mechanisms such as hydration and membrane stabilization [5] and increased or normalized cell energy status [107,108]. In contrast, the findings of Kingsley et al. showed that short-term creatine consumption had no effect on the antioxidant defense or protection against lipid peroxidation caused by the exhaustive cycling among healthy men [109]. Deminice et al. stated that creatine supplementation has no effect on the antioxidant parameters; creatine supplement consumption was inadequate to inhibit oxidative stress induced by acute repeated-sprint exercise. They stated that more studies were needed to confirm the antioxidant effects of creatine consumption in humans [110]. Moreover, Percario et al. stated that creatine supplement consumption along with resistance training stimulates oxidative stress and decreases the overall antioxidant capacity [111]. They stated that total antioxidant status (TAS) values in the creatine + training group were significantly decreased compared to the other groups. Considerable enhancement in strength in the creatine + training group may increase the energy production mechanism due to the high capacity for ATP re-synthesis in cells. This condition is maybe suitable for the manifestation of ischemia-reperfusion syndrome, with enhanced uric acid and hydroxyl radical generation causing the mobilization of antioxidant stores (thereby decreasing TAS) to prevent oxidative stress [111].

**Table 1. Studies on the effects of short-term and long-term creatine supplementation and exercise on oxidative stress.**

| Studies | Subject | Exercise | Intervention | Main Outcome |
|---|---|---|---|---|
| **Human study** | | | | |
| Kingsley et al. (2009) [109] | Active males ($n$ = 18) | Incremental cycling that was continued until the individualized predetermined point of exhaustion | Ingested 22.8 $g{\cdot}d^{-1}$ Cr (equivalent to 5 g Cr × 4 daily) for 5 days. Each supplement dose consisted of 5.7 g Cr and 5 g of glucose polymer dissolved in 500 mL of warm water | = Oxidative stress (as measured by serum hydroperoxide concentrations) |
| Rahimi (2011) [40] | Trained males ($n$ = 27) | 7 sets, 3–6 repetitions, 80–90% 1RM (bench press, lat pull down, and seated rows) | 20 g/day (5 g/serving, 4 serving/day), 7 days before exercise | ↓MDA, 8-OHdG |
| Percario et al. (2012) [111] | Male elite Brazilian handball players ($n$ = 26) | 5 week RT, 50–95% 1RM, 3–12 repetition | First 5 days: a daily dose of 20 g, remaining 27 days: participants were given a dose of 5 g per day, after training | ↓ TAS, =TBARS |

| Studies | Subject | Exercise | Intervention | Main Outcome |
|---|---|---|---|---|
| Deminice et al. (2013) [110] | Male soccer players (*n* = 25) | 2 consecutive running-based anaerobic sprint test, (6 sprints (35 m), maximum speed, 10 s rest between repetition) | 0.3 g/kg, 7 days after first exercise | = MDA, GSH, GSH/GSSG ratio, TAC, CAT, SOD, GPX |
| **Animal study** | | | | |
| Deminice and Jordao. (2012) [105] | Male rats (*n* = 64) | 1 h swimming with load of 4% of total body weight | 2% Cr, 28 days before exercise | ↓TBARS, Lipid hydroperoxide ↑GSH/GSSG ratio, TAC = α-Tocopherol, CAT |
| Silva et al. (2013) [23] | Male rats (*n* = 36) | Exhaustion eccentric running (treadmill, 50–60% $VO_2$max, constant velocity 1.0 km/h) | 300 mg/kg/day, 15 days, dose of initially: 2 serving/day, dose after 6 days: 1 serving/day | = TBARS, PC, TT, SOD, GPX, CAT |
| Araujo et al. (2013) [101] | Male Wistar rats (*n* = 40) | 25 min treadmill at different fixed speeds for each series, 48 h interval between series, 8 weeks | 2% in diet Cr during the maintenance phase equals 20 $g{\cdot}kg^{-1}$ peak in the phase of 13% were used equivalent to 130 $g{\cdot}kg^{-1}$ | T and TCr groups: ↑$H_2O_2$, GSH-GPx CCr and TCr groups: ↑CAT TCr group: ↓SOD Al groups: GSH, GSH/GSSG |
| Stefani et al. (2014) [99] | Male Wistar rats (*n* = 40) | 8 weeks RT (4 series of 10–12 repetitions, 90 s interval, 4 times per week, 65% to 75% of 1 Concurrent Strength and Aerobic Training Order Influence Training-InduceRM) | The first 7 days prior to the initiation of training: dosage of 0.3 g/kg/day, last 7 weeks: the dosage was set at 0.05 g/kg/day | ↓lipoperoxidation, MDA ↑SOD = CAT |

= No significant difference; ↓ significantly decreased responses; ↑ significantly increased responses; creatine (Cr); one repetition maximum (1RM); malondialdehyde (MDA); 8-OH-2-deoxyguanosine (8-OH-dG); thiobarbituric acid-reactive substances (TBARS); glutathione (GSH); oxidized glutathione (GSSG); resistance training (RT); total antioxidant capacity (TAC); catalase (CAT); total antioxidant status (TAS); glutathione peroxidase (GSH-GPx); protein carbonyls (PC); total thiol (TT) superoxide dismutase (SOD); glutathione peroxidase (GPX); hydrogen peroxide ($H_2O_2$); training (T); training + creatine (TCr); and control + creatine (CCr).

According to the existing research (**Table 1**), long-term creatine supplementation along with moderate-intensity resistance and endurance training can probably reduce oxidative stress and increase the antioxidant defense system; however, in the short-term, creatine consumption and its effect on oxidative stress due to endurance exercise is not well known, although it seems that the short-term creatine ingestion possibly reduces oxidative stress due to intense resistance exercise. Considering the antioxidant effects of regular physical activity (PGC-1α, PPARγ) and creatine (maintaining mitochondrial integrity, acting as a cellular energy buffer, reducing extracellular $H_2O_2$ levels, cell membrane stabilization and improvement of cellular energy capacity), it seems that the combined effect of physical activity and creatine consumption can reduce oxidative stress, but further research is needed to conclude more accurately about the intensity of long-term resistance and endurance training with creatine supplementation and the short-term effects of creatine consumption and physical activity on oxidative stress. No research has been conducted on the impact of creatine supplementation in conjunction with contemporaneous exercise; nevertheless, given the antioxidant properties of creatine and the impacts of concurrent exercise, it appears to potentially have beneficial outcomes on oxidative stress. The intensity of exercise can have varying benefits, necessitating further research in this area [112].

## 7. CONCISE SUMMARY

Creatine possesses antioxidant effects and can be useful via both direct and indirect methods. It positively influences oxidative stress and diminishes reactive oxygen species (ROS). Creatine can preserve mitochondrial integrity, enhance CrP reserves, function as a cellular energy buffer, and safeguard two critical cellular targets, mtDNA and RNA, from oxidative damage. The antioxidant properties of creatine may be associated with its constituents: arginine, glycine, and methionine (Figure 3). Creatine supplementation, when paired with prolonged workout, may potentially diminish oxidative stress and enhance the antioxidant system. The ingestion of creatine supplements may have a synergistic effect with training; nevertheless, the intensity and duration of both the training and supplementation period significantly influence antioxidant activity. Limited study has been undertaken regarding the impact of creatine intake in conjunction with both long-term and short-term exercise on oxidative stress; hence, further investigation is required to draw more definitive conclusions in this area.

## AT A GLANCE

Oxidative stress occurs when there is an imbalance between the production of reactive oxygen species (ROS) and their removal by antioxidant systems. Reactive oxygen species (ROS) decompose biogenic compounds, including deoxyribonucleic acid, lipids, and proteins, potentially resulting in oxidative tissue injury. Exercise is presently linked to increased oxidative stress. While a phase of rigorous training may induce oxidative injury to muscle fibers, consistent exercise enhances the cells' capacity to mitigate the over-accumulation of reactive oxygen species (ROS). Consistent moderate-intensity exercise has been demonstrated to enhance antioxidant defense mechanisms. Endogenous antioxidants are incapable of entirely averting oxidative damage under both physiological and pathological situations, such as vigorous exercise and high-altitude exercise. These circumstances may disrupt the natural antioxidant equilibrium and elevate oxidative stress. The administration of antioxidant substances, such as creatine, can positively influence the antioxidant system. Creatine comprises two necessary amino acids, arginine and methionine, together with one non-essential amino acid, glycine. The precise method by which creatine functions as an antioxidant remains unidentified. It has been demonstrated to enhance the activity of antioxidant enzymes and the ability to remove reactive oxygen species (ROS) and reactive nitrogen species (RNS). The antioxidant benefits of creatine appear to stem from multiple processes, including indirect pathways (such as enhanced or normalized cellular energy status) and direct pathways (such as the preservation of mitochondrial integrity). The ingestion of creatine supplements may synergistically enhance training, although the intensity and duration of the workout significantly influence antioxidant activity. This study aimed to examine the literature regarding the impact of creatine supplementation and physical exercise on oxidative stress.

## REFERENCES


1. Cooper, R.; Naclerio, F.; Allgrove, J.; Jimenez, A. Creatine supplementation with specific view to exercise/sports performance: An update. *J. Int. Soc. Sports Nutr.* **2012**, *9*, 33. **[Google Scholar]** **[PubMed]** **[Green Version]**
2. Volek, J.S.; Ratamess, N.A.; Rubin, M.R.; French, D.N.; McGuigan, M.M.; Scheett, T.P.; Sharman, M.J.; Kraemer, W.J. The effects of creatine supplementation on muscular performance and body composition responses to short-term resistance training overreaching. *Graefe Arch. Clin. Exp. Ophthalmol.* **2003**, *91*, 628–637. **[Google Scholar]**
3. Gama, M.S. Efeitos da creatina sobre desempenho aeróbio: Uma revisão sistemática. *Rev. Bras. Nutr. Esport.* **2011**, *5*, 182–190. **[Google Scholar]**
4. Pereira Junior, M.; Moraes, A.J.P.; Ornellas, F.H.; Gonçalves, M.A.; Liberalli, R.; Navarro, F. Eficiência da suplementação de creatina no desempenho físico humano. *Rev. Bras. Prescri. Fisiol. Exer.* **2012**, *6*, 90–97. **[Google Scholar]**
5. Wyss, M.; Schulze, A. Health implications of creatine: Can oral creatine supplementation protect against neurological and atherosclerotic disease? *Neuroscience* **2002**, *112*, 243–260. **[Google Scholar]**
6. Lawler, J.M.; Barnes, W.S.; Wu, G.; Song, W.; Demaree, S. Direct Antioxidant Properties of Creatine. *Biochem. Biophys. Res. Commun.* **2002**, *290*, 47–52. **[Google Scholar]** **[PubMed]**
7. Reardon, T.F.; Allen, D.G. Iron injections in mice increase skeletal muscle iron content, induce oxidative stress and reduce exercise performance. *Exp. Physiol.* **2009**, *94*, 720–730. **[Google Scholar]**
8. Moopanar, T.R.; Allen, D.G. Reactive oxygen species reduce myofibrillar $Ca^{2+}$ sensitivity in fatiguing mouse skeletal muscle at 37 °C. *J. Physiol.* **2005**, *564*, 189–199. **[Google Scholar]**
9. Van Der Poel, C.; Stephenson, D.G. Reversible changes in $Ca^{2+}$—Activation properties of rat skeletal muscle exposed to elevated physiological temperatures. *J. Physiol.* **2002**, *544*, 765–776. **[Google Scholar]**
10. Bloomer, R.J.; Fry, A.C.; Falvo, M.J.; Moore, C.A. Protein carbonyls are acutely elevated following single set anaerobic exercise in resistance trained men. *J. Sci. Med. Sport* **2007**, *10*, 411–417. **[Google

**Scholar]** **[PubMed]**

11. Valko, M.; Leibfritz, D.; Moncol, J.; Cronin, M.T.D.; Mazur, M.; Telser, J. Free radicals and antioxidants in normal physiological functions and human disease. *Int. J. Biochem. Cell Biol.* **2007**, *39*, 44–84. **[Google Scholar]**

12. El Abed, K.; Ammar, A.; Boukhris, O.; Trabelsi, K.; Masmoudi, L.; Bailey, S.J.; Hakim, A.; Bragazzi, N.L. Independent and Combined Effects of All-Out Sprint and Low-Intensity Continuous Exercise on Plasma Oxidative Stress Biomarkers in Trained Judokas. *Front. Physiol.* **2019**, *10*, 842. **[Google Scholar]** **[PubMed]**

13. Matthews, R.T.; Yang, L.; Jenkins, B.G.; Ferrante, R.J.; Rosen, B.R.; Kaddurah-Daouk, R.; Beal, M.F. Neuroprotective Effects of Creatine and Cyclocreatine in Animal Models of Huntington's Disease. *J. Neurosci.* **1998**, *18*, 156–163. **[Google Scholar]** **[PubMed]** **[Green Version]**

14. Suzuki, K.; Tominaga, T.; Ruhee, R.T.; Ma, S. Characterization and Modulation of Systemic Inflammatory Response to Exhaustive Exercise in Relation to Oxidative Stress. *Antioxidants* **2020**, *9*, 401. **[Google Scholar]**

15. Magherini, F.; Fiaschi, T.; Marzocchini, R.; Mannelli, M.; Gamberi, T.; Modesti, P.A.; Modesti, A. Oxidative stress in exercise training: The involvement of inflammation and peripheral signals. *Free Radic. Res.* **2019**, *53*, 1155–1165. **[Google Scholar]** **[PubMed]**

16. Powers, S.K.; Jackson, M.J. Exercise-Induced Oxidative Stress: Cellular Mechanisms and Impact on Muscle Force Production. *Physiol. Rev.* **2008**, *88*, 1243–1276. **[Google Scholar]** **[Green Version]**

17. Henríquez-Olguín, C.; Renani, L.B.; Arab-Ceschia, L.; Raun, S.H.; Bhatia, A.; Li, Z.; Knudsen, J.R.; Holmdahl, R.; Jensen, T.E. Adaptations to high-intensity interval training in skeletal muscle require NADPH oxidase 2. *Redox Biol.* **2019**, *24*, 101188. **[Google Scholar]** **[PubMed]**

18. Fritzen, A.M.; Lundsgaard, A.-M.; Kiens, B. Dietary Fuels in Athletic Performance. *Annu. Rev. Nutr.* **2019**, *39*, 45–73. **[Google Scholar]**

19. Suzuki, K. Involvement of neutrophils in exercise-induced muscle damage and its modulation. *Gen. Intern. Med. Clin. Innov.* **2018**, *3*, 1–8. **[Google Scholar]**

20. McGinley, C.; Shafat, A.; Donnelly, A.E. Does Antioxidant Vitamin Supplementation Protect against Muscle Damage? *Sports Med.* **2009**, *39*, 1011–1032. **[Google Scholar]**

21. Ristow, M.; Zarse, K. How increased oxidative stress promotes longevity and metabolic health: The concept of mitochondrial hormesis (mitohormesis). *Exp. Gerontol.* **2010**, *45*, 410–418. **[Google Scholar]** **[PubMed]**

22. Falone, S.; Mirabilio, A.; Pennelli, A.; Cacchio, M.; Di Baldassarre, A.; Gallina, S.; Passerini, A.; Amicarelli, F. Differential impact of acute bout of exercise on redox- and oxidative damage-related profiles between untrained subjects and amateur runners. *Physiol. Res.* **2010**, *59*, 953. **[Google Scholar]**

23. Silva, L.A.; Tromm, C.B.; Da Rosa, G.; Bom, K.; Luciano, T.F.; Tuon, T.; De Souza, C.T.; Pinho, R.A. Creatine supplementation does not decrease oxidative stress and inflammation in skeletal muscle after eccentric exercise. *J. Sports Sci.* **2013**, *31*, 1164–1176. **[Google Scholar]**

24. Burton, G.J.; Jauniaux, E. Oxidative stress. *Best Pr. Res. Clin. Obstet. Gynaecol.* **2011**, *25*, 287–299. **[Google Scholar]** **[PubMed]** **[Green Version]**

25. Chandrasekaran, A.; Idelchik, M.D.P.S.; Melendez, J.A. Redox control of senescence and age-related disease. *Redox Biol.* **2017**, *11*, 91–102. **[Google Scholar]** **[PubMed]** **[Green Version]**

26. Lobo, V.; Patil, A.; Phatak, A.; Chandra, N. Free radicals, antioxidants and functional foods: Impact on human health. *Pharmacogn. Rev.* **2010**, *4*, 118–126. **[Google Scholar]** **[Green Version]**

27. Salisbury, D.; Bronas, U. Reactive Oxygen and Nitrogen Species. *Nurs. Res.* **2015**, *64*, 53–66. **[Google Scholar]**

28. Phaniendra, A.; Jestadi, D.B.; Periyasamy, L. Free Radicals: Properties, Sources, Targets, and Their Implication in Various Diseases. *Indian J. Clin. Biochem.* **2015**, *30*, 11–26. **[Google Scholar] [PubMed] [Green Version]**

29. Cruzat, V.F.; Rogero, M.M.; Borges, M.C.; Tirapegui, J. Aspectos atuais sobre estresse oxidativo, exercícios físicos e suplementação. *Rev. Bras. Med. Esporte* **2007**, *13*, 336–342. **[Google Scholar] [Green Version]**

30. Genestra, M. Oxyl radicals, redox-sensitive signalling cascades and antioxidants. *Cell. Signal.* **2007**, *19*, 1807–1819. **[Google Scholar]**

31. Liguori, I.; Russo, G.; Curcio, F.; Bulli, G.; Aran, L.; Della-Morte, D.; Gargiulo, G.; Testa, G.; Cacciatore, F.; Bonaduce, D.; et al. Oxidative stress, aging, and diseases. *Clin. Interv. Aging* **2018**, *13*, 757–772. **[Google Scholar] [Green Version]**

32. Dinkova-Kostova, A.T.; Talalay, P. Direct and indirect antioxidant properties of inducers of cytoprotective proteins. *Mol. Nutr. Food Res.* **2008**, *52*, S128–S138. **[Google Scholar] [PubMed]**

33. Dröge, W. Free Radicals in the Physiological Control of Cell Function. *Physiol. Rev.* **2002**, *82*, 47–95. **[Google Scholar] [PubMed]**

34. Wu, G. *Amino Acids: Biochemistry and Nutrition*; CRC Press: Boca Raton, FL, USA, 2013. **[Google Scholar]**

35. Hou, Y.; He, W.; Hu, S.; Wu, G. Composition of polyamines and amino acids in plant-source foods for human consumption. *Amino Acids* **2019**, *51*, 1153–1165. **[Google Scholar] [PubMed]**

36. Wu, G.; Morris, J.S.M. Arginine metabolism: Nitric oxide and beyond. *Biochem. J.* **1998**, *336*, 1–17. **[Google Scholar]**

37. Wu, G. Important roles of dietary taurine, creatine, carnosine, anserine and 4-hydroxyproline in human nutrition and health. *Amino Acids* **2020**, *52*, 329–360. **[Google Scholar] [Green Version]**

38. Hosamani, R.; Ramesh, S.R. Attenuation of Rotenone-Induced Mitochondrial Oxidative Damage and Neurotoxicty in Drosophila melanogaster Supplemented with Creatine. *Neurochem. Res.* **2010**, *35*, 1402–1412. **[Google Scholar] [PubMed]**

39. Sestili, P.; Martinelli, C.; Bravi, G.; Piccoli, G.; Curci, R.; Battistelli, M.; Falcieri, E.; Agostini, D.; Gioacchini, A.M.; Stocchi, V. Creatine supplementation affords cytoprotection in oxidatively injured cultured mammalian cells via direct antioxidant activity. *Free Radic. Biol. Med.* **2006**, *40*, 837–849. **[Google Scholar]**

40. Rahimi, R. Creatine Supplementation Decreases Oxidative DNA Damage and Lipid Peroxidation Induced by a Single Bout of Resistance Exercise. *J. Strength Cond. Res.* **2011**, *25*, 3448–3455. **[Google Scholar]**

41. Clarke, H.; Kim, D.-H.; Meza, C.A.; Ormsbee, M.J.; Hickner, R.C. The Evolving Applications of Creatine Supplementation: Could Creatine Improve Vascular Health? *Nutrients* **2020**, *12*, 2834. **[Google Scholar] [PubMed]**

42. Guidi, C.; Potenza, L.; Sestili, P.; Martinelli, C.; Guescini, M.; Stocchi, L.; Zeppa, S.; Polidori, E.; Annibalini, G.; Stocchi, V. Differential effect of creatine on oxidatively-injured mitochondrial and nuclear DNA. *Biochim. Biophys. Acta Gen. Subj.* **2008**, *1780*, 16–26. **[Google Scholar] [PubMed]**

43. Copeland, W.C. The Mitochondrial DNA Polymerase in Health and Disease. *Alzheimer Dis.* **2009**, *50*, 211–222. **[Google Scholar] [Green Version]**

44. Reddy, P.H. Mitochondrial Medicine for Aging and Neurodegenerative Diseases. *Neuro Mol. Med.* **2008**, *10*, 291–315. **[Google Scholar] [Green Version]**

45. Bender, A.; Beckers, J.; Schneider, I.; Hölter, S.; Haack, T.; Ruthsatz, T.; Vogt-Weisenhorn, D.; Becker, L.; Genius, J.; Rujescu, D.; et al. Creatine improves health and survival of mice. *Neurobiol. Aging* **2008**, *29*, 1404–1411. **[Google Scholar] [PubMed]**

46. Sestili, P.; Martinelli, C.; Colombo, E.; Barbieri, E.; Potenza, L.; Sartini, S.; Fimognari, C. Creatine as an antioxidant. *Amino Acids* **2011**, *40*, 1385–1396. **[Google Scholar]**

47. Fimognari, C.; Sestili, P.; Lenzi, M.; Cantelli-Forti, G.; Hrelia, P. Protective effect of creatine against RNA damage. *Mutat. Res. Mol. Mech. Mutagen.* **2009**, *670*, 59–67. **[Google Scholar]**

48. Louis, M.; Van Beneden, R.; Dehoux, M.; Thissen, J.P.; Francaux, M. Creatine increases IGF-I and myogenic regulatory factor mRNA in C2C12cells. *FEBS Lett.* **2004**, *557*, 243–247. **[Google Scholar]** **[Green Version]**

49. Deldicque, L.; Theisen, D.; Bertrand, L.; Hespel, P.; Hue, L.; Francaux, M. Creatine enhances differentiation of myogenic C2C12 cells by activating both p38 and Akt/PKB pathways. *Am. J. Physiol. Physiol.* **2007**, *293*, C1263–C1271. **[Google Scholar]** **[PubMed]** **[Green Version]**

50. Alfieri, R.R.; Bonelli, M.A.; Cavazzoni, A.; Brigotti, M.; Fumarola, C.; Sestili, P.; Mozzoni, P.; De Palma, G.; Mutti, A.; Carnicelli, D.; et al. Creatine as a compatible osmolyte in muscle cells exposed to hypertonic stress. *J. Physiol.* **2006**, *576*, 391–401. **[Google Scholar]**

51. Almeida, L.S.; Salomons, G.S.; Hogenboom, F.; Jakobs, C.; Schoffelmeer, A.N. Exocytotic release of creatine in rat brain. *Synapse* **2006**, *60*, 118–123. **[Google Scholar]**

52. De Deyn, P.P.; Macdonald, R.L. Guanidino compounds that are increased in cerebrospinal fluid and brain of uremic patients inhibit GABA and glycine responses on mouse neurons in cell culture. *Ann. Neurol.* **1990**, *28*, 627–633. **[Google Scholar]** **[PubMed]** **[Green Version]**

53. Koga, Y.; Takahashi, H.; Oikawa, D.; Tachibana, T.; Denbow, D.; Furuse, M. Brain creatine functions to attenuate acute stress responses through GABAnergic system in chicks. *Neuroscience* **2005**, *132*, 65–71. **[Google Scholar]**

54. Young, J.F.; Larsen, L.B.; Malmendal, A.; Nielsen, N.C.; Straadt, I.K.; Oksbjerg, N.; Bertram, H.C. Creatine-induced activation of antioxidative defence in myotube cultures revealed by explorative NMR-based metabonomics and proteomics. *J. Int. Soc. Sports Nutr.* **2010**, *7*, 9–10. **[Google Scholar]** **[PubMed]** **[Green Version]**

55. Reid, M.B. Invited Review: Redox modulation of skeletal muscle contraction: What we know and what we don't. *J. Appl. Physiol.* **2001**, *90*, 724–731. **[Google Scholar]** **[Green Version]**

56. Grune, T.; Reinheckel, T.; Davies, K.J.A. Degradation of oxidized proteins in mammalian cells. *FASEB J.* **1997**, *11*, 526–534. **[Google Scholar]** **[PubMed]**

57. Gomes, E.C.; Silva, A.N.; De Oliveira, M.R. Oxidants, Antioxidants, and the Beneficial Roles of Exercise-Induced Production of Reactive Species. *Oxidative Med. Cell. Longev.* **2012**, *2012*, 1–12. **[Google Scholar]**

58. Sakellariou, G.K.; Jackson, M.J.; Vasilaki, A. Redefining the major contributors to superoxide production in contracting skeletal muscle. The role of NAD(P)H oxidases. *Free Radic. Res.* **2013**, *48*, 12–29. **[Google Scholar]**

59. Zuo, L.; Zhou, T.; Pannell, B.K.; Ziegler, A.C.; Best, T.M. Biological and physiological role of reactive oxygen species—The good, the bad and the ugly. *Acta Physiol.* **2015**, *214*, 329–348. **[Google Scholar]** **[PubMed]**

60. Mastaloudis, A.; Leonard, S.W.; Traber, M.G. Oxidative stress in athletes during extreme endurance exercise. *Free Radic. Biol. Med.* **2001**, *31*, 911–922. **[Google Scholar]**

61. Jiang, L.; Diaz, P.T.; Best, T.M.; Stimpfl, J.N.; He, F.; Zuo, L. Molecular characterization of redox mechanisms in allergic asthma. *Ann. Allergy Asthma Immunol.* **2014**, *113*, 137–142. **[Google Scholar]**

62. Radak, Z.; Zhao, Z.; Koltai, E.; Ohno, H.; Atalay, M. Oxygen Consumption and Usage During Physical Exercise: The Balance Between Oxidative Stress and ROS-Dependent Adaptive Signaling. *Antioxid. Redox Signal.* **2013**, *18*, 1208–1246. **[Google Scholar]** **[PubMed]** **[Green Version]**

63. He, F.; Li, J.; Liu, Z.; Chuang, C.-C.; Yang, W.; Zuo, L. Redox Mechanism of Reactive Oxygen Species in Exercise. *Front. Physiol.* **2016**, *7*, 486. **[Google Scholar]** **[PubMed]** **[Green Version]**

64. Suzuki, K.; Nakaji, S.; Yamada, M.; Liu, Q.; Kurakake, S.; Okamura, N.; Kumae, T.; Umeda, T.; Sugawara, K. Impact of a Competitive Marathon Race on Systemic Cytokine and Neutrophil Responses. *Med. Sci. Sports Exerc.* **2003**, *35*, 348–355. **[Google Scholar]**

65. Knez, W.L.; Coombes, J.S.; Jenkins, D.G. Ultra-Endurance Exercise and Oxidative Damage. *Sports Med.* **2006**, *36*, 429–441. **[Google Scholar]**

66. Ferraro, E.; Giammarioli, A.M.; Chiandotto, S.; Spoletini, I.; Rosano, G. Exercise-Induced Skeletal Muscle Remodeling and Metabolic Adaptation: Redox Signaling and Role of Autophagy. *Antioxid. Redox Signal.* **2014**, *21*, 154–176. **[Google Scholar]**

67. Zarrindast, S.; Ramezanpour, M.; Moghaddam, M. Effects of eight weeks of moderate intensity aerobic training and training in water on DNA damage, lipid peroxidation and total antioxidant capacity in sixty years sedentary women. *Sci. Sports* **2020**. **[Google Scholar]**

68. Done, A.J.; Traustadóttir, T. Aerobic exercise increases resistance to oxidative stress in sedentary older middle-aged adults. A pilot study. *AGE* **2016**, *38*, 505–512. **[Google Scholar]** **[PubMed]** **[Green Version]**

69. Estébanez, B.; Rodriguez, A.L.; Visavadiya, N.P.; Whitehurst, M.; Cuevas, M.J.; González-Gallego, J.; Huang, C.-J. Aerobic Training Down-Regulates Pentraxin 3 and Pentraxin 3/Toll-Like Receptor 4 Ratio, Irrespective of Oxidative Stress Response, in Elderly Subjects. *Antioxidants* **2020**, *9*, 110. **[Google Scholar]** **[PubMed]** **[Green Version]**

70. Leelarungrayub, D.; Saidee, K.; Pothongsunun, P.; Pratanaphon, S.; Yankai, A.; Bloomer, R.J. Six weeks of aerobic dance exercise improves blood oxidative stress status and increases interleukin-2 in previously sedentary women. *J. Bodyw. Mov. Ther.* **2011**, *15*, 355–362. **[Google Scholar]** **[PubMed]**

71. Inal, M.; Akyüz, F.; Turgut, A.; Getsfrid, W.M. Effect of aerobic and anaerobic metabolism on free radical generation swimmers. *Med. Sci. Sports Exerc.* **2001**, *33*, 564–567. **[Google Scholar]** **[PubMed]**

72. Smith, L.L.; Miles, M.P. *Exercise-Induced Muscle Injury and Inflammation. Exercise and Sport Science*; Lippincott Williams and Wilkins: Philadephia, PA, USA, 2000; pp. 401–411. **[Google Scholar]**

73. Powers, S.K.; Ji, L.L.; Kavazis, A.N.; Jackson, M.J. Reactive Oxygen Species: Impact on Skeletal Muscle. *Compr. Physiol.* **2011**, *1*, 941–969. **[Google Scholar]** **[PubMed]** **[Green Version]**

74. Udensi, U.K.; Tchounwou, P.B. Dual effect of oxidative stress on leukemia cancer induction and treatment. *J. Exp. Clin. Cancer Res.* **2014**, *33*, 1–15. **[Google Scholar]** **[Green Version]**

75. Kozakowska, M.; Pietraszek-Gremplewicz, K.; Jozkowicz, A.; Dulak, J. The role of oxidative stress in skeletal muscle injury and regeneration: Focus on antioxidant enzymes. *J. Muscle Res. Cell Motil.* **2015**, *36*, 377–393. **[Google Scholar]** **[PubMed]** **[Green Version]**

76. Moulin, M.; Ferreiro, A. Muscle redox disturbances and oxidative stress as pathomechanisms and therapeutic targets in early-onset myopathies. *Semin. Cell Dev. Biol.* **2017**, *64*, 213–223. **[Google Scholar]**

77. Gomes, M.J.; Martinez, P.F.; Pagan, L.U.; Damatto, R.L.; Cezar, M.D.D.M.; Lima, A.R.R.; Okoshi, K.; Okoshi, M.P. Skeletal muscle aging: Influence of oxidative stress and physical exercise. *Oncotarget* **2017**, *8*, 20428–20440. **[Google Scholar]** **[PubMed]** **[Green Version]**

78. Parise, G.; Phillips, S.M.; Kaczor, J.J.; Tarnopolsky, M.A. Antioxidant enzyme activity is up-regulated after unilateral resistance exercise training in older adults. *Free Radic. Biol. Med.* **2005**, *39*, 289–295. **[Google Scholar]** **[PubMed]**

79. Peters, P.G.; Alessio, H.M.; Hagerman, A.E.; Ashton, T.; Nagy, S.; Wiley, R.L. Short-term isometric exercise reduces systolic blood pressure in hypertensive adults: Possible role of reactive oxygen species. *Int. J. Cardiol.* **2006**, *110*, 199–205. **[Google Scholar]** **[PubMed]**

80. Da Silva, E.P., Jr.; Soares, E.O.; Malvestiti, R.; Hatanaka, E.; Lambertucci, R.H. Resistance training induces protective adaptation from the oxidative stress induced by an intense-strength session. *Sport Sci. Heal.* **2016**, *12*, 321–328. **[Google Scholar]**

81. Vezzoli, A.; Mrakic-Sposta, S.; Montorsi, M.; Porcelli, S.; Vago, P.; Cereda, F.; Longo, S.; Maggio, M.; Narici, M.; Sposta, M.; et al. Moderate Intensity Resistive Training Reduces Oxidative Stress and Improves Muscle Mass and Function in Older Individuals. *Antioxidants* **2019**, *8*, 431. **[Google Scholar] [PubMed] [Green Version]**

82. Motameni, S.; TaheriChadorneshin, H.; Golestani, A. Comparing the effects of resistance exercise type on serum levels of oxidative stress and muscle damage markers in resistance-trained women. *Sport Sci. Health* **2020**, *16*, 443–450. **[Google Scholar]**

83. Sepehri, M.H.; Nikbakht, M.; Habibi, A.; Moradi, M. Effects of a Single Low-Intensity Resistance Exercise Session on Lipid Peroxidation of Untrained Male Students. *Am. J. Sports Sci.* **2014**, *2*, 87. **[Google Scholar]**

84. Çakir-Atabek, H.; Demir, S.; Pinarba□ili, R.D.; Gündüz, N. Effects of Different Resistance Training Intensity on Indices of Oxidative Stress. *J. Strength Cond. Res.* **2010**, *24*, 2491–2497. **[Google Scholar]**

85. Alves, A.R.; Marta, C.C.; Neiva, H.P.; Izquierdo, M.; Marques, M.C. Does Intrasession Concurrent Strength and Aerobic Training Order Influence Training-Induced Explosive Strength and V.V.$O_2$max in Prepubescent Children? *J. Strength Cond. Res.* **2016**, *30*, 3267–3277. **[Google Scholar] [Green Version]**

86. Creer, A.; Gallagher, P.; Slivka, D.; Jemiolo, B.; Fink, W.; Trappe, S. Influence of muscle glycogen availability on ERK1/2 and Akt signaling after resistance exercise in human skeletal muscle. *J. Appl. Physiol.* **2005**, *99*, 950–956. **[Google Scholar]**

87. Hawley, J.A. Molecular responses to strength and endurance training: Are they incompatible? *Appl. Physiol. Nutr. Metab.* **2009**, *34*, 355–361. **[Google Scholar] [Green Version]**

88. Ammar, A.; Trabelsi, K.; Boukhris, O.; Glenn, J.M.; Bott, N.; Masmoudi, L.; Hakim, A.; Chtourou, H.; Driss, T.; Hoekelmann, A.; et al. Effects of Aerobic-, Anaerobic- and Combined-Based Exercises on Plasma Oxidative Stress Biomarkers in Healthy Untrained Young Adults. *Int. J. Environ. Res. Public Health* **2020**, *17*, 2601. **[Google Scholar] [Green Version]**

89. Turrens, J.F. Mitochondrial formation of reactive oxygen species. *J. Physiol.* **2003**, *552*, 335–344. **[Google Scholar]**

90. Parker, L.; Trewin, A.; Levinger, I.; Shaw, C.S.; Stepto, N.K. Exercise-intensity dependent alterations in plasma redox status do not reflect skeletal muscle redox-sensitive protein signaling. *J. Sci. Med. Sport* **2018**, *21*, 416–421. **[Google Scholar] [Green Version]**

91. Parker, L.; McGuckin, T.A.; Leicht, A.S. Influence of exercise intensity on systemic oxidative stress and antioxidant capacity. *Clin. Physiol. Funct. Imaging* **2014**, *34*, 377–383. **[Google Scholar]**

92. Azizbeigi, K.; Stannard, S.R.; Atashak, S.; Haghighi, M.M. Antioxidant enzymes and oxidative stress adaptation to exercise training: Comparison of endurance, resistance, and concurrent training in untrained males. *J. Exerc. Sci. Fit.* **2014**, *12*, 1–6. **[Google Scholar] [Green Version]**

93. Mota, M.P.; Dos Santos, Z.A.; Soares, J.F.P.; Pereira, A.D.F.; João, P.V.; Gaivão, I.O.; Oliveira, M.M. Intervention with a combined physical exercise training to reduce oxidative stress of women over 40 years of age. *Exp. Gerontol.* **2019**, *123*, 1–9. **[Google Scholar]**

94. McAllister, M.J.; Basham, S.A.; Waldman, H.S.; Smith, J.W.; Mettler, J.A.; Butawan, M.B.; Bloomer, R.J. Effects of psychological stress during exercise on markers of oxidative stress in young healthy, trained men. *Physiol. Behav.* **2019**, *198*, 90–95. **[Google Scholar] [PubMed]**

95. Suzuki, K. Chronic Inflammation as an Immunological Abnormality and Effectiveness of Exercise. *Biomolecules* **2019**, *9*, 223. **[Google Scholar] [Green Version]**

96. Paik, I.-Y.; Jeong, M.-H.; Jin, H.-E.; Kim, Y.-I.; Suh, A.-R.; Cho, S.-Y.; Roh, H.-T.; Jin, C.-H.; Suh, S.-H. Fluid replacement following dehydration reduces oxidative stress during recovery. *Biochem. Biophys. Res. Commun.* **2009**, *383*, 103–107. **[Google Scholar] [PubMed]**

97. Bailey, D.M.; McEneny, J.; Mathieu-Costello, O.; Henry, R.R.; James, P.E.; Mccord, J.M.; Pietri, S.; Young, I.S.; Richardson, R.S. Sedentary aging increases resting and exercise-induced intramuscular free radical formation. *J. Appl. Physiol.* **2010**, *109*, 449–456. **[Google Scholar] [Green Version]**

98. McGinnis, G.; Kliszczewiscz, B.; Barberio, M.; Ballmann, C.; Peters, B.; Slivka, D.; Dumke, C.; Cuddy, J.; Hailes, W.; Ruby, B.; et al. Acute Hypoxia and Exercise-Induced Blood Oxidative Stress. *Int. J. Sport Nutr. Exerc. Metab.* **2014**, *24*, 684–693. **[Google Scholar]**

99. Stefani, G.P.; Nunes, R.B.; Dornelles, A.Z.; Alves, J.P.; Piva, M.O.; Di Domenico, M.; Rhoden, C.R.; Lago, P.D. Effects of creatine supplementation associated with resistance training on oxidative stress in different tissues of rats. *J. Int. Soc. Sports Nutr.* **2014**, *11*, 11. **[Google Scholar] [Green Version]**

100. Zhao, X.; Bey, E.A.; Wientjes, F.B.; Cathcart, M.K. Cytosolic Phospholipase A2 (cPLA2) Regulation of Human Monocyte NADPH Oxidase Activity. *J. Biol. Chem.* **2002**, *277*, 25385–25392. **[Google Scholar] [PubMed] [Green Version]**

101. Araújo, M.B.; Moura, L.P.; Junior, R.C.V.; Junior, M.C.; Dalia, R.A.; Sponton, A.C.; Ribeiro, C.; Mello, M.A.R. Creatine supplementation and oxidative stress in rat liver. *J. Int. Soc. Sports Nutr.* **2013**, *10*, 54. **[Google Scholar] [Green Version]**

102. Tromm, C.B.; Rosa, G.L.; Bom, K.; Mariano, I.; Pozzi, B. Effect of different frequencies weekly training on parameters of oxidative stress. *Rev. Bras. Cineantropom. Desempenho Hum.* **2011**, *14*, 52–60. **[Google Scholar] [Green Version]**

103. Yu, Z.-W.; Li, D.; Ling, W.-H.; Jin, T.-R. Role of nuclear factor (erythroid-derived 2)-like 2 in metabolic homeostasis and insulin action: A novel opportunity for diabetes treatment? *World J. Diabetes* **2012**, *3*, 19–28. **[Google Scholar] [PubMed]**

104. Di Meo, S.; Venditti, P. Mitochondria in Exercise-Induced Oxidative Stress. *Neurosignals* **2001**, *10*, 125–140. **[Google Scholar] [PubMed]**

105. Deminice, R.; Jordão, A.A. Creatine supplementation reduces oxidative stress biomarkers after acute exercise in rats. *Amino Acids* **2011**, *43*, 709–715. **[Google Scholar]**

106. Rochard, P.; Rodier, A.; Casas, F.; Cassar-Malek, I.; Marchal-Victorion, S.; Daury, L.; Wrutniak, C.; Cabello, G. Mitochondrial Activity Is Involved in the Regulation of Myoblast Differentiation through Myogenin Expression and Activity of Myogenic Factors. *J. Biol. Chem.* **2000**, *275*, 2733–2744. **[Google Scholar] [Green Version]**

107. Lenz, H.; Schmidt, M.; Welge, V.; Schlattner, U.; Wallimann, T.; Elsässer, H.-P.; Wittern, K.-P.; Wenck, H.; Stäb, F.; Blatt, T. The Creatine Kinase System in Human Skin: Protective Effects of Creatine Against Oxidative and UV Damage In Vitro and In Vivo. *J. Investig. Dermatol.* **2005**, *124*, 443–452. **[Google Scholar] [PubMed] [Green Version]**

108. Berneburg, M.; Gremmel, T.; Kürten, V.; Schroeder, P.; Hertel, I.; Von Mikecz, A.; Wild, S.; Chen, M.; Declercq, L.; Matsui, M.; et al. Creatine Supplementation Normalizes Mutagenesis of Mitochondrial DNA as Well as Functional Consequences. *J. Investig. Dermatol.* **2005**, *125*, 213–220. **[Google Scholar] [Green Version]**

109. Kingsley, M.I.C.; Cunningham, D.; Mason, L.; Kilduff, L.P.; McEneny, J. Role of Creatine Supplementation on Exercise-Induced Cardiovascular Function and Oxidative Stress. *Oxidative Med. Cell. Longev.* **2009**, *2*, 247–254. **[Google Scholar] [PubMed]**

110. Deminice, R.; Rosa, F.T.; Franco, G.S.; Jordao, A.A.; De Freitas, E.C. Effects of creatine supplementation on oxidative stress and inflammatory markers after repeated-sprint exercise in humans. *Nutrition* **2013**, *29*, 1127–1132. **[Google Scholar] [Green Version]**

111. Percario, S.; Domingues, S.P.D.T.; Teixeira, L.F.M.; Vieira, J.L.F.; De Vasconcelos, F.; Ciarrocchi, D.M.; Almeida, E.D.; Conte, M. Effects of creatine supplementation on oxidative stress profile of athletes. *J. Int. Soc. Sports Nutr.* **2012**, *9*, 56. [**Google Scholar**] [**Green Version**]

112. Suzuki, K.; Hayashida, H. Effect of Exercise Intensity on Cell-Mediated Immunity. *Sports* **2021**, *9*, 8. [**Google Scholar**]

9 Chapter

# EFFECTIVENESS OF COMMON DIETS UTILIZED BY ENDURANCE ATHLETES ON ATHLETIC PERFORMANCE: ADVANTAGEOUS OR HARMFUL?

## 1. INTRODUCTION: AN OVERVIEW

Endurance performance, particularly extended training, necessitates increased metabolic and nutritional requirements from athletes [1]. Endurance athletes encounter challenging conditions while training, prompting them to explore alternate dietary options to enhance endurance performance and metabolic health [2]. A scientifically validated diet is essential prior to its adoption by the athletic population [3]. Vegetarian diets, high-fat diets (HFD), intermittent fasting (IF) diets, gluten-free diets (GFD), and low fermentable oligosaccharides, disaccharides, monosaccharides, and polyols (FODMAP) diets are highly favored by endurance athletes. This review will examine the advantageous and detrimental effects of various diets on metabolic health and endurance performance. Endurance performance, particularly extended training, necessitates increased metabolic and nutritional requirements from athletes [1]. Endurance athletes encounter challenging conditions while training, prompting them to explore alternate dietary options to enhance endurance performance and metabolic health [2]. A scientifically validated diet is essential prior to its adoption by the athletic population [3]. Vegetarian diets, high-fat diets (HFD), intermittent fasting (IF) diets, gluten-free diets (GFD), and low fermentable oligosaccharides, disaccharides, monosaccharides, and polyols (FODMAP) diets are highly favored by endurance athletes. This review will examine the advantageous and detrimental effects of various diets on metabolic health and endurance performance.

## 2. METHODOLOGY

We searched both the PubMed and Cochrane databases for the terms "diet*", "track-and-field", "runner*", "marathoner*", "cyclist", "cycling", "triathlete", "endurance", and "endurance athletes" in the title, abstract, and keywords to detect the most applied diets between 2015 and 2021 in endurance athletes. We obtained 217 results in PubMed and 80 trials in the Cochrane database. We defined the most recurrent diets in endurance athletes, including "High CHO availability", "High-carbohydrate diet", "Ketogenic diet", "Low-CHO diet", "Low-CHO, high-fat diet", "Ketogenic low-carbohydrate, high-fat diet", "Low-carbohydrate ketogenic diet", "Low-carbohydrate, high fat, ketogenic diet", "High-fat, low carbohydrate diet", "Ketone ester supplementation", "time-restrictive eating", "Ketone supplementation", "Intermittent fasting", "fasting during Ramadan", "Vegan diet", "Lacto-Ovo vegetarian diet", "Vegetarian diet", "Low fermentable oligo-, di-, monosaccharide, and polyol diet", and "Gluten-free diet". Since we all know that high-carbohydrate diet is already well proven to enhance endurance performance [**2**], we targeted other diets for in-depth investigation by categorizing them as "vegan/vegetarian diets", "high-fat diets", "intermittent fasting", "low-FODMAP diet, and "gluten-free diet". We included studies on endurance athletes and popular diets, including vegetarian diets, high-fat diets, intermittent fasting, gluten-free diet, and low-FODMAP diet. Using PubMed, Cochrane Library, and Web of Science databases, we aimed to identify studies on races and endurance training. Two researchers (A.D.L and L.H.) independently reviewed the literature. In cases of conflict, a third investigator (B.K.) resolved the disagreement. We identified the studies published from 1983 to 2021. To define the studies on endurance athletes and diets to be included in the current narrative review, we searched MeSH terms (("Diet, Ketogenic" (Majr); "Diet, High-Fat" (Majr); "Diet, Carbohydrate-Restricted" (Majr); "Ketone Bodies" (Majr); "Diet, Vegetarian" (Majr); "Diet, Vegan" (Majr); "Fasting" (Majr); "Diet, Gluten-Free" (Majr); "athletes" (Majr); "physical endurance" (Majr); "Diet Therapy" (Majr); " Oligosaccharides" (Majr), "Disaccharides" (Majr)) and MeSH terms found below this term in the MeSH hierarchy recommended by PubMed and Cochrane Library. We also searched by adding the terms "FODMAP diet", "low-FODMAP diet", "FODMAP*", "Fermentable oligosaccharides, disaccharides and polyols", "Fermentable, poorly absorbed, short chain carbohydrates", "Inulin", "Xylitol", "Mannitol", "Maltitol", "Isomalt", "Fructose", "Fructans", "Galactooligosaccharides", "fructooligosaccharides", and "Polyols" to all databases, as no MeSH terms for the low-FODMAP diet were defined. We discussed the findings after determining the clinical and practical relevance of the studies by considering only human studies. We included studies available in English clearly describing the applied diet and investigating the effect of diet on endurance athletes as the primary goal. In addition, we included studies where diets were applied according to the dietary description. We excluded studies not explicitly addressing the impact of the diet on endurance performance or health-related parameters, that were not written in English, and were conducted on animals or in vitro. Based on our inclusion and exclusion criteria, we identified 57 research articles (**Table 1**). We organized the narrative review by considering both the beneficial and detrimental aspects of all five diets for endurance athletes.

**Table 1. Studies investigating the potential effects of vegetarian, fasting, high-fat, gluten-free, and low-FODMAP diets on athletes' endurance performance.**

| Subjects | Study Design | Diet/Application | Duration | Exercise Protocol(s) | Main Findings | Ref. |
|---|---|---|---|---|---|---|
| **High-Fat Diets** | | | | | | |
| Endurance-trained male athletes (*n* = 20) | A non-randomized control trial | K-LCHF diet (*n* = 9; %CHO:fat:protein = 6:77:17) or HCD (*n* = 11; 65:20:14) | 12 weeks | A 100-km TT performance, a 6-s sprint, and a CPT | ↓ Body mass<br>↓ Body fat percentage<br>↑ Average relative power during the 6 s sprint sprint and CPT<br>↑ Fat oxidation during exercise<br>↔ 100 km TT endurance performance | [14] |
| Recreational male athletes (*n* = 14) | A randomized, crossover design | K-LCHF diet (<10%CHO, 75% fat) and 2 week HCD (>50% CHO), >2 weeks washout period in between | 2 weeks | A 90-min bicycle ergometer exercise test at 60%Wmax | ↓ Exercise-induced cortisol response; however, better results observed in HCD<br>↓ Exercise capacity<br>↑ Fat oxidation during exercise<br>↑ Perceived exertion after exercise<br>↔ Post-exercise s-IgA levels at week 2 | [15] |
| Professional male race walkers (*n* = 25) | A mix of repeated-measures and parallel-group design | K-LCHF diet (*n* = 10; 75–80% FAT, <50 g CHO, 17% protein), HCD (*n* = 8; 60–65% CHO, 20% FAT, 15–20% protein), or PCD, (*n* = 7; 60–65% CHO, 20% FAT, 15–20% protein) | 3 weeks | - A graded walking economy and $VO_2$peak test on treadmill<br>- A 10-km race walk (field)<br>- A 25-km standardized race walk | ↔ $VO_2$peak<br>↓ 10 km race walk performance<br>↑ Perceived exertion after exercise<br>↑ Oxygen cost<br>↑ Fat oxidation during exercise | [16] |

| Subjects | Study Design | Diet/Application | Duration | Exercise Protocol(s) | Main Findings | Ref. |
|---|---|---|---|---|---|---|
| Male and female elite race walkers ($n$ = 24) | A mix of repeated-measures and parallel-group design | K-LCHF diet ($n$ = 9; 75–80% FAT, <50 g CHO, 15–20% protein), HCD ($n$ = 8; 60–65% CHO, 20% FAT, 15–20% protein), or PCD, ($n$ = 7; 60–65% CHO, 20% FAT, 15–20% protein) | 3 weeks | - A graded walking economy and $VO_2$peak test on treadmill | ↔ $VO_2$peak<br>↔ Blood acid-base status | [17] |
| Endurance-trained male athletes ($n$ = 8) | A randomized repeated-measures crossover study | K-LCHF diet (75–80% FAT, <50 g CHO, 15–20% protein), HCD (43% CHO, 38% FAT, 19% protein) | 4.5 weeks | - A graded metabolic test to exhaustion<br>- A TTE performance at 70% $VO_2$max | ↔ TTE performance<br>↔ Perceived exertion after exercise<br>↓ Exercise efficiency above 70% $VO_2$max<br>↔Exercise efficiency above 70% $VO_2$max | [18] |
| Recreationally competitive male runners ($n$ = 8) | A pre–post-test | K-LCHF diet (<50 g CHO, 70% FAT (ad libitum), or HCD (habitual diet defined as moderate to high CHO) | 3 weeks | - Five 10-min running bouts at multiple individual race paces in the heat, 20-min rest, then a 5 km TT performance after 50 min of running in challenging environmental conditions | ↔ 5 km TT performance<br>↔ Perceived exertion after exercise<br>↑ Fat oxidation during exercise<br>↓ Body mass<br>↓ Skinfold thickness<br>↔ Exercise-induced cardiorespiratory, thermoregulatory, or perceptual responses | [19] |
| Elite male cyclists ($n$ = 5) | A pre–post-test | K-LCHF diet (<20 g CHO, 85% FAT, 15% protein) for 3 weeks immediately after a 1 week HCD (66% CHO, 33%FAT, 1.75 g protein/kg BW/d) | 4 weeks (3 weeks LCKD after 1 week HCD) | - A $VO_2$max test on cycle ergometry<br>- A TTE test at 60–65% $VO_2$max at two time points: after HCD and K-LCHF diet | ↔ $VO_2$max<br>↔ TTE performance<br>↑ Fat oxidation<br>↔ Blood glucose levels during TTE performance | [20] |

| Subjects | Study Design | Diet/Application | Duration | Exercise Protocol(s) | Main Findings | Ref. |
|---|---|---|---|---|---|---|
| Recreational athletes ($n$ = 5) | Case study | K-LCHF diet (ad libitum FAT, <50 g CHO, 1.75 g protein/kg BW/d) | 10 weeks | - A TTE performance<br>- A peak power test<br>- A $VO_2$max test | ↓ TTE performance<br>↑ Fat oxidation during exercise even at higher intensities<br>↓ Body mass<br>↓ Skinfold thickness | [21] |
| Endurance-trained male athletes ($n$ = 8) | A randomized, repeated-measures, crossover study | K-LCHF diet (75–80% FAT, <50 g CHO, 15–20% protein), HCD (43% CHO, 38% FAT, 19% protein) | 4.5 weeks | - A graded metabolic test to exhaustion<br>- A TTE performance at 70% $VO_2$max | Preservation of mucosal immunity<br>↑ Both pro- and anti-inflammatory T-cell-related cytokine responses to a multiantigen in vitro | [22] |
| Elite race walkers ($n$ = 25) | A mix of repeated-measures and parallel-group design | K-LCHF diet ($n$ = 10; 75–80% FAT, <50 g CHO, 17% protein), HCD ($n$ = 8; 60–65% CHO, 2% FAT, 15–20% protein), or PCD, ($n$ = 7; 60–65% CHO, 20% FAT, 15–20% protein) | 3.5 weeks | - A graded walking economy and $VO_2$peak test<br>- A 10-km track race After CHO re-adaptation:<br>- A 20-km race walking | ↔ $VO_2$peak<br>↓ 10 km race walk performance<br>↑ Perceived exertion after exercise<br>↑ Oxygen cost<br>↑ Whole-body fat oxidation | [23] |
| Male ultra-endurance runners ($n$ = 20) | A cross-sectional study design | K-LCHF diet ($n$ = 10, 10:19:70) diet or Habitual high-CHO ($n$ = 10, %CHO:protein:fat = 59:14:25) diet | An average of 20 months (range 9–36 months) | - A graded exercise test<br>- A 3-h run at 65% $VO_2$max on a treadmill | ↑ Fat oxidation<br>↔ Muscle glycogen utilization and repletion after 180 min of running and 120 min of recovery | [24] |
| Male competitive recreational distance runners ($n$ = 7) | A randomized counterbalanced, crossover design | K-LCHF diet ($n$ = 10; 75–80% FAT, <50 g CHO, 17% protein), or HCD ($n$ = 8; 60–65% CHO, 20% FAT, 15–20% protein) | 6 weeks | - A $VO_2$max test<br>- A 5-km TT performance (day 4, 14, 28, and 42) | ↔ $VO_2$max<br>↔ TT performance<br>↑ Fat oxidation | [25] |

| Subjects | Study Design | Diet/Application | Duration | Exercise Protocol(s) | Main Findings | Ref. |
|---|---|---|---|---|---|---|
| Endurance-trained male cyclists ($n$ = 5) | Crossover design | A high-fat diet (70% FAT) or an equal-energy, high-carbohydrate diet (70% CHO) | 2×2 weeks, 2 week washout period in between (ad libitum diet during washout period) | - Peak power output test<br>- A cycling exercise to exhaustion at 90% $VO_2$max, 20-min rest, and followed with a cycling exercise to exhaustion at 50% $VO_2$max | ↑ TTE performance during MIE<br>↔ Endurance performance during HIE<br>↑ Fat oxidation | [26] |
| Highly trained male ultra-endurance runners ($n$ = 20) | A cross-sectional study design | Habitual low CHO ($n$ = 10; <20% CHO, >60% FAT) or high CHO ($n$ = 10; >55% CHO) | At least 6 months | | ↑ Circulating total cholesterol, LDL-C, and HDL-C concentrations<br>↑ Fewer small, dense LDL-C particles | [27] |
| Trained male off-road cyclists ($n$ = 8) | A crossover design | A mixed diet (%CHO:fat:protein = 50:30:20) or a NK-LCHF diet (15:70:15) | 4 weeks | A continuous exercise protocol on a cycling ergometer with varied intensity (90 min at 85% LT, then 15 min at 115% LT) | ↑ $VO_2$max<br>↓ Body mass<br>↓ Body fat percentage<br>↑ Fat oxidation<br>↓ Post-exercise muscle damage<br>↓ CK and LDH concentration at rest and during the 105 min exercise protocol in the NK-LCHF diet trial | [28] |
| Endurance trained cyclists ($n$ = 16) | A randomized, controlled study design | A NK-LCHF diet (19:69:10) or a habitual diet (%CHO:fat:protein = 53:30:13) | 15 days | a 2.5-h constant-load ride at 70% $VO_2$peak followed by a simulated 40-km cycling TT while ingesting a 10% 14C-glucose + 3.44% MCT emulsion at a rate of 600 mL/h | ↑ Fat oxidation<br>↔ TT performance | [29] |

| Subjects | Study Design | Diet/Application | Duration | Exercise Protocol(s) | Main Findings | Ref. |
|---|---|---|---|---|---|---|
| Trained male cyclists ($n$ = 9) | A repeated-measures, randomized, crossover study | 2 × 0.35 g/kg KE or placebo (30 min before and 60 min after exercise) | Acute ingestion | A 85-min steady state exercise at 73% $VO_2$max, followed by a 7 kJ/kg TT (~ 30 min) | ↑ Transient type-I T-cell immunity at the gen level | [30] |
| Endurance-trained male and female athletes (male/female, 9/3) | A single-blind, randomized and counterbalanced, crossover design | KE (330 mg/kg BW of βHB containing beverage, or bitter-flavored placebo drink before exercise | Acute ingestion | An incremental bicycle ergometer exercise test to exhaustion | ↔ Blood pH and $HCO_3$ levels<br>↔ TTE performance | [31] |
| Endurance-trained athletes (male/female:5/1) | A single-blind, random order controlled, crossover design | A 400 mL, low-dose β-HB KME 252 mg/kg BW, "low ketosis"; a high-dose βHB KME (752 mg/kg BW, "high ketosis", or a bitter-flavored water (placebo) | Acute ingestion, 60 min prior to exercise | A 60-min continuous cycling exercise, consisting of 20 min intervals at 25%, 50% and 75% Wmax | ↓ Contribution of exogenous βHB to overall energy expenditure<br>↑ Exercise efficiency when blood βHB levels above 2 mmol/L<br>↑ Nausea | [32] |
| High-performance athletes | Study 1:<br>A randomized crossover design<br>Study 2, 3 and 5:<br>A randomized, single-blind, crossover design<br>Study 4:<br>A two-way crossover study | Study 1 ($n$ = 6):<br>A KE (573 mg/kg BW) drink at rest, and during 45 min of cycling exercise 40% and 75% of WMax; with 1 week washout period in between<br>Study 2 ($n$ = 10): - 96% of calories from CHO (dextrose = CHO), KE (573 mg/kg BW), or FAT before test<br>Study 3 ($n$ = 8): | Acute ingestion | Study 1:<br>- A 45-min cycling exercise at 40% and 75% WMax<br>Study 2 and 3:<br>- A fixed-intensity cycling exercise at 75% WMax for 60 min<br>Study 4:<br>- A fixed-intensity bicycle ergometry test at 70%$VO_2$max for 2-h<br>Study 5:<br>- A 60-min steady state workload at 75% WMax followed by a blinded 30-min TT | ↑ TT performance following 1 h of high-intensity exercise<br>↑ Fat oxidation<br>↓ Plasma lactate levels during exercise<br>↑ D-βHB oxidation according to exercise intensity (from 0.35 g/min at 40% WMax to 0.5 g/min at 75% WMax)<br>↔ Blood glucose levels | [33] |

| Subjects | Study Design | Diet/Application | Duration | Exercise Protocol(s) | Main Findings | Ref. |
|---|---|---|---|---|---|---|
| | | - 60% of calories from CHO and 40% of KE (573 mg/kg BW), a mixture of carbohydrates (CHO), or a no-calorie beverage with 1000 mg B3 before test<br>Study 4 ($n$ = 7):<br>- 60% of calories from CHO (dextrose) and 40% from KE, or a mixture of CHOs, 50% of the drink consumed at baseline, the remaining 50% at 30 min, 60 min, and 90 min during exercise as equal aliquots<br>Study 5 ($n$ = 6 male, $n$ = 2 female):<br>- 60% of calories from CHO and KE (573 mg/kg BW), or a mixture of carbohydrates (CHO) | | | | |
| Trained male cyclists ($n$ = 9) | A repeated-measures, randomized, crossover study | A drink containing 0.35 g/kg BW BD or placebo | Acute ingestion (30 min before and 60 min during 85 min of steady state exercise) | A steady state cycling at the power output eliciting 85% of their VT followed by a TT performance equivalent to 7 kJ/kg (~25–35 min) | ↔ TT performance and average power output<br>↔ Blood glucose and lactate levels<br>↑ Fat oxidation<br>↑ GI symptoms | [34] |
| Elite male cyclists ($n$ = 10) | A randomized crossover design | A 1,3-butanediol AcAc diester (2×250 mg/kg BW) or a viscosity and color-matched plasebo drink | Acute ingestion, ~30 min before and immediately prior to commencing the warm up | ~A 31-km laboratory-based TT performance on a cycling ergometer | ↓ TT performance<br>↑ GI symptoms (nausea and reflux)<br>↑ Fat oxidation | [35] |
| Male runners ($n$ = 11) | A randomized crossover design | An energy matched ~650 mL drink containing 60 g CHO + 0.5 g/kg BW 1.3-butanediol (CHO-BD) or 110 g ± 5 g CHO alone | Acute ingestion (50% after baseline measurements + 25% after 30 min of seated rest, + 25% after 10 | A 60-min submaximal running, followed by a 5-km running time trial | ↔ TT performance<br>↔ Overall lactate concentration<br>↑ Blood glucose levels after TT performance | [36] |

| Subjects | Study Design | Diet/Application | Duration | Exercise Protocol(s) | Main Findings | Ref. |
|---|---|---|---|---|---|---|
| Highly trained male cyclists (*n* = 12) | A randomized crossover design | A KE drink (65 g (918,102 mg/kg, range: 722–1072 mg/kg) of KE [ 96% βHB] or a viscosity- and taste-matched placebo | Acute ingestion (at 60 and 20 min before and at 30 min during race) | A simulated cycling race, which consisted of a 3-h intermittent cycling, a 15-min time trial, and a maximal sprint | ↔ High-intensity exercise performance in the final stage of the event<br>↑ Upper-abdominal discomfort<br>↓ Appetite after exercise<br>↔ Net muscle glycogen breakdown | [37] |
| Recreational male distance runners (*n* = 13) | A randomized, double-blind, placebo-controlled, cross- over design | Either one (KS1: 22.1 g) or two (KS2: 44.2 g) servings of the ketone supplement (βHB + MCT) or a flavor-matched placebo drink | Acute ingestion (60 min prior to exercise) | A 5-km running TT on a treadmill | ↔ Post-exercise glucose concentration<br>↔ TT performance<br>↔ Perceived exertion after exercise<br>Dose–response impact on cognitive function | [38] |
| Eight trained, middle- and long-distance runners (male/female, 7/1) | A double-blind, randomized crossover design | An 8% carbohydrate-electrolyte solution before and during exercise, either alone (CHO + PLA), or with 573 mg/kg of a ketone monoester supplement (CHO + KME) | Acute ingestion | A 60-min submaximal exercise at 65%$VO_2$max immediately followed by a 10-km TT | ↔ TT performance<br>↔ $VO_2$max, running economy, RER, HR, perceived exertion<br>↔ Cognitive performance<br>↔ Plasma glucose and lactate levels<br>↑ Fat oxidation | [39] |
| Male and female elite race walkers | A non-randomized clinical trial | A K-LCHF diet (*n* = 18; 75–80% FAT, <50 g CHO, 15–20% PRO) followed by an acute CHO restoration, or HCD (*n* = 14; 60–65% CHO, 20% FAT, 15–20% PRO) | 3.5 weeks | A hybrid laboratory/field test of 25 km (males) or 19 km (females) at around 50 km race pace at 75% $VO_2$max | ↓ Bone resorption markers at rest and post-exercise<br>↑ Bone formation markers at rest and throughout exercise<br>Partial recovery of these effects following CHO restoration | [40] |

| Subjects | Study Design | Diet/Application | Duration | Exercise Protocol(s) | Main Findings | Ref. |
|---|---|---|---|---|---|---|
| Well-trained competitive male cyclists or triathletes ($n = 7$) | A randomized, crossover design | Day 1: a standard CHO diet (%CHO:fat:protein = 58:27:15)<br>Day 2–7: either an HFD (16:69:15) or HCD (70:15:15) for 6 days<br>Day 8: HCD (70:15:15) | 6 day fat adaptation followed by 1 day CHO restoration,<br>a 18 day washout period between | Day 9: A 4-h cycling ergometer at 65% $VO_2$peak, followed by a 60-min TT | ↔ TT performance<br>↑ Fat oxidation | [41] |
| Well-trained competitive male cyclists or triathletes ($n = 8$) | A randomized, crossover design | Day 1–5: either an HFD (%CHO:fat:protein = 19:68:13) or an HCD (74:13:13)<br>Day 6: HCD (74:13:13) | 5 day fat adaptation followed by 1 day CHO restoration,<br>a 2 week washout period between | A 2-h cycling at 70% $VO_2$max; followed by 7 kJ/kg TT | ↔ TT performance<br>↑ Fat oxidation<br>↔ Muscle glycogen utilization<br>↔ Plasma glucose uptake | [42] |
| Well-trained competitive male cyclists or triathletes ($n = 8$) | A randomized, double-blind crossover design | Day 1–5: either an HFD (%CHO:fat:protein = 19:68:13) or an HCD (74:13:13)<br>Day 6: HCD (74:13:13)<br>Pre-exercise: a CHO breakfast (CHO 2 g/kg).<br>During exercise: CHO intake (0.8 g/kg/h) | 5 day fat adaptation followed by 1 day CHO restoration,<br>a 2 week washout period between | A 2-h cycling at 70% $VO_2$max; followed by 7 kJ/kg TT | ↔ TT performance<br>↑ Fat oxidation | [43] |
| Well-trained competitive male cyclists or triathletes ($n = 8$) | A randomized, double-blind crossover design | Day 1–5: either an HFD (%CHO:fat:protein = 19:68:13) or an HCD (74:13:13)<br>Day 6: HCD (74:13:13) | 5 day fat adaptation followed by 1 day CHO restoration,<br>a 2 week washout period between | A 60-min steady state ride<br>at 70% $VO_2$max | ↓ Muscle glycogen utilization<br>↑ Fat oxidation<br>↑ Pre-exercise AMPK-1 and AMPK-2 activity<br>↓ Exercise-induced AMPK-1 and AMPK-2 activity | [44] |
| Endurance-trained male cyclists ($n = 8$) | A randomized, single-blind, crossover design | Day 1–6: either a NK- LCHF diet (%CHO:fat:protein = 16.8:68.2:15.0) or an HCD (67.8:17.1:15.1)<br>Day 6: HCD (16.8:68.2:15.0) | 6 day fat adaptation followed by 1 day CHO restoration,<br>a 2 week washout period between | A 100-km TT on their bicycles;<br>five 1 km sprint distances after 10, 32, 52, 72, and 99 km, four 4 km sprint distances after 20, 40, 60, and 80 km | ↔ TT performance<br>↑ Fat oxidation<br>↓ 1 km sprint power<br>↔ Perceived exertion | [45] |

| Subjects | Study Design | Diet/Application | Duration | Exercise Protocol(s) | Main Findings | Ref. |
|---|---|---|---|---|---|---|
| Endurance-trained male cyclists ($n$ = 5) | Randomized, crossover design | Either 10 day habitual diet (~30% fat), followed with 3 day HCD or 10 day high-fat diet (> 65% fat), followed by 3 day HCD<br>1 h prior to each trial: -400 mL 3.44% MCT ($C_{8-10}$) solution<br>During trial: 600 mL/h 10% glucose ($^{14}C$) + 3.44% MCT solution | 10 day HFD + 3 day HCD vs. 10 day habitual diet + 3 day HCD<br>-<br>Acute ingestion of MCT solution 1 h before trial and glucose + MCT solution during trial | A 150-min cycling at 70% $VO_2$peak, followed immediately by a 20-km TT | ↑ TT performance<br>↑ Fat oxidation<br>↓ Muscle glycogen utilization<br>↔ Body fat, BW | [46] |
| Endurance-trained male cyclists or triathletes ($n$ = 7) | A randomized, double-blind crossover design | Day 1–5: either an HFD (%CHO:fat:protein = 19:68:13) or an HCD (74:13:13)<br>Day 6: HCD (74:13:13) | 5 day fat adaptation, a 2 week washout period between | A 20-min steady state cycling at 70% $VO_2$peak, 1 min rest, a 1 min all-out sprint at 150% PPO, and followed by 4 kJ/kg TT | ↑ Fat oxidation<br>↓ Glycogenolysis and PDH activation<br>↔ Muscle glycogen contents at rest | [47] |
| A lacto-ovo vegetarian athlete who adhered to an LCHF diet for 32 weeks | Case study | An LCHF diet for 32 weeks | 32 weeks | Three professional races while on the LCHF diet in week 21, 24, and 32 (consumption of CHO before and during the race as advised) | ↓ Half-ironman performance at week 21<br>↓ Ironman performance at week 24 and 32<br>↔ Exercise-induced GI symptoms | [48] |
| Trained male cyclists ($n$ = 11) | A reference-controlled crossover (two treatment, two period), balanced, masked, single-center outpatient metabolic trial | HCD (% CHO:protein:fat = 73/14/12) for 2.5 days or HCD for first day and followed by the last 1.5 days with fat-enriched feeding (43/9/48) | 2.5 days (1 day HCD, followed by lipid supplementation for 1.5 day), or 2.5 day HCD | Pre- and post-intervention;<br>-<br>A 3-h exercise on a bicycle ergometer at 50% Wmax post-intervention;<br>-<br>20-km TT | ↔ Perceived exertion after exercise<br>↔ Fat oxidation during prolonged exercise<br>↑ Replenishment of both glycogen content and IMCL stores<br>↔ TT performance | [49] |

| Subjects | Study Design | Diet/Application | Duration | Exercise Protocol(s) | Main Findings | Ref. |
|---|---|---|---|---|---|---|
| Trained male cyclists ($n$ = 22) | A single-blind (clinical trial staff were blinded), 2-treatment crossover randomized clinical trial | An HCD, (CHO 7.4 g/kg BW, FAT 0.5 g/kg BW) for 2.5 days or a high-CHO fat-supplemented (HCF) diet ((first day similar with HCD, followed by 1.5 days with a replication of the HC diet with 240 g surplus fat (30% saturation)) distributed over the last 4 meals of the diet period | 2.5 days (1 day HCD, followed by lipid supplementation for 1.5 day), or 2.5 day HCD | A fixed-task simulated TT lasting approximately 1-h<br>A $VO_2$peak test | ↔ TT performance<br>↔ Fat oxidation during submaximal or 1 h TT exercise<br>↔ Reaction time throughout TT | [50] |
| Male collegiate long-distance athletes ($n$ = 8) | A double-blind, placebo- controlled, crossover study design | 3 days before the trial:<br>an HCD (% CHO:fat:protein = 71:19:10)<br>4 h before exercise:<br>HF meal (% CHO:fat:protein = 30:55:15) or HC meal (% CHO:fat:protein = 70:21:9)<br>Immediately before exercise:<br>-either maltodextrin jelly (M) or a placebo jelly (P) in the HF meal group<br>- a P in the HC group | Acute ingestion (either HF meal or HC meal 4 h before exercise) | An 80-min fixed-load test on a treadmill at ~70 $VO_2$max, followed with continuous endurance running to exhaustion at ~80% $VO_2$max | ↑ TTE performance in pre-exercise HF meal plus M consumption after CHO-loading<br>↑ Fat oxidation | [51] |
| **Vegetarian Diets** | | | | | | |
| Vegan ($n$ = 24), LOV ($n$ = 26) and omnivorous ($n$ = 26) recreational runners | A cross-sectional study design | Omnivorous, LOV or vegan diet for at least half a year | At least 6 months | An incremental exercise test on a bicycle ergometer | ↔ maximum power output<br>↔ Exercise capacity<br>↔ Blood lactate and glucose concentration during incremental exercise | [52] |
| Vegan ($n$ = 23), LOV ($n$ = 25) and omnivorous ($n$ = 25) recreational runners | A cross-sectional study design | Omnivorous, LOV or vegan diet for at least half a year | At least 6 months | An incremental exercise test on a bicycle ergometer | ↑ exercise-induced MDA concentration in the vegan (+15% rise) and LOV (+24% rise) groups<br>↔ NO metabolism | [53] |

| Subjects | Study Design | Diet/Application | Duration | Exercise Protocol(s) | Main Findings | Ref. |
|---|---|---|---|---|---|---|
| Male endurance athletes ($n = 8$) | A crossover design | A mixed meat-rich diet (69% animal protein sources) or a LOV diet (82% vegetable protein sources) | 2 ×6 weeks, 4 week washout period in between (ad libitum diet during washout period) | - A $VO_2$max test | ↔ Immunological parameters<br>↑ Fiber intake<br>↑ P/S ratio of fatty acids<br>↔ $VO_2$max capacity | [54] |
| Omnivorous, lacto-ovo vegetarian, and vegan recreational runners (21–25 subjects, respectively) | A cross-sectional study | Omnivorous, lacto-ovo-vegetarian or vegan diet for at least half a year | At least 6 months | An incremental exercise test on a bicycle ergometer | ↑ exercise-induced MDA concentration<br>↓ Sirtuin activities in vegans | [55] |
| A male vegan ultra-triathlete and a control group of 10 Ironman triathletes | Case report | A vegan ultra-triathlete adhered to a raw vegan diet and a control group of 10 Ironman triathletes adhered to a mixed diet | Vegan athlete living on a raw vegan diet for 6 years, vegan for 9 years and a vegetarian for 13 years | A Triple-Ironman distance (11.4 km swimming, 540 km cycling, and 126 km running) | ↑ $VO_2$max<br>↔ Exercise performance<br>↔ Exercise capacity<br>↔ Systolic and diastolic functions | [56] |
| A female vegan mountain biker | Case report | A vegan athlete living on a vegan diet for approximately 15 years | A vegan diet for approximately 15 years | The Transalp Challenge 2004 (altitude climbed, 22.500 m; total distance, 662 km, lasts approximately 8 days) | Successfully completing ultra-endurance mountain biking with a well-planned and implemented vegan diet | [57] |
| Vegetarian ($n$ = 27) and omnivore ($n = 43$) elite endurance athletes | Cross-sectional study design | Vegetarian and omnivore endurance athletes who adhered to their respective diets for at least three months | At least three months | A $VO_2$max test on the treadmill | ↔ Exercise performance<br>↔ Protein intake (kg BW/day)<br>↑ $VO_2$max (in females)<br>↔ $VO_2$max (in males) | [58] |
| Vegan ($n = 22$) and omnivorous ($n = 30$) amateur runners | Cross-sectional study design | Vegan and omnivore athletes; diet adherence time not reported | - | $VO_2$max and peak power output test on the treadmill | Better systolic and diastolic function<br>↑ $VO_2$max | [59] |
| **Intermittent Fasting Diets** | | | | | | |

| Subjects | Study Design | Diet/Application | Duration | Exercise Protocol(s) | Main Findings | Ref. |
|---|---|---|---|---|---|---|
| Well-trained, middle-distance runners ($n$ = 18) | A non-randomized, controlled study | RIF vs. control | 1 month | Beginning and at the end of Ramadan:<br>- A $VO_2$max test on the treadmill<br>- A MVC testing<br>- A 5-km TT | ↓ TT exercise performance<br>↔ $VO_2$max<br>↔ Running efficiency | **[60]** |
| Middle-distance athletes ($n$ = 8) | Pre–post-test | RIF | 1 month | 5 days before, 7 and 21 days after Ramadan:<br>- A maximal aerobic velocity test | ↓ Nocturnal sleep time<br>↓ Energy intake<br>↔ BW and body fat percentage<br>↔ Testosterone/cortisol ratio<br>↑ Fatigue<br>↑ Transient alteration in circulating IL-6, adrenaline, noradrenaline levels | **[61]** |
| Elite under 23 cyclists ($n$ = 16) | Parallel randomized trial | Time-restrictive eating (TRE) (16 h fasting, 8 h eating periods) or normal diet; both the same energy and macronutrient composition | 4 weeks | Pre- and post-diet:<br>- A $VO_2$max test<br>- A 45-min cycling ergometer at 45% peak power output | ↔ $VO_2$max<br>↔ endurance performance<br>↑ PPO/BW ratio<br>↓ BW and body fat percentage<br>↔ Fat-free mass | **[62]** |
| Male trained cyclists ($n$ = 11) | A non-randomized repeated-measures experimental study design | Ramadan fasting (15 h 15 min fasting period) | 29 days | A slow progressively increasing training load period (endurance training at first, and then intensity training included progressively) | ↑ Perceived exertion<br>↑ DOMS<br>↔ Total sleep time<br>↓ duration of deep and REM sleep stages<br>↔ Cognitive performance | **[63]** |

| Subjects | Study Design | Diet/Application | Duration | Exercise Protocol(s) | Main Findings | Ref. |
|---|---|---|---|---|---|---|
| Adolescent male cyclists ($n$ = 9) | A partially double-blind, placebo-controlled, randomized design | A CHO mouth rinse (with 25 mL of the solution) (CMR), a placebo mouth rinse (PMR), and a no-rinse (NOR) trial during Ramadan fasting state (fasting period ~13.5 h) | The last two weeks of Ramadan | A cycling exercise at 65% $VO_2$peak for 30 min followed by a 10 km TT under hot (32 °C) humid (75%) condition | ↑ TT performance in the CMR and PMR groups<br>↓ Perceived exertion in the CMR compared to the NOR<br>↔ Total sleep time | [64] |
| Trained male middle- and long-distance runners ($n$ = 17) | A randomized, parallel-group, pre-and post-experimental design | A TRE (fasting: 16 h, ad libitum eating: 8 h) ($n$ = 10) or normal diet ($n$ = 7) | 8 weeks | An incremental test until exhaustion | ↓ BW<br>↔ $VO_2$max<br>↔ Running economy<br>↔ Blood lactate, glucose, and insulin<br>↓ Daily energy intake | [65] |
| **Gluten-Free Diet** | | | | | | |
| Non-coeliac or non-IBS competitive endurance cyclists ($n$ = 13) | A controlled, randomized, double-blind, crossover study design | GFD or gluten-containing diet plus additional 2 gluten-free or gluten-containing food bars (total 16 g wheat gluten per day) | 2 × 7 days, a 10 day washout period in between | A steady state cycling at 70% Wmax for 45 min followed by a 15 min TT | ↔ TT performance<br>↔ GI symptoms<br>↔ Intestinal damage<br>↔ Well-being | [66] |
| **Low-FODMAP Diet** | | | | | | |
| Recreationally competitive runners with non-clinical GI symptoms (5 males, 6 females) | A single-blind, crossover design | Either a high-FODMAP or a low-FODMAP (<0.5 g FODMAP/meal) diet | 2×6 days, 1 day washout period in between | - A 5 × 1000-m run on day 4<br>- A 7-km threshold run on day 5 | In the low-FODMAP group;<br>↔ Well-being<br>↓ GI symptoms | [67] |
| A female ultra-endurance runner | Case study | A 4 week low-FODMAP diet, (3.9 g FODMAP/day) | 4 week low-FODMAP diet + 6 week reintroduction of high- FODMAP foods | A 6-day 186.7 km multistage ultra-marathon | Minimal GI symptoms<br>↑ Nausea<br>↓ Energy, protein, CHO, and water intake compared to the recommended guidelines | [68] |

| Subjects | Study Design | Diet/Application | Duration | Exercise Protocol(s) | Main Findings | Ref. |
|---|---|---|---|---|---|---|
| A recreationally competitive multisport athlete | Case study; a single-blind approach | A 6 day low-FODMAP diet (7.2 ± 5.7g FODMAPs/day) vs. habitual diet (81 ± 5 g FODMAPs/day) | 6 days | Same training period both diet trial (Swim 60 min (day 1); cycle 60 min (day 2); rest (day 3); run intervals 70 min (day 4); cycle 180 min and steady state run 65 min (day 5) and; run intervals 65 min (day 6)) | ↓ Exercise-induced GI symptoms | [69] |
| Endurance runners ($n$ = 18) | A double-blind randomized crossover design | A high- (46.9 ± 26.2 g FODMAP/day) or low- (2.0 ± 0.7 FODMAP/day) FODMAP diet | 2 × 1 day; before each experimental trial | A 2-h running at 60% $VO_2max$ in 35 °C ambient temperature | In the low-FODMAP group; ↓ Exercise-associated disruption of GI integrity ↓ Exercise-associated GI symptoms ↓ Breath $H_2$ concentration | [70] |

↓: A significant decrease after the diet manipulation in the experimental group; ↑: A meaningful rise after the diet manipulation in the experimental group; ↔: No change after the diet manipulation in the experimental group. Abbreviations: K-LCHF: ketogenic low-carbohydrate, low-fat diet; NK-LCHF: non-ketogenic low-carbohydrate, low-fat diet CHO: carbohydrate; HCD: high-carbohydrate diet; TT: time trial; CPT: critical power test; s-IgA: serum immunoglobulin A; Wmax: maximal power output; $VO_2peak$: peak oxygen uptake; $VO_2max$: maximal oxygen uptake; PCD: periodized carbohydrate diet; TTE: time-to-exhaustion; MIE: moderate intensity exercise; HIE: high-intensity exercise; LDL-c: low-density lipoprotein; HDL-c: high-density lipoprotein; CK: creatine kinase; LDH: lactate dehydrogenase; SS: steady state; $HCO_3$: hydrogen bicarbonate; KE: ketone ester; KME: ketone monoester; BW: body weight; βHB: (R)-3-hydroxybutyl (R)-3-hydroxybutyrate); VT: ventilatory threshold; GI: gastrointestinal; MCT: medium-chain triglycerides; RER: Respiratory exchange ratio; HR: heart rate; IMCL: Intra myocellular lipid; LOV: lacto-ovo-vegetarian; MDA: malondialdehyde; NO: nitric oxide; P/S ratio: polyunsaturated/saturated fatty acid ratio; MVC: Maximal Voluntary Isometric Contraction; IL-6: interleukine-6; PPO/BW ratio: peak power output/body weight ratio; DOMS: delayed onset muscle soreness; GFD: gluten-free diet; FODMAP: fermentable oligosaccharides, disaccharides, monosaccharides and polyols.

# 3. POPULAR DIETS APPLIED TO IMPROVE SPORTS PERFORMANCE IN ENDURANCE ATHLETES

## 3.1. Vegetarian Diets

Worldwide, it is estimated that around four billion people follow vegetarian diets [**9**]. In addition to many books and documentaries on vegetarian diets along with various types of practice (**Table 1**) and many well-known athletes who have adopted vegan diets and improved their performance [**10**], vegan diets have become more acceptable and feasible in the athletic population [**11**]. Looking at the athletic population, using a survey-based study conducted with 422 marathon runners, approximately 10% (*n* = 39) of the athletes consumed vegetarian/vegan/pescatarian diets [**12**]. However, in the NURMI study, the authors used the prevalence of vegetarian diets in ultra-endurance runners, primarily living in Austria, Germany, and Switzerland [**13**]. The findings revealed that the ratio of vegetarian and vegan athletes was 18.4% and 37.1%, respectively.

### The Impact of Vegetarian Diets on Sports Performance

#### *Benefits of Vegetarian Diets*

With the growing popularity of vegetarian diets in the athletic population, researchers have begun to investigate the role of these diets in sports performance and metabolic profile [**71**].

Studies on vegetarian diets have suggested that these diets may improve endurance performance by increasing exercise capacity and performance, modulating exercise-induced oxidative stress [**72**], inflammatory processes including anti-inflammatory and immunologic responses [**4**], and upper-respiratory tract infections (URTI) [**73**], and providing better cardiovascular function [**59**].

Studies measuring the aerobic capacity of vegetarian and omnivorous athletes reported controversial results [**54,56,58,59**]. Two studies showed that $VO_2$max values were higher in vegetarian athletes compared to omnivore athletes [**56,59**], while a crossover study showed no difference between the groups [**54**]. Studies supported higher $VO_2$max values in vegetarians designed as a case study and two cross-sectional studies [**56,58,59**], which are considered as the lowest level of the etiology hierarchy. A cross-sectional study in amateur runners reported that vegetarian female athletes had higher $VO_2$max values than omnivorous female athletes; however, no difference was observed in $VO_2$max values between vegetarian and omnivorous male athletes [**58**]. We need more high-level studies on the interaction between $VO_2$max and vegetarian diet patterns in endurance athletes.

The availability of studies on vegetarian endurance athletes supports neither a positive nor a negative impact on exercise capacity [**52,56**]. Comparing the exercise capacity of lacto-ovo-vegetarian, vegan and omnivorous athletes, Nebl et al. [**52**] measured maximum power output (Pmax) during incremental exercise as the primary outcome of the study in determining exercise capacity, while maximum power output per lean body weight ($Pmax_{LBW}$), blood lactate and glucose concentration during incremental exercise were evaluated as secondary outcomes. No differences were detected in Pmax, $Pmax_{LBW}$, blood lactate and glucose concentrations between groups during increased exercise, suggesting that there was no difference in exercise capacity compared to the lacto-ovo-vegetarian (LOV), vegan or omnivorous diet pattern in endurance athletes [**52**]. In addition, a case study by Leischik and Spelsberg [**56**] assessed the exercise performance, cardiac status, and nutritional biomarkers of a male vegan ultra-triathlete and a control group of 10 Ironman triathletes during a Triple Iron ultra-triathlon (11.4 km swimming, 540 km cycling, and 126 km running). Apart from a mild thrombopenia with no pathological consequences in laboratory parameters, the vegan athlete did not have weakened nutritional biomarkers or impaired health symptoms. Additionally, the $VO_2$max value of the vegan athlete was greater compared to the omnivorous athletes. Systolic and diastolic functions also did not differ between vegan and omnivorous athletes. The findings indicate that a well-planned vegan diet can provide adequate nutritional support for an ultra-triathlete [**56**].

In addition to these aforementioned benefits, vegetarian diets may also provide advantages for exercise capacity by increasing muscle glycogen levels [**71**], and delaying fatigue [**74**]. As for increasing glycogen stores, carbohydrate intake is considered the cornerstone of a better endurance performance by enhancing muscle glycogen stores, delaying fatigue, and providing athletes to compete at better and higher levels during prolonged periods [**75**]. Given the fact that the vegetarian diets are rich in carbohydrates (CHO) [**71**], such diets may offer more opportunities when considering races or training that can last at least six hours [**2**]. However, these data bring us to the point where foods high in CHO rather than diet types may be responsible for better performance. Taken together, both studies have shown that vegetarian diets neither benefit nor harm exercise capacity and endurance performance compared to omnivorous athletes. However, more studies are needed due to the small number of studies on the topic.

Studies have shown that the beneficial effects of vegetarian diets in alleviating oxidative stress and regulating the anti-inflammatory response are based on their enormous non-nutrient content called phytochemicals [**4**,**76**]. Polyphenols containing flavonoids, phenolic acids, lignans, and stilbenes are the most diverse non-nutrient group of phytochemicals that are produced as secondary metabolites throughout plants and have a broad spectrum of effects on metabolic health [**77**]. Polyphenol research of the athletic population has often been conducted using various fruits and vegetables, mainly berries [**78**], including blueberries [**79**,**80**,**81**,**82**], black currant [**83**], Montgomery cherry [**84**,**85**], and pomegranate [**86**]. Acute polyphenol intake or supplementation of ~300 mg 1–2 h before training or >1000 mg of polyphenol supplementation (equivalent to 450 g blueberries, 120 g blackcurrants or 300 g Montmorency cherries) 3 to more days (1–6 weeks) before and immediately after training is recommended as a countermeasure to improve antioxidant and anti-inflammatory response mechanisms [**87**]. However, only two studies examined the effect of vegetarian diets on exercise-induced oxidative stress in endurance athletes by comparing them with omnivorous diets, revealing contradictory results [**53**,**55**]. An incremental exercise test was applied in both studies. Nebl et al. [**53**] showed that nitric oxide levels, also known as an important biomarker for inflammation, endothelial and vascular function, did not alter between groups. In addition, exercise-induced malondialdehyde (MDA) concentration, an end product of lipid-peroxidation that is commonly measured to detect oxidative stress, significantly increased in vegan athletes in both studies, and in LOV athletes compared to omnivorous athletes [**53**]. Further, Potthast et al. [**55**] found a negative interaction between MDA, and sirtuin activities and antioxidant intakes such as ascorbate and tocopherol. These studies showed opposite results, against expectations, i.e., vegetarian diets increased the antioxidant response while suppressing the oxidant response. One explanation might be that the MDA test may not provide accurate measurement in biological samples due to its high reactivity and cross-reactions with other biochemicals available in the body despite its widely usage as an oxidative stress biomarker [**88**]. Therefore, studies with a greater sample size and including other oxidant parameters are needed to clarify these findings.

In addition to polyphenols, Interleukin 6 (IL-6) has often been identified as an inflammatory biomarker associated with fatigue, skeletal muscle inflammation, and differentiation of immune response, as well as an inducer of the metabolic acute phase response to infection [**4**,**89**,**90**,**91**]. It has been suggested that endurance athletes consuming vegetarian diets may have lower IL-6 concentrations and a lower IL-6 increase in response to endurance performance [**4**]. These data are explained by the positive interaction between muscle glycogen and IL-6 concentration, based on the information that higher muscle glycogen stores cause lower IL-6 elevations [**92**]. The higher CHO content of vegetarian diets may increase muscle glycogen stores, resulting in a down-regulated IL-6 response to endurance performance [**4**]. However, there are no data comparing the vegetarian and omnivorous diets for IL-6 concentration in endurance athletes.

One further point is the possible roles of vegetarian diets in URTI [**73**]. It is well known that endurance athletes are at greater risk for URTI due to prolonged and excessive training or races that cause immunosuppression and immune deficiency [**93**]. The possible link between URTI and a vegetarian diet may be explained with an emphasis on its polyphenolic content [**94**]. Polyphenol supplementation is also preferred in endurance athletes because of its debilitating role in URTI, one of the risk factors that often arise after immunosuppressive endurance exercise. A meta-analysis by Somerville et al. [**73**] reported that flavonoid supplementation reduced the incidence of URTI by 33% compared to a control group. Researchers also examined all factors that may cause a bias between studies, indicating that the risks for sequence generation, allocation concealment, and reporting bias are unclear in the included studies in the systematic review [**73**]. On the other hand, in a crossover design, Richter et al. [**54**] compared the influence of a 6 week LOV diet versus a meat-rich Western diet on in vitro measurements of immunologic parameters in male endurance athletes. The findings reported that no change was detected in $CD3^+$ (pan T-cells), $CD8^+$ (mainly T suppressor cells), $CD4^+$ (mainly T helper cells), $CD16^+$ (natural killer cells), $CD14^+$ (monocytes) after the two diet trials and none of the immunological parameters differed from each other after the two diets. Studies have commonly focused more on diet content rather than diet pattern whether vegetarian or omnivorous. Therefore, the potential immunological benefits of vegetarian diets need to be investigated further.

A review investigating the effect of vegetarian diets on cardiovascular health in endurance athletes highlighted that vegetarian diets can provide better cardiovascular protection by reducing plasma lipid levels, exercise-induced oxidative stress, inflammation and blood pressure, and improving endothelial function and arterial flexibility [**71**]. One cross-sectional study confirmed the information by investigating the difference in heart morphology and function according to the vegan and omnivorous diets in amateur runners [**59**]. The results showed that vegans had better systolic function, determined by longitudinal strain (vegan:-20.5% vs. omnivore:-19.6%), and diastolic function in vegans, determined by higher E-wave velocities (87 cm/s vs. 78 cm/s), compared to omnivorous athletes [**59**]. Therefore, we can confirm that vegetarian diets may have a beneficial impact on cardiovascular function; however, we still need further investigation on endurance athletes.

## Potential Risks of Vegetarian/Vegan Diets

Vegetarian and vegan diets offer several beneficial privileges for athletic populations [**9,71**]. However, the underlying mechanisms linking vegetarian diets to metabolic processes that may lead to undesirable effects on sports performance and, more importantly, metabolic health, should be considered beyond their beneficial functions [**95**]. In cases where athletes follow a vegetarian diet, issues related to the micronutrient deficiency, diet's energy availability [**96**], relative energy deficiency syndrome (RED-S) [**11**], serum hormones [**97,98**], and protein quality/quantity [**99,100**] are topics that need to be addressed first.

Athletes who adhere to vegetarian diets are considered at high risk for deficiency of certain nutrients, especially when their dietary composition is not well-structured [**10**]. These risks are mainly due to the restriction of some food groups with a high nutrient density such as milk, meat, and eggs, the inability to access vegetarian foods when needed, or the development of early satiety and loss of appetite due to the high fiber content of vegetarian foods [**95,101**]. Furthermore, due to these dietary restrictions, athletes are at a higher risk for several micronutrient deficiencies including omega-3, iron, zinc, iodine, calcium, vitamin D, and vitamin $B_{12}$ [**101**].

Nebl et al. [**102**] investigated the food consumption of vegan, lacto-ovo-vegetarian (LOV) and omnivorous (OMN) athletes according to the intake recommendations of the German, Austrian, and Swiss Nutrition Societies for the general population. Most athletes did not reach the recommended energy intake. Although omnivorous athletes consumed lower CHO compared to the recommended intake, vegetarian athletes consumed adequate amounts. For micronutrient intake, vegans achieved adequate iron levels by consuming only foods high in iron, while female LOV and OMN athletes achieved the recommended amount after supplementation. The results showed that all groups consumed enough of most nutrients. However, an analysis of the circulating state of nutrients is also needed to better interpret the effectiveness of dietary intake, particularly for vegetarian athletes [**102**]. A cross-sectional study by the same researchers [**103**] then compared the micronutrient consumption of LOV, vegan, and omnivorous recreational runners and found that 80% of each group had adequate vitamin $B_{12}$ and vitamin D levels, and these parameters were higher in supplement users. Red blood cell folate exceeded the reference range; however, there was no difference in red blood cell folate among all groups [**103**]. No iron deficiency anemia was detected in any group, and less than 30% of each group were found to have depleted iron stores. The results suggest that a well-planned vegetarian diet can meet the athlete's iron, vitamin D, and vitamin $B_{12}$ needs [**103**]. These findings have been confirmed in case reports on vegan mountain bikers and ultra-triathletes [**56,57**]. Additionally, vegetarian diets are often inferior in quality compared to omnivores; this is due to anti-nutritional factors such as trypsin inhibitors, phytate, and tannins in those rich in vegetarian diets [**104**]. However, these challenges can be overcome by applying pre-cooking techniques described in detail in another review [**105**]. Therefore, it is obvious that vegetarian diets require careful monitoring in endurance athletes whose energy, macro and micronutrient needs are higher than their omnivore counterparts. However, with a well-planned diet and close monitoring, the nutritional needs of athletes can be successfully met, even ultra-endurance athletes.

Various metabolic risks such as iron deficiency anemia, menstrual disorders, musculoskeletal injuries, immunity, and hormonal irregularities occur in endurance athletes as a result of insufficient energy and nutrient intake following high-intensity endurance performance [**106,107**]. Relative energy deficiency syndrome has been found more often in vegetarian athletes, which causes endocrine and eating disorders that cause harmful diseases to metabolic health, reduces bone mineral density, and causes menstrual dysfunction [**108,109**]. Relative energy deficiency syndrome was developed to replace the Female Athlete Triad by broadening the definition to include male athletes and impaired physiological function caused by relative energy deficiency [**109**]. The key etiological factor of RED-S is a low energy availability which results in, but is not limited to, impairments of metabolic rate, menstrual function, bone health, immunity, protein synthesis and cardiovascular health [**109**]. In a study, researchers attribute this to either vegetarians' food choices for low-energy-dense, high-fiber foods, even in high-energy situations, or restricted food intake behaviors by indicating dietary rules to mask vegetarians' eating disorders [**110**]. Since low energy availability has already presented a challenging problem for endurance athletes independent of the diet pattern [**111**] and even healthy endurance athletes often cannot fully meet their body energy and vitamin requirements [**112**], nutritional adequacy and the quality of vegetarian diets are often questioned. However, studies examining the nutritional efficiency of vegetarian diets claimed the opposite results. Examining the diet adequacy and performance parameters of a vegan ultra-triathlete with 10 Ironman counterparts, a case report has revealed that a vegan athlete has no nutritional deficiencies or health disorders **[56]**. Researchers examined the spiroergometric, echocardiographic, or hematological parameters of a vegan ultra-endurance triathlete that has been vegetarian for 22 years and vegan for the past nine years. It has been found that a long-term vegetarian diet is not detrimental to metabolic health for a long-distance triathlete, even at micronutrient parameters associated with anemia. Although being a vegan athlete who consumes a well-planned diet does not have a detrimental impact in terms of cardiometabolic health and sports performance **[56]**, findings need to be explored with a larger athletic cohort. These findings are similar to those of Wirnitzer et al. **[57]**, who evaluated the food intake of a vegan mountain biker in the Transalp Challenge race (42 h). The researchers have highlighted that a carefully planned vegan diet strategy ensures that the race goals are achieved, and thus the race is completed in a healthy state **[57]**. Therefore, a well-planned vegan diet can be a great alternative for ultra-endurance athletes who endure extreme conditions such as psychological, physiological, endocrinological, and immunological stress-related metabolic challenges during prolonged training periods. In the last statement by the Academy of Nutrition and Dietetics on vegetarian diets, it was stated that vegetarian diets seemed more sustainable for all stages of life **[113]**. Researchers have suggested that well-planned vegetarian and vegan diets containing certain micronutrients such as high-quality plant protein, iron, n-3 fatty acids, Zn, Ca, iodine, vitamin $B_{12}$, and vitamin D provide various health benefits regarding diseases such as hypertension, ischemic heart disease, diabetes and obesity **[113]**. In addition, given the content of vegetarian diets that can contain milk, eggs, or fish, vegetarian diets may be a better option for providing better nutritional density and quality than a vegan diet **[99]**. It is recommended that vegans carefully monitor blood vitamin $B_{12}$ concentrations and supplement their diets, if necessary, with supplements or fortified foods **[113]**. Vegetarian and vegan nutrition programs should be planned by considering the above-mentioned data.

For many years, there have been claims that vegetarian diets negatively affect serum sex hormones **[97,98]**, but data on the interaction between serum sex hormones and vegetarian diets remain controversial. In a crossover study conducted in 1992, Raben et al. **[114]** studied the effects of a 6 week lacto-ovo-vegetarian and omnivorous diet on serum sex hormones and endurance performance in eight endurance athletes. Although endurance performance did not differ according to the diet model, serum testosterone levels slightly decreased after six weeks of consuming a lacto-ovo-vegetarian diet. The researchers stated that these results may be related to dietary fiber binding to sex hormones and higher fiber intake in the lacto-ovo-vegetarian diet **[114]**. Considering the evidence in the literature that testosterone triggers muscle protein anabolism and lean body mass **[115]**, a decrease in testosterone levels would cause an undesirable situation. However, a recent study in men from the national health and nutrition examination survey (NHANES) database, but not on athletes, found that a vegetarian diet did not link to serum testosterone levels [**116**]. Along with all data, the interpretation of the vegetarian diet as an attenuating factor to sex hormones by disregarding other confounding factors such as age, gender, training intensity, and emotional stress would be inappropriate [**116**] and needs further investigation.

The issue of the protein quality and quantity of vegetarian diets has long been controversial [**99,117**]. While some researchers note that vegetarian proteins have some missing specific amino acids [**118**], others state that including high-quality protein-rich foods such as legumes, seeds, nuts, and grains in a vegetarian diet is sufficient to meet the body's amino acid requirement [**119**]. A vegan diet structure should be created by examining the protein content of the food consumed, especially in terms of quality and quantity. Determining the dietary protein quality using the Digestible Indispensable Amino Acid Score (DIAAS) method in omnivore and vegetarian athletes, Ciuris et al. [**100**] analyzed the diet content of 38 omnivore- and 22 vegetarian athletes. Vegetarian athletes had significantly lower lean body mass (LBM) compared to omnivores (-14%). Available protein was significantly correlated with strength ($r = 0.314$) and LBM ($r = 0.541$). The main findings revealed that vegetarian athletes needed to consume an additional 10 g of protein per day to achieve the recommended protein intake of 1.2 $g{\cdot}kg^{-1}$ body weight (BW) and an additional 22 g of protein to reach 1.4 $g{\cdot}kg^{-1}{\cdot}kg^{-1}$ BW [**100**]. Data on vegetarian proteins such as hemp, soy, potato, and rice proteins highlight that these vegetarian proteins contain sufficient high-quality protein content to increase muscle protein synthesis and post-workout recovery [**119**]. Rogerson [**10**] suggested that vegan athletes could improve their protein intake towards the higher limit of the International Society Of Sports Nutrition's (ISSN) protein recommendation for athletes up to 2.0 $g{\cdot}kg^{-1}$ body mass per day. However, given that there is little evidence in the literature that vegetarian proteins are inadequate to provide an athlete's needs or that vegetarian athletes need a higher protein intake [**11,117**], this recommendation needs further clarification with clinical research.

Additionally, the potential benefits of vegetarian diets are often attributed to their polyphenolic contents [**4**]. The intake of polyphenols with food may be the best choice for regulating body hormesis in the case of antioxidants due to the fact that polyphenol supplements may compromise the body's antioxidant defense metabolism [**87,120**]. However, at this point, the bioavailability of polyphenols taken with food comes into question [**121**]. While some researchers have suggested that the recommended polyphenol intake can be achieved by consuming polyphenol-rich foods or as a polyphenol supplement [**122**], others claimed that some polyphenols, such as quercetin, cannot be taken naturally with food [**123**]. Keeping all this in mind, it is necessary to further clarify the possible mechanisms for how the bioavailability of polyphenols in the body and their effects on sports performance change with their consumption naturally.

With all the data obtained from studies, there is currently no certain evidence that omnivorous or vegetarian diets provide better metabolic health and performance benefits [**52,53,55,56,57,59**]. Therefore, more research is needed to clarify the optimal dietary recommendations for macro and micronutrients, as well as polyphenols, to maintain health and improve performance in endurance athletes following vegetarian diets.

## 3.2. High-Fat Diets

High-fat diets (HFD) have been widely applied for decades as a treatment option for certain diseases such as epilepsy or as an effective dietary strategy for weight loss [**124**]. In recent years, these diets have also become widespread in endurance athletes [**14,15,16,17,18,19,21,22,23,24,38**]. High-fat diets applied in the athletic population are grouped under two main categories: (1) a ketogenic low-CHO high-fat (K-LCHF) diet, and (2) non-ketogenic high-fat (NK-LCHF) diet (described in **Table 2**). While a ketogenic diet aims to increase blood ketone levels from 0.5 to 3.0 mmol/L, non-ketogenic diets aim to provide potential benefits without reaching higher blood ketone concentrations. Ketosis is considered as a survival mechanism for the body to equilibrate blood glucose during a metabolic crisis, such as a lack of calories or glucose, in fasting conditions, or prolonged exercise and to provide energy to the brain, whose survival depends on ketone body (KB) utilization in case of glucose deprivation [**125**].

**Table 2. Types and application processes of new diets applied by endurance athletes.**

| Type | Other Terms Mentioned in Endurance Sport Research | Definition/Application | Ref. |
|---|---|---|---|
| **Vegetarian diets** | | | |
| Vegetarian diet | Vegetarian diet | Excludes all meats but may allow some animal products. | [**99**] |
| Ovo-vegetarian diet | Not detected | Excludes all meat and dairy products from the diet, but allows eggs. | [**99**] |
| Lacto-vegetarian diet | Not detected | Excludes all meat and eggs from the diet, but allows dairy products. | [**99**] |
| Lacto-ovo vegetarian diet | Lacto-ovo vegetarian diet | Excludes all types of meat from the diet, but allows the consumption of eggs and dairy products. | [**99**] |
| Pesco-vegetarian diet | Not detected | Excludes all animal products from the diet except fish. | [**99**] |
| Flexitarian diet | Not detected | A diet that flexible in terms of the consumption of animal products and allow to consume them occasionally. | [**99**] |
| **Vegan diet** | | | |
| Vegan diet | Vegan diet | Excludes all animal products from the diet. | [**99**] |
| **High-fat diets** | | | |

| Type | Other Terms Mentioned in Endurance Sport Research | Definition/Application | Ref. |
|---|---|---|---|
| Ketogenic low-CHO high-fat diet | Ketogenic diet; low-CHO ketogenic diet; ketogenic low-carbohydrate diet; keto-adaptation; high-fat diet; low-carbohydrate diet; low-carbohydrate, high-fat ketogenic diet | Consists of very low-CHO (20–50·g$^{-1}$ day) and high-fat (75–80% of total energy) content with sufficient (15–20%) protein intake, resulting in increased ketone concentrations in blood named ketosis. | [5] |
| Non-ketogenic low-CHO high-fat diet | Non-ketogenic low-CHO high-fat diet, high-fat diet; low-carbohydrate diet | Consists of low-CHO (15–20% of total energy) and high-fat (60–65% of total energy) content with sufficient (15–20%) protein intake. | [5] |
| Acute ketone body supplementation | Ketone ester supplementation, ketone salt supplementation, a ketone monoester supplement, ketone diester ingestion, an exogenous ketone supplement | Creates exogenous ketosis, is applied in forms of either ketone salts or ketone esters. | **[126]** |
| CHO restoration following fat adaptation | Fat adaptation followed by CHO loading, keto-adaptation and glycogen restoration | A diet that is consumed a high-CHO diet for 1–3 days, and followed by a ketogenic or non-ketogenic high-fat diet for 5 to 14 days. | [5] |
| **Intermittent fasting diets** | | | |
| Complete alternate-day fasting | Intermittent fasting | Includes alternate fasting days (does not allow foods and drink consumption), and eating days (allow food and drink consumption ad libitum). | **[127]** |
| Modified fasting | Not detected | Includes a nocturnal fasting period of 16/18/20 h and an ad libitum-eating period of 8/6/4 h, (e.g., 5:2 diet, which includes 5 days (allows for food and drink consumption ad libitum) and 2 non-consecutive days (allows the consumption of 20–25% of energy needs ad libitum)). | **[127]** |

| Type | Other Terms Mentioned in Endurance Sport Research | Definition/Application | Ref. |
|---|---|---|---|
| Time-restricted eating | Time-restrictive eating (16/8) | Allows food or beverages at certain time periods, including regular, extended intervals (e.g., 16:8 diet with 16 h of fasting without energy intake and 8 h of food intake ad libitum). | [127] |
| Religious fasting | Ramadan intermittent fasting, Ramadan fast, Ramadan fasting | Comprises several fasting regimens based on specific religious and spiritual purposes (e.g., Ramadan fasting involving a fasting period from sunrise to sunset). | [127] |
| **Gluten-free diet** | | Complete exclusion of gluten and gluten-containing products. | [128] |
| **Low-FODMAP diet** | | | |
| Long-term FODMAP elimination | A low-FODMAP diet, low-FODMAP foods | - (1) FODMAP restriction for 2 to 6 weeks from the athletes' diet. - (2) reintroduction the restricted high-FODMAP foods step by step. - (3) individualize the athletes' diet according to response against the first and second stages. | [129] |
| Short-term FODMAP elimination | 24 h low-FODMAP diet | A strict FODMAP diet for 1 to 3 days before intensive training or races. | [129] |

CHO: carbohydrate, FODMAP: fermentable oligosaccharides, disaccharides, monosaccharides and polyols.

In HFD studies on endurance athletes, K-LCHF diets have been commonly applied for diet periods ranging from three to 12 weeks [**16,17,18,19,21,22,23,38**]. Two studies, a case report (a 10 week K-LCHF diet) [**21**] and a cross-sectional study (a 20-month K-LCHF diet) [**24**], examined the effects of longer-term ketogenic diets on performance. For NK-LCHF diets, three studies, two crossover (a 2 week NK-LCHF diet) [**26,28**] and a cross-sectional (6-mth NK-LCHF diet) study [**27**], also investigated the impact of NK-LCHF diets on performance and lipoprotein profiles in endurance athletes (Detailed in **Table 1**). Besides these ketogenic diet applications, acute [**30,31,32,33,34,35,36,37,38,39**] or long-term [**130**] administration of KBs (in a ketone ester (KE) or ketone salt (KS) form) and CHO restoration following keto-adaptation [**26,40,41,42,43,45,46,47**] have also been evaluated in endurance athletes. Additionally, studies have been conducted to investigate the effects of an acute pre-exercise high-fat meal [**51**], and a short-term (1.5 days) fat supplementation during high-CHO diet administration [**49,50**]. In this section, we will discuss these high-fat studies in detail, with all their beneficial and harmful consequences for endurance athletes.

### 3.2.1. Potential Beneficial Aspects of High-Fat Diets

High-fat diet administration has taken place in endurance athletes with the aim of improving the utilization of fatty acids and KB [**14,19,20,24,25,26,28,32,33,34,35,36,41,42,43,45,46,47,49,50,51**], sparing muscle glycogen stores [**24,37,42,44,46,47**], increasing weight loss, especially body fat mass [**14,19,21,28**], improving aerobic capacity [**28**], improving time to exhaustion [**26,51**] and time-trial performance [**33,46,131**], regulating performance-related parameters [**34,36,39**], increasing cognitive performance [**38**], regulating exercise-associated immunologic and hormonal response [**15,22,30**], increasing cellular gene expression [**132**], and attenuating overreaching syndrome [**130**].

One of the main goals of applying a high-fat diet to improve performance is to increase the body's ability to use KB and fatty acids as an energy source [**14,19,20,24,25,26,28,32,33,34,35,36,41,42,43,45,46,47,49,50,51**]. The enhancement of the body's ability to use KB as an energy source generally occurs in two type manipulations: (1) By restricting dietary CHO intake for a prolonged time, the body adapts metabolically to using KB instead of glucose; this process is called keto-adaptation [**24**]. (2) Acute KB supplementation instantly changes fuel usage from CHO to KB [**30,31,32,33,34,35,36,37,38,39,130**].

Improvement of fat utilization to fuel, especially during prolonged exercise, may provide advantages for endurance athletes, including the glucose-sparing effect that, in particular, has vital importance for the brain during times of glucose depletion [**133**]. While the intramuscular triglyceride stores are predominantly preferred to provide energy during low- to moderate-intensity exercise (50–75% $VO_2$max), in moderate to vigorous-intensity exercises (>75% $VO_2$max), muscle glycogen is used as the primary substrate to obtain energy provisions [**134**]. However, since the substrate utilization highly depends on the diet pattern, keto-adaptation results in a shift from glycogen to FFA or KBs, even during high-intensity exercises [**21**]. A number of studies such as K-LCHF [**14,15,19,20,21,24,25**] and NK-LCHF trials [**26,28**], acute KB administration [**32,33,34,35,36,39**], keto-adaptation followed by CHO loading [**41,42,43,46**], and pre-workout HF meal administration [**51**] proved that fat oxidation significantly increased at rest and during exercise after HFD applications. Only studies practicing the short-term fat administration during high-CHO diet administration in trained male cyclists revealed that overall fat oxidation did not alter during prolonged exercise and during submaximal or one hour time-trial (TT) exercise training [**49,50**]. However, one of the studies noted that fat oxidation significantly increased regardless of diet [**50**], while another highlighted that intramyocellular lipid utilization increased 3-fold in the fat supplemented group [**49**]. Taking all studies together, it seems that all applications aiming to increase fat ingestion provide better fat and KB utilization in the body, especially during exercise. This metabolic advantage appears to be unique for enhancing endurance performance.

However, along with the changes in substrate utilization towards fatty acids and KBs, KD might not be advantageous for exercise that highly relies on anaerobic metabolism and requires glucose flux such as short-duration exercise or long-duration exercise with interval sprints. In a randomized, crossover study in trained endurance athletes, it was stated that a 5 day fat adaptation followed by 1 day CHO restoration caused a decrease in glycogenolysis and PDH activation [**47**]. The findings suggested that this dietary manipulation could result in an increase in the NADH/NAD+ ratio or the Acetyl-CoA/CoA ratio, which could result in sustained attenuation of PDH activity and impaired glycolysis metabolism. Further research should be elucidated on the possible interaction between impaired glycolysis metabolism and ketogenic diets on prolonged exercise with anaerobic metabolism or high-intensity intermittent exercise.

As it is well known that depleting glycogen stores is one of the major causes of fatigue during endurance exercise [**2**], HFD also aims to reduce muscle glycogen utilization to ensure CHO availability for longer periods of time during endurance training. Although one study on endurance-trained male cyclists showed that muscle glycogen utilization significantly decreased after a 10 day fat adaptation followed by 3 day CHO restoration trial compared to a high-CHO trial [**46**], others investigating muscle glycogen utilization claimed that no difference was observed between the intervention and the control trial [**24,37,42,47**]. In addition, a cross-sectional study on male endurance runners stated that muscle glycogen utilization did not alter after an average of a 20-month K-LCHF or high-carbohydrate (high-CHO) diet. Therefore, studies on HFD and its "muscle glycogen sparing effect" remain controversial. We cannot conclude that HFD provides an advantage to spare muscle glycogen during endurance training. Further work is needed to assess muscle glycogen utilization.

K-LCHF diets might be an effective option for athletes who aim to lose body weight (BW) and body fat while sparing muscle mass [**14,19,21,28**]. A crossover study assessing the effects of a long-term (4 week) K-LCHF diet rich in polyunsaturated fatty acids on aerobic performance and exercise metabolism in trained off-road cyclists revealed that BW and body fat percentage decreased after long-term KD [**28**]. It was also stated that the long-term K-LCHF diet improved maximum oxygen consumption and decreased post-exercise muscle damage. The findings suggest that a long-term K-LCHF diet may provide advantages to both body composition and endurance performance. However, another study claimed that long-term KD (for 12 weeks) caused a decrease in both body fat percentage (5.2%) and body mass (5.9 kg) in endurance-trained athletes [**14**]. However, results also showed that although long-term KD resulted in improved body composition, it had no impact on 100 km TT performance. Consistent with this study, Heatherly et al. [**19**] investigated the impact of a 3 week ad libitum ketogenic diet on markers of endurance performance in recreationally competitive male runners. Results showed that the body composition of subjects positively changed with a decrease of ~2.5 kg BW and skinfold thickness occurring at multiple sites in the trunk region. However, KD did not affect exercise-induced cardiorespiratory, thermoregulatory, and perceptional responses and 5 km TT performance, and perceived exertion [**19**]. Findings indicate that KD may be an alternative strategy for reducing fat mass regardless of endurance performance.

On the other hand, Zinn et al. [**21**] investigated the 10 week ketogenic diet experiences of five endurance athletes and the effects of this diet on body composition and exercise performance. Although body mass and the sum of skinfolds were reduced by an average of 4 kg and 25.9 mm, respectively, endurance athletes experienced an inability to maintain high-intensity exercises during this period [**21**]. These findings raised doubts about the use of KD for weight loss in endurance athletes. In addition to that, a recent study compared the efficiency of two energy-reduced (-500 kcal·day$^{-1}$) diets, including a cyclical ketogenic reduction diet (CKD), defined as a high-fat low-CHO (>30 g·day$^{-1}$) diet for five days, followed by a high carb diet (8–10 g/body FFM) for two days, and a nutritionally balanced reduction diet (RD), a typical diet containing 55% CHO, 15% protein, and 30% fat, on body composition and endurance performance in healthy young males [**135**]. Results revealed that both diets reduced body weight and body fat mass. However, while CKD-related weight loss is due to decreased body fat, body water, and lean body mass, RD leads to a reduction in body weight mainly by reducing body fat mass [**135**]. Among all of these findings, one should note that adherence to a weight loss diet is major factor in achieving a target that does not significantly require KD consumption.

Several studies determined the potential impact of HFD on aerobic capacity [**16,17,20,23,25,28,39**]. It is well known that $VO_2$max is referred to as a gold standard method to measure aerobic fitness [**136**]. Therefore, studies on KD, N-KD, and acute KE ingestion in endurance athletes stated that these diet manipulations had no effect on $VO_2$max performance [**16,17,20,23,25,39**], except for a 4 week KD study on off-road cyclists by Zajac et al. [**28**]. Studies arguing that HFD was ineffective on aerobic capacity also showed that this HFD caused a decrease [**16,23**] or no change [**25,39**] in TT performance, and no alteration in time-to-exhaustion (TTE) performance [**20**]. Therefore, HFD seemed to fail to increase aerobic capacity and endurance in endurance athletes.

Researchers evaluated multiple performance-related factors such as TT performance [**14,19,23,25,29,33,34,35,36,38,39,41,42,43,45,46,48,49,50**], TTE performance [**18,20,21,26,31,37,51**], lactate concentration during exercise [**33,34,36,39**], and post-exercise muscle damage [**28**] to determine the effects of HFD on sports performance. While research on TT and TTE performance in endurance athletes revealed controversial results, the majority of the studies declared that no alterations were observed in TT [**14,19,25,29,34,36,38,39,41,42,43,45,49,50**] and TTE [**18,20,26,31,37**] performance after the HF-associated applications. Additionally, two well-controlled studies of Burke et al. [**16,23**] underlined that a 3.5 week K-LCHF diet not only decreased 10 km race walk performance, but also increased oxygen cost and perceived exertion throughout exercise. These findings suggest that HFD has no advantage or may even negatively affect exercise performance. However, some points should be taken into account when interpreting these findings. Five of eight studies on perceived fatigue during endurance performance revealed that no differences were detected between HFD and control trials [**18,19,38,39,49**]. Similar results were also observed in studies on lactate concentration during exercise [**34,36,39**]. It seems that HFD altered neither perceived exertion nor plasma lactate concentrations. Another important point for endurance performance is the maintenance of blood glucose concentration during exercise [**38**]. Changes in blood glucose levels during exercise were investigated in acute KB ingestion trials [**34,36,38,39**]. Three of four studies indicated that blood glucose concentrations were maintained during endurance exercise and were found to be similar between control groups [**34,38,39**].

Although these results are promising, blood glucose changes should also be examined in studies involving HFD manipulations. Additionally, a crossover study evaluating the efficiency of a 4 week NK-LCHF diet application on off-road cyclists stated that blood CK and LDH concentration, known as muscle damage biomarkers, significantly decreased at rest and during the 105 min exercise protocol in the NK-LCHF diet trial [**28**]. These findings also appear promising. It should be noted that studies reporting that TT or TTE performance did not change after HFD interpreted the study results based on statistical significance. It should also be noted that, although considered as statistically insignificant, a few minutes can be crucial in winning a race. Therefore, this point should be considered when interpreting the study results. Lastly, for post-exercise recovery, Volek et al. [**24**] indicated that long-term (at least 6 months) LCHF diets resulted in an increased fat oxidation rate and a higher peak exercise intensity in endurance athletes compared to counterparts consuming high-CHO low-fat diets. Moreover, although the LCHF diet group consumed 10% CHO, whereas the habitual high-CHO group consumed 59% CHO, there was no difference between the LCHF and high-CHO low-fat diets for 2 h post-exercise recovery [**24**]. These results suggest that long-term LCHF diets can improve post-exercise recovery, especially in ultra-endurance events where the glycogen-sparing effect and adequate post-exercise recovery are crucial for a better performance. Keeping all these findings in mind, although studies on TT and TTE performance mostly found no advantages of HFD or revealed controversial results, performance-related parameters may be positively affecting the HFD. More work is required to clarify this information.

Ketone body consumption in endurance athletes may increase endurance performance by up-regulating physiological parameters and increasing metabolic efficiency [**126**]. For instance, Cox et al. [**33**] conducted comprehensive research including five separate studies on the effect of ketone esters (KE) on the performance of 39 endurance athletes. Twenty minutes after consumption of the ketone ester-based drink, blood ketone concentrations rapidly increased to 2 mmol/L and remained high with a slight drop, reaching a new steady state approximately 30 min following subsequent exercise at 75% Wmax exercise intensity. Findings from the study showed that acute nutritional ketosis caused by the consumption of KE resulted in metabolic improvements in endurance performance by enhancing metabolic flexibility and energy efficiency, rapidly altering substrate utilization towards ketone bodies for oxidative respiration, sparing intramuscular BCAA concentration by reducing BCAA deamination, increasing muscle fat oxidation even though in the presence of glycogen, and decreasing blood lactate levels during exercise [**33**]. On the other hand, most of the studies (6 of 10) applying acute KB intake showed that this practice did not improve TT [**34**,**36**,**38**,**39**] and TTE performance [**31**,**37**]. Study findings remain unclear, and the impact of KB on exercise performance needs further clarification.

The efficacy of HFD on cognitive performance has been investigated in studies on acute KE [**39**] and KS [**38**] administration and fat-enriched feeding during high-CHO diet administration [**50**]. Prins et al. [**38**] administered one (22.1 g) or two (44.2 g) servings of KS or placebo to recreational male distance runners 60 min before a 5 km TT performance, and noted a possible dose–response interaction between KS supplementation and cognitive performance. On the other hand, studies including acute KE administration [**39**] and fat-enriched feeding during high-CHO diet administration [**50**] showed no alteration in cognitive performance. A study applying the high-CHO diet supplemented with fat on trained male cyclists highlighted that a possible explanation for this result is that the study protocol, including 1 h of fixed-task simulated TT performance, may not be sufficient to create mental fatigue [**50**]. However, the study on acute KE intake found similar results despite applying an exercise protocol (1 h submaximal exercise at 65% $VO_2$max followed by a 10 km TT) that caused more fatigue [**39**]. Taken together, studies did not confirm the exact efficiency of HFD on cognitive performance and the interaction needs further investigation.

Few studies investigated the potential influence of HFD on immunologic and hormonal response in endurance athletes [**15**,**22**,**30**]. Assessing the impact of acute (2 day) and prolonged (2 week) adherence to an K-LCHF diet on exercise-induced cortisol, serum immunoglobulin A (s-IgA) responses in a randomized, crossover manner, researchers indicated that a lower cortisol response at week 2 was observed compared to day 2 in the K-LCHF trial (669 ± 243 nmol/L vs. 822 ± 215 nmol/L, respectively) [**15**]. However, a better exercise-induced cortisol response was found in the HCF trial at both day 2 and week 2 (609 ± 208 nmol/L and 555 ± 173 nmol/L, respectively). Additionally, no differences in s-IgA concentrations were observed at week 2 between the K-LCHF diet and high-CHO diet [**15**]. Another study by Shaw et al. [**30**] determined the impact of acute KE supplementation (R,S-1,3-butanediol (BD); 2×0.35 $mg{\cdot}kg^{-1}$ BW; 30 min before and 60 min after exercise) on the T-cell-associated cytokine gene expression within stimulated peripheral blood mononuclear cells (PBMC) following prolonged, strenuous exercise in trained male cyclists. No alteration was detected in serum cortisol, total leukocyte and lymphocyte, and T-cell subset levels, IL-4 and IL-10 mRNA expression, and the IFN-γ/IL-4 mRNA expression ratio between the KE and placebo trials during exercise and recovery. However, a transient increase was observed in T-cell-related IFN-γ mRNA expression throughout exercise and recovery in the KE trial. Results indicated that acute KE supplementation may provide enhanced type-I T-cell immunity at the gene level [**30**]. The same researchers investigated the potential effect of a 4.5 week K-LCHF diet on resting and post-exercise immune biomarkers in endurance-trained male athletes in a randomized, repeated-measures, crossover manner [**22**]. T-cell-related IFN-γ mRNA expression and the IFN-γ/IL-4 mRNA expression ratio within multiantigen-stimulated PBMCs were greater in the K-LCHF trial compared to the high-CHO trial. Furthermore, a significant rise was observed in the multiantigen-stimulated whole-blood IL-10 production, an anti-inflammatory cytokine, post-exercise in the K-LCHF trial. The results indicated that a 4.5 week K-LCHF diet caused an increase in both pro- and anti-inflammatory T-cell-related cytokine response to a multiantigen in vitro [**22**]. Keeping the studies on immunologic and hormonal response to HFD in mind, although post-exercise pro- and anti-inflammatory T-cell-related cytokine response alters after a K-LCHF diet or acute KE supplementation, it remains uncertain how these alterations influence the immunoregulatory response. Therefore, more work is required to elucidate the interaction by adding clinical illness follow-up and tracking immunomodulatory metabolites using metabolomic approaches.

Antioxidant specialties of HFD may be discussed on the basis of KB [**124**]. Antioxidant activity of KBs is one of the multidimensional properties that determine their metabolic activity in the body. The main potential antioxidant properties of KB are mainly explained by its effects on neuroprotection, inhibiting lipid peroxidation and protein oxidation, and improving mitochondrial respiration [**137**]. However, as there is no study investigating the impact of KB on exercise-induced oxidative stress in endurance athletes and the evidence on the impact of KB on exercise-induced oxidative stress is limited, future studies in this field are needed.

Another therapeutic benefit of KD may be linked to increased Fibroblast Growth Factor 21 (FGF21) [**132**]. Fibroblast Growth Factor 21 acts as the primary regulator of skeletal muscle keto-adaptation by increasing activation of the AMP-activated protein kinase (AMPK)—sirtuins 1 (SIRT1)—peroxisome proliferator-activated receptor coactivator 1 (PGC-1) pathway, resulting in increased mitochondrial biogenesis, development of IMTGs, and ketolytic gene expression [**138**]. However, in a study on 5-d fat adaptation followed by 1-d CHO restoration, a significant decrease was observed in the exercise-induced AMPK-1 and AMPK-2 activity in the fat-adapted trial despite the higher AMPK-1 and AMPK-2 activity before exercise. Therefore, more work is required to interpret the possible interaction accurately.

Ketone bodies may have a particular metabolic advantage, not only providing a source of oxidizable carbon to maintain energy needs but also acting as a potential regulator of overtraining by directly regulating autonomic neural output and inflammation [**139,140**]. One study applying three weeks of KE intake during prolonged extreme endurance training investigated the effects of KE on overreaching symptoms [**130**]. Ketone ester ingestion significantly increased sustainable training load (15% higher than the control group), and prevented the increase in nocturnal adrenaline and noradrenaline excretion induced by strenuous training [**130**]. These findings suggest that KE supplementation during exercise substantially reduces the development of overreaching, which is a detrimental factor for endurance performance. In addition, growth differentiation factor (GDF-15), an established biomarker for nutritional and cellular stress, increased 2-fold less in the KE group than the control group. However, this study was conducted on healthy, physically active males, and it is not exactly known whether the same effects can be achieved in endurance athletes [**130**]. For this reason, it is necessary to examine the same mechanism, especially on endurance athletes with intense and frequent training periods.

### 3.2.2. Potential Risks Regarding High-Fat Diets

Some researchers have also investigated HFD's potential risks on endurance, including an increased oxygen cost and an impaired running economy [**16,23**], an altered blood acid-base status [**17,31**], compromised gastrointestinal (GI) symptoms [**32,34,35,37,48**], reduced bone formation markers [**40**], increased cholesterol and lipoprotein levels [**27**], a decreased appetite [**37**], and thereby worsened performance.

The deterioration of the running economy and increased oxygen cost during endurance exercise are considered to be major potential disadvantages of HFD. Burke et al. [**16,23**] demonstrated with two separate studies in elite race-walkers that a 3 week K-LCHF diet during intensity training impaired endurance performance by decreasing exercise economy, which has vital importance in endurance performance, despite enhancing peak aerobic capacity ($VO_2$peak). Another study by Burke et al. claimed that although KD elevated glycogen availability, it still impaired endurance performance mainly by blunting the CHO oxidation rate [**141**]. In addition, LCHF diets can also impair endurance performance by increasing perceived fatigue [**15,16,23**]. The reason why K-LCHF diets cause increased fatigue is thought to be a gradual increase in non-esterified fatty acids (NEFAs) with the LCHF diet [**142**]. Non-esterified fatty acids compete with the tryptophan, a neurotransmitter highly associated with the central fatigue, for binding to albumin, thus resulting in an increase in free tryptophan transfer from the blood–brain barrier towards the brain. However, as we discussed above, the majority of studies found no alteration in perceived exertion during endurance performance [**18,19,38,39,49**].

Studies on well-trained endurance athletes revealed that neither keto-adaptation nor CHO restoration followed by keto-adaptation improves endurance performance, especially at multistage ultra-endurance events with intermittent sprints [**42,45**]. For instance, investigating the impact of a 6 days high-fat (68% fat) diet followed by 1 day CHO loading or high-CHO diet (68% CHO) for seven days on performance parameters during the 100 km time trial, Havemann et al. [**45**] found that 100 km time trial performance assessed by heart rate, perceived exertion, and muscle recruitment did not differ between groups; however, the 1-km sprint power output decreased more in the high-fat diet group than in high-CHO counterparts. Although an improvement was expected in high-intensity sprint bouts after an NK-LCHF diet due to its sparing effect on muscle glycogen, the findings revealed the opposite, decreasing the high-intensity sprint performance, a crucial parameter for endurance performance [**45**]. On the contrary, McSwiney et al. [**14**] also evaluated the impact of K-LCHF diets on 100 km TT performance and 6 s sprint peak power, indicating that although TT performance did not differ between the K-LCHF diet and high-CHO diet groups, 6 s sprint peak power significantly increased (+0.8 $W \cdot kg^{-1}$ rise) compared to the high-CHO group (−0.7 $W \cdot kg^{-1}$ decrease). More research is required to clarify these contradictory results.

Maintaining the acid-base balance in the body during exercise, especially during strenuous exercise, is important to delay acidosis and fatigue and thus to maintain endurance performance [**143**]. Exercise is a well-known factor that alters the acid-base state [**143**]. In addition to exercise, the macronutrient composition of dietary patterns can also affect acid-base balance and systemic pH and $HCO_3$ levels [**31**]. Some researchers claimed that HFD can alter circulating acidity by increasing acidic KB circulation in the body [**144**], while others state that acid-base balance can be well regulated by improving the adaptive mechanisms, regardless of diet [**17**]. The potential effect of HFD on blood acid-base status, blood pH, and $HCO_3$ concentrations was evaluated in only two studies of endurance athletes. The potential effect of HFD on blood acid-base status, blood pH, and $HCO_3$ concentrations was evaluated in two studies, one evaluating a 3 week ketogenic diet [**17**] and the other an acute KE intake in endurance athletes [**31**]. The study findings showed that neither K-LCHF diet nor acute KE intake affected blood pH and $HCO_3$ status and acid-base status [**17,31**]. One explanation is that both studies included well-trained endurance athletes. It is suggested that well-trained athletes can regulate the body acid-base balance well regardless of the diet by developing a metabolic adaptation to strenuous exercise. Therefore, the potential effect of HFD on acid-base status can be interpreted as negligible when applied to well-trained endurance athletes.

Gastrointestinal symptoms triggered by an HFD have commonly been seen during KB consumption [**32,34,35,37**]. A study investigating the kinetics, safety and tolerability of KB revealed that ketone esters may only cause GI symptoms when high doses (2.1 $g \cdot kg^{-1}$) are consumed [**145**]. However, although studies administered a low-dose KE in endurance athletes, the findings stated that acute KE ingestion caused an increase in low to severe GI symptoms, including nausea, reflux, dizziness, euphoria, and upper-abdominal discomfort [**32,34,35,37**]. One study by Dearlove et al. [**32**] compared the dose–response interaction between acute low- or high-dose KE ingestion (0.252 $g \cdot kg^{-1}$ vs. 0.75 $g \cdot kg^{-1}$, respectively) and GI symptoms. Findings showed that no GI discomfort was observed in the low-dose KE ingestion, while nausea symptoms were elevated in the high-dose KE trial. Although the high dose administered in this study (0.75 $g \cdot kg^{-1}$) remained much lower than the high dose (2.1 $g \cdot kg^{-1}$) that was claimed to cause GI symptoms, it still caused exercise-induced nausea in endurance athletes. In addition, Mujika [**48**] investigated the race performance and GI symptoms of a LOV male endurance athlete who adhered to an LCHF diet for 32 weeks. The athlete participated in three professional races while on the LCHF diet in weeks 21, 24, and 32. Although he suffered worse race experiences on the LCHF diet, no alteration was observed in GI symptoms. This result may be due to the athlete's adaptation to the ketogenic diet [**48**]. Taken together, while long-term keto-adaptation may inhibit the increase in GI symptoms, it should be taken into account when applying to endurance athletes that acute KE intake may be disadvantageous on exercise-induced GI symptoms. Interestingly, Zinn et al. [**21**] showed that endurance athletes suffered from constipation during the diet application after a 10 week K-LCHF diet, which might be important for the gut microbiome and well-being. This possibility may also be kept in mind while applying a ketogenic diet. In case of a similar situation, fiber and water intake should be calculated and closely monitored to eliminate constipation-associated problems.

Another less-studied potential disadvantage of HFD is its potential impact on decreasing appetite [**37**], bone formation markers [**40**], and increasing cholesterol and lipoprotein profile [**27**]. A randomized, crossover study evaluating the effects of acute KE ingestion early in a cycling race on glycogen degradation in highly trained cyclists showed a significant attenuation in the perception of hunger, determined using a validated 10-point visual analog scale [**37**]. This potential effect of HFD on appetite should be taken into account, especially during HFD administration planned for long-term application.

Heikura et al. [**40**] investigated the effects of a 3.5 week K-LCHF diet followed by CHO restoration on bone biomarkers in male and female race walkers. Their findings showed a meaningful increase in bone resorption markers at rest and post-exercise while a significant attenuation in bone formation markers at rest and throughout exercise in K-LCHF diet trial occurred. However, these alterations partially recovered after CHO restoration [**40**]. As only one study investigated the interaction between bone markers and ketogenic diets in endurance athletes, and a recent narrative review on ketogenic diets and bone health noted that we do not have enough high-quality experimental research to adequately clarify the potential disadvantages of ketogenic diets on bone health, we need more high-quality research on this topic.

Only one cross-sectional study of 20 competitive ultra-endurance athletes investigated the interaction between a long-term low-CHO diet and the circulating lipoprotein and cholesterol profiles [**27**]. Although a higher level of exercise tended to lower total and LDL-C concentrations, a hypercholesterolemic profile was observed in ultra-endurance athletes who adhered to a low-CHO diet, suggesting that a possible explanation may involve an expansion of the endogenous cholesterol pool during keto-adaptation and may remain higher on a low-CHO diet. Further, a higher consumption of saturated fat (86 vs. 21 g·day$^{-1}$) and cholesterol (844 vs. 251 mg·day$^{-1}$), and lower fiber intake (23 vs. 57 g·day$^{-1}$) may be another cause of these hypercholesterolemic profiles of ultra-endurance athletes [**27**]. However, due to the small sample size ($n$ = 20) and the lack of checking for familial hypercholesterolemia or specific polymorphisms [**27**], future work is needed to evaluate this interaction in depth.

Another possible pathway is that KD high in protein causes an increase in ammonia, thereby altering both brain energy metabolism and neuronal pathways, thus triggering central fatigue [**146**]. Both NEFA and ammonia may lead to increased central fatigue during exercise in endurance athletes adopting KD [**142**]. The interaction between the gut–brain axis can have critical importance to reveal performance- and, especially, fatigue-related metabolism during endurance events [147]. However, none of the HFD studies on endurance athletes studied the gut–brain axis, increased ammonia concentration, or endurance performance. Another point regarding a high protein intake during KD is that a high protein consumption can disrupt ketosis by providing gluconeogenic precursors, thus inducing gluconeogenesis [148]. Therefore, moderate protein consumption is generally recommended during KDs. As we know that endurance athletes tend to consume more protein intake (1.2–2.0 $g·kg^{-1}$ $BW·day^{-1}$) [149], this important effect of protein on ketosis should be kept in mind during the KD administration periods.

There are some important points that need to be considered before applying an HFD in endurance athletes. During NK-LCHF diet applications, the metabolic adaptation of muscle may evolve towards oxidation of fat as the primary energy source (maximum fat oxidation rate (fat max) from 0.4–0.6 $g·min^{-1}$ to 1.2–1.3 $g·min^{-1}$) [139]. However, glycogen stores may not provide enough glucose to power the brain, thus increasing fatigue [150] and decreasing endurance performance. For this reason, the adaptation period should be chosen carefully in order to alleviate the side effects of transition periods. Phinney et al. [20] noted that ketogenic high-fat diets may impair performance at first (a reduction of approximately 20%), but improvements in performance (up to a 155% increase) can be observed after metabolic adaptation to the ketogenic state.

Another important point that needs to be considered while planning further studies on HFD is to evaluate blood ketone concentration at frequent intervals during the study application period [151]. A review investigating the role of ketone bodies on physical performance found that 7 out of 10 studies included in the review failed to reach BOHB concentrations at the 2 mmol/L threshold, but only caused an acute ketosis state (B-OHB > 0.5 mmol/L) [151]. Another significant point is which KB type should be used [152]. The impact of ketone bodies on metabolism differs according to the type (ester-based form or salt-based form), and optical isoform (e.g., L or D isoforms of BOHB) consumed [137]. For example, D-βOHB is produced from acetoacetate (AcAc), released by the liver, and is actively used in metabolic pathways [153], while L-OHB is an intracellular metabolite known for having less activity in oxidative metabolism [150]. Therefore, L-βOHB supplementation may not provide the performance-related benefits of ketone bodies. These results explain that the specific effect of KD or KB on physical performance awaits further investigation, as most studies of KB failed to achieve the required ketone concentrations or applied ineffective KB to enhance endurance performance [152].

To conclude, there are several HFD strategies, as discussed in detail above, practiced by endurance athletes. However, while these diets may provide performance and health benefits, they are sometimes not effective at all or create many problems for endurance athletes. In addition, the physiological response to acute (exogenous) or endogenous nutritional ketosis may vary between highly trained endurance athletes and untrained individuals [140]. Therefore, it should be noted that these strategies may not be suitable for all endurance athletes. At first glance, while high-fat diets may seem like a promising approach to endurance performance, more research is needed to keep in mind all study results.

## 3.3. Intermittent Fasting

Intermittent fasting (IF) is defined as a period of voluntary withdrawal from food and beverages. It is an ancient approach that is implemented in different formats by different populations around the world [**154**]. Intermittent fasting diets have become more prevalent in recent years, including the scientific literature investigating the metabolic interaction between IF and health, as well as in the media and among the public [**127**]. Intermittent fasting diets are divided into four groups: (1) complete alternate-day fasting, (2) modified fasting, (3) time-restrictive eating and (4) religious fasting such as Ramadan IF (R-IF) (explained in detail in **Table 2**) [**127**].

### Intermittent Fasting and Sports Performance

#### *Possible Benefits of Intermittent Fasting in Endurance Athletes*

Studies on IF in endurance athletes have often been conducted during the religious fasting period (R-IF) [**60,61,63,64**], with few studies investigating the effects of time-restrictive eating (16:8) on endurance performance and health-related effects [**62,65**]. Fasting diets may alter metabolic pathways in the body by acting as a potential physiological stimulus for ketogenesis [**155**], regulating metabolic, hormonal and inflammatory responses [**61**], and stimulating mitochondrial biogenesis and suppressing mTOR activity [**155**], and regulating body composition [**62,65**].

Energy restriction/fasting for more than 12 to 16 h leads to a metabolic switch in basic energy fuels from carbohydrates to fats, resulting in metabolic ketosis, the same as the ketogenic diets [**155**]. These KD-like alterations in substrate uses are believed to serve as an inductor for fat oxidation, and a preservative for muscle mass and function [**156**].

The effect of fasting diets on muscle cells is generally known to be similar to aerobic exercise, including stimulation of mitochondrial biogenesis and suppression of mTOR activity [**157**]. However, the main mechanism on fasting diets is driven by fatty acid metabolism and peroxisome proliferator-activated receptor delta (PPAR-d), instead of $Ca^{2+}$, which is known to be effective in aerobic exercise [**155**]. Although the main mechanism on muscle cells differs between exercise and fasting diets, research findings suggest that application of a fasting diet along with exercise could switch cellular metabolism from glucose to ketone bodies [**156**], thereby inducing ketone utilization, which might, in turn, trigger mitochondrial biogenesis and preserve muscle mass [**158**]. Although the potential benefits of IF on mitochondrial biogenesis and mTOR activity appear promising, no study has investigated these metabolic interactions in endurance athletes adhering to IF.

The impact of R-IF on hormonal, metabolic and inflammatory responses is a less-studied point in terms of IF diets. In a study on middle-distance runners, Chennaoui et al. [**61**] examined the effects on R-IF on the hormonal, metabolic and inflammatory responses in a pre–post-test study design. Researchers applied a maximal aerobic velocity test 5 days before, 7 and 21 days after Ramadan. No change was observed in the testosterone/cortisol ratio during the RIF trial. A significant rise was reported in IL-6, adrenaline, and noradrenaline concentrations after the RIF; however, all parameters returned to baseline levels 7 days after exercise [**61**]. More work is needed to interpret these results effectively.

Another aspect of IF is its impact on the body composition of endurance athletes. Studies on endurance athletes and TRE (16:8) revealed that TRE caused a meaningful decrease in BW and body fat percentage in endurance athletes [**62,65**]. Moro et al. [**62**] claimed that although $VO_2$max and endurance performance did not change after a 4 week TRE, a meaningful rise in the peak power output/BW ratio was due to the BW loss. However, another study showed a decrease in TT performance (-25%) and no improvement in running efficiency after R-IF in well-trained middle-distance runners [**65**]. Taking these studies into account, although IF may provide some benefits by decreasing BW and body fat percentage, we cannot assume that it positively affects endurance performance.

### *Risks to Be Considered When Applying Fasting Diets*

Potential risks of IF diets are reduced endurance capacity [**60**], increased fatigue [**61,63**], altered sleep habits (i.e., delayed bedtime, decreased sleep time) [**61,63,64**], and dehydration [**159**] in endurance athletes.

Studies on IF diets and endurance capacity and performance-related parameters have produced conflicting results in endurance athletes [**60,62,64**]. Both R-IF and TRE studies on endurance athletes stated that IF diets had no influence on the aerobic capacity, determined by $VO_2$max [**60,62,64**]. Additionally, one study on TT performance and R-IF in well-trained middle-distance runners showed that R-IF caused a decrease in TT performance [**60**]. However, another study determining the impact of the CHO mouth rising technique on 10 km TT performance declared that the CHO mouth rising technique provided benefits by increasing 10 km TT performance [**64**]. For TRE and endurance performance, Moro et al. [**62**] revealed that a 4 week TRE had no impact on endurance performance. As for evaluating performance-related parameters, several researchers investigated the exercise-induced fatigue, blood lactate, glucose, and insulin concentrations in endurance athletes [**61,63,64,65**]. Exercise-induced fatigue, as determined by the Fatigue score [**61**] and the Rated Perceived Exertion (RPE) Scale [**63**], increased after a maximum aerobic speed test and an intensive endurance training, while it decreased significantly in an R-IF trial applying mouth rising during a 10 km TT performance [**64**]. One TRE study also showed that blood lactate, glucose and insulin concentrations did not alter during an incremental test [**65**]. We know that endurance exercise lasts more than an incremental test duration. Therefore, although blood parameters were well-maintained during an incremental test, we cannot interpret the study as the parameters will be preserved during prolonged strenuous exercise. Since there are few studies on endurance performance and IF, further studies should be conducted with an exercise protocol similar to races and competitions, including all performance-related parameters.

One study assessed the effect of R-IF on cognitive function in a non-randomized, repeated-measures, experimental design manner [**63**]. No difference was observed in cognitive performance, measured using reaction time and mean latency times on simple and complex tasks during Ramadan in trained male cyclists. Therefore, the implementation of IF diets to increase endurance capacity, improve performance-related parameters or cognitive performance does not appear to be a well-approved strategy. On the other hand, it would be wrong to refer the IF diet as a detrimental strategy due to the controversial findings of studies. Further, a review of the role of R-IF in sports performance, which included well-controlled studies, reported that although R-IF generally affected athletic performance with a few declines in physical fitness at a modest level, including perceived exertion, feelings of fatigue, and mood fluctuations, these negative effects may not cause a decrease in sports performance [**160**]. Furthermore, while prolonged fasting has detrimental effects on endurance performance by decreasing endurance time and causing carbohydrate depletion, hyperthermia, and severe dehydration [**161,162,163,164**], IF causes preventable adverse effects on performance [**160**].

An important factor among the difficulties that IF can cause is the alterations in sleeping habits of endurance athletes who practice R-IF [**61,63,64**]. During R-IF, in contrary to other IF diets, sleeping periods alter due to the difference of fasting/feeding cycle, thereby disturbing the circadian sleep/waking rhythm [**160**]. These changes may trigger general fatigue, mood, and mental and physical performance in endurance athletes. A study on 8 middle-distance athletes who maintained training during Ramadan revealed that R-IF affected physical performance by disturbing sleeping habits, creating energy deficiency, and fatigue [**61**]. Another study on cyclists showed a significant reduction in the duration of deep and REM sleep two weeks after starting R-IF, although total sleep time was unchanged [**63**]. On the other hand, a study on adolescent cyclists also reported no change in total sleep time following R-IF [**64**]. As sleep is one of the major components for maintaining metabolic health and performance [**165**], during Ramadan IF, the sleep cycle of endurance athletes should be carefully monitored and effective sleep strategies should be developed for this period. Further, in order to determine the effects of Ramadan IF on sleep patterns more accurately, more objective sleep measurements should be applied.

Another adverse effect of R-IF on endurance athletes is the deterioration of hydration conditions before, during and after exercise [**159**]. Starting competition in euhydrated state is one of the key factors for greater performance [**166**]. Further, providing adequate fluid ingestion during exercise, especially prolonged strenuous training, has a major impact on body fluid homeostasis. Although glycogen breakdown provides an average of 1.2 L water [**155**], it is still not enough to meet the body fluid need during the marathon, especially in hot weather conditions [**156**]. Therefore, fasting due to lack of water/fluid consumption can create adverse health problems beyond performance detriments [146]. Although TRE diets allow the consumption of water and unsweetened coffee and tea, R-IF has restrictive rules that forbid the consumption of anything during the fasting state [127]. Therefore, the water balance and fluid strategy of endurance athletes should be carefully planned, especially for endurance athletes applying R-IF diets.

The adverse effects of the IF diets also vary according to the weather conditions during fasting, training severity, training load, and training level of athletes [159]. These factors and, more importantly, endurance athletes' ability to cope with these metabolic changes determines how their sports performance will be during Ramadan. Evidence suggests that the performance success of athletes following an IF diet depends on their energy availability and macro and micronutrient intake, as well as training load and sleep length and quality [167]. Chennaoui et al. [61] suggested that athletes struggling with R-IF can reduce the negative effects of IF by reducing their training load and taking daytime naps.

Taking all studies into account, the efficiency of IF to improve exercise capacity and performance-related parameters still remains uncertain. Therefore, as we consistently repeat in the review, more work is needed before recommending these diets, especially in hot environments or during intense training periods. Since many Muslim athletes follow a month-long R-IF diet for religious reasons, even if there is a major competition or tournament [160], we need to develop effective strategies to maintain endurance performance and inhibit any decrease in endurance capacity during Ramadan.

## 3.4. Gluten-Free Diet

Exercise-induced GI symptoms in endurance athletes share common characteristics with Irritable Bowel Syndrome (IBS), including altered bowel functions (e.g., diarrhea, constipation), bloating, intestinal cramps, urge to defecate, and flatulence without any known organic disease [168]. These symptoms strongly affect the quality of life, psychological well-being, and also have quite a detrimental influence on exercise performance [1,168]. Therefore, several therapies have been developed for manipulating and attenuating these GI symptoms [169]. While drug-based treatments can be of benefit, certain foods are thought to trigger GI symptoms. In a research study, 63% of patients with IBS reported that some foods trigger their IBS symptoms [170]. Therefore, diet therapies gain more interest than other therapy options in patients with IBS and endurance athletes with GI symptoms. For example, a gluten-free diet (GFD) [128] and a low Fermentable Oligo-, Di-, Mono-saccharides, and Polyols (FODMAP) diet [171] are classified as elimination diets that both exclude or limit certain foods or nutrients that may cause undesirable GI problems such as abdominal bloating, cramps, flatulence or urge to defecate.

### 3.4.1. Why Do Endurance Athletes Consider a Gluten-Free Diet to Be Beneficial?

A gluten-free diet is a strict elimination diet that requires the complete exclusion of gluten, a storage protein found in wheat, rye, barley seeds, and includes gluten-free foods and food products that do not contain gluten or have a gluten content of less than

20 ppm, as per European legislation [172]. It has been used for decades as a treatment for celiac disease (CD) or to treat other gluten-related disorders that require strict gluten elimination from the diet [173]. However, recently, gluten has been considered to be an inducer that triggers the pathophysiology of various conditions. Based on this theory, endurance athletes have widely practiced GFD even if CD or non-celiac gluten sensitivity (NCGS) has not been diagnosed [7]. Although they applied GFD as a possible dietary therapy because of their belief in a diet that could improve metabolic health and performance or alleviate exercise-induced GI symptoms, the results show no significant improvement in performance with GFD in non-celiac athletes [129].

A study of 910 athletes (male = 377, female = 528, no gender selected = 5) found that 41% of the athletes reduced their gluten consumption by approximately 50% to 100% due to their belief that gluten causes GI symptoms, inflammation, and decreased performance [7]. Endurance athletes in particular (70%) tend to exclude gluten from their diet. Almost half of the athletes who consumed GFD reported that at least one of their GI symptoms was attenuated with ongoing GFD [7]. Inconsistent with the study, a randomized controlled, double-blind, crossover study of 13 endurance cyclists with no known gluten-related disease who followed GFD or gluten-containing diet for a short period (7 days) showed that gluten elimination did not alleviate GI symptoms [66]. Additionally, neither plasma intestinal fatty acid binding protein (I-FABP), a marker of intestinal damage, nor TT performance differed between the groups. This is the only randomized-controlled study investigating the influence of GFD vs. gluten-containing diet on endurance performance and intestinal injury, and perceived well-being in endurance athletes [66]. Further research is required to elucidate the GFD, endurance performance and GI symptoms.

The best technique for identifying gluten-related issues is to remove gluten from the diet and check it for health effects in clinical practice [174]. With this gluten-related practice, athletes often self-diagnose that they have gluten-related disorders, resulting in gluten being excluded from the diet [129]. Assessing the presence of celiac symptoms, prevalence, and comorbidities in 141 collegiate athletes, Leone et al. [175] found that athletes reported being 3.85 times more likely to be diagnosed with CD and 18.36 times more likely to be associated with CD than the general population. This close association negatively alters the athlete' health, leading to several detrimental consequences, including higher depression and perceived stress levels [175]. A possible explanation is that CD can be diagnosed faster as athletes monitor their health on a regular basis and work with an interdisciplinary team. The rapid detection of CD can provide an advantage to begin treatment as soon as possible, thereby reducing other harmful consequences associated with celiac disease.

A study on endurance athletes showed that they generally believed in GFD and its benefits to GI stress and exercise performance [176]. It is well known that the "belief effect" in athletes is an influential factor that can increase sports performance by 1 to 3% [177]. Whether gluten triggers exercise-related GI symptoms or whether endurance athletes with GI issues have a higher rate of NCGS remains unclear [66]. Additionally, switching to GFD can cause some healthy dietary changes in athletes, such as increased consumption of fruits, vegetables, legumes, and whole grains, and these changes may have more significant benefits on the GFD than gluten elimination [**96**]. Therefore, the gluten-free diet should not be recommended to non-celiac athletes (NCAs), as there is no evidence in the literature about its benefits to GI stress, immune response, and athletic performance [**8**,**66**].

### 3.4.2. Possible Risks of a Gluten-Free Diet

The main concerns of GFD for endurance athletes can be classified as low energy availability [**96**] and the potential to create an energy deficit, micronutrients and fiber, leading to the RED-S [**3**]. Although GFD limits the consumption of certain gluten-containing foods rich in CHO that could lead to an energy deficiency [**173**], there is insufficient data to investigate the effect of GFD on energy deficiency in endurance athletes. We recommend that more studies are required on this topic, especially with a well-planned GFD for endurance athletes.

In addition, athletes consuming GFD need to greatly consider their diet as they need to control all foods for gluten content, which can negatively affect psychology [**128**]. For athletes with CD or other gluten-related clinical conditions, removing gluten from the diet is the only effective treatment [**173**]. In endurance athletes with CD, an increase in exercise performance and a decrease in GI problems were found after a gluten-free diet was adopted [**178**]. However, it is worth noting that endurance athletes need more energy to perform better in prolonged training and races, and gluten is present in carbohydrate-rich foods, which are the primary common source to meet their energy needs [**112**]. Gluten-free products are also known for their high cost and can sometimes be difficult to find [**128**]. Therefore, dietary gluten elimination may be an effective strategy for athletes with CD [**173**]. However, when applied to non-celiac athletes, it can create a large energy deficit and low energy availability, impairing both metabolic health and performance.

## 3.5. Low-FODMAP Diet

Exercise-related GI problems affect performance and health conditions in approximately 70% of endurance athletes [**179**]. Several foods are believed to trigger these GI symptoms, including foods high in fructose, lactose, digestible fibers, and undigested fermentable carbohydrates such as inulin and oligofructose, named "prebiotics" [**180**]. These fermentable short-chain carbohydrates are classified as FODMAP, including animal milk (lactose), legumes (galactooligosaccharides; GOS), wheat (fructans), fruits (high in fructose), and prebiotic foods (high in inulin, fructooligosaccharides (FOS) and oligofructose) [**180**,**181**]. Prebiotics are known for their beneficial effects on health, including reducing disease risks by increasing the microbial abundance of beneficial bacteria such as Bifidobacterium and butyrate producers [**182**]. However, they reach the colon and are fermented by colonic bacteria [**183**]. Thus, they can cause GI symptoms such as abdominal distress, bloating and gas, resulting in gas production, including hydrogen and methane and osmotic water translocation [**184**]. As a result, luminal distention and GI symptoms such as bloating, and cramps, can increase, impairing well-being and athletic performance [**185**]. Therefore, endurance athletes tend to remove high-FODMAP foods from their diets to eliminate their undesirable effects on the GI system [**67**]. In endurance athletes with exercise-induced GI symptoms, low-FODMAP diets could apply in two different processes, including the long or short term (both described in detail in **Table 2**) [**8**].

### 3.5.1. Several Points Indicating That a Low-FODMAP Diet Is Advantageous

Endurance athletes' expectations of a low-FODMAP diet are the same as those they have of GFD, including reduced GI symptoms, and thereby increased performance [**8**]. It is estimated that approximately 22% of endurance athletes have IBS [**186**]. Exercise-induced oxidative stress and physiological changes in the body can lead to impaired GI motility and intestinal permeability, which also occur as a result of IBS [**147**]. Foods rich in FODMAPs can further trigger GI symptoms in athletes with impaired GI function or in IBS patients [**187**]. In addition, foods high in FODMAPs can also cause upper-GI symptoms, such as stomach swelling due to the high consumption of fructose and glucose [**184**]. For example, upper-GI distress syndromes such as bloating, nausea, and stomach pain/cramps are common in cyclists, which can impair performance and well-being during exercise and daily life [**188**]. The potential efficiency of a low-FODMAP diet on exercise-induced GI symptoms has been studied in four studies, two randomized controlled crossover studies [**67,70**], and two case reports [**68,69**]. All studies suggested the low-FODMAP diet as an efficient treatment for reducing exercise-associated GI symptoms. A case study investigating a multisport athlete with exercise-induced GI symptoms showed that a short-term (6 day) restriction of foods high in FODMAPs (from 81.0 ± 5.0 g to 7.2 ± 5.7 g·day$^{-1}$) resulted in a decrease in GI symptoms both during exercise and daily life of the athlete [**69**]. Another case report evaluated a long-term (4 week restriction of foods high in FODMAPs followed by reintroduction of foods high in FODMAPs for 6 weeks) low-FODMAP application before an aggressive multistage ultra-marathon race [**68**]. Apart from severe nausea, minimal GI symptoms including bloating and flatulence were observed throughout the race. Examining the influence of a 6-day low-FODMAP diet on recreationally competitive athletes with non-clinical GI symptoms in a single-blind, crossover design, Lis et al. [**67**] reported a significant decrease in exercise-induced GI symptoms, particularly in flatulence, urge to defecate, loose stool, and diarrhea, in nine of 11 athletes after the low-FODMAP trial. Another well-designed crossover study also applied 1 day low-FODMAP or high-FODMAP diet before exertional-heat stress to evaluate its impact on GI integrity, functions, and discomfort [**70**]. An exercise protocol that includes 2 h of work at 65% $VO_2max$ at 35 °C ambient temperature was applied after the diet applications. The study findings indicated that lower exercise-induced GI symptoms and I-FABP concentrations were observed after 1 day low-FODMAP diet, suggesting that 1 day low-FODMAP diet provided a crucial advantage by decreasing exercise-associated disruption of GI integrity, and attenuating GI symptoms [**70**]. Therefore, studies evaluating exertional-heat stress during long-term exercise have administered a 24 h low-FODMAP diet as a control diet to eliminate GI symptoms associated with food and fluid intake [**189,190,191**].

It should be noted that endurance athletes typically eat foods high in FODMAPs [**8**]. A study investigating the content of FODMAPs in various sports foods has shown that FODMAPs are often included in sports foods, such as dry dates (fructans), fructose, inulin (fructans), honey (fructose), and chicory root (oligosaccharides) [**8**]. Therefore, sports food alternatives low in FODMAPs could be a better choice for endurance athletes, in particular, those who have previously experienced GI symptoms.

A meta-analysis of nine randomized trials reported the administration of a low-FODMAP diet for short-term attenuated GI symptoms, abdominal pain, and quality of life in patients with IBS [**192**]. However, 25% of patients did not respond to the diet, and responders experienced the diarrhea-predominant type of IBS. These findings suggest that the higher response rate of diarrhea-type IBS may be due to osmotic changes in the gut following a low-FODMAP diet [**192**]. Note that runner's diarrhea is known to be one of the most common exercise-related GI problems [**168**]; the chances of responding positively to a low-FODMAP diet are high in endurance athletes, especially athletes with runner's diarrhea.

Exercise-induced GI symptoms may become detectable after intense exercise, affecting recovery and refueling periods [**188**]. The management of this process becomes crucial in multistage events that last multiple stages in a day or over multiple days [**112,193**]. In endurance athletes with exercise-induced GI symptoms, the FODMAPs restriction may also be needed for the post-exercise period [**129**], which is crucial to provide optimal nutrient delivery to the body after exercise, particularly intense training periods.

Taken together, as all studies on a low-FODMAP diet and exercise-associated GI symptoms confirmed the efficiency of the diet, we can consider a low-FODMAP diet as an efficient therapy to attenuate exercise-associated GI symptoms. However, the response rate to the low-FODMAP diet should also be determined before planning any long-term low-FODMAP diet application for endurance athletes.

### 3.5.2. Potential Risks to Consider When Applying a Low-FODMAP Diet

A low-FODMAP diet may result in decreased consumption of prebiotics, which is highly recommended for maintaining a healthy gut microbiome [**178**]. Additionally, adherence to the diet may be problematic for athletes due to difficulties during the application process [**3**].

By assessing the low-FODMAP diet based on nutrients instead of general composition, we can realize that complex polysaccharides, the most significant prebiotic metabolites, are restricted with the diet, thus negatively affecting microbiome composition [**194**]. Although highlighted in several studies on humans with IBS [**195,196,197**], randomized controlled studies are needed to investigate the gut microbiome and low-FODMAP diet to evaluate the potential effects of a low-FODMAP diet in endurance athletes.

A low-FODMAP diet should not only attenuate GI problems but provide sports-specific nutrients and energy intake efficiently as well [**171**]. Subjects that fail to show any improvement during the first phase of long-term FODMAP application should not continue the diet [**3**]. Additionally, the reintroduction phase should be carefully applied to subjects by trained dietitians and professionals to identify which foods high in FODMAPs cause these symptoms, and personalize the diet to attenuate IBS symptoms, and thereby maintain healthy gut functions [**8**].

A general recommendation to reduce the FODMAP content of the diet consists of reducing FODMAP intake from 15–30 g FODMAP·day$^{-1}$ to 5–18 g FODMAP·day$^{-1}$ [**198**]. It is recommended for patients with IBS that less than 0.5 g FODMAP per meal or less than 3 g per day be consumed [**199**]. However, endurance athletes with exercise-induced GI symptoms consume 2-fold higher FODMAPs than the diet classified as high in FODMAPs in clinical research (up to 43 g·day$^{-1}$) [**67**]. Therefore, foods high in FODMAPs could be a contributing factor for exercise-induced GI symptoms. A recent study on athletes reported that 55% ($n$ = 910) of athletes removed at least one high FODMAP from their diet to attenuate exercise-induced GI symptoms, and approximately 85% reduced GI symptoms by removing food from their diet [**171**]. Lactose is often reported as the most problematic nutrient high in FODMAPs [**163**]. The most frequently eliminated foods are reported as lactose (86%), GOS (23.9%), fructose (23.0%), fructans (6.2%), and polyols (5.4%). Therefore, before strict FODMAP restriction, it should be considered that lactose and fructose are the most common inductors for GI distress [**200**]. Lactose consumption of athletes may be greater than that in the general population due to high protein ingredients, good sources of calcium, and rehydration [**69**]. Furthermore, higher fructose consumption may be greater in endurance athletes, especially during exercise due to sufficient energy supply during long-duration (> 90 min.) events or training [**201**]. Higher fructose intake may be more likely to trigger exercise-induced GI symptoms [**202**]. Therefore, just reducing or eliminating lactose and fructose instead of all high FODMAPs may inhibit the detrimental gut alterations and may solve the GI problems in endurance athletes.

## 4. CONCISE SUMMARY

This chapter examines the efficacy of five prevalent diets—vegetarian diets, high-fat diets (HFD), intermittent fasting (IF), gluten-free diets (GFD), and low-FODMAP diets—on endurance performance and metabolic function. Upon reviewing the findings, all five diets examined exhibit both advantageous and adverse effects on endurance performance. For vegetarian diets, we recommend that a sports dietitian (a) identify the specific vegetarian diet the athlete follows; (b) assess the athlete's micronutrient levels and associated biomarkers, particularly vitamin B12, folate, vitamin D, and iron; (c) evaluate the athlete's energy requirements along with all macro- and micronutrient needs to avert deficiencies; and (d) oversee dietary intake and modify it according to individual and sport-specific requirements. Although assessments of the HFD and athletic performance yield mixed outcomes, the scientific data supporting the efficacy of HFD for endurance performance is insufficient to endorse these diets for endurance athletes. Further inquiry is required to enhance the evidence regarding intermittent fasting diets, endurance performance, and health-related indicators. Additional research is required prior to endorsing the IF diet for endurance athletes. Based on the pertinent study findings [66,68,69,70], it may be concluded that a low-FODMAP diet may be more advantageous than a gluten-free diet, except for athletes diagnosed with celiac disease. It is essential to recognize that the implementation of the low-FODMAP diet involves intricate procedures and necessitates meticulous oversight by a qualified dietitian. Furthermore, the exclusion of lactose and fructose from the diet should be contemplated for endurance athletes before implementing a low-FODMAP diet. We recommend initially using a short-term (1–6 days) low-FODMAP diet prior to formulating a long-term strategy, particularly before endurance racing or intense physical activity. In conclusion, all five diets examined in the review are applicable to endurance athletes based on their current metabolic requirements. Prior to selecting a prevalent diet, evaluating the existing metabolic and sport-specific conditions of endurance athletes will yield healthier and more advantageous outcomes.

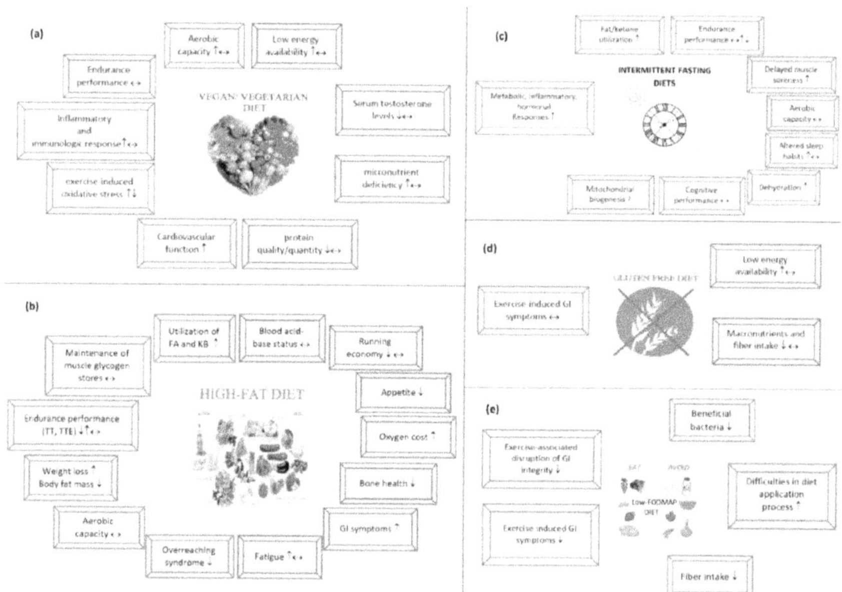


**Figure 1. Possible beneficial and detrimental effects of popular diets on endurance athletes. Statements presented in green boxes show the beneficial effects of diets, while red boxes indicate the potential risks of diets. (a): Vegetarian diets; (b) high-fat diets; (c) Intermittent Fasting; (d) Gluten-free diet; (e) low-FODMAP diet. Abbreviations: URTI: Upper-respiratory tract infections; RED-S: relative energy deficiency syndrome; FA: fatty acids; KB: Ketone bodies; GI: Gastrointestinal; FODMAP: fermentable oligosaccharides, disaccharides, monosaccharides and polyols.**

## AT A GLANCE

Endurance athletes require a comprehensive and meticulously structured nutrition regimen to replenish their energy reserves prior to training or competition, to offer nutritional support that enables them to withstand challenging conditions while training or racing, and to facilitate good recovery post-training or racing. Given that exercise-induced gastrointestinal disturbances can considerably impact performance, it is imperative to create measures to mitigate these concerns. These characteristics compel endurance athletes to always pursue an improved nutritional strategy. Consequently, numerous novel nutritional strategies have attracted attention from endurance athletes in recent decades. This study presents a contemporary analysis of five prevalent dietary approaches: (a) vegetarian diets, (b) high-fat diets, (c) intermittent fasting diets, (d) gluten-free diets, and (e) low fermentable oligosaccharides, disaccharides, monosaccharides, and polyols (FODMAP) diets. We examined scholarly research published from 1983 to January 2021 that explored the effects of these prevalent diets on the endurance performance and health of endurance athletes. We examine both the advantageous and detrimental elements of these diets and provide essential recommendations for endurance athletes to contemplate while adhering to them.

## REFERENCES


1. Knechtle, B.; Nikolaidis, P.T. Physiology and pathophysiology in Ultra-Marathon Running. *Front. Physiol.* **2018**, *9*, 634. **[Google Scholar]** **[PubMed]** **[Green Version]**
2. Nikolaidis, P.T.; Veniamakis, E.; Rosemann, T.; Knechtle, B. Nutrition in ultra-endurance: State of the art. *Nutrients* **2018**, *10*, 1995. **[Google Scholar]** **[PubMed]** **[Green Version]**
3. Lis, D.M.; Kings, D.; Larson-Meyer, D.E. Dietary practices adopted by track-and-field athletes: Gluten-free, low FODMAP, vegetarian, and fasting. *Int. J. Sport Nutr. Exerc. Metab.* **2019**, *29*, 236–245. **[Google Scholar]** **[PubMed]**
4. Craddock, J.C.; Neale, E.P.; Peoples, G.E.; Probst, Y.C. Plant-based eating patterns and endurance performance: A focus on inflammation, oxidative stress and immune responses. *Nutr. Bull.* **2020**, *45*, 123–132. **[Google Scholar]**
5. Burke, L.M. Ketogenic low-CHO, high-fat diet: The future of elite endurance sport? *J. Physiol.* **2020.** **[Google Scholar]**
6. Levy, E.; Chu, T. Intermittent fasting and its effects on athletic performance: A review. *Curr. Sports Med. Rep.* **2019**, *18*, 266–269. **[Google Scholar]**
7. Lis, D.M.; Stellingwerff, T.; Shing, C.M.; Ahuja, K.D.K.; Fell, J.W. Exploring the popularity, experiences, and beliefs surrounding gluten-free diets in nonceliac athletes. *Int. J. Sport Nutr. Exerc. Metab.* **2015**, *25*, 37–45. **[Google Scholar]**
8. Lis, D.M. Exit Gluten-Free and Enter Low FODMAPs: A Novel Dietary Strategy to Reduce Gastrointestinal Symptoms in Athletes. *Sports Med.* **2019**, *49*, 87–97. **[Google Scholar]** **[Green Version]**
9. Pimentel, D.; Pimentel, M. Sustainability of meat-based and plant-based diets and the environment. *Am. J. Clin. Nutr.* **2003**, *78*, 660S–663S. **[Google Scholar]**
10. Rogerson, D. Vegan diets: Practical advice for athletes and exercisers. *J. Int. Soc. Sports Nutr.* **2017**, *14*, 36. **[Google Scholar]** **[Green Version]**
11. Larson-Meyer, E. Vegetarian and Vegan Diets for Athletic Training and Performance. *Sports Sci. Exch.* **2018**, *29*, 1–7. **[Google Scholar]**
12. Wilson, P.B. Nutrition behaviors, perceptions, and beliefs of recent marathon finishers. *Phys. Sportsmed.* **2016**, *44*, 242–251. **[Google Scholar]** **[PubMed]**

13. Wirnitzer, K.; Seyfart, T.; Leitzmann, C.; Keller, M.; Wirnitzer, G.; Lechleitner, C.; Rüst, C.A.; Rosemann, T.; Knechtle, B. Prevalence in running events and running performance of endurance runners following a vegetarian or vegan diet compared to non-vegetarian endurance runners: The NURMI Study. *Springerplus* **2016**, *5*, 1–7. **[Google Scholar]** **[PubMed]** **[Green Version]**

14. McSwiney, F.T.; Wardrop, B.; Hyde, P.N.; Lafountain, R.A.; Volek, J.S.; Doyle, L. Keto-adaptation enhances exercise performance and body composition responses to training in endurance athletes. *Metabolism* **2018**, *81*, 25–34. **[Google Scholar]**

15. Terink, R.; Witkamp, R.F.; Hopman, M.T.E.; Siebelink, E.; Savelkoul, H.F.J.; Mensink, M. A 2 week cross-over intervention with a low carbohydrate, high fat diet compared to a high carbohydrate diet attenuates exercise-induced cortisol response, but not the reduction of exercise capacity, in recreational athletes. *Nutrients* **2021**, *13*, 157. **[Google Scholar]** **[PubMed]**

16. Burke, L.M.; Ross, M.L.; Garvican-Lewis, L.A.; Welvaert, M.; Heikura, I.A.; Forbes, S.G.; Mirtschin, J.G.; Cato, L.E.; Strobel, N.; Sharma, A.P.; et al. Low carbohydrate, high fat diet impairs exercise economy and negates the performance benefit from intensified training in elite race walkers. *J. Physiol.* **2017**, *595*, 2785–2807. **[Google Scholar]** **[Green Version]**

17. Carr, A.J.; Sharma, A.P.; Ross, M.L.; Welvaert, M.; Slater, G.J.; Burke, L.M. Chronic ketogenic low carbohydrate high fat diet has minimal effects on acid–base status in elite athletes. *Nutrients* **2018**, *10*, 236. **[Google Scholar]** **[Green Version]**

18. Shaw, D.M.; Merien, F.; Braakhuis, A.; Maunder, E.D.; Dulson, D.K. Effect of a Ketogenic Diet on Submaximal Exercise Capacity and Efficiency in Runners. *Med. Sci. Sports Exerc.* **2019**, *51*, 2135–2146. **[Google Scholar]**

19. Heatherly, A.J.; Killen, L.G.; Smith, A.F.; Waldman, H.S.; Seltmann, C.L.; Hollingsworth, A.; O'Neal, E.K. Effects of Ad libitum Low-Carbohydrate High-Fat Dieting in Middle-Age Male Runners. *Med. Sci. Sports Exerc.* **2018**, *50*, 570–579. **[Google Scholar]**

20. Phinney, S.D.; Bistrian, B.R.; Evans, W.J.; Gervino, E.; Blackburn, G.L. The human metabolic response to chronic ketosis without caloric restriction: Preservation of submaximal exercise capability with reduced carbohydrate oxidation. *Metabolism* **1983**, *32*, 769–776. **[Google Scholar]**

21. Zinn, C.; Wood, M.; Williden, M.; Chatterton, S.; Maunder, E. Ketogenic diet benefits body composition and well-being but not performance in a pilot case study of New Zealand endurance athletes. *J. Int. Soc. Sports Nutr.* **2017**, *14*, 22–31. **[Google Scholar]** **[PubMed]** **[Green Version]**

22. Shaw, D.M.; Merien, F.; Braakhuis, A.; Keaney, L.; Dulson, D.K. Adaptation to a ketogenic diet modulates adaptive and mucosal immune markers in trained male endurance athletes. *Scand. J. Med. Sci. Sports* **2020**, *31*, 140–152. **[Google Scholar]** **[PubMed]**

23. Burke, L.M.; Sharma, A.P.; Heikura, I.A.; Forbes, S.F.; Holloway, M.; McKay, A.K.A.; Bone, J.L.; Leckey, J.J.; Welvaert, M.; Ross, M.L. Crisis of confidence averted: Impairment of exercise economy and performance in elite race walkers by ketogenic low carbohydrate, high fat (LCHF) diet is reproducible. *PLoS ONE* **2020**, *15*, e0234027. **[Google Scholar]**

24. Volek, J.S.; Freidenreich, D.J.; Saenz, C.; Kunces, L.J.; Creighton, B.C.; Bartley, J.M.; Davitt, P.M.; Munoz, C.X.; Anderson, J.M.; Maresh, C.M.; et al. Metabolic characteristics of keto-adapted ultra-endurance runners. *Metabolism* **2016**, *65*, 100–110. **[Google Scholar]** **[PubMed]** **[Green Version]**

25. Prins, P.J.; Noakes, T.D.; Welton, G.L.; Haley, S.J.; Esbenshade, N.J.; Atwell, A.D.; Scott, K.E.; Abraham, J.; Raabe, A.S.; Buxton, J.D.; et al. High rates of fat oxidation induced by a low-carbohydrate, high-fat diet, do not impair 5-km running performance in competitive recreational athletes. *J. Sports Sci. Med.* **2019**, *18*, 738–750. **[Google Scholar]**

26. Lambert, E.V.; Speechly, D.P.; Dennis, S.C.; Noakes, T.D. Enhanced endurance in trained cyclists during moderate intensity exercise following 2 weeks adaptation to a high fat diet. *Eur. J. Appl. Physiol. Occup. Physiol.* **1994**, *69*, 287–293. **[Google Scholar]**

27. Creighton, B.C.; Hyde, P.N.; Maresh, C.M.; Kraemer, W.J.; Phinney, S.D.; Volek, J.S. Paradox of hypercholesterolaemia in highly trained, keto-adapted athletes. *BMJ Open Sport Exerc. Med.* **2018**, *4*, e000429. **[Google Scholar] [Green Version]**

28. Zajac, A.; Poprzecki, S.; Maszczyk, A.; Czuba, M.; Michalczyk, M.; Zydek, G. The Effects of a Ketogenic Diet on Exercise Metabolism and Physical Performance in Off-Road Cyclists. *Nutrients* **2014**, *6*, 2493–2508. **[Google Scholar]**

29. Goedecke, J.H.; Christie, C.; Wilson, G.; Dennis, S.C.; Noakes, T.D.; Hopkins, W.G.; Lambert, E.V. Metabolic adaptations to a high-fat diet in endurance cyclists. *Metabolism* **1999**, *48*, 1509–1517. **[Google Scholar]**

30. Shaw, D.M.; Merien, F.; Braakhuis, A.; Keaney, L.; Dulson, D.K. Acute hyperketonaemia alters T-cell-related cytokine gene expression within stimulated peripheral blood mononuclear cells following prolonged exercise. *Eur. J. Appl. Physiol.* **2020**, *120*, 191–202. **[Google Scholar]**

31. Dearlove, D.J.; Faull, O.K.; Rolls, E.; Clarke, K.; Cox, P.J. Nutritional ketoacidosis during incremental exercise in healthy athletes. *Front. Physiol.* **2019**, *10*, 290. **[Google Scholar] [PubMed]**

32. Dearlove, D.J.; Harrison, O.K.; Hodson, L.; Jefferson, A.; Clarke, K.; Cox, P.J. The Effect of Blood Ketone Concentration and Exercise Intensity on Exogenous Ketone Oxidation Rates in Athletes. *Med. Sci. Sports Exerc.* **2020. [Google Scholar] [PubMed]**

33. Cox, P.J.; Kirk, T.; Ashmore, T.; Willerton, K.; Evans, R.; Smith, A.; Murray, A.J.; Stubbs, B.; West, J.; McLure, S.W.; et al. Nutritional Ketosis Alters Fuel Preference and Thereby Endurance Performance in Athletes. *Cell Metab.* **2016**, *24*, 256–268. **[Google Scholar] [PubMed] [Green Version]**

34. Shaw, D.M.; Merien, F.; Braakhuis, A.; Plews, D.; Laursen, P.; Dulson, D.K. The effect of 1,3-butanediol on cycling time-trial performance. *Int. J. Sport Nutr. Exerc. Metab.* **2019**, *29*, 466–473. **[Google Scholar] [Green Version]**

35. Leckey, J.J.; Ross, M.L.; Quod, M.; Hawley, J.A.; Burke, L.M. Ketone Diester Ingestion Impairs Time-Trial Performance in Professional Cyclists. *Front. Physiol.* **2017**, *8*, 806. **[Google Scholar] [Green Version]**

36. Scott, B.E.; Laursen, P.B.; James, L.J.; Boxer, B.; Chandler, Z.; Lam, E.; Gascoyne, T.; Messenger, J.; Mears, S.A. The effect of 1,3-butanediol and carbohydrate supplementation on running performance. *J. Sci. Med. Sport* **2019**, *22*, 702–706. **[Google Scholar] [Green Version]**

37. Poffé, C.; Ramaekers, M.; Bogaerts, S.; Hespel, X.P. Exogenous ketosis impacts neither performance nor muscle glycogen breakdown in prolonged endurance exercise. *J. Appl. Physiol.* **2020**, *128*, 1643–1653. **[Google Scholar]**

38. Prins, P.J.; D'Agostino, D.P.; Rogers, C.Q.; Ault, D.L.; Welton, G.L.; Jones, D.W.; Henson, S.R.; Rothfuss, T.J.; Aiken, K.G.; Hose, J.L.; et al. Dose response of a novel exogenous ketone supplement on physiological, perceptual and performance parameters. *Nutr. Metab.* **2020**, *17*, 81. **[Google Scholar]**

39. Evans, M.; McSwiney, F.T.; Brady, A.J.; Egan, B. No Benefit of Ingestion of a Ketone Monoester Supplement on 10-km Running Performance. *Med. Sci. Sports Exerc.* **2019**, *51*, 2506–2515. **[Google Scholar]**

40. Heikura, I.A.; Burke, L.M.; Hawley, J.A.; Ross, M.L.; Garvican-Lewis, L.; Sharma, A.P.; McKay, A.K.A.; Leckey, J.J.; Welvaert, M.; McCall, L.; et al. A Short-Term Ketogenic Diet Impairs Markers of Bone Health in Response to Exercise. *Front. Endocrinol.* **2020**, *10*, 880. **[Google Scholar] [Green Version]**

41. Carey, A.L.; Staudacher, H.M.; Cummings, N.K.; Stepto, N.K.; Nikolopoulos, V.; Burke, L.M.; Hawley, J.A. Effects of fat adaptation and carbohydrate restoration on prolonged endurance exercise. *J. Appl. Physiol.* **2001**, *91*, 115–122. **[Google Scholar] [PubMed] [Green Version]**

42. Burke, L.M.; Angus, D.J.; Cox, G.R.; Cummings, N.K.; Febbraio, M.A.; Gawthorn, K.; Hawley, J.A.; Minehan, M.; Martin, D.T.; Hargreaves, M.; et al. Effect of fat adaptation and carbohydrate

restoration on metabolism and performance during prolonged cycling. *J. Appl. Physiol.* **2000**, *89*, 2413–2421. **[Google Scholar] [PubMed] [Green Version]**

43. Burke, L.M.; Hawley, J.A.; Angus, D.J.; Cox, G.R.; Clark, S.A.; Cummings, N.K.; Desbrow, B.; Hargreaves, M. Adaptations to short-term high-fat diet persist during exercise despite high carbohydrate availability. *Med. Sci. Sports Exerc.* **2002**, *34*, 83–91. **[Google Scholar] [PubMed]**

44. Yeo, W.K.; Lessard, S.J.; Chen, Z.P.; Garnham, A.P.; Burke, L.M.; Rivas, D.A.; Kemp, B.E.; Hawley, J.A. Fat adaptation followed by carbohydrate restoration increases AMPK activity in skeletal muscle from trained humans. *J. Appl. Physiol.* **2008**, *105*, 1519–1526. **[Google Scholar] [Green Version]**

45. Havemann, L.; West, S.J.; Goedecke, J.H.; Macdonald, I.A.; St Clair Gibson, A.; Noakes, T.D.; Lambert, E.V. Fat adaptation followed by carbohydrate loading compromises high-intensity sprint performance. *J. Appl. Physiol.* **2006**, *100*, 194–202. **[Google Scholar]**

46. Lambert, E.V.; Goedecke, J.H.; Van Zyl, C.; Murphy, K.; Hawley, J.A.; Dennis, S.C.; Noakes, T.D. High-fat diet versus habitual diet prior to carbohydrate loading: Effects on exercise metabolism and cycling performance. *Int. J. Sport Nutr.* **2001**, *11*, 209–225. **[Google Scholar]**

47. Stellingwerff, T.; Spriet, L.L.; Watt, M.J.; Kimber, N.E.; Hargreaves, M.; Hawley, J.A.; Burke, L.M. Decreased PDH activation and glycogenolysis during exercise following fat adaptation with carbohydrate restoration. *Am. J. Physiol. Endocrinol. Metab.* **2006**, *290*, 380–388. **[Google Scholar] [Green Version]**

48. Mujika, I. Case study: Long-term low-carbohydrate, high-fat diet impairs performance and subjective well-being in a world-class vegetarian long-distance triathlete. *Int. J. Sport Nutr. Exerc. Metab.* **2019**, *29*, 339–344. **[Google Scholar]**

49. Zehnder, M.; Christ, E.R.; Ith, M.; Acheson, K.J.; Pouteau, E.; Kreis, R.; Trepp, R.; Diem, P.; Boesch, C.; Décombaz, J. Intramyocellular lipid stores increase markedly in athletes after 1.5 days lipid supplementation and are utilized during exercise in proportion to their content. *Eur. J. Appl. Physiol.* **2006**, *98*, 341–354. **[Google Scholar]**

50. Décombaz, J.; Grathwohl, D.; Pollien, P.; Schmitt, J.A.J.; Borrani, F.; Lecoultre, V. Effect of short-duration lipid supplementation on fat oxidation during exercise and cycling performance. *Appl. Physiol. Nutr. Metab.* **2013**, *38*, 766–772. **[Google Scholar]**

51. Murakami, I.; Sakuragi, T.; Uemura, H.; Menda, H.; Shindo, M.; Tanaka, H. Significant Effect of a Pre-Exercise High-Fat Meal after a 3-Day High-Carbohydrate Diet on Endurance Performance. *Nutrients* **2012**, *4*, 625–637. **[Google Scholar] [PubMed] [Green Version]**

52. Nebl, J.; Haufe, S.; Eigendorf, J.; Wasserfurth, P.; Tegtbur, U.; Hahn, A. Exercise capacity of vegan, lacto-ovo-vegetarian and omnivorous recreational runners. *J. Int. Soc. Sports Nutr.* **2019**, *16*, 23. **[Google Scholar] [PubMed] [Green Version]**

53. Nebl, J.; Drabert, K.; Haufe, S.; Wasserfurth, P.; Eigendorf, J.; Tegtbur, U.; Hahn, A.; Tsikas, D. Exercise-Induced Oxidative Stress, Nitric Oxide and Plasma Amino Acid Profile in Recreational Runners with Vegetarian and Non-Vegetarian Dietary Patterns. *Nutrients* **2019**, *11*, 1875. **[Google Scholar] [Green Version]**

54. Richter, E.A.; Kiens, B.; Raben, A.; Tvede, N.; Pedersen, B.K. Immune parameters in male atheletes after a lacto-ovo vegetarian diet and a mixed Western diet. *Med. Sci. Sports Exerc.* **1991**, *23*, 517–521. **[Google Scholar] [PubMed]**

55. Potthast, A.B.; Nebl, J.; Wasserfurth, P.; Haufe, S.; Eigendorf, J.; Hahn, A.; Das, A. Impact of Nutrition on Short-Term Exercise-Induced Sirtuin Regulation: Vegans Differ from Omnivores and Lacto-Ovo Vegetarians. *Nutrients* **2020**, *12*, 1004. **[Google Scholar] [Green Version]**

56. Leischik, R.; Spelsberg, N. Vegan Triple-Ironman (Raw Vegetables/Fruits). *Case Rep. Cardiol.* **2014**, *2014*, 1–4. **[Google Scholar] [Green Version]**

57. Wirnitzer, K.C.; Kornexl, E. Energy and Macronutrient Intake of a Female Vegan Cyclist During an 8-Day Mountain Bike Stage Race. *Baylor Univ. Med. Cent. Proc.* **2014**, *27*, 42–45. **[Google Scholar]**

58. Lynch, H.M.; Wharton, C.M.; Johnston, C.S. Cardiorespiratory fitness and peak torque differences between vegetarian and omnivore endurance athletes: A cross-sectional study. *Nutrients* **2016**, *8*, 726. **[Google Scholar]** **[Green Version]**

59. Król, W.; Price, S.; Śliż, D.; Parol, D.; Konopka, M.; Mamcarz, A.; Wełnicki, M.; Braksator, W. A Vegan Athlete's Heart—Is It Different? Morphology and Function in Echocardiography. *Diagnostics* **2020**, *10*, 477. **[Google Scholar]**

60. Brisswalter, J.; Bouhlel, E.; Falola, J.M.; Abbiss, C.R.; Vallier, J.M.; Hauswirth, C. Effects of ramadan intermittent fasting on middle-distance running performance in well-trained runners. *Clin. J. Sport Med.* **2011**, *21*, 422–427. **[Google Scholar]**

61. Chennaoui, M.; Desgorces, F.; Drogou, C.; Boudjemaa, B.; Tomaszewski, A.; Depiesse, F.; Burnat, P.; Chalabi, H.; Gomez-Merino, D. Effects of Ramadan fasting on physical performance and metabolic, hormonal, and inflammatory parameters in middle-distance runners. *Appl. Physiol. Nutr. Metab.* **2009**, *34*, 587–594. **[Google Scholar]** **[PubMed]**

62. Moro, T.; Tinsley, G.; Longo, G.; Grigoletto, D.; Bianco, A.; Ferraris, C.; Guglielmetti, M.; Veneto, A.; Tagliabue, A.; Marcolin, G.; et al. Time-restricted eating effects on performance, immune function, and body composition in elite cyclists: A randomized controlled trial. *J. Int. Soc. Sports Nutr.* **2020**, *17*, 65. **[Google Scholar]** **[PubMed]**

63. Chamari, K.; Briki, W.; Farooq, A.; Patrick, T.; Belfekih, T.; Herrera, C.P. Impact of Ramadan intermittent fasting on cognitive function in trained cyclists: A pilot study. *Biol. Sport* **2016**, *33*, 49–56. **[Google Scholar]** **[PubMed]**

64. Che Muhamed, A.M.; Mohamed, N.G.; Ismail, N.; Aziz, A.R.; Singh, R. Mouth rinsing improves cycling endurance performance during Ramadan fasting in a hot humid environment. *Appl. Physiol. Nutr. Metab.* **2014**, *39*, 458–464. **[Google Scholar]** **[PubMed]**

65. Brady, A.J.; Langton, H.M.; Mulligan, M.; Egan, B. Effects of Eight Weeks of 16:8 Time-restricted Eating in Male Middle- and Long-Distance Runners. *Med. Sci. Sports Exerc.* **2020**. **[Google Scholar]**

66. Lis, D.; Stellingwerff, T.; Kitic, C.M.; Ahuja, K.D.; Fell, J. No Effects of a Short-Term Gluten-free Diet on Performance in Nonceliac Athletes. *Med. Sci. Sports Exerc.* **2015**, *47*, 2563–2570. **[Google Scholar]**

67. Lis, D.; Stellingwerff, T.; Kitic, C.M.; Fell, J.W.; Ahuja, K.D.K. Low FODMAP: A Preliminary Strategy to Reduce Gastrointestinal Distress in Athletes. *Med. Sci. Sports Exerc.* **2018**, *50*, 116–123. **[Google Scholar]**

68. Gaskell, S.K.; Costa, R.J.S. Applying a Low-FODMAP dietary intervention to a female ultraendurance runner with irritable bowel syndrome during a multistage ultramarathon. *Int. J. Sport Nutr. Exerc. Metab.* **2019**, *29*, 61–67. **[Google Scholar]**

69. Lis, D.; Ahuja, K.D.K.; Stellingwerff, T.; Kitic, C.M.; Fell, J. Case study: Utilizing a low FODMAP diet to combat exercise-induced gastrointestinal symptoms. *Int. J. Sport Nutr. Exerc. Metab.* **2016**, *26*, 481–487. **[Google Scholar]**

70. Gaskell, S.K.; Taylor, B.; Muir, J.; Costa, R.J.S. Impact of 24-h high and low fermentable oligo-, di-, monosaccharide, and polyol diets on markers of exercise-induced gastrointestinal syndrome in response to exertional heat stress. *Appl. Physiol. Nutr. Metab.* **2020**, *45*, 569–580. **[Google Scholar]**

71. Barnard, N.D.; Goldman, D.M.; Loomis, J.F.; Kahleova, H.; Levin, S.M.; Neabore, S.; Batts, T.C. Plant-based diets for cardiovascular safety and performance in endurance sports. *Nutrients* **2019**, *11*, 130. **[Google Scholar]** **[PubMed]** **[Green Version]**

72. Trapp, D.; Knez, W.; Sinclair, W. Could a vegetarian diet reduce exercise-induced oxidative stress? A review of the literature. *J. Sports Sci.* **2010**, *28*, 1261–1268. **[Google Scholar]** **[PubMed]**

73. Somerville, V.S.; Braakhuis, A.J.; Hopkins, W.G. Effect of flavonoids on upper respiratory tract infections and immune function: A systematic review and meta-analysis. *Adv. Nutr.* **2016**, *7*, 488–497. **[Google Scholar] [PubMed] [Green Version]**

74. Borrione, P.; Grasso, L.; Quaranta, F.; Parisi, A. Vegetarian diet and athletes. *Int. SportMed J.* **2009**, *10*, 20–24. **[Google Scholar]**

75. Marquet, L.-A.; Brisswalter, J.; Louis, J.; Tiollier, E.; Burke, L.M.; Hawley, J.A.; Hausswirth, C. Enhanced Endurance Performance by Periodization of Carbohydrate Intake. *Med. Sci. Sports Exerc.* **2016**, *48*, 663–672. **[Google Scholar]**

76. Kennedy, D.O. Phytochemicals for Improving Aspects of Cognitive Function and Psychological State Potentially Relevant to Sports Performance. *Sports Med.* **2019**, *49*, 39–58. **[Google Scholar] [Green Version]**

77. D'Angelo, S. Polyphenols: Potential Beneficial Effects of These Phytochemicals in Athletes. *Curr. Sports Med. Rep.* **2020**, *19*, 260–265. **[Google Scholar]**

78. Cook, M.D.; Willems, M.E.T. Dietary anthocyanins: A review of the exercise performance effects and related physiological responses. *Int. J. Sport Nutr. Exerc. Metab.* **2019**, *29*, 322–330. **[Google Scholar] [Green Version]**

79. McAnulty, S.R.; McAnulty, L.S.; Nieman, D.C.; Dumke, C.L.; Morrow, J.D.; Utter, A.C.; Henson, D.A.; Proulx, W.R.; George, G.L. Consumption of blueberry polyphenols reduces exercise-induced oxidative stress compared to vitamin C. *Nutr. Res.* **2004**, *24*, 209–221. **[Google Scholar]**

80. Nieman, D.C.; Gillitt, N.D.; Knab, A.M.; Shanely, R.A.; Pappan, K.L.; Jin, F.; Lila, M.A. Influence of a Polyphenol-Enriched Protein Powder on Exercise-Induced Inflammation and Oxidative Stress in Athletes: A Randomized Trial Using a Metabolomics Approach. *PLoS ONE* **2013**, *8*, 72215. **[Google Scholar]**

81. Park, C.H.; Kwak, Y.S.; Seo, H.K.; Kim, H.Y. Assessing the Values of Blueberries Intake on Exercise Performance, TAS, and Inflammatory Factors. *Iran. J. Public Health* **2018**, *47*, 27–32. **[Google Scholar] [PubMed]**

82. Nieman, D.C.; Gillitt, N.D.; Chen, G.-Y.; Zhang, Q.; Sha, W.; Kay, C.D.; Chandra, P.; Kay, K.L.; Lila, M.A. Blueberry and/or Banana Consumption Mitigate Arachidonic, Cytochrome P450 Oxylipin Generation during Recovery from 75-km Cycling: A Randomized Trial. *Front. Nutr.* **2020**, *7*, 121. **[Google Scholar] [PubMed]**

83. Braakhuis, A.J.; Somerville, V.X.; Hurst, R.D. The effect of New Zealand blackcurrant on sport performance and related biomarkers: A systematic review and meta-analysis. *J. Int. Soc. Sports Nutr.* **2020**, *17*, 25. **[Google Scholar] [PubMed]**

84. Vitale, K.C.; Hueglin, S.; Broad, E. Tart Cherry Juice in Athletes: A Literature Review and Commentary. *Curr. Sports Med. Rep.* **2017**, *16*, 230–239. **[Google Scholar]**

85. Alba, C.M.-A.; Daya, M.; Franck, C. Tart Cherries and health: Current knowledge and need for a better understanding of the fate of phytochemicals in the human gastrointestinal tract. *Crit. Rev. Food Sci. Nutr.* **2019**, *59*, 626–638. **[Google Scholar]**

86. Torregrosa-García, A.; Ávila-Gandía, V.; Luque-Rubia, A.J.; Abellán-Ruiz, M.S.; Querol-Calderón, M.; López-Román, F.J. Pomegranate extract improves maximal performance of trained cyclists after an exhausting endurance trial: A randomised controlled trial. *Nutrients* **2019**, *11*, 721. **[Google Scholar] [Green Version]**

87. Bowtell, J.; Kelly, V. Fruit-Derived Polyphenol Supplementation for Athlete Recovery and Performance. *Sports Med.* **2019**, *49*, 3–23. **[Google Scholar] [Green Version]**

88. Khoubnasabjafari, M.; Ansarin, K.; Jouyban, A. Reliability of malondialdehyde as a biomarker of oxidative stress in psychological disorders. *BioImpacts* **2015**, *5*, 123–127. **[Google Scholar]**

89. Smith, K.A.; Kisiolek, J.N.; Willingham, B.D.; Morrissey, M.C.; Leyh, S.M.; Saracino, P.G.; Baur, D.A.; Cook, M.D.; Ormsbee, M.J. Ultra-endurance triathlon performance and markers of whole-body and gut-specific inflammation. *Eur. J. Appl. Physiol.* **2020**, *120*, 349–357. **[Google Scholar]**

90. Welc, S.S.; Clanton, T.L. The regulation of interleukin-6 implicates skeletal muscle as an integrative stress sensor and endocrine organ. *Exp. Physiol.* **2013**, *98*, 359–371. **[Google Scholar] [Green Version]**

91. Neubauer, O.; König, D.; Wagner, K.H. Recovery after an Ironman triathlon: Sustained inflammatory responses and muscular stress. *Eur. J. Appl. Physiol.* **2008**, *104*, 417–426. **[Google Scholar] [PubMed]**

92. Keller, C.; Steensberg, A.; Hansen, A.K.; Fischer, C.P.; Plomgaard, P.; Pedersen, B.K. Effect of exercise, training, and glycogen availability on IL-6 receptor expression in human skeletal muscle. *J. Appl. Physiol.* **2005**, *99*, 2075–2079. **[Google Scholar] [PubMed] [Green Version]**

93. Nieman, D.C. Risk of upper respiratory tract infection in athletes: An epidemiologic and immunologic perspective. *J. Athl. Train.* **1997**, *32*, 344–349. **[Google Scholar] [PubMed]**

94. González-Gallego, J.; García-Mediavilla, M.V.; Sánchez-Campos, S.; Tuñó, M.J. Fruit polyphenols, immunity and inflammation. *Br. J. Nutr.* **2010**, *104*, S15–S27. **[Google Scholar] [PubMed] [Green Version]**

95. Barr, S.I.; Rideout, C.A. Nutritional considerations for vegetarian athletes. *Nutrition* **2004**, *20*, 696–703. **[Google Scholar]**

96. Cialdella-Kam, L.; Kulpins, D.; Manore, M. Vegetarian, Gluten-Free, and Energy Restricted Diets in Female Athletes. *Sports* **2016**, *4*, 50. **[Google Scholar] [Green Version]**

97. Howie, B.J.; Shultz, T.D. Dietary and hormonal interrelationships among vegetarian Seventh-Day Adventists and nonvegetarian men. *Am. J. Clin. Nutr.* **1985**, *42*, 127–134. **[Google Scholar] [Green Version]**

98. Allen, N.E.; Appleby, P.N.; Davey, G.K.; Key, T.J. Hormones and diet: Low insulin-like growth factor-1 but normal bioavailable androgens in vegan men. *Br. J. Cancer* **2000**, *83*, 95–97. **[Google Scholar] [Green Version]**

99. Clarys, P.; Deliens, T.; Huybrechts, I.; Deriemaeker, P.; Vanaelst, B.; de Keyzer, W.; Hebbelinck, M.; Mullie, P. Comparison of nutritional quality of the vegan, vegetarian, semi-vegetarian, pesco-vegetarian and omnivorous diet. *Nutrients* **2014**, *6*, 1318–1332. **[Google Scholar]**

100. Ciuris, C.; Lynch, H.M.; Wharton, C.; Johnston, C.S. A comparison of dietary protein digestibility, based on diaas scoring, in vegetarian and non-vegetarian athletes. *Nutrients* **2019**, *11*, 3016. **[Google Scholar] [Green Version]**

101. Fuhrman, J.; Ferreri, D.M. Fueling the vegetarian (vegan) athlete. *Curr. Sports Med. Rep.* **2010**, *9*, 233–241. **[Google Scholar] [PubMed]**

102. Nebl, J.; Schuchardt, J.P.; Wasserfurth, P.; Haufe, S.; Eigendorf, J.; Tegtbur, U.; Hahn, A. Characterization, dietary habits and nutritional intake of omnivorous, lacto-ovo vegetarian and vegan runners—A pilot study. *BMC Nutr.* **2019**, *5*, 51. **[Google Scholar] [PubMed] [Green Version]**

103. Nebl, J.; Schuchardt, J.P.; Ströhle, A.; Wasserfurth, P.; Haufe, S.; Eigendorf, J.; Tegtbur, U.; Hahn, A. Micronutrient status of recreational runners with vegetarian or non-vegetarian dietary patterns. *Nutrients* **2019**, *11*, 1146. **[Google Scholar] [PubMed] [Green Version]**

104. Gilani, G.S.; Xiao, C.W.; Cockell, K.A. Impact of antinutritional factors in food proteins on the digestibility of protein and the bioavailability of amino acids and on protein quality. *Br. J. Nutr.* **2012**, *108*, S315–S332. **[Google Scholar]**

105. Samtiya, M.; Aluko, R.E.; Dhewa, T. Plant food anti-nutritional factors and their reduction strategies: An overview. *Food Prod. Process. Nutr.* **2020**, *2*, 1–14. **[Google Scholar]**

106. Williamson, E. Nutritional implications for ultra-endurance walking and running events. *Extrem. Physiol. Med.* **2016**, *5*, 13. **[Google Scholar]** **[Green Version]**

107. Black, K.; Slater, J.; Brown, R.C.; Cooke, R. Low energy availability, plasma lipids, and hormonal profiles of recreational athletes. *J. Strength Cond. Res.* **2018**, *32*, 2816–2824. **[Google Scholar]**

108. Mountjoy, M.; Sundgot-Borgen, J.; Burke, L.; Carter, S.; Constantini, N.; Lebrun, C.; Meyer, N.; Sherman, R.; Steffen, K.; Budgett, R.; et al. The IOC consensus statement: Beyond the Female Athlete Triad-Relative Energy Deficiency in Sport (RED-S). *Br. J. Sports Med.* **2014**, *48*, 491–497. **[Google Scholar]**

109. Mountjoy, M.; Sundgot-Borgen, J.; Burke, L.; Ackerman, K.E.; Blauwet, C.; Constantini, N.; Lebrun, C.; Lundy, B.; Melin, A.; Torstveit, M.K.; et al. International Olympic Committee (IOC) Consensus statement on relative energy deficiency in sport (red-s): 2018 update. *Int. J. Sport Nutr. Exerc. Metab.* **2018**, *28*, 316–331. **[Google Scholar]** **[Green Version]**

110. Brytek-Matera, A.; Czepczor-Bernat, K.; Jurzak, H.; Kornacka, M.; Kołodziejczyk, N. Strict health-oriented eating patterns (orthorexic eating behaviours) and their connection with a vegetarian and vegan diet. *Eat. Weight Disord.* **2019**, *24*, 441–452. **[Google Scholar]** **[Green Version]**

111. Melin, A.; Tornberg, Å.; Skouby, S.; Møller, S.S.; Faber, J.; Sundgot-Borgen, J.; Sjödin, A. Low-energy density and high fiber intake are dietary concerns in female endurance athletes. *Scand. J. Med. Sci. Sports* **2016**, *26*, 1060–1071. **[Google Scholar]** **[PubMed]**

112. Hough, P.A.; Earle, J. Energy Balance during a Self-Sufficient, Multistage Ultramarathon. *J. Hum. Perform. Extrem. Environ.* **2017**, *13*, 5. **[Google Scholar]** **[Green Version]**

113. Melina, V.; Craig, W.; Levin, S. Position of the Academy of Nutrition and Dietetics: Vegetarian Diets. *J. Acad. Nutr. Diet.* **2016**, *116*, 1970–1980. **[Google Scholar]** **[PubMed]**

114. Raben, A.; Kiens, B.; Richter, E.A.; Rasmussen, L.B.; Svenstrup, B.; Micic, S.; Benett, P. Serum sex hormones and endurance performance after a lacto-ovo vegetarian and a mixed diet—Publications. *Med. Sci. Sports Exerc.* **1992**, *24*, 1290–1297. **[Google Scholar]** **[PubMed]**

115. Wolfe, R.; Ferrando, A.; Sheffield-Moore, M.; Urban, R. Testosterone and muscle protein metabolism. *Mayo Clin. Proc.* **2000**, *75*, S55–S60. **[Google Scholar]**

116. Kuchakulla, M.; Nackeeran, S.; Blachman-Braun, R.; Ramasamy, R. The association between plant-based content in diet and testosterone levels in US adults. *World J. Urol.* **2020**, *2020*, 1–5. **[Google Scholar]**

117. Lynch, H.; Johnston, C.; Wharton, C. Plant-Based Diets: Considerations for Environmental Impact, Protein Quality, and Exercise Performance. *Nutrients* **2018**, *10*, 1841. **[Google Scholar]** **[Green Version]**

118. Berrazaga, I.; Micard, V.; Gueugneau, M.; Walrand, S. The role of the anabolic properties of plant- versus animal-based protein sources in supporting muscle mass maintenance: A critical review. *Nutrients* **2019**, *11*, 1825. **[Google Scholar]** **[Green Version]**

119. Mariotti, F.; Gardner, C.D. Dietary protein and amino acids in vegetarian diets—A review. *Nutrients* **2019**, *11*, 2661. **[Google Scholar]** **[Green Version]**

120. Visioli, F. *Polyphenols in Sport: Facts or Fads?* CRC Press/Taylor & Francis: Boca Raton, FL, USA, 2015; ISBN 9781466567573. **[Google Scholar]**

121. Sorrenti, V.; Fortinguerra, S.; Caudullo, G.; Buriani, A. Deciphering the Role of Polyphenols in Sports Performance: From Nutritional Genomics to the Gut Microbiota toward Phytonutritional Epigenomics. *Nutrients* **2020**, *12*, 1265. **[Google Scholar]**

122. D'angelo, S. Polyphenols and Athletic Performance: A Review on Human Data. In *Plant Physiological Aspects of Phenolic Compounds*; IntechOpen: London, UK, 2019. **[Google Scholar]**

123. Kawabata, K.; Yoshioka, Y.; Terao, J. Role of intestinal microbiota in the bioavailability and physiological functions of dietary polyphenols. *Molecules* **2019**, *24*, 370. **[Google Scholar] [PubMed] [Green Version]**

124. Yang, H.; Shan, W.; Zhu, F.; Wu, J.; Wang, Q. Ketone bodies in neurological diseases: Focus on neuroprotection and underlying mechanisms. *Front. Neurol.* **2019**, *10*, 585. **[Google Scholar] [PubMed] [Green Version]**

125. Paoli, A.; Bianco, A.; Grimaldi, K.A. The Ketogenic Diet and Sport: A Possible Marriage? *Exerc. Sport Sci. Rev.* **2015**, *43*, 153–162. **[Google Scholar] [PubMed] [Green Version]**

126. Pinckaers, P.J.M.; Churchward-Venne, T.A.; Bailey, D.; Van Loon, L.J.C. Ketone Bodies and Exercise Performance: The Next Magic Bullet or Merely Hype? *Sports Med.* **2017**, *47*, 383–391. **[Google Scholar] [Green Version]**

127. Patterson, R.E.; Laughlin, G.A.; LaCroix, A.Z.; Hartman, S.J.; Natarajan, L.; Senger, C.M.; Martínez, M.E.; Villaseñor, A.; Sears, D.D.; Marinac, C.R.; et al. Intermittent Fasting and Human Metabolic Health. *J. Acad. Nutr. Diet.* **2015**, *115*, 1203–1212. **[Google Scholar] [Green Version]**

128. Niland, B.; Cash, B.D. Health Benefits and Adverse Effects of a Gluten-Free Diet in Non-Celiac Disease Patients. Gastroenterol. *Hepatol.* **2018**, *14*, 82–91. **[Google Scholar]**

129. Lis, D. From Celiac Disease, Gluten-Sensitivity vs Gluten Sensationalism, to Fodmap Reduction as a Tool to Manage Gastrointestinal Symptoms in Athletes. Exercise-Induced Gastrointestinal Syndrome and Diet. *Sports Sci. Exch.* **2018**, *29*, 1–6. **[Google Scholar]**

130. Poffé, C.; Ramaekers, M.; van Thienen, R.; Hespel, P. Ketone ester supplementation blunts overreaching symptoms during endurance training overload. *J. Physiol.* **2019**, *597*, 3009–3027. **[Google Scholar]**

131. Webster, C.C.; Swart, J.; Noakes, T.D.; Smith, J.A. A carbohydrate ingestion intervention in an elite athlete who follows a low-carbohydrate high-fat diet. *Int. J. Sports Physiol. Perform.* **2018**, *13*, 957–960. **[Google Scholar]**

132. Martínez-Garza, Ú.; Torres-Oteros, D.; Yarritu-Gallego, A.; Marrero, P.F.; Haro, D.; Relat, J. Fibroblast growth factor 21 and the adaptive response to nutritional challenges. *Int. J. Mol. Sci.* **2019**, *20*, 4692. **[Google Scholar] [Green Version]**

133. Yeo, W.K.; Carey, A.L.; Burke, L.; Spriet, L.L.; Hawley, J.A. Fat adaptation in well-trained athletes: Effects on cell metabolism. *Appl. Physiol. Nutr. Metab.* **2011**, *36*, 12–22. **[Google Scholar] [PubMed]**

134. Hargreaves, M.; Spriet, L.L. Skeletal muscle energy metabolism during exercise. *Nat. Metab.* **2020**, *2*, 817–828. **[Google Scholar] [PubMed]**

135. Kysel, P.; Haluzíková, D.; Doležalová, R.P.; Laňková, I.; Lacinová, Z.; Kasperová, B.J.; Trnovská, J.; Hrádková, V.; Mráz, M.; Vilikus, Z.; et al. The influence of cyclical ketogenic reduction diet vs. Nutritionally balanced reduction diet on body composition, strength, and endurance performance in healthy young males: A randomized controlled trial. *Nutrients* **2020**, *12*, 2832. **[Google Scholar] [PubMed]**

136. Edvardsen, E.; Hem, E.; Anderssen, S.A. End criteria for reaching maximal oxygen uptake must be strict and adjusted to sex and age: A cross-sectional study. *PLoS ONE* **2014**, *9*, e85276. **[Google Scholar] [PubMed] [Green Version]**

137. Puchalska, P.; Crawford, P.A. Multi-dimensional Roles of Ketone Bodies in Fuel Metabolism, Signaling, and Therapeutics. *Cell Metab.* **2017**, *25*, 262–284. **[Google Scholar] [Green Version]**

138. Chau, M.D.L.; Gao, J.; Yang, Q.; Wu, Z.; Gromada, J. Fibroblast growth factor 21 regulates energy metabolism by activating the AMPK-SIRT1-PGC-1α pathway. *Proc. Natl. Acad. Sci. USA* **2010**, *107*, 12553–12558. **[Google Scholar] [Green Version]**

139. Sansone, M.; Sansone, A.; Borrione, P.; Romanelli, F.; Di Luigi, L.; Sgrò, P. Effects of Ketone Bodies on Endurance Exercise. *Curr. Sports Med. Rep.* **2018**, *17*, 444–453. **[Google Scholar]**

140. Evans, M.; Cogan, K.E.; Egan, B. Metabolism of ketone bodies during exercise and training: Physiological basis for exogenous supplementation. *J. Physiol.* **2017**, *595*, 2857–2871. **[Google Scholar] [Green Version]**

141. Burke, L.M.; Whitfield, J.; Heikura, I.A.; Ross, M.L.R.; Tee, N.; Forbes, S.F.; Hall, R.; McKay, A.K.A.; Wallett, A.M.; Sharma, A.P. Adaptation to a low carbohydrate high fat diet is rapid but impairs endurance exercise metabolism and performance despite enhanced glycogen availability. *J. Physiol.* **2020**. **[Google Scholar]**

142. Chang, C.K.; Borer, K.; Lin, P.J. Low-Carbohydrate-High-Fat Diet: Can it Help Exercise Performance? *J. Hum. Kinet.* **2017**, *56*, 81–92. **[Google Scholar]**

143. Baranauskas, M.; Jablonskienė, V.; Abaravičius, J.A.; Samsonienė, L.; Stukas, R. Dietary Acid-Base Balance in High-Performance Athletes. *Int. J. Environ. Res. Public Health* **2020**, *17*, 5332. **[Google Scholar] [PubMed]**

144. Hietavala, E.M.; Stout, J.R.; Hulmi, J.J.; Suominen, H.; Pitkänen, H.; Puurtinen, R.; Selänne, H.; Kainulainen, H.; Mero, A.A. Effect of diet composition on acid-base balance in adolescents, young adults and elderly at rest and during exercise. *Eur. J. Clin. Nutr.* **2015**, *69*, 399–404. **[Google Scholar] [PubMed]**

145. Clarke, K.; Tchabanenko, K.; Pawlosky, R.; Carter, E.; Todd King, M.; Musa-Veloso, K.; Ho, M.; Roberts, A.; Robertson, J.; VanItallie, T.B.; et al. Kinetics, safety and tolerability of (R)-3-hydroxybutyl (R)-3-hydroxybutyrate in healthy adult subjects. *Regul. Toxicol. Pharmacol.* **2012**, *63*, 401–408. **[Google Scholar] [PubMed] [Green Version]**

146. Wilkinson, D.J.; Smeeton, N.J.; Watt, P.W. Ammonia metabolism, the brain and fatigue; Revisiting the link. *Prog. Neurobiol.* **2010**, *91*, 200–219. **[Google Scholar] [PubMed]**

147. Clark, A.; Mach, N. Exercise-induced stress behavior, gut-microbiota-brain axis and diet: A systematic review for athletes. *J. Int. Soc. Sports Nutr.* **2016**, *13*, 43–64. **[Google Scholar] [Green Version]**

148. Fromentin, C.; Tomé, D.; Nau, F.; Flet, L.; Luengo, C.; Azzout-Marniche, D.; Sanders, P.; Fromentin, G.; Gaudichon, C. Dietary proteins contribute little to glucose production, even under optimal gluconeogenic conditions in healthy humans. *Diabetes* **2013**, *62*, 1435–1442. **[Google Scholar] [Green Version]**

149. Jäger, R.; Kerksick, C.M.; Campbell, B.I.; Cribb, P.J.; Wells, S.D.; Skwiat, T.M.; Purpura, M.; Ziegenfuss, T.N.; Ferrando, A.A.; Arent, S.M.; et al. International Society of Sports Nutrition Position Stand: Protein and exercise. *J. Int. Soc. Sports Nutr.* **2017**, *14*, 20. **[Google Scholar] [Green Version]**

150. White, A.M.; Johnston, C.S.; Swan, P.D.; Tjonn, S.L.; Sears, B. Blood Ketones Are Directly Related to Fatigue and Perceived Effort during Exercise in Overweight Adults Adhering to Low-Carbohydrate Diets for Weight Loss: A Pilot Study. *J. Am. Diet. Assoc.* **2007**, *107*, 1792–1796. **[Google Scholar]**

151. Harvey, K.L.; Holcomb, L.E.; Kolwicz, S.C. Ketogenic Diets and Exercise Performance. *Nutrients* **2019**, *11*, 2296. **[Google Scholar] [Green Version]**

152. Margolis, L.M.; O'Fallon, K.S. Utility of Ketone Supplementation to Enhance Physical Performance: A Systematic Review. *Adv. Nutr.* **2020**, *2*, 412–419. **[Google Scholar] [Green Version]**

153. Puchalska, P.; Martin, S.E.; Huang, X.; Nagy, L.; Patti, G.J.; Correspondence, P.A.C.; Lengfeld, J.E.; Daniel, B.; Graham, M.J.; Han, X.; et al. Hepatocyte-Macrophage Acetoacetate Shuttle Protects against Tissue Fibrosis Article Hepatocyte-Macrophage Acetoacetate Shuttle Protects against Tissue Fibrosis. *Cell Metab.* **2019**, *29*, 383–398. **[Google Scholar] [PubMed] [Green Version]**

154. Carrero, K. A Literature Review on Intermittent Fasting. Senior Honors Thesis, Liberty University, Lynchburg, Virginia, 2020. **[Google Scholar]**

155. Anton, S.D.; Moehl, K.; Donahoo, W.T.; Marosi, K.; Lee, S.A.; Mainous, A.G.; Leeuwenburgh, C.; Mattson, M.P. Flipping the Metabolic Switch: Understanding and Applying the Health Benefits of Fasting. *Obesity* **2018**, *26*, 254–268. **[Google Scholar] [PubMed]**

156. Maughan, R.J.; Fallah, J.S.; Coyle, E.F. The effects of fasting on metabolism and performance. *Br. J. Sports Med.* **2010**, *44*, 490–494. **[Google Scholar]** **[PubMed]**

157. Hoppeler, H.; Baum, O.; Lurman, G.; Mueller, M. Molecular Mechanisms of Muscle Plasticity with Exercise. In *Comprehensive Physiology*; John Wiley & Sons, Inc.: Hoboken, NJ, USA, 2011; Volume 1, pp. 1383–1412. **[Google Scholar]**

158. Marosi, K.; Moehl, K.; Navas-Enamorado, I.; Mitchell, S.J.; Zhang, Y.; Lehrmann, E.; Aon, M.A.; Cortassa, S.; Becker, K.G.; Mattson, M.P. Metabolic and molecular framework for the enhancement of endurance by intermittent food deprivation. *FASEB J.* **2018**, *32*, 3844–3858. **[Google Scholar]** **[PubMed]** **[Green Version]**

159. Chaouachl, A.; Leiper, J.B.; Souissi, N.; Coutts, A.J.; Chamari, K. Effects of ramadan intermittent fasting on sports performance and training: A review. *Int. J. Sports Physiol. Perform.* **2009**, *4*, 419–434. **[Google Scholar]**

160. Chaouachi, A.; Leiper, J.B.; Chtourou, H.; Aziz, A.R.; Chamari, K. The effects of Ramadan intermittent fasting on athletic performance: Recommendations for the maintenance of physical fitness. *J. Sports Sci.* **2012**, *30*, S53–S73. **[Google Scholar]**

161. Loy, S.F.; Conlee, R.K.; Winder, W.W.; Nelson, A.G.; Arnall, D.A.; Fisher, A.G. Effects of 24-h fast on cycling endurance time at two different intensities. *J. Appl. Physiol.* **1986**, *61*, 654–659. **[Google Scholar]**

162. Nieman, D.C.; Carlson, K.A.; Brandstater, M.E.; Naegele, R.T.; Blankenship, J.W. Running endurance in 27-h-fasted humans. *J. Appl. Physiol.* **1987**, *63*, 2502–2509. **[Google Scholar]**

163. Zinker, B.A.; Britz, K.; Brooks, G.A. Effects of a 36-h fast on human endurance and substrate utilization. *J. Appl. Physiol.* **1990**, *69*, 1849–1855. **[Google Scholar]**

164. Dohm, G.L.; Beeker, R.T.; Israel, R.G.; Tapscott, E.B. Metabolic responses to exercise after fasting. *J. Appl. Physiol.* **1986**, *61*, 1363–1368. **[Google Scholar]**

165. Watson, A.M. Sleep and Athletic Performance. *Curr. Sports Med. Rep.* **2017**, *16*, 413–418. **[Google Scholar]** **[PubMed]**

166. Rehrer, N.J. Fluid and Electrolyte Balance in Ultra-Endurance Sport. *Sports Med.* **2001**, *31*, 701–715. **[Google Scholar]** **[PubMed]**

167. Shephard, R.J. The impact of Ramadan observance upon athletic performance. *Nutrients* **2012**, *4*, 491–505. **[Google Scholar]** **[PubMed]**

168. Parnell, J.A.; Wagner-Jones, K.; Madden, R.F.; Erdman, K.A. Dietary restrictions in endurance runners to mitigate exercise-induced gastrointestinal symptoms. *J. Int. Soc. Sports Nutr.* **2020**, *17*, 32. **[Google Scholar]** **[PubMed]**

169. Chong, P.P.; Chin, V.K.; Looi, C.Y.; Wong, W.F.; Madhavan, P.; Yong, V.C. The microbiome and irritable bowel syndrome—A review on the pathophysiology, current research and future therapy. *Front. Microbiol.* **2019**, *10*, 1136. **[Google Scholar]** **[Green Version]**

170. Simrén, M.; Månsson, A.; Langkilde, A.M.; Svedlund, J.; Abrahamsson, H.; Bengtsson, U.; Björnsson, E.S. Food-related gastrointestinal symptoms in the irritable bowel syndrome. *Digestion* **2001**, *63*, 108–115. **[Google Scholar]**

171. Lis, D.; Ahuja, K.D.K.; Stellingwerff, T.; Kitic, C.M.; Fell, J. Food avoidance in athletes: FODMAP foods on the list. *Appl. Physiol. Nutr. Metab.* **2016**, *41*, 1002–1004. **[Google Scholar]**

172. Ciacci, C.; Ciclitira, P.; Hadjivassiliou, M.; Kaukinen, K.; Ludvigsson, J.F.; McGough, N.; Sanders, D.S.; Woodward, J.; Leonard, J.N.; Swift, G.L. The gluten-Free diet and its current application in coeliac disease and dermatitis Herpetiformis. *United Eur. Gastroenterol. J.* **2015**, *3*, 121–135. **[Google Scholar]**

173. Sharma, N.; Bhatia, S.; Chunduri, V.; Kaur, S.; Sharma, S.; Kapoor, P.; Kumari, A.; Garg, M. Pathogenesis of Celiac Disease and Other Gluten Related Disorders in Wheat and Strategies for Mitigating Them. *Front. Nutr.* **2020**, *7*, 6. **[Google Scholar]** **[Green Version]**

174. Osorio, C.E.; Mejías, J.H.; Rustgi, S. Gluten detection methods and their critical role in assuring safe diets for celiac patients. *Nutrients* **2019**, *11*, 2920. **[Google Scholar] [Green Version]**

175. Leone, J.E.; Wise, K.A.; Mullin, E.M.; Gray, K.A.; Szlosek, P.A.; Griffin, M.F.; Jordan, C.A. Celiac Disease Symptoms in Athletes: Prevalence Indicators of Perceived Quality of Life. *Sports Health* **2020**, *12*, 246–255. **[Google Scholar] [PubMed]**

176. D'angelo, S.; Cusano, P.; Di Palma, D. Gluten-free diets in athletes. *J. Phys. Educ. Sport* **2020**, *20*, 2330–2336. **[Google Scholar]**

177. Halson, S.L.; Martin, D.T. Lying to win—Placebos and sport science. *Int. J. Sports Physiol. Perform.* **2013**, *8*, 597–599. **[Google Scholar] [PubMed] [Green Version]**

178. Dieterich, W.; Zopf, Y. Gluten and FODMAPS—Sense of a Restriction/When Is Restriction Necessary? *Nutrients* **2019**, *11*, 1957. **[Google Scholar] [Green Version]**

179. Peters, H.P.F.; Bos, M.; Seebregts, L.; Akkermans, L.M.A.; Van Berge Henegouwen, G.P.; Bol, E.; Mosterd, W.L.; de Vries, W.R. Gastrointestinal symptoms in long-distance runners, cyclists, and triathletes: Prevalence, medication, and etiology. *Am. J. Gastroenterol.* **1999**, *94*, 1570–1581. **[Google Scholar]**

180. Tuck, C.J.; Muir, J.G.; Barrett, J.S.; Gibson, P.R. Fermentable oligosaccharides, disaccharides, monosaccharides and polyols: Role in irritable bowel syndrome. *Expert Rev. Gastroenterol. Hepatol.* **2014**, *8*, 819–834. **[Google Scholar]**

181. Hill, P.; Muir, J.G.; Gibson, P.R. Controversies and recent developments of the low-FODMAP diet. *Gastroenterol. Hepatol.* **2017**, *13*, 36–45. **[Google Scholar]**

182. Shortt, C.; Hasselwander, O.; Meynier, A.; Nauta, A.; Noriega Fernández, E.; Putz, P.; Rowland, I.; Swann, J.; Türk, J.; Vermeiren, J.; et al. Systematic review of the effects of the intestinal microbiota on selected nutrients and non-nutrients. *Eur. J. Nutr.* **2018**, *57*, 25–49. **[Google Scholar] [Green Version]**

183. Yan, Y.L.; Hu, Y.; Gänzle, M.G. Prebiotics, FODMAPs and dietary fiber—Conflicting concepts in development of functional food products? *Curr. Opin. Food Sci.* **2018**, *20*, 30–37. **[Google Scholar]**

184. Sloan, T.J.; Jalanka, J.; Major, G.A.D.; Krishnasamy, S.; Pritchard, S.; Abdelrazig, S.; Korpela, K.; Singh, G.; Mulvenna, C.; Hoad, C.L.; et al. A low FODMAP diet is associated with changes in the microbiota and reduction in breath hydrogen but not colonic volume in healthy subjects. *PLoS ONE* **2018**, *13*, e0201410. **[Google Scholar] [Green Version]**

185. Roberfroid, M.; Gibson, G.R.; Hoyles, L.; McCartney, A.L.; Rastall, R.; Rowland, I.; Wolvers, D.; Watzl, B.; Szajewska, H.; Stahl, B.; et al. Prebiotic effects: Metabolic and health benefits. *Br. J. Nutr.* **2010**, *104*, S1–S63. **[Google Scholar] [PubMed] [Green Version]**

186. Killian, L.; Lee, S.-Y. Nutritional Habits and FODMAPs in Relation to Gastrointestinal Issues of Endurance Athletes. *Gastroenterology* **2017**, *152*, S751. **[Google Scholar]**

187. Staudacher, H.M.; Lomer, M.C.E.; Farquharson, F.M.; Louis, P.; Fava, F.; Franciosi, E.; Scholz, M.; Tuohy, K.M.; Lindsay, J.O.; Irving, P.M.; et al. A Diet Low in FODMAPs Reduces Symptoms in Patients With Irritable Bowel Syndrome and A Probiotic Restores Bifidobacterium Species: A Randomized Controlled Trial. *Gastroenterology* **2017**, *153*, 936–947. **[Google Scholar] [PubMed] [Green Version]**

188. De Oliveira, E.P.; Jeukendrup, A. Nutritional Recommendations to Avoid Gastrointestinal Distress during Exercise. Available online: **https://www.gssiweb.org/sports-science-exchange/article/sse-114-nutritional-recommendations-to-avoid-gastrointestinal-distress-during-exercise** (accessed on 28 October 2019).

189. Costa, R.J.S.; Gaskell, S.K.; McCubbin, A.J.; Snipe, R.M.J. Exertional-heat stress-associated gastrointestinal perturbations during Olympic sports: Management strategies for athletes preparing and competing in the 2020 Tokyo Olympic Games. *Temperature* **2020**, *7*, 58–88. **[Google Scholar] [Green Version]**

190. Snipe, R.M.J.; Costa, R.J.S. Does the temperature of water ingested during exertional-heat stress influence gastrointestinal injury, symptoms, and systemic inflammatory profile? *J. Sci. Med. Sport* **2018**, *21*, 771–776. **[Google Scholar]**

191. Costa, R.J.S.; Camões-Costa, V.; Snipe, R.M.J.; Dixon, D.; Russo, I.; Huschtscha, Z. Impact of exercise-induced hypohydration on gastrointestinal integrity, function, symptoms, and systemic endotoxin and inflammatory profile. *J. Appl. Physiol.* **2019**, *126*, 1281–1291. **[Google Scholar]**

192. Schumann, D.; Klose, P.; Lauche, R.; Dobos, G.; Langhorst, J.; Cramer, H. Low fermentable, oligo-, di-, mono-saccharides and polyol diet in the treatment of irritable bowel syndrome: A systematic review and meta-analysis. *Nutrition* **2018**, *45*, 24–31. **[Google Scholar]**

193. Knechtle, B. Nutrition in ultra-endurance racing—aspects of energy balance, fluid balance and exercise-associated hyponatremia. *Med. Sport.* **2013**, *17*, 200–210. **[Google Scholar]**

194. Barrett, J.S. Extending Our Knowledge of Fermentable, Short-Chain Carbohydrates for Managing Gastrointestinal Symptoms. *Nutr. Clin. Pract.* **2013**, *28*, 300–306. **[Google Scholar]**

195. Valeur, J.; Småstuen, M.C.; Knudsen, T.; Lied, G.A.; Røseth, A.G. Exploring Gut Microbiota Composition as an Indicator of Clinical Response to Dietary FODMAP Restriction in Patients with Irritable Bowel Syndrome. *Dig. Dis. Sci.* **2018**, *63*, 429–436. **[Google Scholar]**

196. Halmos, E.P.; Christophersen, C.T.; Bird, A.R.; Shepherd, S.J.; Gibson, P.R.; Muir, J.G. Diets that differ in their FODMAP content alter the colonic luminal microenvironment. *Gut* **2015**, *64*, 93–100. **[Google Scholar]**

197. McIntosh, K.; Reed, D.E.; Schneider, T.; Dang, F.; Keshteli, A.H.; de Palma, G.; Madsen, K.; Bercik, P.; Vanner, S. FODMAPs alter symptoms and the metabolome of patients with IBS: A randomised controlled trial. *Gut* **2017**, *66*, 1241–1251. **[Google Scholar]** **[PubMed]**

198. Böhn, L.; Störsrud, S.; Liljebo, T.; Collin, L.; Lindfors, P.; Törnblom, H.; Simrén, M. Diet Low in FODMAPs Reduces Symptoms of Irritable Bowel Syndrome as Well as Traditional Dietary Advice: A Randomized Controlled Trial. *Gastroenterology* **2015**, *149*, 1399–1407.e2. **[Google Scholar]** **[PubMed]** **[Green Version]**

199. Barrett, J.S. How to institute the low-FODMAP diet. *J. Gastroenterol. Hepatol.* **2017**, *32*, 8–10. **[Google Scholar]** **[PubMed]** **[Green Version]**

200. Lacy, B.E.; Gabbard, S.L.; Crowell, M.D. Pathophysiology, evaluation, and treatment of bloating: Hope, hype, or hot air? *Gastroenterol. Hepatol.* **2011**, 7, 729–739. **[Google Scholar]**

201. Thomas, D.T.; Erdman, K.A.; Burke, L.M. Position of the Academy of Nutrition and Dietetics, Dietitians of Canada, and the American College of Sports Medicine: Nutrition and Athletic Performance. *J. Acad. Nutr. Diet.* **2016**, *116*, 501–528. **[Google Scholar]** **[PubMed]**

202. Jeukendrup, A.E. Carbohydrate intake during exercise and performance. *Nutrition* **2004**, *20*, 669–677. **[Google Scholar]** **[PubMed]**

# 10 Chapter

# IRON METABOLISM: ATHLETE-RELEVANT PROCESSES

## 1. INTRODUCTION: AN OVERVIEW

Strategies that enhance athlete health and training accessibility are crucial for maximizing training outcomes and competitive preparedness. Nutrition is recognized as a vital component in attaining these goals, as it provides energy, macronutrients, and micronutrients necessary for health and performance. Energy supply is a crucial component of sports nutrition, as athletes experience both intentional and unintentional changes in the balance between intake and expenditure when modifying body composition and training loads. Although energy balance has historically been the standard for assessing such changes, the modern notion of energy availability has become a crucial topic in conversations about athlete health, training consistency, and competitive performance. Energy availability (EA) is calculated by deducting an athlete's energy expenditure during training from their nutritional energy intake, indicating the energy accessible for maintaining the body's essential physiological functions (e.g., reproductive system, bone metabolism, and endocrine function) [2]. Low energy availability (LEA), caused by a reduction in an athlete's caloric intake and/or an escalation in exercise intensity, is associated with the downregulation and dysfunction of critical physiological processes due to inadequate energy provision. LEA addresses the clinical consequences associated with the conditions recognized as the Female Athlete Triad [4] and Relative Energy Deficiency in Sport (RED-S) [5,6]. Historically, the focus was on the disturbance of the menstrual cycle and bone health in female athletes; however, contemporary models acknowledge that Low Energy Availability (LEA) is also a critical issue for male athletes [7].The availability of carbohydrates (CHO) has become a significant focus, referring to the equilibrium between the CHO demands of the muscles and central nervous system, as well as potentially other organs and systems, during an exercise session in relation to both endogenous and exogenous CHO supply. Substantial data indicates that measures ensuring high carbohydrate availability (i.e., balancing supply with demand) correlate with improved exercise capacity and athletic performance, especially in lengthy endurance events necessitating high-intensity efforts [9,10]. These results have prompted recommendations that, to achieve optimal performance, endurance athletes should implement daily carbohydrate consumption and/or ensure high carbohydrate availability during critical exercise periods to satisfy the fuel requirements of those sessions [8]. The utilization of advanced analytical techniques to examine exercise-nutrient interactions has demonstrated that strategies achieving low carbohydrate availability (i.e., acute carbohydrate restriction surrounding an exercise session) can enhance cellular adaptations in skeletal muscle during and post-exercise [11]. Integrating the modulation of carbohydrate availability into the training cycle, aligning it with the demands and objectives of each session, could provide a strategic combination of enhanced adaption workouts and focused quality sessions, resulting in improved performance outcomes [8,12]. Conversely, a different strategy for metabolic preparation for endurance exercise involves chronic dietary carbohydrate restriction, which enables muscle to attain a 2–3 fold enhancement in fat oxidation while concurrently reducing carbohydrate utilization, thereby transitioning its fuel dependence from limited carbohydrate stores to the comparatively abundant body fat reserves. The overall efficacy of these tactics must be evaluated in relation to an athlete's performance objectives and their need for metabolic flexibility [8,16,17]. Moreover, they must be meticulously incorporated into the athlete's periodized training regimen to achieve particular training objectives and performance results [8].Although initial apprehensions regarding LEA were centered on reproductive and bone health, there is now heightened awareness of its potential to disrupt other physiological systems [5,6]. There is a growing interest in the effects of modifying carbohydrate availability, which extends beyond its impact on metabolic changes in muscle or performance results to the future goals of inter-organ communication. Iron metabolism is becoming acknowledged as a system influenced by both factors. Insufficient iron status is often associated with Low Energy Availability (LEA), as a recent study including 1,000 female athletes revealed an odds ratio of 1.64 for a history of anemia, reduced hemoglobin, or depleted iron reserves in those diagnosed with LEA. Moreover, mechanisms exist by which exercising with diminished carbohydrate availability can interfere with iron control [19,20]. This review aims to synthesize current understanding of the impact of energy and carbohydrate availability on iron metabolism, including the dietary habits of elite endurance athletes. This study functions as a narrative review, recognizing the complexity and preliminary stage of these notions' development. We intend to leverage insights from our extensive research on certain themes, alongside contributions from others, to underscore issues that require further investigation through a structured series of observational and intervention studies.

## 2. IMPORTANCE OF ADEQUATE IRON RESERVES FOR ATHLETES

Iron is essential for the best performance of endurance athletes due to its critical involvement in oxygen delivery, cellular energy production, cognitive function, and immunological response. Depleted iron reserves can hinder essential physiological functions, adversely affecting athlete health and performance. High levels of aerobic fitness, often essential for peak endurance performance, may be constrained by the oxygen-delivery capacity to the muscles [23]. In iron-compromised individuals with anemia, the impairment of hemoglobin production results in decrements to aerobic performance [**24**]. However, in such cases, once iron stores are restored via oral or intravenous supplementation, increases in $VO_{2max}$ [**25**], exercise time-trial performance

[26] and exercise efficiency [27,28] have been reported.

Despite research and clinical knowledge, iron deficiency in athlete populations remains a common issue. To understand the prevalence, various thresholds used to classify the severity of iron deficiency must be established. Accordingly, three stages of iron deficiency have been proposed: (1) Iron depletion, where iron stores are depleted without hematological consequences; (2) Iron deficiency non-anemia, where erythropoiesis diminishes as the iron supply to the erythroid marrow is reduced; and (3) Iron deficiency anemia, where hemoglobin production falls, resulting in anemia [29]. At a minimum, quantification of serum ferritin, hemoglobin and transferrin concentrations are required to diagnose an iron deficiency, with additional variables such as serum soluble transferrin receptor, hemoglobin mass, or C-reactive protein presenting as potential beneficial adjunct markers of detection [20]. While there is general agreement that iron deficiency can negatively impact performance, there is less conformity surrounding the classification criteria of these categories. Iron deficiency non-anemia has been commonly defined in athletic populations as a serum ferritin of <20 μg·L$^{-1}$ and transferrin <16% [20,29]; however, variations in the literature range from serum ferritin values of <12 μg·L$^{-1}$ through to <40 μg·L$^{-1}$ [29,30,31]. Iron deficiency anemia is thought to be apparent once hemoglobin concentrations become compromised, with diagnostic thresholds below 11.5–12 g·dL$^{-1}$ commonly used. The incidence of iron deficiency non-anemia is reported as 24–47% of female and 0–17% of male athletes [32]; however, rates as high as 86% of female youth athletes from a mixed-sport cohort have been reported [33]. The higher incidence of iron deficiency observed in females has been attributed to the increased iron losses associated with menstruation [34]. The elevated incidence of diminished iron reserves frequently observed in athletes can be partially attributed to the integration of iron into newly formed tissues and cells resulting from training adaptations, alongside exerciserelated iron losses through mechanisms such as hemolysis, hematuria, perspiration, gastrointestinal bleeding, and acute transient elevations in the iron regulatory hormone, hepcidin [3 The elevated incidence of diminished iron reserves frequently observed in athletes can be partially attributed to the integration of iron into newly formed tissues and cells resulting from training adaptations, alongside exercise-related iron losses through mechanisms such as hemolysis, hematuria, perspiration, gastrointestinal bleeding, and acute transient elevations in the iron regulatory hormone, hepcidin [35].5].

## 3. HEPCIDIN AND IRON REGULATION

The body methodically regulates iron status through homeostatic control of iron transport across the gastrointestinal tract and intercellularly. Homeostasis is essential for promoting iron absorption during deficiency and for preventing iron toxicity and overload.Iron regulation is governed by the primary regulatory hormone, hepcidin, released by the liver to modulate the availability of iron for biological functions. [36]. Hepcidin primarily functions by binding to and internalizing the body's cellular iron export channels, ferroportin, which are situated on the cell surfaces of macrophages in the reticuloendothelial system, enterocytes in the duodenum, and hepatocytes.

Interactions between hepcidin and ferroportin diminish the quantity of dietary iron absorbed by duodenal enterocytes and the volume of iron recycled by macrophages. Hepcidin regulates transferrin and intracellular iron reserves in a homeostatic manner through this mechanism. In persons with iron deficiency, hepcidin levels are diminished to promote iron absorption and facilitate the restoration of iron reserves. Excess iron, however, induces the liver to produce hepcidin to mitigate subsequent increases in iron availability [38].While iron status appears to be a dominant factor in hepcidin regulation, inflammation is also known to impact hepcidin levels, and subsequently, iron balance [**39**]. The inflammatory cytokine interleukin-6 (IL-6) directly stimulates hepcidin production via an increase in signal transducer and activator of transcription 3 (STAT 3) production, resulting in increased transcription of hepcidin from hepatocytes [**40**]. This mechanism was highlighted through administration of 30 $\mu g{\cdot}L^{-1}$ recombinant IL-6, which elicited a 7.5-fold increase in hepcidin concentrations 2 h post-infusion [**41**]. This outcome was replicated in a study using a 2 $ng{\cdot}kg^{-1}$ body mass (BM) injection of lipopolysaccharide (i.e., stimulating an inflammatory response), in which IL-6 was increased 3 h post-injection, followed by an increase in hepcidin levels 3 h later (i.e., 6 h post-injection, but 3 h post-IL-6 response) [**42**]. Since exercise is known to be a potent inflammatory stimulus, the relationship between exercise, inflammation, and hepcidin activity has attracted attention. Indeed, IL-6 is released from the skeletal muscle in response to exercise, playing a key role in mediating the acute phase response [**43**]. The duration of exercise appears to be the largest determinant of the post-exercise IL-6 response, with increases occurring in a time-dependent exponential manner, peaking immediately post-exercise [**44**]. Furthermore, exercise intensity and modality can also influence the IL-6 response, with higher intensity and weight-bearing modes (i.e., running vs. cycling) yielding greater increases in post-exercise cytokine levels [**43,45**]. An early investigation of the link between exercise, IL-6 and hepcidin tracked the time course of changes in these two variables following 60 min of treadmill running (15 min at 75–80% HRpeak, followed by 45 min at 85–90% HRpeak) [**46**]. Here, a 6.9-fold increase in IL-6 was evident immediately post-exercise, followed by a subsequent peak in hepcidin levels 3–6 h later (5.2-fold increase). This was the first study to demonstrate that increases in hepcidin levels occur subsequent to an exercise-induced inflammatory stimulus. This sequence is important, as it is likely that iron absorption is impaired during the post-exercise period, when hepcidin levels are elevated. This outcome could have negative implications for athletes' iron balance, particularly when performing frequent high-volume training. Within the exercise literature in particular, hepcidin levels have been used as a surrogate marker of iron bioavailability, with interest in strategies that minimize the hepcidin response to exercise.

Multiple regression analysis of both physiological and biochemical markers has shown that the increase in IL-6 concentrations is a small, yet significant contributor to the magnitude of subsequent hepcidin increase at 3 h post-exercise [**47**]. Interestingly, nutritional manipulation of the magnitude of the IL-6 response to exercise may provide a mechanism to improve iron absorption during the post-exercise period. Factors that influence the release of IL-6 during exercise include the task duration, mode, intensity, training status, and of importance in the context of sports nutrition, muscle glycogen stores [**19,48**]. Although an increased production of IL-6 has been demonstrated in response to running or cycling for ≥2 h at moderate to high intensities, this response can be attenuated when CHO is consumed throughout the exercise task to maintain blood glucose concentrations and decrease the reliance on/depletion of muscle glycogen stores [**19**]. However, studies utilizing exercise bouts <2 h in duration have shown CHO supplementation has minimal impact on IL-6 concentrations, unless exercise is commenced with low muscle glycogen stores, in which case the response is augmented [**19**]. In this low muscle glycogen scenario, CHO ingestion during exercise bouts of 30–90 min in duration can promote the attenuation of the IL-6 response to exercise [**49,50**]. The correlation between IL-6 and hepcidin activity suggests that an elevated IL-6 response due to training under conditions of reduced carbohydrate availability and/or diminished muscle glycogen stores may elevate hepcidin levels three hours post-exercise, potentially adversely affecting iron homeostasis in athletic populations. Consequently, methods that enhance carbohydrate availability may mitigate the post-exercise reduction in iron absorption by alleviating exercise-induced inflammation and subsequently reducing post-exercise hepcidin levels. The amount and timing of carbohydrate intake are critical determinants in modulating this response.

## 4. AVAILABILITY OF CARBOHYDRATES AND REGULATION OF IRON

### 4.1. Post-Exercise Carbohydrate Intake

Post-exercise CHO consumption is an important nutritional strategy to optimize recovery, particularly for endurance athletes. When an athlete's goal is to maximize post-exercise muscle glycogen restoration to support subsequent training/competition sessions, CHO ingestion should occur as soon as practical after exercise, to take advantage of the higher rates of muscle glycogen synthesis in the early phases of recovery, and maximize the duration of the period when exogenous substrate is available for muscle storage [**51**]. CHO intake targets for rapid refueling during the 1–4 h following exercise have been set at 1.0–1.2 $g{\cdot}kg{\cdot}h^{-1}$, consumed as small regular meals [**52**]. Several studies have investigated whether such practices also influence iron metabolism. Initial work by Badenhorst et al. [**53**] examined the effect of consuming 12 $mL{\cdot}kg^{-1}$ body mass (BM) of a 10% CHO beverage at different stages of recovery following a 60 min interval running task on post-exercise inflammation and hepcidin levels. There were no differences in either IL-6 or hepcidin activity for up to 5 h post-exercise between immediate (15 and 120 min post-exercise) and delayed (120 and 240 min post-exercise) ingestion of CHO [**53**]. Since peak IL-6 concentrations occur immediately after exercise and return rapidly to baseline within 1–2 h [**54**], it is likely that this finding reflects the inability of CHO ingestion to affect hepcidin levels when IL-6 concentrations are already elevated. Indeed, similar findings were reported by Dahlquist et al. [**55**], who investigated the IL-6 and hepcidin response to different post-exercise nutrition support approaches following interval-based cycling sessions (8 × 3 min intervals at 85% of power output at $VO_{2max}$). This study found similar post-exercise IL-6 and hepcidin responses to a recovery beverage containing 75 g CHO and 25 g of protein, the same beverage with the addition of a vitamin D (5000 UI) and vitamin $K_2$ (1000 mcg) complex, or a taste-matched placebo. Therefore, it appears that the post-exercise consumption of CHO occurs too late to influence post-exercise IL-6 or hepcidin levels, raising the prospect that CHO intake may need to occur prior to, or during the exercise session, to be of benefit to this response. Of course, post-exercise CHO consumption should still be emphasized for its other contributions to recovery, such as the restoration of muscle glycogen stores, particularly following strenuous exercise [**52**].

## 4.2. Carbohydrate Feeding during Exercise

Given the lack of a substantial post-exercise effect from CHO consumption on inflammatory responses and iron regulation, attention turns to the impact of consumption during exercise. Robson-Ansley et al. [**56**] studied the ingestion of either a 8% CHO solution or a placebo beverage prior to and during a 2 h submaximal run (60% $vVO_{2max}$), at a rate of 2 mL·kg$^{-1}$ BM consumed every 20 min. Immediately following the 2 h run, a 5 km running time-trial was performed. Despite attenuation of the IL-6 response immediately post-exercise when the CHO beverage was consumed, no differences in hepcidin concentration were reported between conditions. Unfortunately, in this study, post-exercise hepcidin concentrations were measured immediately after, and at 24 h of recovery; timings that would likely not reflect the key periods during which hepcidin is elevated (i.e., 3–6 h post-exercise [**46**]). In a follow-up study, participants ran for 90 min on a motorized treadmill at 75% $VO_{2peak}$, while consuming either a 6% CHO or placebo beverage at a rate of 3 mL·kg$^{-1}$ BM every 20 min [**57**]. Despite using more appropriate sampling time points (e.g., measuring hepcidin concentrations 3 h post-exercise), no differences in either IL-6 or hepcidin levels were evident between the CHO or placebo beverage trials. One explanation for the absence of an effect is that the selected exercise protocol was too short for muscle glycogen stores to become sufficiently different in terms of eliciting increased IL-6 production. Accordingly, scenarios which involve exercise in the presence of muscle glycogen depletion could elicit a greater influence on iron regulation. On this basis, the manipulation of CHO in the hours prior to exercise is of interest.

## 4.3. Implications of Acute Carbohydrate Restriction

Badenhorst et al. [**50**] assessed the impact of muscle glycogen stores on iron regulation by implementing an exercise task known to deplete muscle glycogen stores by ~50% [**58**]. Here, participants performed a 16 km run at 80% $vVO_{2peak}$, followed by 5 × 1 min efforts at 130% $vVO_{2peak}$ with 2 min recovery between efforts. This task was followed by 24 h of diets of either low (3 g kg$^{-1}$ BM) or high (10 g kg$^{-1}$ BM) CHO intake with similar energy support (4100 and 4500 kcal, respectively) [**50**]. Participants then performed an interval-based running task (8 × 3 min at 85% $vVO_{2peak}$) 24 h later, with

IL-6 and hepcidin concentrations measured pre/post-exercise and at 3 h post-exercise, respectively. The results showed that the high CHO trial was associated with an attenuated post-exercise IL-6 response (2-fold vs. 3-fold increase) with a trend towards lower hepcidin levels 3 h post-exercise compared to low CHO trial (4.1 vs. 6.4 nM; d = 0.72). While differences in the hepcidin response did not reach statistical significance, this study demonstrated the potential for a moderately greater increase in hepcidin following exercise undertaken with theoretical (albeit not quantified) depletion of muscle glycogen stores. This study provides some evidence of an association between macronutrient intake, inflammation and iron regulation, especially when considered in the context of the athlete's pre-exercise nutritional state.

These outcomes become important in light of the contemporary interest in strategies to periodize CHO availability around specific training sessions. It is likely that periodic glycogen depletion occurs within the training programs of high performance endurance athletes, with the high frequency and load (intensity and volume) of their sessions preventing a full glycogen restoration between each workout. However, more recent practices that deliberately manipulate low CHO availability have evolved as a strategy to enhance endurance training adaptations. For example, in a survey of the self-reported practices of elite runners and race walkers, a majority (62%) of the distance athletes reported training in a fasted state, typically 1–3 times/week around easier sessions [**59**], where low liver glycogen stores and low exogenous CHO availability would be expected [**8**]. Although some athletes identified "practical" reasons for this behavior (e.g., to allow them to get more sleep before training or to reduce the risk of gut discomfort during training), the majority identified a strategic rationale for the approach (e.g., to assist with body composition changes or enhance the training response). Furthermore, 44% of the total cohort reported an occasional restriction of CHO intake around or between some training sessions, theoretically creating a scenario of training with low muscle glycogen availability, which would upregulate the accompanying cell signaling and gene expression response [**60**]. Although many of the athletes who reported such practices identified that they were underpinned by a strategic rationale, a significant number of the group who identified the absence of CHO restriction strategies noted a lack of overall performance improvement, or an increase in illness/injury, among their experiences [**59**]. Indeed, given the potential exacerbation of inflammation and hepcidin activity following exercise with low muscle glycogen stores, the implications to iron balance become an interesting point for consideration.

Recent work from our group investigated this question of dietary manipulation in an applied setting, with elite triathletes performing four 48 h manipulations of diet and exercise [**61**]. Here, two trials involved a 'train-high, sleep-low, train-low' sequence [**8**], which restricted CHO intake between the two training sessions to achieve low glycogen training on the session of interest. The remaining two trials involving exercise performed under consistently high CHO availability (8 g kg $BM^{-1}$ $day^{-1}$ CHO). The final session of the sequence involved a 45 min running protocol, or a 60 min cycling protocol, with the cycling trials of higher intensity (evidenced by increased heart rate and RER). During the running trials, no differences in hepcidin concentrations were evident between conditions of high or low CHO availability. However, during cycling trials, when exercise intensity was increased, a ~72% greater hepcidin response was evident during the 'train-high, sleep-low, train-low' dietary condition. Taken together, it appears that muscle glycogen availability and exercise intensity are both critical factors in determining the magnitude of the post-exercise hepcidin response, and that alterations in iron regulation may only occur once a critical level of metabolic stress is achieved. An important practical outcome of this study was the demonstration that strategies of acute CHO periodization can be implemented throughout the training cycle without altering iron regulation if applied to sessions of short duration and low intensity. This outcome supports previous suggestions to maximize the efficacy of targeted approaches [**8**], where low CHO availability should be periodized around lighter training sessions to enhance the molecular adaptations to training, while high CHO availability can be used to support training when quality and/or high intensity are required.

## 4.4. Implications of Long Term Carbohydrate Manipulation

Although it may be possible to integrate acute restriction of CHO into the training program with minimal influence on post-exercise iron regulation, longer-term manipulation of CHO can yield unavoidable or larger alterations to iron metabolism, which, over time, could eventually deplete iron stores with negative effects to an athlete's health, wellbeing and performance. To explore this chronic effect, Badenhorst et al. [**62**] had trained endurance runners complete two structured 7 day training blocks while consuming diets of either low (3 $g{\cdot}kg^{-1}$ BM) or high (8 $g{\cdot}kg^{-1}$ BM) CHO content. On days 1 and 7 of each training week, athletes performed a 45 min treadmill run at 65% $VO_{2max}$ to measure the IL-6 and hepcidin response to exercise. Contrary to expectations, there were no clear differences in post-exercise IL-6 or hepcidin concentrations between Days 1 and 7, or between dietary conditions. However, interrogation of the study protocol notes that it scheduled five days of key training sessions, followed by a rest day on Day 6, then the post-intervention test on Day 7. As such, it is possible that the day of rest, combined with a higher (22%) protein intake in the isocaloric low CHO condition, could have allowed both diets to achieve sufficient restoration of muscle glycogen on Day 7. Consequently, any differences in inflammatory and iron regulatory markers to the observed exercise session were likely negated.

The ketogenic low CHO high fat (LCHF) diet represents another model of chronic CHO restriction of current interest. Ketogenic diets are characterized by CHO intakes of <50 $g{\cdot}day^{-1}$ and low to moderate protein intake (~15% energy intake), with the remaining daily energy consumed in the form of dietary fat [**63**]. Adherence to a LCHF diet increases blood ketone concentrations, while re-tooling the muscle to substantially increase fat oxidation, including an increase in the exercise intensity at which maximal rates of fat oxidation occur [**17,63**]. Studies of medium term (e.g., 4 weeks) adherence to such diets show reduced resting muscle glycogen content and reduced utilization of glycogen during exercise [**64**]. It is of interest to note that even with extreme restriction of dietary CHO intake, gluconeogenesis and the storage of muscle glycogen is enabled from precursors such as lactate, glycerol and some amino acids [**17,64**]. Of note, the time course of adaptation to a LCHF diet remains a contentious issue, largely due to the absence of a clear definition of the processes and outcomes of keto-adaptions. Although it has been argued that 2–3 months, or even longer, may be needed for complete keto-adaptation to occur [**17**], substantial alterations in substrate utilization and ketone concentrations have been demonstrated in as little as 5 days adherence to a ketogenic LCHF diet [**15,65**]. Controversially, and of importance to the current review, it has been proposed that long-term adherence to a ketogenic diet enhances glycogenesis, restoring or "normalizing" muscle glycogen content to levels similar to that of athletes adhering to high CHO diets [**66**]. However, this theory is only supported by evidence from a single cross-sectional study, where endurance athletes who reported (and had confirmed) long-term adherence to a ketogenic LCHF diet (>6 months; <50 g·day$^{-1}$ CHO), were compared to a similar cohort who consumed diets with higher CHO availability [**66**]. Meanwhile, studies with similar methodology [**67**] and other lines of interrogation contradict this theory, justifying that further scrutiny is warranted [**17**]. Nevertheless, with the majority of studies supporting the notion that ketogenic LCHF diets are associated with chronically reduced muscle glycogen content, it is possible that such nutritional approaches can result in a cumulative increase in hepcidin levels (both at baseline and post-exercise), with negative implications to iron status. Of course, there may also exist other iron-related issues from such diets, on the basis of the food choice changes, which would impact the quantity and sources of dietary iron intake.

To explore such issues, our group recently examined the effect of 3 weeks adherence to a LCHF diet (<50 g·day$^{-1}$ CHO, ~80% fat) during a period of intensified training on iron metabolism in elite race walkers [**68**]. The dietary iron content of the LCHF diet was ~25% lower than that of the CHO-rich diet (13.7 vs. 17.8 mg·day$^{-1}$; $p$ = 0.005) due to the exclusion of fortified grains and cereals, which provide a substantial source of non-heme iron in the Western diet. Despite a lower dietary iron intake, the LCHF group exhibited a smaller decrement in serum ferritin levels (23% decrease) than athletes adhering to CHO-rich diets (37% decrease; $p$ = 0.021) [**68**]. While this outcome seems contradictory, we propose that the greater decrease in serum ferritin may reflect a larger, more adaptive hematological response to training in the group exposed to consistently or strategically high CHO availability. Here, iron may have been used for adaptive processes such as increases in the production of hemoglobin or iron-associated enzyme activity, outcomes that benefits aerobic performance. Indeed, these athletes experienced a mean 4.8–6.0% improvement in 10 km race walk performance, as compared to the 1.6–2.3% decrement evident in athletes adhering to a LCHF diet [**13,14**]. However, there are multiple factors that can influence performance, and unfortunately, hematological adaptation (i.e., hemoglobin mass) was not quantified to confirm this hypothesis. Another investigation of moderately trained individuals (defined as endurance training >7 h per week), assessed the impact of a 12-week LCHF dietary intervention on hematological parameters [**69**]. In a free-living situation where participants self-selected all their foods, athletes adhering to the LCHF diet consumed significantly less dietary iron than athletes adhering to a high CHO diet (12.0 vs. 18.2 mg·day$^{-1}$). However, in this instance no changes in serum ferritin were evident after 12 weeks in either the high CHO or LCHF dietary groups. Differences between our work and that of McSwinney and colleagues **[69]** may be attributed to the caliber of athlete and level of the training stimulus. It is likely that the elite athlete cohort from our work completed a more demanding training schedule than the moderately-trained participants engaged by McSwinney et al. **[69]**, which in combination with the highly hemolytic nature of race walking, may have elicited larger exercise-associated iron losses **[35]**, and therefore, reductions in iron stores.

We also studied the impact of a LCHF diet on the iron regulatory response to exercise **[68]**. Here, a greater IL-6 and hepcidin response occurred following a 25 km exercise protocol in athletes who had adapted to a LCHF diet, compared to athletes that remained on a high CHO diet. This result presents the possibility that iron absorption may have been impaired in keto-adapted athletes in the hours following exercise. Importantly, however, the differences in serum ferritin levels need to be considered, as they have a strong homeostatic influence on the magnitude of the post-exercise hepcidin increase **[47,70]**. Accordingly, the higher serum ferritin levels evident in the LCHF group post-intervention, may have contributed to the greater hepcidin outcomes reported at 3 h post-exercise. This question prompted examination of the iron regulatory response in a subset of athletes, matched for serum ferritin levels, to remove any influence of baseline iron status **[71]**. This follow-up study revealed no differences in post-exercise hepcidin concentrations between keto-adapted athletes (<50 g·day$^{-1}$ CHO) and those adhering to CHO-rich diets (~8·g·kg$^{-1}$ BM·day$^{-1}$ CHO). Therefore, it collectively appears that iron status may have been a confounding factor in our initial study **[68]**, and that an athlete's initial iron status may exert a more dominant influence over hepcidin expression than dietary manipulation. In conclusion, while acute studies manipulating muscle glycogen content can alter hepcidin activity, evidence of altered iron regulation resulting from chronic CHO restriction is yet to be clearly demonstrated. It is possible that prolonged adherence to a low CHO diet may result in an adaptive state, whereby these acute alterations subside as the dietary adherence is maintained over time. However, this assertion is speculative, and future research is required to confirm this prospect.

Finally, given the potential for negative implications to iron metabolism when training with low CHO availability, it was speculated that sustained high CHO availability may exert a positive influence on iron metabolism. A recent investigation had elite race walkers adhere to a novel dietary strategy aimed at optimizing endogenous and exogenous CHO availability for 2 weeks **[72]**. This dietary approach strategically incorporated a number strategies to promote high CHO availability, which included high CHO intake (10–12 g·kg$^{-1}$ BM), gut training strategies **[73]**, low residue foods, and sucralose ingestion. The combination of such strategies was intended to increase CHO availability and oxidation during prolonged high intensity exercise, in an attempt to improve exercise economy and gut tolerance [**74**], whilst positively influencing athletic performance. However, these outcomes may also improve the ability to better sustain blood glucose concentrations and muscle glycogen stores, which could attenuate the IL-6 response to exercise and minimize post-exercise hepcidin levels. Regardless, no differences in serum ferritin, inflammation or hepcidin concentrations were evident in athletes adhering to the novel, very high CHO dietary approach, compared to athletes consuming a more moderate CHO intake (6–8 $g{\cdot}kg^{-1}$ BM). Therefore, it appears that there is no additional benefit to iron regulation from increasing CHO intake to very high levels, leaving us to conclude that a moderate CHO intake appears sufficient to mediate the various factors we know have an impact on iron regulation.

## 5. ENERGY ACCESSIBILITY AND IRON REGULATION

While CHO has received significant attention as a potential moderator of iron metabolism, a more recent focal point has been the impact of inadequate energy availability. LEA in athletes, which can arise from restrictions in energy intake, excessive energy expenditure, or a combination of both, is thought to impair key physiological processes that underpin health and performance [**6**]. Interestingly, it has been suggested that low iron stores may contribute to LEA or its clinical manifestations, yet it is also acknowledged that LEA may itself contribute to low iron status in athletes [**75**]. With no innate mechanism available for the body to synthesize iron, humans are solely reliant on dietary iron sources to replace incidental daily [**76**] and exercise-induced [**35**] iron losses, including the replacement of iron used for adaptive purposes. Absolute restriction of energy intake, which is commonly involved in scenarios of LEA in weight restricted or weight sensitive sports [**77**], may contribute to reduced intake of micronutrients, exacerbated by disordered eating or other restrictions of dietary range. Furthermore, scenarios of LEA can also be accompanied by very high energy expenditures resulting from excessive training loads, which potentially increase exercise-induced iron losses via mechanisms such as hemolysis, sweating, gastrointestinal bleeding, inflammation and hepcidin elevations [**35**]. This mismatch between iron losses and iron intake may partially explain the high rate of iron deficiency commonly observed in athletes with LEA [**18**].

The action of the iron regulatory hormone hepcidin may also be influenced by LEA. Increases in resting hepcidin concentrations have been reported in physically active military personnel completing a 4 day military training exercise, that elicited a 55% energy deficit and 2.7 kg decrease in body mass (EI = ~2200 $kcal{\cdot}day^{-1}$; EE = ~6100 $kcal{\cdot}day^{-1}$) [**78**]. Here, the increase in resting hepcidin levels seen was positively associated with energy expenditure ($r = 0.40$), and negatively correlated with energy balance ($r = -0.43$). However, the macronutrient content of the diet had no influence on either IL-6 or hepcidin levels. Collectively these data indicate a link between hepcidin expression and energy provision, occurring independently of an inflammatory stimulus, highlighting the importance of maintaining energy availability to avoid unnecessary elevations in hepcidin concentrations. Similar findings were reported in a crossover study of highly trained endurance athletes, where resting hepcidin concentrations were increased by a 3 day exposure to LEA (18 kcal·kg·FFM$^{-1}$) compared to a diet of sustained adequate energy availability diet (52 kcal·kg·FFM$^{-1}$) [**79**]. In this same study, 75 min of treadmill running at 70% $VO_{2max}$ yielded a significantly larger post-exercise IL-6 response in the LEA trial, compared to the adequate EA condition. Here, a steady decline (-28%) in muscle glycogen content was evident over the 3-day LEA period, which is likely responsible for the augmented inflammatory response reported. However, despite differences in IL-6 between dietary conditions, no significant differences in hepcidin levels at 3 h post-exercise were reported. Taken together, the differences in resting hepcidin concentrations between dietary conditions (without changes to inflammation), in addition to a similar post-exercise hepcidin increase (occurring despite differences in IL-6 levels), provides further evidence that LEA may be influencing hepcidin activity via a non-inflammatory mechanism that is independent of the STAT-3 pathway primarily responsible for CHO induced alterations in hepcidin levels [**40**].

The precise mechanism underpinning the observed alterations to hepcidin concentrations associated with LEA are still in question. One prospect is the regulation of hepcidin via gluconeogenic signaling [**80**]. For instance, in response to metabolic disturbances induced by food deprivation, a ~5-fold increase in transcription of the hepcidin gene (hepcidin antimicrobial peptide; HAMP) has been reported. This upregulation was followed by a ~2-fold increase in hepcidin concentrations, attributed to activation of cyclic adenosine monophosphate response binding protein (CREBH) [**80**]. This study demonstrated the ability for hepcidin to be a gluconeogenic sensor during times of starvation, potentially making this pathway a candidate to explain the increased hepcidin expression in athletes with LEA. Alternatively, the expression of another key regulator of iron metabolism, erythroferrone (ERFE), can also be regulated by nutrient availability [**81**]. Increases in ERFE act as an inhibitor of hepcidin expression, and therefore, ERFE reductions that occur in response to starvation result in an increase in hepcidin concentrations [**81**]. Irrespective of the current lack of knowledge surrounding the precise mechanistic pathway relevant here, the increase in hepcidin levels that are evident in scenarios of LEA has led to the proposition that hepcidin could be a useful biomarker for early identification of LEA in athletes [**82**]. Although this is an intriguing prospect, it is noted that the majority of evidence supporting this association has been largely drawn from animal studies, or models of starvation. Therefore, it remains to be determined whether LEA in athletes creates metabolic perturbations of sufficient magnitude to alter these signaling pathways. Accordingly, future research should identify the exact mechanism(s) responsible for alterations in hepcidin expression caused by LEA before it can be considered as a useful biomarker in the early identification of this issue in athletes.

Interestingly, it is also possible that hepcidin concentrations may be indirectly affected by LEA as a secondary response to other hormonal perturbations. A study of exercising military personnel had participants placed into a 55% energy deficit for 28 days, while receiving either a weekly 200 mg testosterone injection, or an isovolumetric placebo

[**83**]. Participants receiving placebo injections reported no changes to serum ferritin or hepcidin levels over the 28-day energy deficit period, however, a decline in hemoglobin concentrations and erythropoiesis was noted. In comparison, participants that were supplemented with testosterone reported a 41% decline in hepcidin levels, which increased iron availability to support a 34% increase in erythropoietin concentrations, allowing erythropoiesis and hemoglobin concentrations to be sustained during the energy deficit. These outcomes indicate that testosterone has suppressive effects on hepcidin expression, which is particularly important in scenarios of LEA where hepcidin may otherwise be elevated. Moreover, the key female sex hormone, estrogen, can have a similar suppressive effect on hepcidin concentrations [**84,85**]. Such findings become interesting in the context of athletes, where low sex hormone concentrations are a common outcome of sustained LEA and part of the clinical sequalae of RED-S [**7,86**]. Therefore, an increase in hepcidin expression may indirectly occur in response to declining estrogen or testosterone concentrations, which may subsequently implicate poor iron stores as a secondary outcome of LEA.

While we have primarily reviewed mechanisms by which LEA can augment hepcidin levels, potentially leading to a state of iron deficiency, there is also evidence of a bi-directional relationship in which low iron stores contribute to an energy deficit (**Figure 1**). For instance, the oxidative production of adenosine triphosphate (ATP) through the electron transport chain requires non-heme iron sulphur enzymes and heme-containing cytochromes [**22**]. In cases where iron stores are compromised, an athlete may become metabolically inefficient, characterized by a shift from ATP production via oxidative phosphorylation towards anaerobic metabolism. This effect increases the energy expenditure for a given exercise task, potentially reducing energy availability [**6**]. Additionally, low iron stores may exacerbate some of the other negative health outcomes associated with LEA (**Figure 1**) [**75**]. For example, associations between iron status and bone mineral density have been reported in non-athletic populations [**87**], leading to the assertion that chronic iron deficiency can induce bone resorption [**88**]. Impairments in bone turnover markers have been demonstrated in studies where LEA has been induced [**89,90**], which over time, may lead to poor bone health. In athletes with both depleted iron stores and LEA, the negative impact on markers of bone turnover may be amplified, potentially accelerating the progression towards undesirable and irreversible conditions such as osteopenia. Another key system possibly influenced by LEA is the immune system [**6**], with evidence of an increased incidence of illness reported in athletes with LEA [**91**]. However, it has also been proposed that LEA has minimal impact on immunity, and studies demonstrating this association may instead be mediated by poor mental health (e.g., anxiety or perceived stress) [**92**], another proposed consequence (and cause) of LEA in athletes [**6**]. Nevertheless, iron plays an important role in mounting an effective immune response to invading pathogens, and iron deficiency may contribute to decreased immune resistance and increased susceptibility to infection [**93**]. It may be that when LEA and depleted iron stores occur simultaneously in athletes, that immune resistance is further compromised, potentially via the indirect effect of LEA on psychological health, which is known to impact immune resistance [**94**]. Finally, iron deficiency can reduce thyroid functioning [**95**], and decrease the release of growth hormone and insulin-like growth factor [**96**]. These alterations (which also occur in scenarios of LEA to preserve energy [**6**]) can have wide-reaching effects, including interfering with growth, reproduction, bone health, and metabolism [**75,97**]. Accordingly, it may be that the identification of an iron deficiency can serve as an early indicator of LEA, and therefore, dieticians working with athletes wishing to correct an iron deficiency might also consider screening for LEA and clinical signs of RED-S. Furthermore, correcting an iron deficiency may be an important first step in minimizing some of the other negative health consequences that can result from LEA.

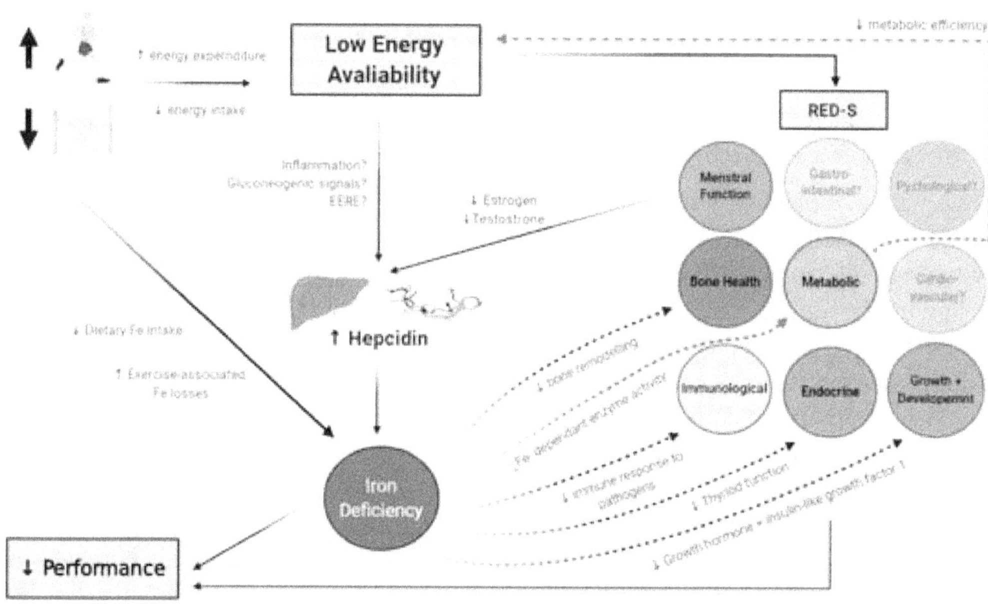


**Figure 1. Schematic representation of the interactions between low energy availability (LEA) and iron status in athletes. Solid lines identify pathways where LEA is thought to affect iron status, often mediated by hepcidin expression. Broken lines indicate how iron deficiency can exacerbate other health consequences associated with LEA in relation to the Relative Energy Deficiency in Sport syndrome (RED-S) [6].**

## 6. CONCISE SUMMARY

Nutrient availability seems to influence the iron regulatory response to exercise. Concerning carbohydrate availability, the abrupt alteration in muscle glycogen levels, which prompts the athlete to "train low," seems to elevate hepcidin levels during post-exercise recovery. Athletes aiming to incorporate this specialized training strategy into a periodized training and nutrition program should concentrate nutrient manipulation on low-intensity, short-duration training sessions to mitigate any potential effects on hepcidin levels and iron regulation. As of now, chronic studies on carbohydrate restriction (i.e., ketogenic low-carbohydrate high-fat diets) have not demonstrated definitive evidence of adverse effects on iron status or control. Nevertheless, the iron level in LCHF diets is generally inferior to that in carbohydrate-rich diets, a factor that athletes should contemplate when adopting these dietary strategies for the long term. Research on animal models and military personnel suggests a correlation between low energy availability (LEA) and iron metabolism; nevertheless, existing studies involving athletes are scarce. Future study should focus on elucidating the impact of energy deficiency, both acute and chronic, on hematological functions and their interplay with other health systems.

## AT A GLANCE

The inclusion or exclusion of specific nutrients in an athlete's diet can induce various alterations in fuel usage, training adaptation, and performance results. Moreover, dietary availability can impact athlete health, particularly regarding iron metabolism. This study aimed to summarize existing research on the effects of dietary modifications on the iron regulatory response to exercise. We evaluated the effects of acute and chronic carbohydrate (CHO) restriction on iron metabolism, pertinent to modern sports nutrition strategies, including periodized CHO availability models and ketogenic low CHO high fat diets. Furthermore, we examined the existing evidence connecting inadequate iron status and modified hepcidin activity with diminished energy availability in athletes. A comprehensive understanding of these interactions informs nutritional guidelines for athletes facing challenges in sustaining adequate iron levels, and underscores prospective research avenues and knowledge deficiencies pertinent to elite athletes.

## REFERENCES


1. Loucks, A.B. Energy balance and body composition in sports and exercise. *J. Sports Sci.* **2004**, *22*, 1–14. **[Google Scholar]**

2. Loucks, A.B.; Kiens, B.; Wright, H.H. Energy availability in athletes. *J. Sports Sci.* **2011**, *29* (Suppl. S1), S7–S15. **[Google Scholar]**

3. Logue, D.; Madigan, S.M.; Delahunt, E.; Heinen, M.; Mc Donnell, S.J.; Corish, C.A. Low energy availability in athletes: A review of prevalence, dietary patterns, physiological health, and sports performance. *Sports Med.* **2018**, *48*, 73–96. **[Google Scholar]**

4. Nattiv, A.; Loucks, A.B.; Manore, M.M.; Sanborn, C.F.; Sundgot-Borgen, J.; Warren, M.P. American College of Sports Medicine position stand. The female athlete triad. *Med. Sci. Sports Exerc.* **2007**, *39*, 1867–1882. **[Google Scholar]**

5. Mountjoy, M.; Sundgot-Borgen, J.; Burke, L.; Carter, S.; Constantini, N.; Lebrun, C.; Meyer, N.; Sherman, R.; Steffen, K.; Budgett, R.; et al. The IOC consensus statement: Beyond the Female Athlete Triad-Relative Energy Deficiency in Sport (RED- S). *Br. J. Sports Med.* **2014**, *48*, 491–497. **[Google Scholar] [PubMed]**

6. Mountjoy, M.; Sundgot-Borgen, J.; Burke, L.; Ackerman, K.E.; Blauwet, C.; Constantini, N.; Lebrun, C.; Lundy, B.; Melin, A.; Meyer, N.; et al. International Olympic Committee (IOC) consensus statement on Relative Energy Deficiency in Sport (RED-S): 2018 update. *Int. J. Sport Nutr. Exerc. Metab.* **2018**, *28*, 316–331. **[Google Scholar] [PubMed] [Green Version]**

7. Tenforde, A.S.; Barrack, M.T.; Nattiv, A.; Fredericson, M. Parallels with the female athlete triad in male athletes. *Sports Med.* **2016**, *46*, 171–182. **[Google Scholar] [PubMed]**

8. Burke, L.M.; Hawley, J.A.; Jeukendrup, A.; Morton, J.P.; Stellingwerff, T.; Maughan, R.J. Toward a common understanding of diet-exercise strategies to manipulate fuel availability for training and competition preparation in endurance sport. *Int. J. Sport Nutr. Exerc. Metab.* **2018**, *28*, 451–463. **[Google Scholar] [Green Version]**

9. Burke, L.M.; Hawley, J.A.; Wong, S.H.; Jeukendrup, A.E. Carbohydrates for training and competition. *J. Sports Sci.* **2011**, *29*, S17–S27. **[Google Scholar]**

10. Stellingwerff, T.; Cox, G.R. Systematic review: Carbohydrate supplementation on exercise performance or capacity of varying durations. *Appl. Physiol. Nutr. Metab.* **2014**, *39*, 998–1011. **[Google Scholar]**

11. Bartlett, J.D.; Hawley, J.A.; Morton, J.P. Carbohydrate availability and exercise training adaptation: Too much of a good thing? *Eur. J. Sport Sci.* **2015**, *15*, 3–12. **[Google Scholar] [PubMed]**

12. Impey, S.G.; Hearris, M.A.; Hammond, K.M.; Bartlett, J.D.; Louis, J.; Close, G.L.; Morton, J.P. Fuel for the work required: A theoretical framework for carbohydrate periodization and the glycogen threshold hypothesis. *Sports Med.* **2018**, *48*, 1031–1048. **[Google Scholar] [PubMed] [Green Version]**

13. Burke, L.M.; Ross, M.L.; Garvican-Lewis, L.A.; Welvaert, M.; Heikura, I.A.; Forbes, S.G.; Mirtschin, J.G.; Cato, L.E.; Strobel, N.; Sharma, A.P.; et al. Low carbohydrate, high fat diet impairs exercise economy and negates the performance benefit from intensified training in elite race walkers. *J. Physiol.* **2017**, *595*, 2785–2807. **[Google Scholar] [PubMed] [Green Version]**

14. Burke, L.M.; Sharma, A.P.; Heikura, I.A.; Forbes, S.F.; Holloway, M.; McKay, A.K.A.; Bone, J.L.; Leckey, J.J.; Welvaert, M.; Ross, M.L. Crisis of confidence averted: Impairment of exercise economy and performance in elite race walkers by ketogenic low carbohydrate, high fat (LCHF) diet is reproducible. *PLoS ONE* **2020**, *15*, e0234027. **[Google Scholar]**

15. Burke, L.M.; Whitfield, J.; Heikura, I.A.; Ross, M.L.R.; Tee, N.; Forbes, S.F.; Hall, R.; McKay, A.K.A.; Wallett, A.M.; Sharma, A.P. Adaptation to a low carbohydrate high fat diet is rapid but impairs endurance exercise metabolism and performance despite enhanced glycogen availability. *J. Physiol.* **2020**. **[Google Scholar]**

16. Hawley, J.A.; Leckey, J.J. Carbohydrate dependence during prolonged, intense endurance exercise. *Sports Med.* **2015**, *45* (Suppl. S1), S5–S12. **[Google Scholar] [Green Version]**

17. Burke, L.M. Ketogenic low CHO, high fat diet: The future of elite endurance sport? *J. Physiol.* **2020**. **[Google Scholar]**

18. Ackerman, K.E.; Holtzman, B.; Cooper, K.M.; Flynn, E.F.; Bruinvels, G.; Tenforde, A.S.; Popp, K.L.; Simpkin, A.J.; Parziale, A.L. Low energy availability surrogates correlate with health and performance consequences of Relative Energy Deficiency in Sport. *Br. J. Sports Med.* **2019**, *53*, 628–633. **[Google Scholar]**

19. Hennigar, S.R.; McClung, J.P.; Pasiakos, S.M. Nutritional interventions and the IL-6 response to exercise. *FASEB J.* **2017**, *31*, 3719–3728. **[Google Scholar] [Green Version]**

20. Sim, M.; Garvican-Lewis, L.A.; Cox, G.R.; Govus, A.; McKay, A.K.A.; Stellingwerff, T.; Peeling, P. Iron considerations for the athlete: A narrative review. *Eur. J. Appl. Physiol.* **2019**, *119*, 1463–1478. **[Google Scholar]**

21. Beard, J.L. Iron biology in immune function, muscle metabolism and neuronal functioning. *J. Nutr.* **2001**, *131* (Suppl. S2), 568S–580S. **[Google Scholar]**

22. Beard, J.; Tobin, B. Iron status and exercise. *Am. J. Clin. Nutr.* **2000**, *72*, 594S–597S. **[Google Scholar] [Green Version]**

23. Joyner, M.J.; Coyle, E.F. Endurance exercise performance: The physiology of champions. *J. Physiol.* **2008**, *586*, 35–44. **[Google Scholar]**

24. Myhre, K.E.; Webber, B.J.; Cropper, T.L.; Tchandja, J.N.; Ahrendt, D.M.; Dillon, C.A.; Haas, R.W.; Guy, S.L.; Pawlak, M.T.; Federinko, S.P. Prevalence and impact of anemia on basic trainees in the US air force. *Sports Med. Open* **2016**, *2*, 23. **[Google Scholar]** **[PubMed]** **[Green Version]**

25. Friedmann, B.; Weller, E.; Mairbaurl, H.; Bartsch, P. Effects of iron repletion on blood volume and performance capacity in young athletes. *Med. Sci. Sports Exerc.* **2001**, *33*, 741–746. **[Google Scholar]** **[PubMed]**

26. Hinton, P.S.; Giordano, C.; Brownlie, T.; Haas, J.D. Iron supplementation improves endurance after training in iron-depleted, nonanemic women. *J. Appl. Physiol.* **2000**, *88*, 1103–1111. **[Google Scholar]** **[PubMed]**

27. Hinton, P.S.; Sinclair, L.M. Iron supplementation maintains ventilatory threshold and improves energetic efficiency in iron-deficient nonanemic athletes. *Eur. J. Clin. Nutr.* **2007**, *61*, 30–39. **[Google Scholar]** **[Green Version]**

28. DellaValle, D.M.; Haas, J.D. Iron supplementation improves energetic efficiency in iron-depleted female rowers. *Med. Sci. Sports Exerc.* **2014**, *46*, 1204–1215. **[Google Scholar]**

29. Peeling, P.; Blee, T.; Goodman, C.; Dawson, B.; Claydon, G.; Beilby, J.; Prins, A. Effect of iron injections on aerobic-exercise performance of iron-depleted female athletes. *Int. J. Sport Nutr. Exerc. Metab.* **2007**, *17*, 221–231. **[Google Scholar]**

30. Clénin, G.; Cordes, M.; Huber, A.; Schumacher, Y.O.; Noack, P.; Scales, J.; Kriemler, S. Iron deficiency in sports-definition, influence on performance and therapy. *Swiss Med. Wkly.* **2015**, *145*, w14196. **[Google Scholar]** **[Green Version]**

31. Burden, R.J.; Pollock, N.; Whyte, G.P.; Richards, T.; Moore, B.; Busbridge, M.; Srai, S.K.; Otto, J.; Pedlar, C.R. Effect of intravenous iron on aerobic capacity and iron metabolism in elite athletes. *Med. Sci. Sports Exerc.* **2015**, *47*, 1399–1407. **[Google Scholar]** **[PubMed]**

32. Rowland, T. Iron deficiency in athletes: An update. *Am. J. Lifestyle Med.* **2012**, *6*, 319–327. **[Google Scholar]**

33. Shoemaker, M.E.; Gillen, Z.M.; McKay, B.D.; Koehler, K.; Cramer, J.T. High prevalence of poor iron status among 8-to 16-year-old youth athletes: Interactions among biomarkers of iron, dietary intakes, and biological maturity. *J. Am. Coll. Nutr.* **2020**, *39*, 155–162. **[Google Scholar]** **[PubMed]**

34. McClung, J.P. Iron status and the female athlete. *J. Trace Elem. Med. Biol.* **2012**, *26*, 124–126. **[Google Scholar]**

35. Peeling, P.; Dawson, B.; Goodman, C.; Landers, G.; Trinder, D. Athletic induced iron deficiency: New insights into the role of inflammation, cytokines and hormones. *Eur. J. Appl. Physiol.* **2008**, *103*, 381–391. **[Google Scholar]** **[PubMed]**

36. Ganz, T. Hepcidin, a key regulator of iron metabolism and mediator of anemia of inflammation. *Blood* **2003**, *102*, 783–788. **[Google Scholar]** **[PubMed]** **[Green Version]**

37. Nemeth, E.; Tuttle, M.S.; Powelson, J.; Vaughn, M.B.; Donovan, A.; Ward, D.M.; Ganz, T.; Kaplan, J. Hepcidin regulates cellular iron efflux by binding to ferroportin and inducing its internalization. *Science* **2004**, *306*, 2090–2093. **[Google Scholar]** **[Green Version]**

38. Ganz, T. Hepcidin and iron regulation, 10 years later. *Blood* **2011**, *117*, 4425–4433. **[Google Scholar]** **[Green Version]**

39. Hintze, K.J.; McClung, J.P. Hepcidin: A critical regulator of iron metabolism during hypoxia. *Adv. Hematol.* **2011**, *2011*, 510304. **[Google Scholar]**

40. Wrighting, D.M.; Andrews, N.C. Interleukin-6 induces hepcidin expression through STAT3. *Blood* **2006**, *108*, 3204–3209. **[Google Scholar]**

41. Nemeth, E.; Rivera, S.; Gabayan, V.; Keller, C.; Taudorf, S.; Pedersen, B.K.; Ganz, T. IL-6 mediates hypoferremia of inflammation by inducing the synthesis of the iron regulatory hormone hepcidin. *J. Clin. Investig.* **2004**, *113*, 1271–1276. **[Google Scholar]** **[PubMed]** **[Green Version]**

42. Kemna, E.; Pickkers, P.; Nemeth, E.; van der Hoeven, H.; Swinkels, D. Time-course analysis of hepcidin, serum iron, and plasma cytokine levels in humans injected with LPS. *Blood* **2005**, *106*, 1864–1866. **[Google Scholar] [PubMed]**

43. Fischer, C.P. Interleukin-6 in acute exercise and training: What is the biological relevance? *Exerc. Immunol. Rev.* **2006**, *12*, 6–33. **[Google Scholar] [PubMed]**

44. Pedersen, B.K.; Steensberg, A.; Schjerling, P. Exercise and interleukin-6. *Curr. Opin. Hematol.* **2001**, *8*, 137–141. **[Google Scholar] [PubMed]**

45. Newlin, M.K.; Williams, S.; McNamara, T.; Tjalsma, H.; Swinkels, D.W.; Haymes, E.M. The effects of acute exercise bouts on hepcidin in women. *Int. J. Sport Nutr. Exerc. Metab.* **2012**, *22*, 79–88. **[Google Scholar]**

46. Peeling, P.; Dawson, B.; Goodman, C.; Landers, G.; Wiegerinck, E.T.; Swinkels, D.W.; Trinder, D. Effects of exercise on hepcidin response and iron metabolism during recovery. *Int. J. Sport Nutr. Exerc. Metab.* **2009**, *19*, 583–597. **[Google Scholar] [Green Version]**

47. Peeling, P.; McKay, A.K.A.; Pyne, D.B.; Guelfi, K.J.; McCormick, R.H.; Laarakkers, C.M.; Swinkels, D.W.; Garvican-Lewis, L.A.; Ross, M.L.R.; Sharma, A.P.; et al. Factors influencing the post-exercise hepcidin-25 response in elite athletes. *Eur. J. Appl. Physiol.* **2017**, *117*, 1233–1239. **[Google Scholar]**

48. Steensberg, A.; Febbraio, M.A.; Osada, T.; Schjerling, P.; van Hall, G.; Saltin, B.; Pedersen, B.K. Interleukin-6 production in contracting human skeletal muscle is influenced by pre-exercise muscle glycogen content. *J. Physiol.* **2001**, *537*, 633–639. **[Google Scholar]**

49. Li, T.L.; Gleeson, M. The effects of carbohydrate supplementation during the second of two prolonged cycling bouts on immunoendocrine responses. *Eur. J. Appl. Physiol.* **2005**, *95*, 391–399. **[Google Scholar]**

50. Badenhorst, C.E.; Dawson, B.; Cox, G.R.; Laarakkers, C.M.; Swinkels, D.W.; Peeling, P. Acute dietary carbohydrate manipulation and the subsequent inflammatory and hepcidin responses to exercise. *Eur. J. Appl. Physiol.* **2015**, *115*, 2521–2530. **[Google Scholar]**

51. Thomas, D.T.; Erdman, K.A.; Burke, L.M. Position of the academy of nutrition and dietetics, dietitians of Canada, and the American college of sports medicine: Nutrition and athletic performance. *J. Acad. Nutr. Diet.* **2016**, *116*, 501–528. **[Google Scholar] [PubMed]**

52. Burke, L.M.; van Loon, L.J.C.; Hawley, J.A. Postexercise muscle glycogen resynthesis in humans. *J. Appl. Physiol.* **2017**, *122*, 1055–1067. **[Google Scholar] [PubMed] [Green Version]**

53. Badenhorst, C.E.; Dawson, B.; Cox, G.R.; Laarakkers, C.M.; Swinkels, D.W.; Peeling, P. Timing of post-exercise carbohydrate ingestion: Influence on IL-6 and hepcidin responses. *Eur. J. Appl. Physiol.* **2015**, *115*, 2215–2222. **[Google Scholar] [PubMed]**

54. Pedersen, B.K.; Steensberg, A.; Fischer, C.; Keller, C.; Ostrowski, K.; Schjerling, P. Exercise and cytokines with particular focus on muscle-derived IL-6. *Exerc. Immunol. Rev.* **2001**, *7*, 18–31. **[Google Scholar] [PubMed]**

55. Dahlquist, D.T.; Stellingwerff, T.; Dieter, B.P.; McKenzie, D.C.; Koehle, M.S. Effects of macro- and micronutrients on exercise-induced hepcidin response in highly trained endurance athletes. *Appl. Physiol. Nutr. Metab.* **2017**, *42*, 1036–1043. **[Google Scholar] [PubMed] [Green Version]**

56. Robson-Ansley, P.; Walshe, I.; Ward, D. The effect of carbohydrate ingestion on plasma interleukin-6, hepcidin and iron concentrations following prolonged exercise. *Cytokine* **2011**, *53*, 196–200. **[Google Scholar] [PubMed]**

57. Sim, M.; Dawson, B.; Landers, G.; Wiegerinck, E.T.; Swinkels, D.W.; Townsend, M.A.; Trinder, D.; Peeling, P. The effects of carbohydrate ingestion during endurance running on post-exercise inflammation and hepcidin levels. *Eur. J. Appl. Physiol.* **2012**, *112*, 1889–1898. **[Google Scholar] [PubMed]**

58. Costill, D.L.; Sherman, W.M.; Fink, W.J.; Maresh, C.; Witten, M.; Miller, J.M. The role of dietary carbohydrates in muscle glycogen resynthesis after strenuous running. *Am. J. Clin. Nutr.* **1981**, *34*, 1831–1836. **[Google Scholar]** **[Green Version]**

59. Heikura, I.A.; Stellingwerff, T.; Burke, L.M. Self-reported periodization of nutrition in elite female and male runners and race walkers. *Front. Physiol.* **2018**, *9*, 1732. **[Google Scholar]**

60. Jeukendrup, A.E. Periodized nutrition for athletes. *Sports Med.* **2017**, *47* (Suppl. S1), 51–63. **[Google Scholar]** **[Green Version]**

61. Mckay, A.K.A.; Heikura, I.A.; Burke, L.M.; Peeling, P.; Pyne, D.B.; van Swelm, R.P.L.; Laarakkers, C.M.; Cox, G.R. Influence of periodizing dietary carbohydrate on iron regulation and immune function in elite triathletes. *Int. J. Sport Nutr. Exerc. Metab.* **2020**, *30*, 34–41. **[Google Scholar]** **[PubMed]**

62. Badenhorst, C.E.; Dawson, B.; Cox, G.R.; Sim, M.; Laarakkers, C.M.; Swinkels, D.W.; Peeling, P. Seven days of high carbohydrate ingestion does not attenuate post-exercise IL-6 and hepcidin levels. *Eur. J. Appl. Physiol.* **2016**, *116*, 1715–1724. **[Google Scholar]** **[PubMed]**

63. Volek, J.S.; Noakes, T.; Phinney, S.D. Rethinking fat as a fuel for endurance exercise. *Eur. J. Sport Sci.* **2015**, *15*, 13–20. **[Google Scholar]** **[PubMed]**

64. Phinney, S.D.; Bistrian, B.R.; Evans, W.J.; Gervino, E.; Blackburn, G.L. The human metabolic response to chronic ketosis without caloric restriction—Preservation of submaximal exercise capability with reduced carbohydrate oxidation. *Metabolism* **1983**, *32*, 769–776. **[Google Scholar]**

65. Whitfield, J.; Burke, L.M.; McKay, A.K.A.; Heikura, I.A.; Hall, R.; Fensham, N.; Sharma, A.P. Acute ketogenic diet and ketone ester supplementation impairs race wak performance. *Med. Sci. Sports Exerc.* **2020**. **[Google Scholar]**

66. Volek, J.S.; Freidenreich, D.J.; Saenz, C.; Kunces, L.J.; Creighton, B.C.; Bartley, J.M.; Davitt, P.M.; Munoz, C.X.; Anderson, J.M.; Maresh, C.M.; et al. Metabolic characteristics of keto-adapted ultra-endurance runners. *Metabolism* **2016**, *65*, 100–110. **[Google Scholar]** **[Green Version]**

67. Webster, C.C.; Noakes, T.D.; Chacko, S.K.; Swart, J.; Kohn, T.A.; Smith, J.A. Gluconeogenesis during endurance exercise in cyclists habituated to a long-term low carbohydrate high-fat diet. *J. Physiol.* **2016**, *594*, 4389–4405. **[Google Scholar]**

68. McKay, A.K.A.; Peeling, P.; Pyne, D.B.; Welvaert, M.; Tee, N.; Leckey, J.J.; Sharma, A.P.; Ross, M.L.R.; Garvican-Lewis, L.A.; Swinkels, D.W.; et al. Chronic adherence to a ketogenic diet modifies iron metabolism in elite athletes. *Med. Sci. Sports Exerc.* **2019**, *51*, 548–555. **[Google Scholar]**

69. McSwiney, F.T.; Doyle, L. Low-carbohydrate ketogenic diets in male endurance athletes demonstrate different micronutrient contents and changes in corpuscular haemoglobin over 12 weeks. *Sports* **2019**, *7*, 201. **[Google Scholar]** **[Green Version]**

70. Peeling, P.; Sim, M.; Badenhorst, C.E.; Dawson, B.; Govus, A.D.; Abbiss, C.R.; Swinkels, D.W.; Trinder, D. Iron status and the acute post-exercise hepcidin response in athletes. *PLoS ONE* **2014**, *9*, e93002. **[Google Scholar]**

71. McKay, A.K.A.; Peeling, P.; Pyne, D.B.; Welvaert, M.; Tee, N.; Leckey, J.J.; Sharma, A.P.; Ross, M.L.R.; Garvican-Lewis, L.A.; van Swelm, R.P.L.; et al. Acute carbohydrate ingestion does not influence the post-exercise iron-regulatory response in elite keto-adapted race walkers. *J. Sci. Med. Sport* **2019**, *22*, 635–640. **[Google Scholar]** **[PubMed]**

72. McKay, A.K.A.; Peeling, P.; Pyne, D.B.; Tee, N.; Welveart, M.; Heikura, I.A.; Sharma, A.P.; Whitfield, J.; Ross, M.L.; van Swelm, R.P.L.; et al. Sustained exposure to high carbohydrate availability does not influence iron regulatory responses in elite endurance athletes. *Int. J. Sport Nutr. Exerc. Metab.* **2020**, in press. **[Google Scholar]**

73. Jeukendrup, A.E. Training the gut for athletes. *Sports Med.* **2017**, *47*, 101–110. **[Google Scholar]** **[PubMed]** **[Green Version]**

74. Costa, R.J.S.; Miall, A.; Khoo, A.; Rauch, C.; Snipe, R.; Camões-Costa, V.; Gibson, P. Gut-training: The impact of two weeks repetitive gut-challenge during exercise on gastrointestinal status, glucose availability, fuel kinetics, and running performance. *Appl. Physiol. Nutr. Metab.* **2017**, *42*, 547–557. **[Google Scholar] [PubMed] [Green Version]**

75. Petkus, D.L.; Murray-Kolb, L.E.; de Souza, M.J. The unexplored crossroads of the female athlete triad and iron deficiency: A narrative review. *Sports Med.* **2017**, *47*, 1721–1737. **[Google Scholar] [PubMed]**

76. Nielsen, P.; Nachtigall, D. Iron supplementation in athletes. Current recommendations. *Sports Med.* **1998**, *26*, 207–216. **[Google Scholar]**

77. Wells, K.R.; Jeacocke, N.A.; Appaneal, R.; Smith, H.D.; Vlahovich, N.; Burke, L.M.; Hughes, D. The Australian Institute of Sport (AIS) and National Eating Disorders Collaboration (NEDC) position statement on disordered eating in high performance sport. *Br. J. Sports Med.* **2020**, *54*, 1247–1258. **[Google Scholar]**

78. Pasiakos, S.M.; Margolis, L.M.; Murphy, N.E.; McClung, H.L.; Martini, S.; Gundersen, Y.; Castellani, J.W.; Karl, J.P.; Teien, H.K.; Madslien, E.H.; et al. Effects of exercise mode, energy, and macronutrient interventions on inflammation during military training. *Physiol. Rep.* **2016**, *4*, e12820. **[Google Scholar] [Green Version]**

79. Ishibashi, A.; Kojima, C.; Tanabe, Y.; Iwayama, K.; Hiroyama, T.; Tsuji, T.; Kamei, A.; Goto, K.; Takahashi, H. Effect of low energy availability during three consecutive days of endurance training on iron metabolism in male long distance runners. *Physiol. Rep.* **2020**, *8*, e14494. **[Google Scholar]**

80. Vecchi, C.; Montosi, G.; Garuti, C.; Corradini, E.; Sabelli, M.; Canali, S.; Pietrangelo, A. Gluconeogenic signals regulate iron homeostasis via hepcidin in mice. *Gastroenterology* **2014**, *146*, 1060–1069. **[Google Scholar] [Green Version]**

81. Coffey, R.; Ganz, T. Erythroferrone: An erythroid regulator of hepcidin and iron metabolism. *HemaSphere* **2018**, *2*, e35. **[Google Scholar] [PubMed]**

82. Badenhorst, C.E.; Black, K.E.; O'Brien, W.J. Hepcidin as a prospective individualized biomarker for individuals at risk of low energy availability. *Int. J. Sport Nutr. Exerc. Metab.* **2019**, *29*, 671–681. **[Google Scholar] [PubMed]**

83. Hennigar, S.R.; Berryman, C.E.; Harris, M.N.; Karl, J.P.; Lieberman, H.R.; McClung, J.P.; Rood, J.C.; Pasiakos, S.M. Testosterone administration during energy deficit suppresses hepcidin and increases iron availability for erythropoiesis. *J. Clin. Endocrinol. Metab.* **2020**, *105*. **[Google Scholar] [PubMed] [Green Version]**

84. Yang, Q.; Jian, J.; Katz, S.; Abramson, S.B.; Huang, X. 17β-Estradiol inhibits iron hormone hepcidin through an estrogen responsive element half-site. *Endocrinology* **2012**, *153*, 3170–3178. **[Google Scholar] [PubMed] [Green Version]**

85. Hou, Y.L.; Zhang, S.P.; Wang, L.; Li, J.P.; Qu, G.B.; He, J.Y.; Rong, H.Q.; Ji, H.; Liu, S.J. Estrogen regulates iron homeostasis through governing hepatic hepcidin expression via an estrogen response element. *Gene* **2012**, *511*, 398–403. **[Google Scholar] [PubMed]**

86. De Souza, M.J.; Koltun, K.J.; Williams, N.I. The role of energy availability in reproductive function in the female athlete triad and extension of its effects to men: An initial working model of a similar syndrome in male athletes. *Sports Med.* **2019**, *49* (Suppl. S2), 125–137. **[Google Scholar] [Green Version]**

87. Lu, M.; Liu, Y.; Shao, M.; Tesfaye, G.C.; Yang, S. Associations of iron intake, serum iron and serum ferritin with bone mineral density in women: The national health and nutrition examination survey, 2005–2010. *Calcif. Tissue Int.* **2020**, *106*, 232–238. **[Google Scholar]**

88. Toxqui, L.; Vaquero, M.P. Chronic iron deficiency as an emerging risk factor for osteoporosis: A hypothesis. *Nutrients* **2015**, *7*, 2324–2344. **[Google Scholar] [Green Version]**

89. Papageorgiou, M.; Elliott-Sale, K.J.; Parsons, A.; Tang, J.C.Y.; Greeves, J.P.; Fraser, W.D.; Sale, C. Effects of reduced energy availability on bone metabolism in women and men. *Bone* **2017**, *105*, 191–199. **[Google Scholar]** **[Green Version]**

90. Ihle, R.; Loucks, A.B. Dose-response relationships between energy availability and bone turnover in young exercising women. *J. Bone Miner. Res.* **2004**, *19*, 1231–1240. **[Google Scholar]**

91. Drew, M.; Vlahovich, N.; Hughes, D.; Appaneal, R.; Burke, L.M.; Lundy, B.; Rogers, M.; Toomey, M.; Watts, D.; Lovell, G.; et al. Prevalence of illness, poor mental health and sleep quality and low energy availability prior to the 2016 Summer Olympic Games. *Br. J. Sports Med.* **2017**, *52*, 47–53. **[Google Scholar]** **[PubMed]**

92. Walsh, N.P. Nutrition and athlete immune health: New perspectives on an old paradigm. *Sports Med.* **2019**, *49* (Suppl. S2), 153–168. **[Google Scholar]** **[PubMed]** **[Green Version]**

93. Ward, R.J.; Crichton, R.R.; Taylor, D.L.; Della Corte, L.; Srai, S.K.; Dexter, D.T. Iron and the immune system. *J. Neural Transm.* **2011**, *118*, 315–328. **[Google Scholar]** **[PubMed]**

94. Cohen, S.; Tyrrell, D.A.; Smith, A.P. Psychological stress and susceptibility to the common cold. *N. Engl. J. Med.* **1991**, *325*, 606–612. **[Google Scholar]** **[PubMed]**

95. Zimmermann, M.B.; Kohrle, J. The impact of iron and selenium deficiencies on iodine and thyroid metabolism: Biochemistry and relevance to public health. *Thyroid* **2002**, *12*, 867–878. **[Google Scholar]** **[PubMed]**

96. Ashraf, T.S.; De Sanctis, V.; Yassin, M.; Adel, A. Growth and growth hormone-insulin like growth factor-I (GH-IGF-I) axis in chronic anemias. *Acta Bio Med. Atenei Parm.* **2017**, *88*, 101. **[Google Scholar]**

97. Elliott-Sale, K.J.; Tenforde, A.S.; Parziale, A.L.; Holtzman, B.; Ackerman, K.E. Endocrine effects of relative energy deficiency in sport. *Int. J. Sport Nutr. Exerc. Metab.* **2018**, *28*, 335–349. **[Google Scholar]**

# 11 Chapter

# PRE-EXERCISE NUTRITION AND THE RESPONSE TO ENDURANCE EXERCISE: CURRENT PERSPECTIVES AND FUTURE DIRECTIONS

## 1. INTRODUCTION: AN OVERVIEW

Regardless of their degree, from Olympians to recreational exercisers, athletes universally confront the identical inquiries: what should I consume before to exercise, and how does it influence my training? Although pertinent to all individuals engaging in exercise, numerous inquiries regarding the impact of dietary consumption on endurance training responses and adaptations remain unresolved.

The length and intensity of exercise are the primary parameters affecting the adaptive response to endurance training [1]. Nevertheless, techniques that modify food availability before to and during exercise can influence training adaptations by adjusting the exercise stimulus and/or cellular responses to exercise-induced disturbances [2]. Strategies to modify nutritional availability may encompass exercising in a fasted state overnight, limiting carbohydrate intake between training sessions, and augmenting carbohydrate consumption prior to or during exercise [3]. While performance may enhance after pre-exercise carbohydrate ingestion [4,5], exercising with diminished carbohydrate availability can elevate the activation of critical signaling proteins compared to exercise conducted with ample carbohydrate availability [6], potentially affecting long-term training adaptations. Among the intracellular signals comprising the endurance training response are mechanical stretch, reactive oxygen and nitrogen species (RONS), calcium flux, AMP:ATP ratio, and the availability of endogenous CHO and free fatty acids (FFA) [7,**8**]. These signals are affected by both the duration and intensity of an exercise session, and by the pre-exercise nutrition choices of an athlete (i.e., the size, type, and timing of the pre-exercise meal(s), **Figure 1**). Although some lines of evidence suggest ingesting CHO before exercise can negatively influence endurance training adaptations, contrasting findings have been reported. For example, ingesting CHO has decreased [9], increased [10], or had no effect [11] on the activity of the 5′ AMP-activated protein kinase (AMPK) following exercise. Similarly, training-induced improvements in maximal oxygen consumption ($VO_{2max}$) have been reported to increase [12], decrease [13], or remain unchanged [14] following 4–6 weeks of CHO-fed compared with fasted-state training. These contrasting findings can be a source of confusion and may explain why the beliefs and practices relating to the role and influence of pre-exercise nutrition vary so widely among coaches and athletes [15,16]. This study aims to elucidate the existing understanding of how pre-exercise nutritional intake affects metabolic, physiological, and performance outcomes in endurance training. We emphasize areas for practitioners where data is insufficient, especially with trained athletes, and provide avenues for future research.

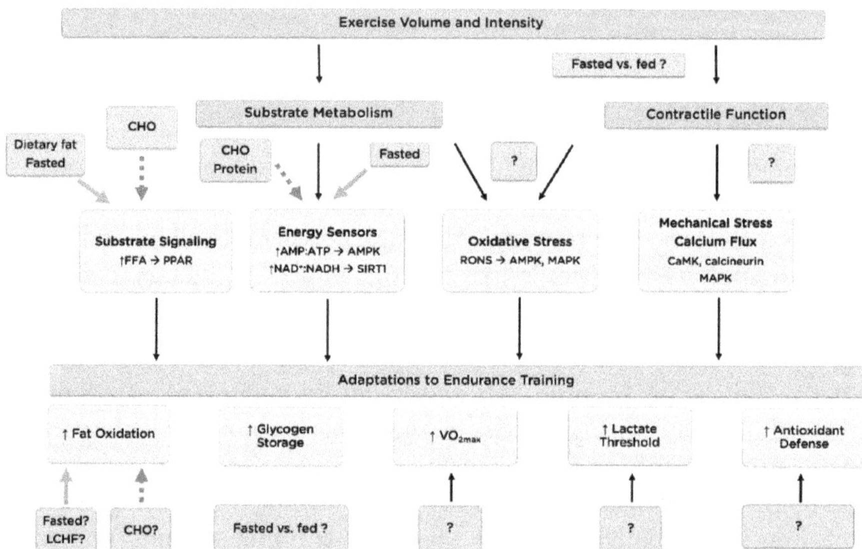


**Figure 1. Schematic of areas where pre-exercise nutrition has the potential to impact the adaptive responses to endurance training. Green arrows suggest the potential to increase or augment specific signaling, and red dashed arrows suggest the potential to decrease or impair specific signaling. Abbreviations: AMPK, AMP-activated protein kinase; CaMK, calcium/calmodulin-stimulated protein kinase; CHO, carbohydrate; FFA, free fatty acids; LCHF, low-CHO high-fat; MAPK, mitogen-activated protein kinase; $VO_{2max}$, maximal oxygen consumption.**

## 2. IMMEDIATE REACTIONS TO PRE-EXERCISE NUTRITIONAL CONSUMPTION

The predominant number of pre-exercise nutritional therapies have been executed in an acute environment. While immediate reactions to training do not consistently align with long-term adaptations, the cumulative effect of temporary, exercise-induced alterations in gene expression is believed to be a primary contributor to several training adaptations. Consequently, it is crucial to examine the immediate impacts of pre-exercise diet alongside the long-term adaptations.

## 2.1. Metabolism and Substrate Oxidation

The liver is essential for metabolic control during prolonged exercise [20]. Notwithstanding the approximately 40% decrease in liver glycogen after an overnight fast [21], blood glucose levels can remain within acceptable ranges during exercise due to enhanced gluconeogenesis and/or reduced glucose use in skeletal muscle [22,23]. The liver is essential for metabolic control during prolonged exercise [20]. Notwithstanding the approximately 40% decrease in liver glycogen after an overnight fast [21], blood glucose levels can remain within acceptable ranges during exercise due to enhanced gluconeogenesis and/or reduced glucose use in skeletal muscle [22,23]. Fatigue after prolonged exercise is frequently linked to diminished blood glucose levels, underscoring the essential function of liver glycogen in attaining peak performance during sustained physical activity.

Exercising in a fasting state typically facilitates more fat oxidation compared to exercising in a carbohydrate-fed state during low-to-moderate intensity workouts and can elevate the relative intensity at which maximal fat oxidation transpires. Consuming carbohydrates prior to exercise elevates plasma glucose and insulin concentrations, resulting in decreased hepatic glucose production and enhanced glucose absorption by skeletal muscles during exercise [27]. This can reduce fat oxidation by diminishing plasma free fatty acid availability through insulin-mediated suppression of lipolysis, and by inhibiting fat oxidation in the muscle due to an elevated glycolytic flux. Intramuscular triglycerides (IMTG) serve as a crucial substrate for fat oxidation, predominantly during exercise in a fasting state [30,31]. However, their utilization diminishes with prolonged exercise, while the oxidation of plasma free fatty acids (FFA) escalates [32]. Following a carbohydrate-rich breakfast, up to 6 hours may be necessary for substrate oxidation and glucose homeostasis to revert to levels seen during fasted-state exercise [33].

Unlike exercise conducted in a fasted overnight condition, which diminishes hepatic glycogen without affecting muscle glycogen [34], carbohydrate restriction between training sessions enables exercise to occur with diminished muscle glycogen levels [35]. During exercise with diminished muscle glycogen, there is an elevation in the oxidation of fat and amino acids, accompanied by a decrease in muscle glycogen degradation. In activity conducted with standard muscle glycogen levels, the breakdown of muscle glycogen is comparable between fed and fasted states [31,42,43,44], and may be diminished when carbohydrates are consumed during exercise [45].

Most studies examining fat oxidation have contrasted carbohydrates with a placebo, although the role of pre-exercise protein consumption is a compelling and under-explored domain. The intake of protein before to and during steady-state activity did not influence free fatty acid availability or overall fat oxidation in comparison to fasted-state exercise initiated with normal or reduced muscle glycogen levels, despite increased insulin concentrations. This may pertain to elevated catecholamine levels during exercise, which significantly influence the lipolytic rate of adipose tissue and can surpass insulin's inhibitory effects [48]. While protein consumption before to exercise in a low-glycogen condition does not influence muscle protein synthesis rates, it may potentially diminish muscle protein degradation during exercise [49]. Pre-exercise protein consumption may enhance amino acid oxidation during exercise [49], however additional measurement of its effects is required.

To compare the influence of pre-exercise CHO ingestion, muscle glycogen levels, and glycemic index on substrate oxidation and AMPK activity, we pooled the results of 125 studies (available as **supplementary online files**) that included the relevant intervention groups (**Figure 2, Figure 3, Figure 4, Figure 5, Figure 6** and **Figure 7**). Together, these studies included 1245 subjects (12.8% female), with an average age, BMI, and $VO_{2max}$ of 25.4 ± 3.1 years, 23.2 ± 1.4 kg $m^2$, and 56.7 ± 8.2 mL $kg^{-1}$ $min^{-1}$. Linear correlation analysis was used to calculate the correlation coefficient between variables, according to Pearson's product moment (r) using R statistical software. Pooled data are reported as mean ± SD, with the level of statistical significance set at $p < 0.05$.

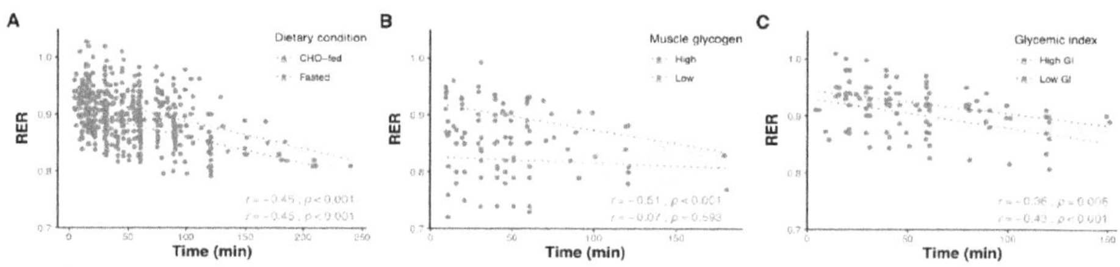


**Figure 2. Substrate oxidation in relation to exercise duration for studies reporting respiratory exchange ratio (RER) at multiple time points comparing overnight-fasted and/or CHO-fed exercise with normal muscle glycogen levels (A), exercise undertaken with high (471 ± 208 mmol $kg^{-1}$ dry mass) and low (232 ± 112 mmol $kg^{-1}$ dry mass) muscle glycogen levels (B), and following high (82 ± 10) and low (36 ± 9) glycemic index meals (C). Shaded areas represent 95% confidence intervals. Data were obtained by pooling results from 60 studies (see supplementary files for references).**

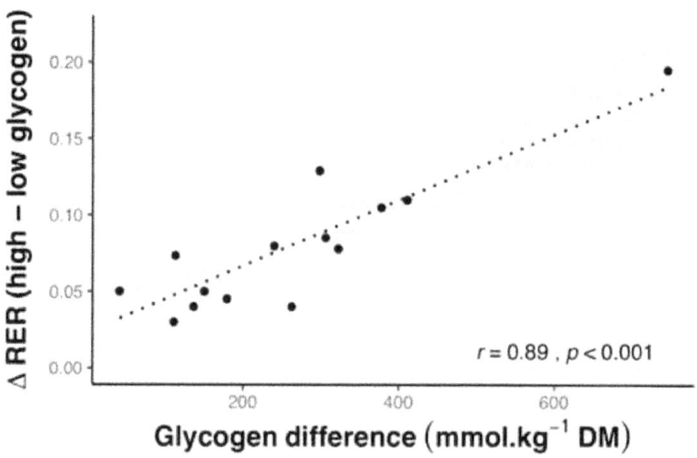


**Figure 3. Correlation between differences in respiratory exchange ratio (RER) during exercise and differences in pre-exercise glycogen levels. Shaded area represents**

**95% confidence intervals. Data were obtained by pooling results from 13 studies that manipulated glycogen levels and reported RER for high- and low-glycogen trials (see supplementary files for references). DM = dry mass.**

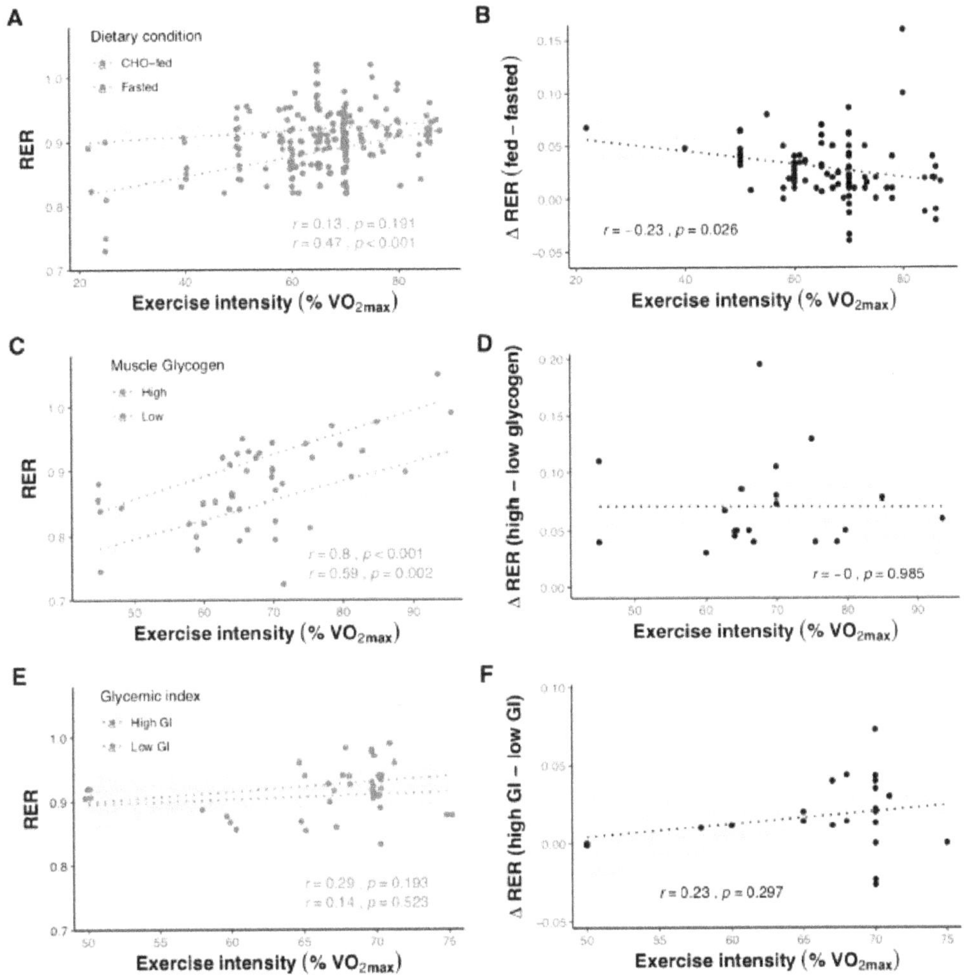


**Figure 4. Substrate oxidation in relation to exercise intensity for studies comparing overnight-fasted and CHO-fed exercise with normal muscle glycogen levels (A,B), exercise undertaken with high (471 ± 208 mmol kg$^{-1}$ dry mass) and low (232 ± 112 mmol kg$^{-1}$ dry mass) muscle glycogen levels (C,D), and following high (82 ± 10) and low (36 ± 9) glycemic index meals (E,F). Shaded areas represent 95% confidence intervals. Data were obtained by pooling results from 103 studies (see supplementary files for references).**

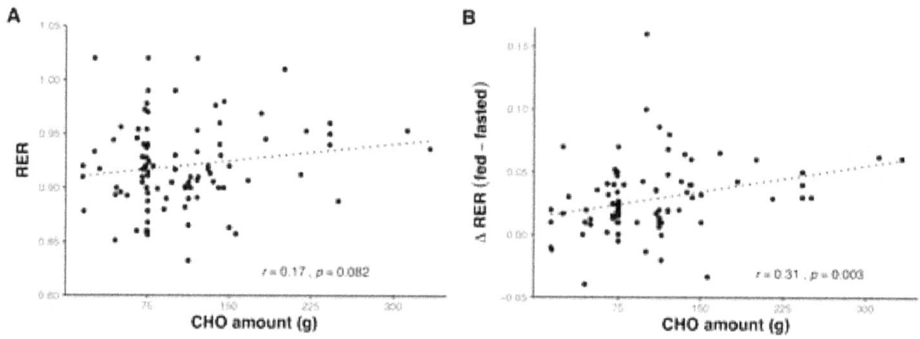


**Figure 5.** Substrate oxidation in relation to amount of carbohydrate (CHO) consumed before exercise, as absolute RER value during exercise (A) and difference in RER between fed and fasted-state exercise (B). Shaded areas represent 95% confidence intervals. Data were obtained by pooling results from 76 studies (see supplementary files for references).

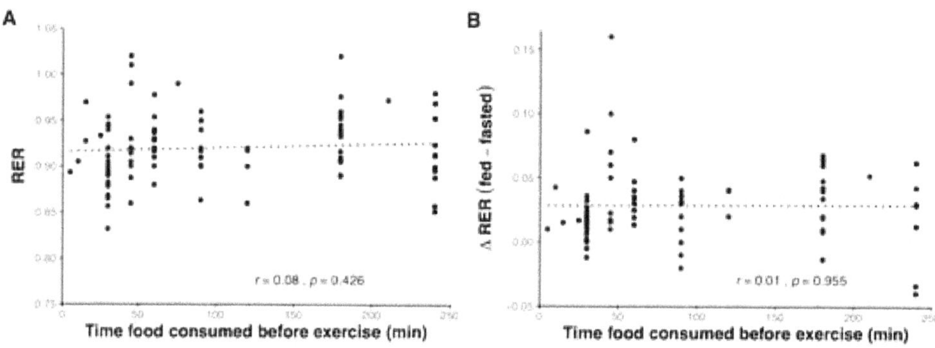


**Figure 6.** Substrate oxidation in relation to the time food was consumed before exercise, as absolute RER value during exercise (A) and difference in RER between CHO-fed and fasted-state exercise (B). Shaded areas represent 95% confidence intervals. Data were obtained by pooling results from 76 studies (see supplementary files for references).

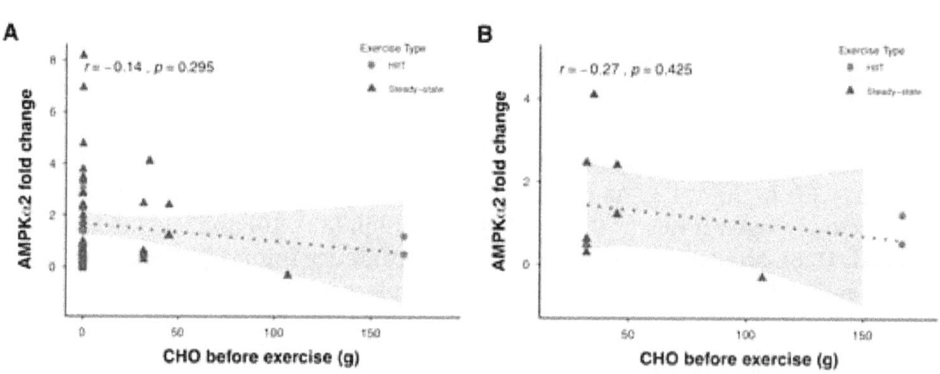


**Figure 7.** Relationship between AMPKα2 activity during exercise (measured as fold-change from pre-exercise resting levels to immediately post-exercise) and carbohydrate (CHO) intake before exercise including (A) and excluding (B) studies that tested in the overnight-fasted state. HIIT: high-intensity interval training. Shaded areas represent

**95% confidence intervals. Data were obtained by pooling results from 22 studies (see supplementary files for references), which included 265 participants (6.0% female), 25.1 ± 2.8 years, $VO_{2max}$ 52.9 ± 11.0 mL $kg^{-1}$ $min^{-1}$.**

### 2.1.1. Effect of Exercise Duration

The respiratory exchange ratio (RER—a measure of substrate oxidation) decreases with exercise duration, indicating an increasing reliance on fat oxidation as the duration of exercise extends [**50**]. Differences in RER between exercising in the fed vs. fasted state and following low vs. high glycemic index CHO remain largely similar throughout exercise, while the differences in RER between high and low starting muscle glycogen decrease as exercise duration extends (**Figure 2**). The latter could presumably be related to the greater utilization of muscle glycogen during exercise undertaken with higher levels of glycogen, leading to more similar levels during the later stages of exercise. This idea is supported by the pooled data, which show a strong correlation ($r = 0.89$, $p < 0.001$) between the differences in pre-exercise glycogen levels and differences in RER during exercise (**Figure 3**).

### 2.1.2. Effect of Exercise Intensity

Exercise intensity is well-established to influence substrate oxidation during exercise, with RER increasing with intensity [**51**]. Differences in RER between fed and fasted-state exercise are larger at lower intensities and decrease as intensity increases (**Figure 4**A,B). In contrast, exercise undertaken with low muscle glycogen maintains lower RER values compared with normal glycogen, despite increasing exercise intensity (**Figure 4**C,D). The glycemic index of the pre-exercise meal appears to have minimal effects on the relationship between intensity and substrate oxidation (**Figure 4**E,F).

### 2.1.3. Effect of Carbohydrate Amount

Several studies have directly compared varying amounts of CHO ingested before exercise, either showing no differences in substrate oxidation with varying amounts of pre-exercise CHO [**5,52,53,54**], or differences throughout all [**55**] or portions [**56,57**] of the exercise bout. When pooling a number of studies together, there is a weak positive relationship between the amount of CHO ingested and RER during subsequent exercise, while differences in RER between CHO-fed and fasted-state exercise increase as the amount of CHO ingested is increased (**Figure 5**).

### 2.1.4. Effect of Pre-Exercise Meal Timing

The amount of time before exercise food is consumed is another factor that can influence metabolism and substrate oxidation, and studies have undertaken exercise in the fed state between 5 [**58**] and 240 min [**59,60**] post-prandial. Although direct comparisons of the influence of meal-timing are limited, no differences in substrate oxidation were found when the same meals were ingested 15, 45, or 75 min [**61**] and 30, 60, or 90 min [**62**] before exercise. When consumed within 4 h of exercise, the amount of time prior to exercise does not have a meaningful impact on substrate oxidation (**Figure 6**).

### 2.1.5. Summary and Future Directions

During submaximal steady-state exercise, fat oxidation is generally higher in the overnight-fasted compared with CHO-fed state. Although fat oxidation increases with exercise duration, fasted-state exercise increases fat burning throughout the duration of exercise compared with consuming CHO before exercise. However, as exercise intensity increases the difference in fat oxidation between CHO-fed and fasted-state exercise diminishes. Fat oxidation is also higher when undertaking exercise with low, compared with normal muscle glycogen levels, with the differences maintained across varying exercise intensities but diminishing as the duration of exercise extends. While the amount of time before exercise food is consumed does not meaningfully influence substrate oxidation, greater amounts of CHO in the pre-exercise meal leads to greater differences in substrate oxidation between fed and fasted-state exercise. These findings are most applicable to moderately-trained males, who made up ~87% of study participants. Substrate metabolism may differ between males and females [**63**], with differences further affected by the female menstrual cycle [**64**] and the use of oral contraceptives [**65**]. Additionally, sedentary populations typically show no differences in post-exercise glucose, insulin, or FFAs between fasted and fed conditions [**66**], which is in contrast with trained athletes [**67**,**68**,**69**] who also show a greater capacity for fat oxidation compared with untrained or recreationally active populations [**70**].

Despite fasted-state training being performed by a large number of endurance athletes [**15**], there are potential negative implications from its use. Particularly for athletes doing a high volume of training, exercising in the overnight-fasted state could more likely lead to a negative energy balance, which can be associated with hormonal and immune dysfunction [**71**]. As a method of providing energy intake while still allowing higher levels of fat oxidation, future studies should examine the effects of a protein-rich breakfast on fat oxidation during exercise, in direct comparison with exercise following a CHO-rich breakfast and in the overnight-fasted state. As this approach is currently utilized by few endurance athletes [**16**], it could be a useful tool for those who want to increase fat burning without incurring a large caloric deficit. The influence of various pre-exercise meals on gut comfort should also be investigated, as a large number of athletes perform fasted-state training to avoid gut discomfort [**15**]. Exercise-induced gastrointestinal distress is beyond the scope of this review but has been reviewed elsewhere [**72**,**73**].

## 2.2. Cell Signaling

Among the key intracellular signals influencing skeletal muscle adaptations to endurance training are changes in the AMP:ATP ratio, contraction-induced changes in mechanical strain, increased calcium flux, an increase in RONS, and the availability of endogenous CHO and FFA [**7**,**8**,**74**]. Nutritional intake has the potential to modify signaling across several of these pathways, primarily related to energy sensing and nutrient availability.

### 2.2.1. Energy Sensing and the AMP-Activated Protein Kinase

The 5′ AMP-activated protein kinase (AMPK) is a cellular energy sensor that regulates cellular and whole-body energy balance by inhibiting ATP-consuming pathways and activating ATP-producing pathways [**75**]. Activation of AMPK can lead to a range of metabolic adaptations including increases in glucose uptake, glycolytic flux, fat oxidation, and mitochondrial biogenesis [**76**]. The degree of AMPK activation during exercise can be influenced by exercise intensity [**77**], training status [**78**], muscle glycogen [**79**], and nutrient availability [**80**].

When starting exercise with normal muscle glycogen levels, studies that have shown a blunting effect of CHO ingestion on AMPK-α2 activity [**9,81**] have been at lower intensities than those showing no differences between CHO-fed and fasted-state exercise [**11,82**]. Conversely, exercise that is undertaken with low, compared with normal muscle glycogen levels, has resulted in greater increases in the activity of AMPK-α2 following 1 h of steady-state endurance exercise at 65–70% $VO_{2max}$ [**83,84,85**], but similar increases in AMPK activity and/or phosphorylation were seen following both exhaustive and non-exhaustive high-intensity exercise undertaken with high and low muscle glycogen levels [**86,87,88**]. Therefore, ingesting CHO before exercise may dampen AMPK activity during low but not high-intensity exercise, and an intensity threshold may exist below which CHO ingestion could blunt AMPK signaling.

The CHO content of the pre-exercise meal size could also influence molecular signaling. Compared with exercising in the fasted state, consumption of <70 g CHO prior to exercise had no effect [**11,82**] or even increased [**10**] skeletal muscle AMPK signaling following exercise compared with exercise performed in the fasted state. In contrast, ingesting 130–160 g of CHO before exercise reduced the exercise-induced increases in $AMPK^{Thr172}$ phosphorylation [**89**], with the phosphorylation of acetyl-CoA carboxylase (ACC) decreased [**36**] or unaffected [**89**]. When pooling a number of studies together, non-significant correlations can be observed between the exercise-induced increases in AMPK-α2 activation and CHO intake before exercise (**Figure** 7). Future studies that are designed to examine the relationships between meal size, exercise type and intensity, and AMPK activity are warranted.

Interpretation of the research comparing pre-exercise nutrition choices on AMPK activity during exercise is complicated by the small number of studies available, training status of participants, and specific markers being reported. For example, AMPK-α2 activity during exercise is reduced by short- and longer-term endurance training, making it difficult to compare between trained and untrained subjects [**78,90,91**]. Additionally, some studies report the phosphorylation of $AMPK^{Thr172}$, which reflects phosphorylation of both AMPK-α1 and -α2 subunits and may be less sensitive for detecting changes in AMPK activity that are only occurring in the -α2 subunit that is more responsive to exercise [**81,82,86**]. Further complicating interpretation of the available literature, several studies have shown a blunting effect of CHO ingestion on AMPK-α2 activity or $AMPK^{Thr172}$ phosphorylation, yet similar increases in phosphorylation of ACC, a downstream substrate of AMPK [**81,83,92**]. Similar increases in PGC-1α mRNA expression following HIIT performed with low or high CHO availability have also been reported, despite phosphorylation of ACC being reduced by high CHO availability [**36,93**]. Furthermore, despite an attenuation of exercise-induced AMPK activation when ingesting CHO during a single bout of exercise [**81**], no differences in training adaptations were observed following 10 weeks of training with or without CHO ingestion during exercise [**94**]. These apparent discrepancies could be due to crosstalk between signaling pathways and/or the wide variability in exercise-induced changes in mRNA expression [**95**] and highlight the importance of looking at longer-term changes in mitochondrial content or function rather than acute changes in specific proteins.

#### 2.2.2. Contraction-Induced Signaling

Another key intramuscular signal comes from increased calcium released during muscle contraction. Calcium-dependent transcriptional pathways play important roles in regulating fat oxidation, mitochondrial biogenesis, and muscle fiber-type changes via myocyte enhancer factor 2 (MEF2) and p38 mitogen-activated protein kinase (MAPK) [**96,97,98,99**]. Few studies have compared the effects of nutrition interventions on calcium-dependent, contraction-induced signaling pathways. There appear to be minimal effects of exercise performed in the fed vs. fasted-state or with varying levels of muscle glycogen [**36,87,89,100**], but some evidence suggests p38 may be sensitive to nutrient status [**101,102**]. Although more research is needed, the independence of these pathways from nutritional influence could help to explain why similar longer-term changes could be observed when training under differing nutritional conditions.

#### 2.2.3. Substrate Signaling

Exercise performed in the overnight-fasted state generally results in higher levels of FFA compared with CHO-fed exercise, and an inverse relationship is seen between FFA concentration and CHO oxidation during exercise [**33**]. In addition to acting as substrate for β-oxidation in the mitochondria, FFA also play a role in molecular signaling cascades that regulate fatty acid metabolism and mitochondrial biogenesis, via activation of peroxisome proliferator-activated receptors (PPAR), MAPKs, and sirtuin 1 [**7,103,104,105**]. Some studies have found differences in FFA between fed and fasted state throughout an entire bout of exercise [**50,106**], while others have shown differences appearing from 20 [**59**], 30 [**107**], 45 [**4**], or 60 min [**108**] into exercise. These differences do not appear to show any pattern related to meal size, time of ingestion, or exercise intensity. Similar levels of FFA are found during exercise in the fasted-state and following ingestion of a high-fat meal [**60,109**] or following pre-exercise protein ingestion with normal [**46**] and low [**47**] muscle glycogen levels. Although a high-fat diet, in the absence of exercise, can increase rates of fat oxidation during exercise, a high-fat intake by itself does not increase mitochondrial content or exercise performance without simultaneously engaging in exercise training [**105**]. Future studies are needed to determine if differences in FFA during CHO-fed vs. fasted-state can significantly alter training adaptations.

#### 2.2.4. Reactive Oxygen and Nitrogen Species

Rather than simply being a byproduct of oxidative stress, RONS play a direct role in regulating the response to both acute exercise (e.g., muscle contractile function, glucose uptake, blood flow, and cell bioenergetics) and longer-term exercise training (e.g., mitochondrial biogenesis, muscle hypertrophy, angiogenesis, and redox homeostasis) **[110]**. Very little research exists looking at the influence of a pre-exercise meal on the oxidative stress response to a bout of exercise. At rest, a high-CHO meal can evoke a greater postprandial oxidative stress response compared with a high-fat meal **[111]**, while the addition of olive oil to a meal reduced post-meal increases in oxidative stress markers, such as NADPH oxidase and 8-isoprostane, both of which have been associated with endurance training adaptations **[112,113,114]**. Acute and chronic fruit ingestion can dampen lipid oxidation during exercise **[115]**, and fruit-derived phenolic compounds may promote muscle fiber-type transformation **[116]**. Whey protein can also impact the antioxidant defense system by enhancing activity of the endogenous antioxidant enzymes **[117]**. It is currently unknown how various pre-exercise meals affect oxidative stress in response to exercise and if there are any longer-term training implications.

#### 2.2.5. Summary and Future Directions

Overall, it appears that ingesting small amounts of CHO (<75 g) does not meaningfully impair mitochondrial signaling, but lower-intensity exercise may be more influenced by CHO ingestion than high-intensity exercise. Beyond the differences in exercise intensity and duration, interpretation of the existing literature is further challenged by several studies comparing the effects of fasted and CHO-fed exercise that have provided CHO both before and during exercise **[9,30,118,119]**. This is relevant because CHO ingestion during exercise can reduce muscle glycogen breakdown **[45]**, which itself may be a key signal for AMPK activity **[79]** and alter levels of TCA cycle intermediates **[120]**.

Although crosstalk between signaling pathways exists, higher-volume endurance training is more likely to influence training adaptations through the contraction-induced signaling pathways, while higher-intensity training, which increases the AMP:ATP ratio, appears more likely to signal for mitochondrial biogenesis through energy-sensing pathways **[121]**. It is possible that there may be a threshold for the amount of CHO ingested before exercise (~75 g), above which may impair intracellular (e.g., AMPK) signaling, independent of muscle glycogen levels. This is relevant as a large number of endurance athletes report consuming a small amount of CHO-based foods before training **[15]**. It is also possible that the influence of CHO ingestion on AMPK signaling may be related to exercise intensity. Future research could seek to better understand the interplay between exercise intensity and the amount of CHO ingested before and/or during exercise, bearing in mind that interactions between CHO ingestion and exercise intensity may be different during continuous and intermittent exercise **[122]**. Additionally, a better understanding of the influence of pre-exercise nutrition on RONS signaling during exercise is needed.

## 2.3. Performance

Pre-exercise CHO ingestion has been found to generally enhance prolonged (>60 min), but not shorter duration aerobic exercise performance [**66**]. However, ingesting CHO during exercise minimizes the differences between consuming CHO or a placebo prior to exercise [**123,124,125,126**]. The vast majority of studies comparing performance in the fed or fasted state have used steady-state endurance exercise [**66**], but similar effects of exercise duration are found with HIIT, as performance was improved in the fed state for 90 min of high-intensity intermittent running [**68,127**], but not short-duration HIIT [**128,129,130**]. However, one study showed a benefit of pre-exercise CHO ingestion on an exercise capacity test lasting ~8–10 min [**67**]. Several studies have compared high-fat and high-CHO pre-exercise meals with minimal performance differences observed [**57,60,125,131**].

### 2.3.1. Amount, Type, and Timing of the Pre-Exercise Meal

The amount of CHO (25–312 g) consumed prior to exercise does not have a meaningful influence on time trial performance [**5,52,53,55**], while the glycemic index appears to have only a small impact that is more likely to be observed in time-to-exhaustion, but not time-trial performance tests [**132**]. No differences in performance have been observed following pre-exercise ingestion of solid vs. liquid CHO [**43**], solid vs. gel-based CHO [**133,134**], or fast-food vs. sport supplements [**135**]. Timing of the pre-exercise meal has minimal effects when consumed 15, 45, or 75 min [**61**], 15 or 60 min [**129**], or 5 or 35 min [**58**] before exercise, but CHO ingested 30 min before exercise resulted in better performance than 120 min before exercise [**67**]. Taken together, performing fed vs. fasted exercise appears to have a far larger effect on exercise performance than the amount or timing of the meals, unless the difference in meal timing is at least 90 min. There is some fear of hypoglycemia from consuming CHO between 30–60 min prior to exercise; however, despite occurring in a small number of cases, there does not appear to be any detrimental performance effects or any relationship between low blood glucose concentrations and performance [**136**].

### 2.3.2. Athlete Perceptions and Behavior

The perception of breakfast is also a consideration when comparing the acute performance effects of pre-exercise CHO intake and fasted exercise. Trained cyclists completed a ~20 min cycling time-trial more quickly when they perceived that they had consumed breakfast (CHO or placebo) prior to the start of the exercise, compared with a fasted exercise session [**137**], and there was a 4% improvement in ~1 h time-trial performance when cyclists were told the placebo drink actually contained CHO compared with a blinded trial [**138**]. However, when a time-trial was preceded by 2 h of steady-state cycling, there were no placebo effects observed [**139**], suggesting placebo effects may be minimized with longer exercise durations. When undertaking exercise with reduced muscle glycogen levels, the perception of CHO availability augmented HIIT capacity, although performance was not restored to that of CHO consumption [**140**]. In a survey of endurance athletes, 26% agreed and 51% disagreed with the statement, "the quality of my workout is the same whether I eat or do not eat beforehand" [**15**], making it likely that a large inter-individual variation exists with regard to the perception of breakfast and its influence on performance.

### 2.3.3. Future Directions

Overall, the importance of consuming CHO before exercise increases as the exercise duration increases and exercising in the fed vs. fasted state appears to have a far greater effect on performance than the size or timing of the meals. To better understand the influence of pre-exercise energy availability vs. CHO availability and its effects on HIIT, future studies should compare fed vs. fasted exercise, along with pre-exercise protein ingestion, in the absence of CHO, prior to both HIIT and steady-state performance tests.

## 3. TRAINING ADAPTATIONS

The majority of research looking at pre-exercise nutrition interventions has been in relation to a single exercise session, with far fewer studies looking at the impact on training adaptations. This is relevant because acute responses to exercise do not always correspond with long-term adaptations. For example, increased fat oxidation observed when training with low vs. high CHO availability does not translate into longer-term increases in fat-burning capacity [**141,142**]. Likewise, blunting key mitochondrial signaling proteins with CHO ingestion during acute exercise did not impair training-induced improvements in performance or mitochondrial biogenesis [**81,94**]. Therefore, it is important to understand the changes that occur with chronic training rather than an acute bout of exercise alone.

### 3.1. Skeletal Muscle Adaptation

Of the studies examining the effects of longer-term (>4 weeks) training in the fasted state on endurance adaptations [**12,13,14,143,144,145**], only one [**144**] has used endurance-trained subjects. Furthermore, almost all studies using moderate-intensity continuous endurance training in the fasted state also provided the fed groups with CHO during exercise, which can independently influence both acute [**120**] and chronic [**93**] responses to exercise. Other studies have examined pre-exercise CHO supplementation, though not necessarily in the overnight-fasted state and using untrained subjects [**146,147**]. Additionally, fasted state training has been used as part of studies comparing low vs. high muscle glycogen [**148**] and once vs. twice daily training [**149**]. Therefore, making comparisons across studies is challenged by the variety of methods that have been used to compare high vs. low CHO availability around training sessions (**Figure 8**).

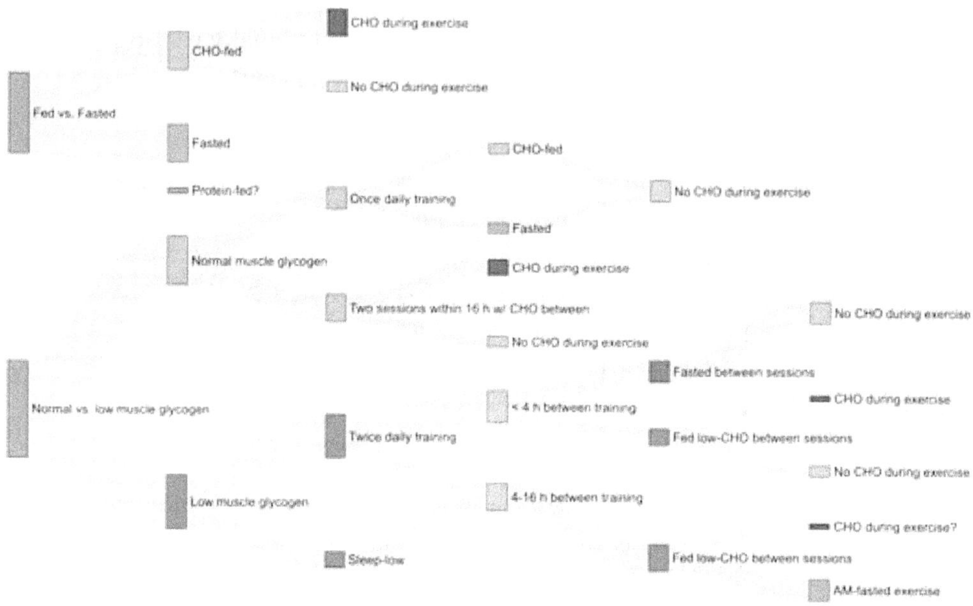


**Figure 8. Comparison of the various methods of altering CHO availability used in training studies. Protocols used to commence training with a reduced availability of endogenous carbohydrate include overnight fasting, and training twice within a 24 h period consuming low-CHO nutrition between sessions or remaining in the fasted state. Some studies have fed carbohydrate during exercise, while others have not. Thickness of the line is related to the number of studies using a given approach. Question marks represent areas yet to be studied. Created from [12,13,14,31,35,93,141,142,143,144,145,148,149,150,151,152,153 ], which included 307 participants (10.7% female), 26.3 ± 4.2 years, $VO_{2max}$ 53.2 ± 11.0 mL $kg^{-1}$ $min^{-1}$.**

### 3.1.1. Substrate Usage

One of the reasons athletes perform training sessions in the fasted state is a desire to increase fat oxidation during exercise [**15**]. As discussed above (**Section 2.1**), fat oxidation is higher during an acute bout of exercise performed in the overnight-fasted, compared with the CHO-fed state, and with low compared with high muscle glycogen. Despite these differences, most studies have found no differences in fat oxidation following 4–6 weeks of fed or fasted-state training when tested in the fed [**13,14,145**] or fasted [**31,146**] state. Similar findings have been reported in the "sleep-low" context, where fat oxidation is increased during fasted training sessions performed with low muscle glycogen compared with exercising in the fed-state, but no differences in fat oxidation were observed following one [**148**], three [**142**], or four [**141**] weeks of training when tested in the fed state. However, it is possible that longer time periods of fasted training may be needed before relevant differences in fat oxidation would be observed, as proteins involved in fat oxidation have been increased following fasted, but not fed-state training [**12,14**]. Studies that have reported improvements in fat oxidation following training with low compared with normal muscle glycogen tested subjects in the fasted state and trained twice-daily with only water ingested between the sessions [**149,150**]. Though speculative, these differences could be related to FFA signaling, which are increased during exercise and increased even further if no food is ingested in the hours following exercise [**105**]. Finally, IMTG usage during exercise was increased after 6 weeks of fasted (but not fed) training when tested in the fasted state [**145**], but there were no differences when tested in a fed state, while also providing additional CHO [**14**]. Taken together, it appears that increases in fat oxidation following fasted-state or low-glycogen training may not be relevant during typical racing conditions when consuming CHO before and during exercise, but more studies in endurance-trained athletes are needed to compare acute and chronic changes.

### 3.1.2. Mitochondrial Markers

A key feature of the adaptive response to endurance training are changes in the activity of enzymes involved in the tricarboxylic acid (TCA) cycle and the β-oxidative pathway [**154**]. Activity of citrate synthase (CS) is the most widely used biomarker of mitochondrial content in skeletal muscle because of the strong correlation between resting CS activity and resting mitochondrial content when measured using the "gold standard" transmission electron microscopy (TEM) [**155**]. Similar changes in CS activity have been observed between fasted and fed-state training following 4–6 weeks of moderate-intensity training [**12,13**] and HIIT [**143,146**]. A key enzyme of the β-oxidative pathway, β-hydroxyacyl coenzyme A dehydrogenase (β-HAD), is also generally not impacted by pre-exercise nutrition [**12,13,143**]. However, one study has shown an increase in both CS and β-HAD only with fasted, but not CHO-fed training [**145**]. It is possible that this difference may be related to the very large amount of CHO ingested in the fed-training group (~2 g $kg^{-1}$ 90 min prior and 1 g $kg^{-1}$ $h^{-1}$ during exercise), as other studies showing similar adaptations between fed and fasted training used smaller (e.g., 1–1.5 g $kg^{-1}$ CHO) pre-training meals [**13,143**]. Increases in succinate dehydrogenase activity following twice-daily training were blunted when ingesting CHO before and during the second workout, which was commenced with lowered muscle glycogen [**93**], suggesting a strong, and potentially underappreciated influence of ingesting CHO during exercise that adds complexity when interpreting the current literature.

Greater increases in CS have been reported in two studies that had subjects train twice-daily every other day, inducing low muscle glycogen during the second bout of exercise, compared with once-daily training with normal muscle glycogen [**35,150**]. In these studies, the two sessions were 1–2 h apart and subjects received only water between sessions. In contrast, other studies using twice-daily training but feeding low- or high-CHO meals between sessions found similar training-induced increases in CS activity between groups [**151,153**]. When comparing two different "train-low" protocols (2 h vs. 15 h between low-glycogen training sessions), greater elevations in acute signaling and mitochondrial adaptations were observed when training with 2 h between sessions without ingesting any food [**152,156**]. Thus, it appears that remaining in the fasted state following the first bout of exercise may be an important factor in the augmented adaptations observed following twice-daily training.

Overall, the exercise training itself seems to be the primary driver of changes in mitochondrial content, though very large pre-exercise meals (>1.5 g/kg CHO) and CHO ingestion during exercise may have blunting effects on some signaling pathways, possibly related to the interactions between AMPK and glycogen [**79**]. Future research should explore the effects of pre-exercise nutrition choices on contraction-induced and RONS signaling pathways.

### 3.1.3. $VO_{2max}$ and Peak Aerobic Power

Studies comparing fasted and fed training have reported no differences in $VO_{2max}$ following 4 weeks of sprint interval training (SIT) [**144**], 6 weeks of aerobic training [**14,145**], and 3 weeks of mixed intensity training [**157**]. However, greater training-induced increases in $VO_{2max}$ have also been reported following both fasted vs. fed-state training [**13**] and fed vs. fasted-state training [**12**]. Reasons for these divergent findings are unclear, as both studies used untrained participants performing 4–6 weeks of steady-state aerobic training. Similar improvements in $VO_{2max}$ and peak power were seen in untrained men following 8 weeks of HIIT with or without prior CHO [**146**], and following exercise undertaken with low or high muscle glycogen levels in trained and untrained athletes [**35,93,153,158,159**].

### 3.1.4. Future Directions

Pre-exercise nutrition intake would not be expected to have an effect on $VO_{2max}$ (which is largely affected by central adaptations [**160**]), but may affect peripheral adaptations that are influenced by fuel availability such as the substrate usage and mitochondrial size, particularly in untrained participants. Although there is some potential for pre-exercise nutrition intake to influence adaptations to endurance training, the lack of research in endurance-trained subjects, the very large amounts of CHO ingested before exercise in some studies, and the provision of CHO both before and during exercise in other studies makes extrapolating results to trained athletes challenging. Additionally, some of the strongest evidence suggesting low-glycogen training can magnify signaling responses to exercise is based on studies performing the experimental exercise session a few hours after a glycogen-lowering exercise bout [**149,150,151**], and some of these effects might simply be attributable to performing two exercise sessions in close proximity [**156**].

Future training studies should compare fasted-state training against low-CHO and moderate-CHO pre-exercise meals, with both normal and low muscle glycogen, and in the context of both HIIT and steady-state continuous endurance training to determine if there are differential effects on fat oxidation and/or mitochondrial biogenesis. It would also be of interest to investigate if there is a threshold for the amount of pre-exercise CHO ingested, independent of muscle glycogen levels [**161**], above which adaptations may be negatively impacted but below which adaptations are not impaired. Additionally, sex-based differences in the response to training programs should be investigated, as females accounted for just ~10% of participants in the training studies discussed.

## 3.2. Performance Changes

Studies comparing fed vs. fasted training have reported similar improvements in time-to-exhaustion during a maximal incremental test [**145,162**] and 1-h time-trial performance [**145**] following 6 weeks of endurance training. In contrast, time-to-fatigue at 85% $VO_{2max}$ improved more in trained cyclists performing SIT in the fasted state compared to those that consumed CHO (>2.5 g $kg^{-1}$ CHO prior and CHO drink during exercise), despite performing less work during training sessions [**144**]. Trained endurance athletes had greater improvements in a 12 min running time-trial following 3 weeks of aerobic training while consuming a low-GI compared with moderate GI diet [**163**].

Some studies comparing high vs. low glycogen training have reported similar performance improvements between groups [**93,141,149,150,153**], however greater improvements were seen following one and three weeks of sleep-low training [**142,148**], twice-daily training with low-CHO vs. high-CHO consumption between sessions [**151**], and twice- vs. once-daily training [**35**]. Two studies using a combination of tactics to vary CHO availability around training sessions (i.e., periodized-CHO) found similar improvements between chronic high-CHO and periodized-CHO diets, both of which resulted in greater improvements than a chronic low-CHO diet [**158,159**]. Future training studies should compare pre-exercise protein ingestion against CHO-fed and fasted-state training in the context of both HIIT and steady-state continuous endurance training. Additionally, it would be of interest to study whether a delayed CHO ingestion strategy [**164**] in the context of low glycogen or fasted-state training has any influence on the adaptive response and whether it is training specific (e.g., high- vs. low-intensity training).

# 4. SCIENCE TO PRACTICE

In an attempt to optimize both training adaptations and acute performance during key training sessions, current sport nutrition guidelines suggest training be performed both with high CHO availability, in order to enhance glycolytic and CHO oxidation pathways, and low CHO availability to increase the activation of acute cell signaling pathways related to mitochondrial biogenesis and fat oxidation [**3**].

Despite the rationale for a periodized approach to nutrition, whereby CHO availability for each workout is varied according to the type of session and its goals within a periodized training cycle [**161**], many athletes are not following these recommendations and/or are unclear on the current best-practice guidelines. For example, only 17–27% of elite athletes report following a periodized-CHO diet, and less than half of endurance athletes report varying their pre-exercise nutrition choices based on exercise duration or intensity [**16,165**]. Although training in the overnight-fasted state is performed by nearly two-thirds of endurance athletes (63%), many are doing it because they think it is beneficial, while others avoid it because they think it is not beneficial [15]. Furthermore, nearly all beliefs and practices relating to pre-exercise nutrition appear to vary based on sex, competitive level, and habitual dietary pattern [15,16]. Taken together, this highlights the need for more research in trained athletes as well as improved communication of the available research to athletes and coaches. From the standpoint of practical application, the duration and intensity of the exercise session should be considered when considering the best pre-exercise nutrition choices, along with the personal preferences of each individual athlete, as described in **Figure 9**. While the principles behind these recommendations should be applicable to a broad population, the relative influence of nutrition on training adaptations may vary based on sex, BMI, and training status.

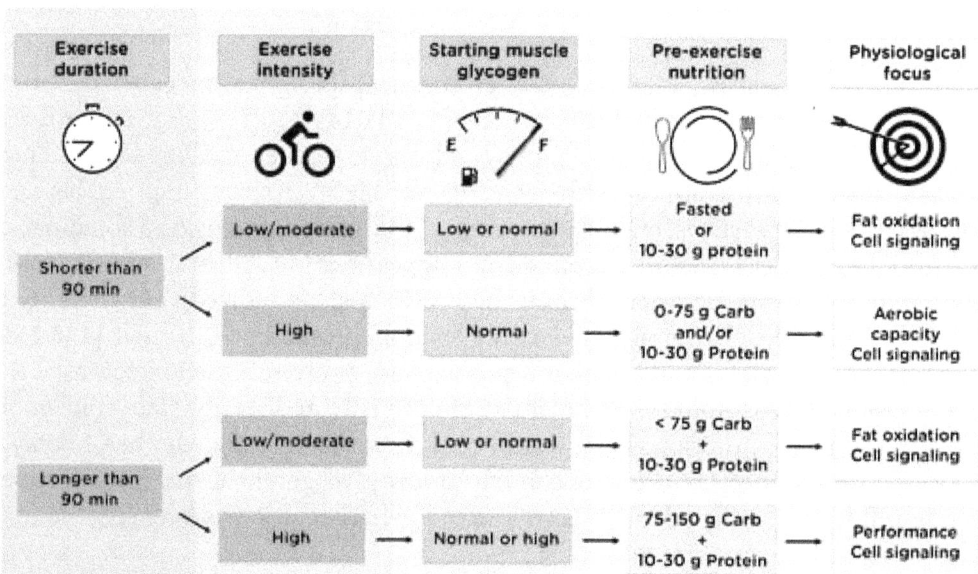


**Figure 9. Practical application of pre-exercise nutrition to optimize training adaptations. The duration and intensity of the exercise session should be considered when considering the best pre-exercise nutrition choices. Before shorter duration exercise sessions that focus on lower intensity steady-state training, it may be beneficial to withhold CHO, while there is little evidence supporting CHO restriction before high-intensity exercise. When consuming less than ~75 g CHO, food choices before HIIT can be left to personal preference. For longer duration exercise (>90 min), there is little evidence to suggest fasted-state training offers any additional benefit, although this is still practiced by approximately one-third of endurance athletes [16]. Ingesting less than ~75 g CHO is unlikely to impair mitochondrial signaling adaptations from longer-duration, low-intensity exercise, while consuming 75–150 g CHO prior to extended high-intensity exercise is suggested to increase endogenous fuel storage.**

## 5. CONCISE SUMMARY

The availability of endogenous and exogenous CHO, fat, and protein before and during exercise can influence the acute and longer-term responses to endurance exercise.

Acutely, CHO ingestion inhibits fat burning, however evidence showing enhanced fat burning capacity following long-term training in the fasted state is lacking. Contrasting findings related to the influence of CHO ingestion on mitochondrial signaling may be related to the amount of carbohydrate consumed and the intensity of exercise. Consumption of >120 g CHO before submaximal, steady-state exercise has blunted mitochondrial signaling, while <70 g CHO has not, yet CHO availability appears to have minimal effects following HIIT exercise. Performance is improved following pre-exercise CHO ingestion for longer but not shorter duration exercise, while training-induced performance changes following various pre-exercise nutrition strategies vary based on the type of nutrition protocol used. Caution should be used when generalizing these findings to wider populations, as the majority of research participants have been trained males between 20–30 years of age. In addition to wider participant demographics, more research is needed on the acute and longer-term effects of pre-exercise protein ingestion, studies in endurance-trained subjects performing fasted-state training compared with ingesting moderate and low-CHO meals before exercise, and fasted vs. fed-state training without CHO ingestion during exercise.

## AT A GLANCE

The principal factors affecting the adaptive response to endurance training are the time and intensity of the activity. Nevertheless, modifying food availability prior to and during exercise can influence the training response by adjusting the exercise stimulus and/or the physiological and molecular reactions to the exercise-induced disruptions. This study aims to elucidate the existing understanding of the impact of pre-exercise nutritional intake on metabolic, physiological, and performance outcomes in endurance training, while proposing avenues for future investigation. Carbohydrate consumption significantly diminishes fat oxidation; nevertheless, there is scant data indicating improved fat-burning capacity after prolonged training in a fasting condition. Performance enhancement occurs after pre-exercise carbohydrate consumption for prolonged activity, but not for brief durations; additionally, training-related performance gains from nutritional techniques that adjust carbohydrate availability differ according to the specific nutrition plan implemented. Discrepant results on the impact of acute carbohydrate consumption on mitochondrial signaling may be attributed to the quantity of carbohydrate ingested and the intensity of the exercise performed. This review can assist athletes, coaches, and nutritionists in tailoring pre-exercise nutrition regimens and in formulating research projects to further clarify the function of nutrition in endurance training adaptations.

## REFERENCES


1. Seiler, S. What is best practice for training intensity and duration distribution in endurance athletes? *Int. J. Sports Physiol. Perform.* **2010**, 5, 276–291. **[Google Scholar] [PubMed]**
2. Earnest, C.P.; Rothschild, J.; Harnish, C.R.; Naderi, A. Metabolic adaptations to endurance training and nutrition strategies influencing performance. *Res. Sports Med.* **2019**, *27*, 134–146. **[Google Scholar] [PubMed]**

3. Stellingwerff, T.; Morton, J.P.; Burke, L.M. A Framework for Periodized Nutrition for Athletics. *Int. J. Sport Nutr. Exerc. Metab.* **2019**, *29*, 141–151. **[Google Scholar]** **[PubMed]** **[Green Version]**

4. Tokmakidis, S.P.; Karamanolis, I.A. Effects of carbohydrate ingestion 15 min before exercise on endurance running capacity. *Appl. Physiol. Nutr. Metab.* **2008**, *33*, 441–449. **[Google Scholar]**

5. Sherman, W.M.; Peden, M.C.; Wright, D.A. Carbohydrate feedings 1 h before exercise improves cycling performance. *Am. J. Clin. Nutr.* **1991**, *54*, 866–870. **[Google Scholar]** **[Green Version]**

6. Hawley, J.A.; Morton, J.P. Ramping up the signal: Promoting endurance training adaptation in skeletal muscle by nutritional manipulation. *Clin. Exp. Pharmacol. Physiol.* **2014**, *41*, 608–613. **[Google Scholar]**

7. Philp, A.; Burke, L.M.; Baar, K. Altering endogenous carbohydrate availability to support training adaptations. *Nestle Nutr. Inst. Workshop Ser.* **2011**, *69*, 19–31. **[Google Scholar]** **[Green Version]**

8. Coffey, V.G.; Hawley, J.A. The molecular bases of training adaptation. *Sports Med.* **2007**, *37*, 737–763. **[Google Scholar]**

9. Civitarese, A.E.; Hesselink, M.K.; Russell, A.P.; Ravussin, E.; Schrauwen, P. Glucose ingestion during exercise blunts exercise-induced gene expression of skeletal muscle fat oxidative genes. *Am. J. Physiol. Endocrinol. Metab.* **2005**, *289*, E1023–E1029. **[Google Scholar]** **[Green Version]**

10. Edinburgh, R.M.; Hengist, A.; Smith, H.A.; Travers, R.L.; Koumanov, F.; Betts, J.A.; Thompson, D.; Walhin, J.P.; Wallis, G.A.; Hamilton, D.L.; et al. Preexercise breakfast ingestion versus extended overnight fasting increases postprandial glucose flux after exercise in healthy men. *Am. J. Physiol. Endocrinol. Metab.* **2018**, *315*, E1062–E1074. **[Google Scholar]** **[Green Version]**

11. Lee-Young, R.S.; Palmer, M.J.; Linden, K.C.; LePlastrier, K.; Canny, B.J.; Hargreaves, M.; Wadley, G.D.; Kemp, B.E.; McConell, G.K. Carbohydrate ingestion does not alter skeletal muscle AMPK signaling during exercise in humans. *Am. J. Physiol. Endocrinol. Metab.* **2006**, *291*, E566–E573. **[Google Scholar]** **[PubMed]** **[Green Version]**

12. Van Proeyen, K.; Szlufcik, K.; Nielens, H.; Pelgrim, K.; Deldicque, L.; Hesselink, M.; Van Veldhoven, P.; Hespel, P. Training in the fasted state improves glucose tolerance during fat-rich diet. *J. Physiol.* **2010**, *588*, 4289–4302. **[Google Scholar]** **[PubMed]**

13. Stannard, S.R.; Buckley, A.J.; Edge, J.A.; Thompson, M.W. Adaptations to skeletal muscle with endurance exercise training in the acutely fed versus overnight-fasted state. *J. Sci. Med. Sport* **2010**, *13*, 465–469. **[Google Scholar]** **[PubMed]**

14. De Bock, K.; Derave, W.; Eijnde, B.O.; Hesselink, M.K.; Koninckx, E.; Rose, A.J.; Schrauwen, P.; Bonen, A.; Richter, E.A.; Hespel, P. Effect of training in the fasted state on metabolic responses during exercise with carbohydrate intake. *J. Appl. Physiol. (1985)* **2008**, *104*, 1045–1055. **[Google Scholar]** **[Green Version]**

15. Rothschild, J.A.; Kilding, A.E.; Plews, D.J. Prevalence and determinants of fasted training in endurance athletes: A survey analysis. *Int. J. Sport Nutr. Exerc. Metab.* **2020**, *30*, 345–356. **[Google Scholar]**

16. Rothschild, J.; Kilding, A.E.; Plews, D.J. Pre-exercise nutrition habits and beliefs of endurance athletes vary by sex, competitive level and diet. *J. Am. Coll. Nutr.* **2020**, in press. **[Google Scholar]**

17. Wadley, G.D.; Nicolas, M.A.; Hiam, D.; McConell, G.K. Xanthine oxidase inhibition attenuates skeletal muscle signaling following acute exercise but does not impair mitochondrial adaptations to endurance training. *Am. J. Physiol.-Endocrinol. Metab.* **2013**, *304*, E853–E862. **[Google Scholar]** **[Green Version]**

18. Cochran, A.J.; Percival, M.E.; Tricarico, S.; Little, J.P.; Cermak, N.; Gillen, J.B.; Tarnopolsky, M.A.; Gibala, M.J. Intermittent and continuous high-intensity exercise training induce similar acute but different chronic muscle adaptations. *Exp. Physiol.* **2014**, *99*, 782–791. **[Google Scholar]** **[Green Version]**

19. Perry, C.G.; Lally, J.; Holloway, G.P.; Heigenhauser, G.J.; Bonen, A.; Spriet, L.L. Repeated transient mRNA bursts precede increases in transcriptional and mitochondrial proteins during training in human skeletal muscle. *J. Physiol.* **2010**, *588*, 4795–4810. **[Google Scholar]**

20. Trefts, E.; Williams, A.S.; Wasserman, D.H. Exercise and the Regulation of Hepatic Metabolism. *Prog. Mol. Biol. Transl. Sci.* **2015**, *135*, 203–225. **[Google Scholar] [Green Version]**

21. Nilsson, L.H.; Hultman, E. Liver glycogen in man--the effect of total starvation or a carbohydrate-poor diet followed by carbohydrate refeeding. *Scand. J. Clin. Lab. Investig.* **1973**, *32*, 325–330. **[Google Scholar] [PubMed]**

22. Dohm, G.L.; Beeker, R.T.; Israel, R.G.; Tapscott, E.B. Metabolic responses to exercise after fasting. *J. Appl. Physiol.* **1986**, *61*, 1363–1368. **[Google Scholar] [PubMed]**

23. Margolis, L.M.; Wilson, M.A.; Whitney, C.C.; Carrigan, C.T.; Murphy, N.E.; Hatch, A.M.; Montain, S.J.; Pasiakos, S.M. Exercising with low muscle glycogen content increases fat oxidation and decreases endogenous, but not exogenous carbohydrate oxidation. *Metabolism* **2019**, *97*, 1–8. **[Google Scholar] [PubMed]**

24. Coggan, A.R.; Coyle, E.F. Carbohydrate ingestion during prolonged exercise: Effects on metabolism and performance. *Exerc. Sport Sci. Rev.* **1991**, *19*, 1–40. **[Google Scholar]**

25. Vieira, A.F.; Costa, R.R.; Macedo, R.C.O.; Coconcelli, L.; Kruel, L.F.M. Effects of aerobic exercise performed in fasted v. fed state on fat and carbohydrate metabolism in adults: A systematic review and meta-analysis. *Br. J. Nutr.* **2016**, *116*, 1153–1164. **[Google Scholar] [Green Version]**

26. Andersson Hall, U.; Edin, F.; Pedersen, A.; Madsen, K. Whole-body fat oxidation increases more by prior exercise than overnight fasting in elite endurance athletes. *Appl. Physiol. Nutr. Metab.* **2015**, *41*, 430–437. **[Google Scholar] [PubMed] [Green Version]**

27. Marmy-Conus, N.; Fabris, S.; Proietto, J.; Hargreaves, M. Preexercise glucose ingestion and glucose kinetics during exercise. *J. Appl. Physiol.* **1996**, *81*, 853–857. **[Google Scholar]**

28. Horowitz, J.F.; Mora-Rodriguez, R.; Byerley, L.O.; Coyle, E.F. Lipolytic suppression following carbohydrate ingestion limits fat oxidation during exercise. *Am. J. Physiol.* **1997**, *273*, E768–E775. **[Google Scholar] [PubMed]**

29. Coyle, E.F.; Jeukendrup, A.E.; Wagenmakers, A.; Saris, W. Fatty acid oxidation is directly regulated by carbohydrate metabolism during exercise. *Am. J. Physiol.-Endocrinol. Metab.* **1997**, *273*, E268–E275. **[Google Scholar]**

30. De Bock, K.; Richter, E.A.; Russell, A.; Eijnde, B.O.; Derave, W.; Ramaekers, M.; Koninckx, E.; Leger, B.; Verhaeghe, J.; Hespel, P. Exercise in the fasted state facilitates fibre type-specific intramyocellular lipid breakdown and stimulates glycogen resynthesis in humans. *J. Physiol.* **2005**, *564*, 649–660. **[Google Scholar]**

31. Edinburgh, R.M.; Bradley, H.E.; Abdullah, N.-F.; Robinson, S.L.; Chrzanowski-Smith, O.J.; Walhin, J.-P.; Joanisse, S.; Manolopoulos, K.N.; Philp, A.; Hengist, A.; et al. Lipid metabolism links nutrient-exercise timing to insulin sensitivity in men classified as overweight or obese. *J. Clin. Endocrinol. Metab.* **2020**, *105*, 660–676. **[Google Scholar] [Green Version]**

32. Van Loon, L.J.; Koopman, R.; Stegen, J.H.; Wagenmakers, A.J.; Keizer, H.A.; Saris, W.H. Intramyocellular lipids form an important substrate source during moderate intensity exercise in endurance-trained males in a fasted state. *J. Physiol.* **2003**, *553*, 611–625. **[Google Scholar] [Green Version]**

33. Montain, S.J.; Hopper, M.; Coggan, A.R.; Coyle, E.F. Exercise metabolism at different time intervals after a meal. *J. Appl. Physiol.* **1991**, *70*, 882–888. **[Google Scholar] [PubMed]**

34. Knapik, J.J.; Meredith, C.N.; Jones, B.H.; Suek, L.; Young, V.R.; Evans, W.J. Influence of fasting on carbohydrate and fat metabolism during rest and exercise in men. *J. Appl. Physiol. (1985)* **1988**, *64*, 1923–1929. **[Google Scholar] [PubMed]**

35. Hansen, A.K.; Fischer, C.P.; Plomgaard, P.; Andersen, J.L.; Saltin, B.; Pedersen, B.K. Skeletal muscle adaptation: Training twice every second day vs. training once daily. *J. Appl. Physiol.* **2005**, *98*, 93–99. **[Google Scholar] [PubMed] [Green Version]**

36. Bartlett, J.D.; Louhelainen, J.; Iqbal, Z.; Cochran, A.J.; Gibala, M.J.; Gregson, W.; Close, G.L.; Drust, B.; Morton, J.P. Reduced carbohydrate availability enhances exercise-induced p53 signaling in human skeletal muscle: Implications for mitochondrial biogenesis. *Am. J. Physiol. Regul. Integr. Comp. Physiol.* **2013**, *304*, R450–R458. **[Google Scholar] [PubMed] [Green Version]**

37. Gillen, J.B.; West, D.W.D.; Williamson, E.P.; Fung, H.J.W.; Moore, D.R. Low-Carbohydrate Training Increases Protein Requirements of Endurance Athletes. *Med. Sci. Sports Exerc.* **2019**, *51*, 2294–2301. **[Google Scholar]**

38. Howarth, K.R.; Phillips, S.M.; MacDonald, M.J.; Richards, D.; Moreau, N.A.; Gibala, M.J. Effect of glycogen availability on human skeletal muscle protein turnover during exercise and recovery. *J. Appl. Physiol. (1985)* **2010**, *109*, 431–438. **[Google Scholar] [Green Version]**

39. Lemon, P.W.; Mullin, J.P. Effect of initial muscle glycogen levels on protein catabolism during exercise. *J. Appl. Physiol. Respir. Environ. Exerc. Physiol.* **1980**, *48*, 624–629. **[Google Scholar]**

40. Weltan, S.M.; Bosch, A.N.; Dennis, S.C.; Noakes, T.D. Preexercise muscle glycogen content affects metabolism during exercise despite maintenance of hyperglycemia. *Am. J. Physiol.* **1998**, *274*, E83–E88. **[Google Scholar]**

41. Hargreaves, M.; McConell, G.; Proietto, J. Influence of muscle glycogen on glycogenolysis and glucose uptake during exercise in humans. *J. Appl. Physiol.* **1995**, *78*, 288–292. **[Google Scholar] [PubMed]**

42. Devlin, J.T.; Calles-Escandon, J.; Horton, E.S. Effects of preexercise snack feeding on endurance cycle exercise. *J. Appl. Physiol.* **1986**, *60*, 980–985. **[Google Scholar] [PubMed]**

43. Neufer, P.D.; Costill, D.L.; Flynn, M.G.; Kirwan, J.P.; Mitchell, J.B.; Houmard, J. Improvements in exercise performance: Effects of carbohydrate feedings and diet. *J. Appl. Physiol.* **1987**, *62*, 983–988. **[Google Scholar] [PubMed]**

44. Febbraio, M.A.; Stewart, K.L. CHO feeding before prolonged exercise: Effect of glycemic index on muscle glycogenolysis and exercise performance. *J. Appl. Physiol.* **1996**, *81*, 1115–1120. **[Google Scholar] [PubMed]**

45. Tsintzas, K.; Williams, C. Human muscle glycogen metabolism during exercise. Effect of carbohydrate supplementation. *Sports Med.* **1998**, *25*, 7–23. **[Google Scholar] [PubMed]**

46. Impey, S.G.; Smith, D.; Robinson, A.L.; Owens, D.J.; Bartlett, J.D.; Smith, K.; Limb, M.; Tang, J.; Fraser, W.D.; Close, G.L. Leucine-enriched protein feeding does not impair exercise-induced free fatty acid availability and lipid oxidation: Beneficial implications for training in carbohydrate-restricted states. *Amino Acids* **2015**, *47*, 407–416. **[Google Scholar]**

47. Taylor, C.; Bartlett, J.D.; van de Graaf, C.S.; Louhelainen, J.; Coyne, V.; Iqbal, Z.; MacLaren, D.P.; Gregson, W.; Close, G.L.; Morton, J.P. Protein ingestion does not impair exercise-induced AMPK signalling when in a glycogen-depleted state: Implications for train-low compete-high. *Eur. J. Appl. Physiol.* **2013**, *113*, 1457–1468. **[Google Scholar]**

48. Enevoldsen, L.; Simonsen, L.; Macdonald, I.; Bülow, J. The combined effects of exercise and food intake on adipose tissue and splanchnic metabolism. *J. Physiol.* **2004**, *561*, 871–882. **[Google Scholar]**

49. Larsen, M.S.; Holm, L.; Svart, M.V.; Hjelholt, A.J.; Bengtsen, M.B.; Dollerup, O.L.; Dalgaard, L.B.; Vendelbo, M.H.; van Hall, G.; Moller, N.; et al. Effects of protein intake prior to carbohydrate-restricted endurance exercise: A randomized crossover trial. *J. Int. Soc. Sports Nutr.* **2020**, *17*, 7. **[Google Scholar] [Green Version]**

50. Wright, D.; Sherman, W.; Dernbach, A. Carbohydrate feedings before, during, or in combination improve cycling endurance performance. *J. Appl. Physiol.* **1991**, *71*, 1082–1088. **[Google Scholar]**

51. Romijn, J.A.; Coyle, E.F.; Sidossis, L.S.; Gastaldelli, A.; Horowitz, J.F.; Endert, E.; Wolfe, R.R. Regulation of endogenous fat and carbohydrate metabolism in relation to exercise intensity and duration. *Am. J. Physiol.* **1993**, *265*, E380–E391. [Google Scholar] [Green Version]

52. Sherman, W.M.; Brodowicz, G.; Wright, D.A.; Allen, W.K.; Simonsen, J.; Dernbach, A. Effects of 4 h preexercise carbohydrate feedings on cycling performance. *Med. Sci. Sports Exerc.* **1989**, *21*, 598–604. [Google Scholar] [PubMed]

53. Jentjens, R.L.; Cale, C.; Gutch, C.; Jeukendrup, A.E. Effects of pre-exercise ingestion of differing amounts of carbohydrate on subsequent metabolism and cycling performance. *Eur. J. Appl. Physiol.* **2003**, *88*, 444–452. [Google Scholar] [PubMed]

54. Calles-Escandón, J.; Devlin, J.T.; Whitcomb, W.; Horton, E.S. Pre-exercise feeding does not affect endurance cycle exercise but attenuates post-exercise starvation-like response. *Med. Sci. Sports Exerc.* **1991**, *23*, 818–824. [Google Scholar] [PubMed]

55. Cramp, T.; Broad, E.; Martin, D.; Meyer, B.J. Effects of preexercise carbohydrate ingestion on mountain bike performance. *Med. Sci. Sports Exerc.* **2004**, *36*, 1602–1609. [Google Scholar] [PubMed]

56. Khong, T.K.; Selvanayagam, V.S.; Hamzah, S.H.; Yusof, A. Effect of quantity and quality of pre-exercise carbohydrate meals on central fatigue. *J. Appl. Physiol.* **2018**, *125*, 1021–1029. [Google Scholar]

57. Okano, G.; Sato, Y.; Takumi, Y.; Sugawara, M. Effect of 4h preexercise high carbohydrate and high fat meal ingestion on endurance performance and metabolism. *Int. J. Sports Med.* **1996**, *17*, 530–534. [Google Scholar]

58. Smith, G.J.; Rhodes, E.C.; Langill, R.H. The effect of pre-exercise glucose ingestion on performance during prolonged swimming. *Int. J. Sport Nutr. Exerc. Metab.* **2002**, *12*, 136–144. [Google Scholar]

59. Coyle, E.F.; Coggan, A.R.; Hemmert, M.K.; Lowe, R.C.; Walters, T.J. Substrate usage during prolonged exercise following a preexercise meal. *J. Appl. Physiol.* **1985**, *59*, 429–433. [Google Scholar]

60. Whitley, H.A.; Humphreys, S.M.; Campbell, I.T.; Keegan, M.A.; Jayanetti, T.D.; Sperry, D.A.; MacLaren, D.P.; Reilly, T.; Frayn, K.N. Metabolic and performance responses during endurance exercise after high-fat and high-carbohydrate meals. *J. Appl. Physiol.* **1998**, *85*, 418–424. [Google Scholar] [Green Version]

61. Moseley, L.; Lancaster, G.I.; Jeukendrup, A.E. Effects of timing of pre-exercise ingestion of carbohydrate on subsequent metabolism and cycling performance. *Eur. J. Appl. Physiol.* **2003**, *88*, 453–458. [Google Scholar] [PubMed]

62. Willcutts, K.F.; Wilcox, A.; Grunewald, K. Energy metabolism during exercise at different time intervals following a meal. *Int. J. Sports Med.* **1988**, *9*, 240–243. [Google Scholar] [PubMed] [Green Version]

63. Wismann, J.; Willoughby, D. Gender differences in carbohydrate metabolism and carbohydrate loading. *J. Int. Soc. Sports Nutr.* **2006**, 3, 28–34. [Google Scholar] [PubMed] [Green Version]

64. Ashley, C.D.; Kramer, M.L.; Bishop, P. Estrogen and substrate metabolism: A review of contradictory research. *Sports Med.* **2000**, *29*, 221–227. [Google Scholar]

65. Sims, S.T.; Heather, A.K. Myths and Methodologies: Reducing scientific design ambiguity in studies comparing sexes and/or menstrual cycle phases. *Exp. Physiol.* **2018**, *103*, 1309–1317. [Google Scholar] [Green Version]

66. Aird, T.P.; Davies, R.W.; Carson, B.P. Effects of fasted vs. fed state exercise on performance and post-exercise metabolism: A systematic review & meta-analysis. *Scand. J. Med. Sci. Sports* **2018**, *28*, 1476–1493. [Google Scholar]

67. Galloway, S.D.; Lott, M.J.; Toulouse, L.C. Preexercise carbohydrate feeding and high-intensity exercise capacity: Effects of timing of intake and carbohydrate concentration. *Int. J. Sport Nutr. Exerc. Metab.* **2014**, *24*, 258–266. [Google Scholar] [Green Version]

68. Little, J.P.; Chilibeck, P.D.; Ciona, D.; Forbes, S.; Rees, H.; Vandenberg, A.; Zello, G.A. Effect of low- and high-glycemic-index meals on metabolism and performance during high-intensity, intermittent exercise. *Int. J. Sport Nutr. Exerc. Metab.* **2010**, *20*, 447–456. **[Google Scholar] [Green Version]**

69. Scott, J.P.; Sale, C.; Greeves, J.P.; Casey, A.; Dutton, J.; Fraser, W.D. Effect of fasting versus feeding on the bone metabolic response to running. *Bone* **2012**, *51*, 990–999. **[Google Scholar]**

70. Hetlelid, K.J.; Plews, D.J.; Herold, E.; Laursen, P.B.; Seiler, S. Rethinking the role of fat oxidation: Substrate utilisation during high-intensity interval training in well-trained and recreationally trained runners. *BMJ Open Sport Exerc. Med.* **2015**, *1*, e000047. **[Google Scholar] [Green Version]**

71. Tenforde, A.S.; Barrack, M.T.; Nattiv, A.; Fredericson, M. Parallels with the Female Athlete Triad in Male Athletes. *Sports Med.* **2016**, *46*, 171–182. **[Google Scholar] [PubMed]**

72. Wilson, P.B. 'I think I'm gonna hurl': A Narrative Review of the Causes of Nausea and Vomiting in Sport. *Sports* **2019**, *7*, 162. **[Google Scholar] [PubMed] [Green Version]**

73. De Oliveira, E.P.; Burini, R.C.; Jeukendrup, A. Gastrointestinal complaints during exercise: Prevalence, etiology, and nutritional recommendations. *Sports Med.* **2014**, *44* (Suppl. 1), S79–S85. **[Google Scholar] [PubMed] [Green Version]**

74. Egan, B.; Zierath, J.R. Exercise metabolism and the molecular regulation of skeletal muscle adaptation. *Cell Metab.* **2013**, *17*, 162–184. **[Google Scholar] [PubMed] [Green Version]**

75. Hardie, D.G.; Ross, F.A.; Hawley, S.A. AMPK: A nutrient and energy sensor that maintains energy homeostasis. *Nat. Rev. Mol. Cell Biol.* **2012**, *13*, 251–262. **[Google Scholar] [PubMed] [Green Version]**

76. Steinberg, G.R.; Kemp, B.E. AMPK in Health and Disease. *Physiol. Rev.* **2009**, *89*, 1025–1078. **[Google Scholar]**

77. Wojtaszewski, J.F.; Nielsen, P.; Hansen, B.F.; Richter, E.A.; Kiens, B. Isoform-specific and exercise intensity-dependent activation of 5′-AMP-activated protein kinase in human skeletal muscle. *J. Physiol.* **2000**, *528*, 221–226. **[Google Scholar]**

78. McConell, G.K.; Wadley, G.D.; Le Plastrier, K.; Linden, K.C. Skeletal muscle AMPK is not activated during 2 h of moderate intensity exercise at~ 65% VO2 peak in endurance trained men. *J. Physiol.* **2020**, *598*, 3859–3870. **[Google Scholar]**

79. Janzen, N.R.; Whitfield, J.; Hoffman, N.J. Interactive Roles for AMPK and Glycogen from Cellular Energy Sensing to Exercise Metabolism. *Int. J. Mol. Sci.* **2018**, *19*, 3344. **[Google Scholar] [Green Version]**

80. Bartlett, J.D.; Hawley, J.A.; Morton, J.P. Carbohydrate availability and exercise training adaptation: Too much of a good thing? *Eur. J. Sport Sci.* **2015**, *15*, 3–12. **[Google Scholar]**

81. Akerstrom, T.C.; Birk, J.B.; Klein, D.K.; Erikstrup, C.; Plomgaard, P.; Pedersen, B.K.; Wojtaszewski, J. Oral glucose ingestion attenuates exercise-induced activation of 5′-AMP-activated protein kinase in human skeletal muscle. *Biochem. Biophys. Res. Commun.* **2006**, *342*, 949–955. **[Google Scholar]**

82. Treebak, J.T.; Pehmoller, C.; Kristensen, J.M.; Kjobsted, R.; Birk, J.B.; Schjerling, P.; Richter, E.A.; Goodyear, L.J.; Wojtaszewski, J.F. Acute exercise and physiological insulin induce distinct phosphorylation signatures on TBC1D1 and TBC1D4 proteins in human skeletal muscle. *J. Physiol.* **2014**, *592*, 351–375. **[Google Scholar]**

83. Roepstorff, C.; Halberg, N.; Hillig, T.; Saha, A.K.; Ruderman, N.B.; Wojtaszewski, J.F.; Richter, E.A.; Kiens, B. Malonyl-CoA and carnitine in regulation of fat oxidation in human skeletal muscle during exercise. *Am. J. Physiol. Endocrinol. Metab.* **2005**, *288*, E133–E142. **[Google Scholar] [Green Version]**

84. Steinberg, G.R.; Watt, M.J.; McGee, S.L.; Chan, S.; Hargreaves, M.; Febbraio, M.A.; Stapleton, D.; Kemp, B.E. Reduced glycogen availability is associated with increased AMPKα2 activity, nuclear AMPKα2 protein abundance, and GLUT4 mRNA expression in contracting human skeletal muscle. *Appl. Physiol. Nutr. Metab.* **2006**, *31*, 302–312. **[Google Scholar] [Green Version]**

85. Wojtaszewski, J.F.; MacDonald, C.; Nielsen, J.N.; Hellsten, Y.; Hardie, D.G.; Kemp, B.E.; Kiens, B.; Richter, E.A. Regulation of 5′ AMP-activated protein kinase activity and substrate utilization in exercising human skeletal muscle. *Am. J. Physiol. Endocrinol. Metab.* **2003**, *284*, E813–E822. **[Google Scholar] [Green Version]**

86. Impey, S.G.; Hammond, K.M.; Shepherd, S.O.; Sharples, A.P.; Stewart, C.; Limb, M.; Smith, K.; Philp, A.; Jeromson, S.; Hamilton, D.L.; et al. Fuel for the work required: A practical approach to amalgamating train-low paradigms for endurance athletes. *Physiol. Rep.* **2016**, *4*. **[Google Scholar]**

87. Hearris, M.A.; Hammond, K.M.; Seaborne, R.A.; Stocks, B.; Shepherd, S.O.; Philp, A.; Sharples, A.P.; Morton, J.P.; Louis, J.B. Graded reductions in preexercise muscle glycogen impair exercise capacity but do not augment skeletal muscle cell signaling: Implications for CHO periodization. *J. Appl. Physiol.* **2019**, *126*, 1587–1597. **[Google Scholar]**

88. Hearris, M.A.; Owens, D.J.; Strauss, J.A.; Shepherd, S.O.; Sharples, A.P.; Morton, J.P.; Louis, J.B. Graded reductions in pre-exercise glycogen concentration do not augment exercise-induced nuclear AMPK and PGC-1α protein content in human muscle. *Exp. Physiol.* **2020**. in Press. **[Google Scholar]**

89. Stocks, B.; Dent, J.R.; Ogden, H.B.; Zemp, M.; Philp, A. Postexercise skeletal muscle signaling responses to moderate- to high-intensity steady-state exercise in the fed or fasted state. *Am. J. Physiol. Endocrinol. Metab.* **2019**, *316*, E230–E238. **[Google Scholar]**

90. McConell, G.K.; Lee-Young, R.S.; Chen, Z.P.; Stepto, N.K.; Huynh, N.N.; Stephens, T.J.; Canny, B.J.; Kemp, B.E. Short-term exercise training in humans reduces AMPK signalling during prolonged exercise independent of muscle glycogen. *J. Physiol.* **2005**, *568*, 665–676. **[Google Scholar]**

91. Mortensen, B.; Hingst, J.R.; Frederiksen, N.; Hansen, R.W.; Christiansen, C.S.; Iversen, N.; Friedrichsen, M.; Birk, J.B.; Pilegaard, H.; Hellsten, Y.; et al. Effect of birth weight and 12 weeks of exercise training on exercise-induced AMPK signaling in human skeletal muscle. *Am. J. Physiol. Endocrinol. Metab.* **2013**, *304*, E1379–E1390. **[Google Scholar] [PubMed] [Green Version]**

92. Guerra, B.; Guadalupe-Grau, A.; Fuentes, T.; Ponce-Gonzalez, J.G.; Morales-Alamo, D.; Olmedillas, H.; Guillen-Salgado, J.; Santana, A.; Calbet, J.A. SIRT1, AMP-activated protein kinase phosphorylation and downstream kinases in response to a single bout of sprint exercise: Influence of glucose ingestion. *Eur. J. Appl. Physiol.* **2010**, *109*, 731–743. **[Google Scholar] [PubMed]**

93. Morton, J.P.; Croft, L.; Bartlett, J.D.; MacLaren, D.P.; Reilly, T.; Evans, L.; McArdle, A.; Drust, B. Reduced carbohydrate availability does not modulate training-induced heat shock protein adaptations but does upregulate oxidative enzyme activity in human skeletal muscle. *J. Appl. Physiol.* **2009**, *106*, 1513–1521. **[Google Scholar] [PubMed] [Green Version]**

94. Akerstrom, T.C.; Fischer, C.P.; Plomgaard, P.; Thomsen, C.; Van Hall, G.; Pedersen, B.K. Glucose ingestion during endurance training does not alter adaptation. *J. Appl. Physiol.* **2009**, *106*, 1771–1779. **[Google Scholar]**

95. Islam, H.; Edgett, B.A.; Bonafiglia, J.T.; Shulman, T.; Ma, A.; Quadrilatero, J.; Simpson, C.A.; Gurd, B.J. Repeatability of exercise-induced changes in mRNA expression and technical considerations for qPCR analysis in human skeletal muscle. *Exp. Physiol.* **2019**, *104*, 407–420. **[Google Scholar]**

96. Chin, E.R. The role of calcium and calcium/calmodulin-dependent kinases in skeletal muscle plasticity and mitochondrial biogenesis. *Proc. Nutr. Soc.* **2004**, *63*, 279–286. **[Google Scholar] [Green Version]**

97. Wright, D.C. Mechanisms of calcium-induced mitochondrial biogenesis and GLUT4 synthesis. *Appl. Physiol. Nutr. Metab.* **2007**, *32*, 840–845. **[Google Scholar]**

98. Margolis, L.M.; Pasiakos, S.M. Optimizing intramuscular adaptations to aerobic exercise: Effects of carbohydrate restriction and protein supplementation on mitochondrial biogenesis. *Adv. Nutr.* **2013**, *4*, 657–664. **[Google Scholar] [Green Version]**

99. Jordy, A.B.; Kiens, B. Regulation of exercise-induced lipid metabolism in skeletal muscle. *Exp. Physiol.* **2014**, *99*, 1586–1592. **[Google Scholar]** **[Green Version]**

100. Yeo, W.K.; McGee, S.L.; Carey, A.L.; Paton, C.D.; Garnham, A.P.; Hargreaves, M.; Hawley, J.A. Acute signalling responses to intense endurance training commenced with low or normal muscle glycogen. *Exp. Physiol.* **2010**, *95*, 351–358. **[Google Scholar]**

101. Cochran, A.J.; Little, J.P.; Tarnopolsky, M.A.; Gibala, M.J. Carbohydrate feeding during recovery alters the skeletal muscle metabolic response to repeated sessions of high-intensity interval exercise in humans. *J. Appl. Physiol.* **2010**, *108*, 628–636. **[Google Scholar]** **[PubMed]** **[Green Version]**

102. Chan, M.S.; McGee, S.L.; Watt, M.J.; Hargreaves, M.; Febbraio, M.A. Altering dietary nutrient intake that reduces glycogen content leads to phosphorylation of nuclear p38 MAP kinase in human skeletal muscle: Association with IL-6 gene transcription during contraction. *FASEB J.* **2004**, *18*, 1785–1787. **[Google Scholar]** **[PubMed]**

103. Zbinden-Foncea, H.; Van Loon, L.J.; Raymackers, J.-M.; Francaux, M.; Deldicque, L. Contribution of nonesterified fatty acids to mitogen-activated protein kinase activation in human skeletal muscle during endurance exercise. *Int. J. Sport Nutr. Exerc. Metab.* **2013**, *23*, 201–209. **[Google Scholar]** **[PubMed]**

104. Garcia-Roves, P.; Huss, J.M.; Han, D.H.; Hancock, C.R.; Iglesias-Gutierrez, E.; Chen, M.; Holloszy, J.O. Raising plasma fatty acid concentration induces increased biogenesis of mitochondria in skeletal muscle. *Proc. Natl. Acad. Sci. USA* **2007**, *104*, 10709–10713. **[Google Scholar]** **[Green Version]**

105. Fritzen, A.M.; Lundsgaard, A.M.; Kiens, B. Tuning fatty acid oxidation in skeletal muscle with dietary fat and exercise. *Nat. Rev. Endocrinol.* **2020**, *16*, 683–696. **[Google Scholar]**

106. Gleeson, M.; Maughan, R.J.; Greenhaff, P.L. Comparison of the effects of pre-exercise feeding of glucose, glycerol and placebo on endurance and fuel homeostasis in man. *Eur. J. Appl. Physiol. Occup. Physiol.* **1986**, *55*, 645–653. **[Google Scholar]**

107. Foster, C.; Costill, D.; Fink, W. Effects of preexercise feedings on endurance performance. *Med. Sci. Sports* **1979**, *11*, 1–5. **[Google Scholar]**

108. Febbraio, M.A.; Chiu, A.; Angus, D.J.; Arkinstall, M.J.; Hawley, J.A. Effects of carbohydrate ingestion before and during exercise on glucose kinetics and performance. *J. Appl. Physiol.* **2000**, *89*, 2220–2226. **[Google Scholar]** **[Green Version]**

109. Paul, D.; Jacobs, K.A.; Geor, R.J.; Hinchcliff, K.W. No effect of pre-exercise meal on substrate metabolism and time trial performance during intense endurance exercise. *Int. J. Sport Nutr. Exerc. Metab.* **2003**, *13*, 489–503. **[Google Scholar]**

110. Margaritelis, N.V.; Paschalis, V.; Theodorou, A.A.; Kyparos, A.; Nikolaidis, M.G. Redox basis of exercise physiology. *Redox Biol.* **2020**, *35*, 101499. **[Google Scholar]**

111. Gregersen, S.; Samocha-Bonet, D.; Heilbronn, L.K.; Campbell, L.V. Inflammatory and oxidative stress responses to high-carbohydrate and high-fat meals in healthy humans. *J. Nutr. Metab.* **2012**, *2012*, 238056. **[Google Scholar]**

112. Margaritelis, N.V.; Theodorou, A.A.; Paschalis, V.; Veskoukis, A.S.; Dipla, K.; Zafeiridis, A.; Panayiotou, G.; Vrabas, I.S.; Kyparos, A.; Nikolaidis, M.G. Adaptations to endurance training depend on exercise-induced oxidative stress: Exploiting redox interindividual variability. *Acta Physiol.* **2018**, *222*, e12898. **[Google Scholar]** **[PubMed]**

113. Henriquez-Olguin, C.; Renani, L.B.; Arab-Ceschia, L.; Raun, S.H.; Bhatia, A.; Li, Z.; Knudsen, J.R.; Holmdahl, R.; Jensen, T.E. Adaptations to high-intensity interval training in skeletal muscle require NADPH oxidase 2. *Redox Biol.* **2019**, *24*, 101188. **[Google Scholar]** **[PubMed]**

114. Carnevale, R.; Pignatelli, P.; Nocella, C.; Loffredo, L.; Pastori, D.; Vicario, T.; Petruccioli, A.; Bartimoccia, S.; Violi, F. Extra virgin olive oil blunt post-prandial oxidative stress via NOX2 down-regulation. *Atherosclerosis* **2014**, *235*, 649–658. **[Google Scholar]** **[PubMed]**

115. Nieman, D.C.; Gillitt, N.D.; Chen, G.-Y.; Zhang, Q.; Sha, W.; Kay, C.D.; Chandra, P.; Kay, K.L.; Lila, M.A. Blueberry and/or Banana Consumption Mitigate Arachidonic, Cytochrome P450 Oxylipin Generation During Recovery From 75-Km Cycling: A Randomized Trial. *Front. Nutr.* **2020**, *7*, 121. **[Google Scholar] [PubMed]**

116. Chen, X.; Jia, G.; Liu, G.; Zhao, H.; Huang, Z. Effects of apple polyphenols on myofiber-type transformation in longissimus dorsi muscle of finishing pigs. *Anim. Biotechnol.* **2020**, 1–8. **[Google Scholar] [PubMed]**

117. Draganidis, D.; Karagounis, L.G.; Athanailidis, I.; Chatzinikolaou, A.; Jamurtas, A.Z.; Fatouros, I.G. Inflammaging and skeletal muscle: Can protein intake make a difference? *J. Nutr.* **2016**, *146*, 1940–1952. **[Google Scholar]**

118. Cluberton, L.J.; McGee, S.L.; Murphy, R.M.; Hargreaves, M. Effect of carbohydrate ingestion on exercise-induced alterations in metabolic gene expression. *J. Appl. Physiol.* **2005**, *99*, 1359–1363. **[Google Scholar] [Green Version]**

119. Akerstrom, T.C.; Krogh-Madsen, R.; Petersen, A.M.; Pedersen, B.K. Glucose ingestion during endurance training in men attenuates expression of myokine receptor. *Exp. Physiol.* **2009**, *94*, 1124–1131. **[Google Scholar]**

120. Spencer, M.K.; Yan, Z.; Katz, A. Carbohydrate supplementation attenuates IMP accumulation in human muscle during prolonged exercise. *Am. J. Physiol.* **1991**, *261*, C71–C76. **[Google Scholar]**

121. Laursen, P.B. Training for intense exercise performance: High-intensity or high-volume training? *Scand. J. Med. Sci. Sports* **2010**, *20* (Suppl. 2), 1–10. **[Google Scholar] [PubMed]**

122. Combes, A.; Dekerle, J.; Webborn, N.; Watt, P.; Bougault, V.; Daussin, F.N. Exercise-induced metabolic fluctuations influence AMPK, p38-MAPK and CaMKII phosphorylation in human skeletal muscle. *Physiol. Rep.* **2015**, *3*, e12462. **[Google Scholar] [PubMed]**

123. Chryssanthopoulos, C.; Williams, C.; Wilson, W.; Asher, L.; Hearne, L. Comparison between carbohydrate feedings before and during exercise on running performance during a 30-km treadmill time trial. *Int. J. Sport Nutr. Exerc. Metab.* **1994**, *4*, 374–386. **[Google Scholar] [PubMed] [Green Version]**

124. Burke, L.M.; Claassen, A.; Hawley, J.A.; Noakes, T.D. Carbohydrate intake during prolonged cycling minimizes effect of glycemic index of preexercise meal. *J. Appl. Physiol.* **1998**, *85*, 2220–2226. **[Google Scholar] [PubMed]**

125. Rowlands, D.S.; Hopkins, W.G. Effect of high-fat, high-carbohydrate, and high-protein meals on metabolism and performance during endurance cycling. *Int. J. Sport Nutr. Exerc. Metab.* **2002**, *12*, 318–335. **[Google Scholar]**

126. Learsi, S.K.; Ghiarone, T.; Silva-Cavalcante, M.D.; Andrade-Souza, V.A.; Ataide-Silva, T.; Bertuzzi, R.; de Araujo, G.G.; McConell, G.; Lima-Silva, A.E. Cycling time trial performance is improved by carbohydrate ingestion during exercise regardless of a fed or fasted state. *Scand. J. Med. Sci. Sports* **2019**, *29*, 651–662. **[Google Scholar]**

127. Little, J.P.; Chilibeck, P.D.; Ciona, D.; Vandenberg, A.; Zello, G.A. The effects of low- and high-glycemic index foods on high-intensity intermittent exercise. *Int. J. Sports Physiol. Perform.* **2009**, *4*, 367–380. **[Google Scholar] [Green Version]**

128. Coffey, V.G.; Moore, D.R.; Burd, N.A.; Rerecich, T.; Stellingwerff, T.; Garnham, A.P.; Phillips, S.M.; Hawley, J.A. Nutrient provision increases signalling and protein synthesis in human skeletal muscle after repeated sprints. *Eur. J. Appl. Physiol.* **2011**, *111*, 1473–1483. **[Google Scholar]**

129. Pritchett, K.; Bishop, P.; Pritchett, R.; Kovacs, M.; Davis, J.; Casaru, C.; Green, M. Effects of timing of pre-exercise nutrient intake on glucose responses and intermittent cycling performance. *S. Afr. J. Sports Med.* **2008**, *20*, 86–90. **[Google Scholar]**

130. Astorino, T.A.; Sherrick, S.; Mariscal, M.; Jimenez, V.C.; Stetson, K.; Courtney, D. No effect of meal intake on physiological or perceptual responses to self-selected high intensity interval exercise (HIIE). *Biol. Sport* **2019**, *36*, 225. **[Google Scholar]**

131. Murakami, I.; Sakuragi, T.; Uemura, H.; Menda, H.; Shindo, M.; Tanaka, H. Significant effect of a pre-exercise high-fat meal after a 3-day high-carbohydrate diet on endurance performance. *Nutrients* **2012**, *4*, 625–637. **[Google Scholar] [PubMed] [Green Version]**

132. Burdon, C.A.; Spronk, I.; Cheng, H.L.; O'Connor, H.T. Effect of Glycemic Index of a Pre-exercise Meal on Endurance Exercise Performance: A Systematic Review and Meta-analysis. *Sports Med.* **2017**, *47*, 1087–1101. **[Google Scholar] [PubMed]**

133. Kern, M.; Heslin, C.J.; Rezende, R.S. Metabolic and performance effects of raisins versus sports gel as pre-exercise feedings in cyclists. *J. Strength Cond. Res.* **2007**, *21*, 1204–1207. **[Google Scholar] [PubMed]**

134. Campbell, C.; Prince, D.; Braun, M.; Applegate, E.; Casazza, G.A. Carbohydrate-supplement form and exercise performance. *Int. J. Sport Nutr. Exerc. Metab.* **2008**, *18*, 179–190. **[Google Scholar] [PubMed]**

135. Cramer, M.J.; Dumke, C.L.; Hailes, W.S.; Cuddy, J.S.; Ruby, B.C. Postexercise Glycogen Recovery and Exercise Performance is Not Significantly Different Between Fast Food and Sport Supplements. *Int. J. Sport Nutr. Exerc. Metab.* **2015**, *25*, 448–455. **[Google Scholar]**

136. Jeukendrup, A.E.; Killer, S.C. The myths surrounding pre-exercise carbohydrate feeding. *Ann. Nutr. Metab.* **2010**, *57* (Suppl. 2), 18–25. **[Google Scholar]**

137. Mears, S.A.; Dickinson, K.; Bergin-Taylor, K.; Dee, R.; Kay, J.; James, L.J. Perception of Breakfast Ingestion Enhances High-Intensity Cycling Performance. *Int. J. Sports Physiol. Perform.* **2018**, *13*, 504–509. **[Google Scholar] [Green Version]**

138. Clark, V.R.; Hopkins, W.G.; Hawley, J.A.; Burke, L.M. Placebo effect of carbohydrate feedings during a 40-km cycling time trial. *Med. Sci. Sports Exerc.* **2000**, *32*, 1642–1647. **[Google Scholar]**

139. Hulston, C.J.; Jeukendrup, A.E. No placebo effect from carbohydrate intake during prolonged exercise. *Int. J. Sport Nutr. Exerc. Metab.* **2009**, *19*, 275–284. **[Google Scholar]**

140. Waterworth, S.P.; Spencer, C.C.; Porter, A.L.; Morton, J.P. Perception of Carbohydrate Availability Augments High-Intensity Intermittent Exercise Capacity Under Sleep-Low, Train-Low Conditions. *Int. J. Sport Nutr. Exerc. Metab.* **2020**, *30*, 105–111. **[Google Scholar]**

141. Riis, S.; Moller, A.B.; Dollerup, O.; Hoffner, L.; Jessen, N.; Madsen, K. Acute and sustained effects of a periodized carbohydrate intake using the sleep-low model in endurance-trained males. *Scand. J. Med. Sci. Sports* **2019**, *29*, 1866–1880. **[Google Scholar] [PubMed]**

142. Marquet, L.-A.; Brisswalter, J.; Louis, J.; Tiollier, E.; Burke, L.; Hawley, J.; Hausswirth, C. Enhanced Endurance Performance by Periodization of CHO Intake:" sleep low" strategy. *Med. Sci. Sports Exerc.* **2016**, *48*, 663–672. **[Google Scholar] [PubMed]**

143. Gillen, J.B.; Percival, M.E.; Ludzki, A.; Tarnopolsky, M.A.; Gibala, M. Interval training in the fed or fasted state improves body composition and muscle oxidative capacity in overweight women. *Obesity* **2013**, *21*, 2249–2255. **[Google Scholar] [PubMed]**

144. Terada, T.; Toghi Eshghi, S.R.; Liubaoerjijin, Y.; Kennedy, M.; Myette-Cote, E.; Fletcher, K.; Boule, N.G. Overnight fasting compromises exercise intensity and volume during sprint interval training but improves high-intensity aerobic endurance. *J. Sports Med. Phys. Fit.* **2019**, *59*, 357–365. **[Google Scholar]**

145. Van Proeyen, K.; Szlufcik, K.; Nielens, H.; Ramaekers, M.; Hespel, P. Beneficial metabolic adaptations due to endurance exercise training in the fasted state. *J. Appl. Physiol.* **2011**, *110*, 236–245. **[Google Scholar] [Green Version]**

146. Nybo, L.; Pedersen, K.; Christensen, B.; Aagaard, P.; Brandt, N.; Kiens, B. Impact of carbohydrate supplementation during endurance training on glycogen storage and performance. *Acta Physiol.* **2009**, *197*, 117–127. **[Google Scholar]**

147. Beaudouin, F.; Joerg, F.; Hilpert, A.; Meyer, T.; Hecksteden, A. Carbohydrate intake and training efficacy—a randomized cross-over study. *J. Sports Sci.* **2018**, *36*, 942–948. **[Google Scholar]**

148. Marquet, L.A.; Hausswirth, C.; Molle, O.; Hawley, J.A.; Burke, L.M.; Tiollier, E.; Brisswalter, J. Periodization of Carbohydrate Intake: Short-Term Effect on Performance. *Nutrients* **2016**, *8*, 755. **[Google Scholar]** **[Green Version]**

149. Hulston, C.J.; Venables, M.C.; Mann, C.H.; Martin, C.; Philp, A.; Baar, K.; Jeukendrup, A.E. Training with low muscle glycogen enhances fat metabolism in well-trained cyclists. *Med. Sci. Sports Exerc.* **2010**, *42*, 2046–2055. **[Google Scholar]** **[Green Version]**

150. Yeo, W.K.; Paton, C.D.; Garnham, A.P.; Burke, L.M.; Carey, A.L.; Hawley, J.A. Skeletal muscle adaptation and performance responses to once a day versus twice every second day endurance training regimens. *J. Appl. Physiol.* **2008**, *105*, 1462–1470. **[Google Scholar]** **[Green Version]**

151. Cochran, C.A.J.R.; Myslik, F.; MacInnis, M.J.; Percival, M.E.; Bishop, D.; Tarnopolsky, M.A.; Gibala, M.J. Manipulating carbohydrate availability between twice-daily sessions of high-intensity interval training over 2 weeks improves time-trial performance. *Int. J. Sport Nutr. Exerc. Metab.* **2015**, *25*, 463–470. **[Google Scholar]** **[PubMed]**

152. Ghiarone, T.; Andrade-Souza, V.A.; Learsi, S.K.; Tomazini, F.; Ataide-Silva, T.; Sansonio, A.; Fernandes, M.P.; Saraiva, K.L.; Figueiredo, R.C.; Tourneur, Y. Twice-a-day training improves mitochondrial efficiency, but not mitochondrial biogenesis, compared with once-daily training. *J. Appl. Physiol.* **2019**, *127*, 713–725. **[Google Scholar]** **[PubMed]**

153. Gejl, K.D.; Thams, L.B.; Hansen, M.; Rokkedal-Lausch, T.; Plomgaard, P.; Nybo, L.; Larsen, F.J.; Cardinale, D.A.; Jensen, K.; Holmberg, H.-C. No Superior Adaptations to Carbohydrate Periodization in Elite Endurance Athletes. *Med. Sci. Sports Exerc.* **2017**, *49*, 2486–2497. **[Google Scholar]** **[PubMed]** **[Green Version]**

154. Holloszy, J.O.; Coyle, E.F. Adaptations of skeletal muscle to endurance exercise and their metabolic consequences. *J. Appl. Physiol. Respir. Environ. Exerc. Physiol.* **1984**, *56*, 831–838. **[Google Scholar]** **[PubMed]**

155. Larsen, S.; Nielsen, J.; Hansen, C.N.; Nielsen, L.B.; Wibrand, F.; Stride, N.; Schroder, H.D.; Boushel, R.; Helge, J.W.; Dela, F.; et al. Biomarkers of mitochondrial content in skeletal muscle of healthy young human subjects. *J. Physiol.* **2012**, *590*, 3349–3360. **[Google Scholar]**

156. Andrade-Souza, V.A.; Ghiarone, T.; Sansonio, A.; Santos Silva, K.A.; Tomazini, F.; Arcoverde, L.; Fyfe, J.; Perri, E.; Saner, N.; Kuang, J.; et al. Exercise twice-a-day potentiates markers of mitochondrial biogenesis in men. *FASEB J.* **2020**, *34*, 1602–1619. **[Google Scholar]** **[Green Version]**

157. Charlot, K.; Pichon, A.; Chapelot, D. Effets de l'entraînement à jeun sur la V˙ O2max, l'oxydation des lipides et la performance aérobie chez des jeunes hommes modérément entraînés. *Sci. Sports* **2016**, *31*, 166–171. **[Google Scholar]**

158. Burke, L.M.; Ross, M.L.; Garvican-Lewis, L.A.; Welvaert, M.; Heikura, I.A.; Forbes, S.G.; Mirtschin, J.G.; Cato, L.E.; Strobel, N.; Sharma, A.P.; et al. Low carbohydrate, high fat diet impairs exercise economy and negates the performance benefit from intensified training in elite race walkers. *J. Physiol.* **2017**, *595*, 2785–2807. **[Google Scholar]** **[Green Version]**

159. Burke, L.M.; Sharma, A.P.; Heikura, I.A.; Forbes, S.F.; Holloway, M.; McKay, A.K.A.; Bone, J.L.; Leckey, J.J.; Welvaert, M.; Ross, M.L. Crisis of confidence averted: Impairment of exercise economy and performance in elite race walkers by ketogenic low carbohydrate, high fat (LCHF) diet is reproducible. *PLoS ONE* **2020**, *15*, e0234027. **[Google Scholar]**

160. Lundby, C.; Montero, D.; Joyner, M. Biology of VO2max: Looking under the physiology lamp. *J. Acta Physiol.* **2017**, *220*, 218–228. **[Google Scholar]**

161. Impey, S.G.; Hearris, M.A.; Hammond, K.M.; Bartlett, J.D.; Louis, J.; Close, G.L.; Morton, J.P. Fuel for the work required: A theoretical framework for carbohydrate periodization and the glycogen threshold hypothesis. *Sports Med.* **2018**, *48*, 1031–1048. **[Google Scholar] [PubMed] [Green Version]**

162. Van Proeyen, K.; Szlufcik, K.; Nielens, H.; Deldicque, L.; Van Dyck, R.; Ramaekers, M.; Hespel, P. High-fat diet overrules the effects of training on fiber-specific intramyocellular lipid utilization during exercise. *J. Appl. Physiol. (1985)* **2011**, *111*, 108–116. **[Google Scholar] [PubMed] [Green Version]**

163. Durkalec-Michalski, K.; Zawieja, E.E.; Zawieja, B.E.; Jurkowska, D.; Buchowski, M.S.; Jeszka, J. Effects of Low Versus Moderate Glycemic Index Diets on Aerobic Capacity in Endurance Runners: Three-Week Randomized Controlled Crossover Trial. *Nutrients* **2018**, *10*, 370. **[Google Scholar] [PubMed] [Green Version]**

164. Podlogar, T.; Free, B.; Wallis, G.A. High rates of fat oxidation are maintained after the sleep low approach despite delayed carbohydrate feeding during exercise. *Eur. J. Sport Sci.* **2020**, 1–11. **[Google Scholar] [PubMed]**

165. Heikura, I.A.; Stellingwerff, T.; Burke, L.M. Self-reported periodization of nutrition in elite female and male runners and race walkers. *Front. Physiol.* **2018**, *9*, 1732. **[Google Scholar] [PubMed]**

12

Chapter

# BETAINE SUPPLEMENTATION MAY ENHANCE HEAT TOLERANCE: POTENTIAL MECHANISMS IN HUMANS

## 1. INTRODUCTION : AN OVERVIEW

In the contemporary global civilization, the necessity for individuals to engage in labor under high temperatures is escalating [1,2]. Heat stress impacts manual laborers, military people, and athletes, resulting in around 620 fatalities annually in the United States and thousands worldwide. Consequently, techniques to mitigate heat stress and extend exercise or activity duration in high temperatures have been thoroughly investigated [7,8,9,10]. Broadly, these strategies can be categorized into *physical* and *nutritional* strategies. Physical strategies may include pre-cooling, cold water immersion, misting fans, and/or altering clothing [**11**]. These strategies have gained popularity among sports medical personnel and shown various levels of efficacy. Nutritional methods, mostly focused on preserving plasma volume through the consumption of substantial amounts of electrolytes, carbohydrates, and cold drinks, are also crucial in mitigating heat stress. One of the nutritional treatments for managing heat stress is the intake of betaine. The articles for this review were obtained through the PubMed. gov search engine by querying the phrase "Betaine" both independen These strategies have gained popularity among sports medical personnel and shown various levels of efficacy. Nutritional methods, mostly focused on preserving plasma volume through the consumption of substantial amounts of electrolytes, carbohydrates, and cold drinks, are also crucial in mitigating heat stress. One of the nutritional treatments for managing heat stress is the intake of betaine.

The articles for this review were obtained through the PubMed.gov search engine by querying the phrase "Betaine" both independently and in combination with "Heat Stress," "Heat Shock Proteins," "Hydration," "Gut Permeability," "Osmolytes," "Performance," and "Thermoregulation." Searches were concluded in July 2020.tly and in combination with "Heat Stress," "Heat Shock Proteins," "Hydration," "Gut Permeability," "Osmolytes," "Performance," and "Thermoregulation." Searches were concluded in July 2020.

## 2. BETAINE

Trimethylglycine (betaine) is a derivative of the amino acid glycine. Betaine can be endogenously synthesized through the metabolism of choline, or exogenously consumed through dietary intake [12]. Although betaine concentrations in foods vary depending on cooking and preparation methods, grain products and vegetables such as wheat bran (1340 mg·100 $g^{-1}$), wheat germ (1240 mg·100 $g^{-1}$), spinach (600–645 mg·100 $g^{-1}$), and beets (114–297 mg·100 $g^{-1}$) are the best sources of dietary betaine [13]. Average dietary intake for Western culture typically ranges from 100 to 400 mg·$day^{-1}$, with a mean of 208 ± 90 mg·$day^{-1}$ and results in an average resting plasma betaine concentration of 0.02–0.07 mmol·$L^{-1}$ [14,15]. As betaine is a short-chain, neutral, amino acid derivative, absorption across the enterocyte is thought to primarily use the sodium-dependent Amino Acid Transport System A, however sodium-independent absorption is also known to occur [12,16]. A single dose of betaine (50 mg·$kg^{-1}$) in healthy young men (mean age: 28 years old) free of any known diseases resulted in a peak concentration of ~1 mmol·$L^{-1}$, in ~1 h [15]. The elimination half-life of a single dose of betaine is ~14 ± 7 h, with <5% of the original dose present in 72 h [15]. However, a loading strategy of 50 mg·$kg^{-1}$ per 12 h for 5 days in the same population resulted in a peak concentration of ~1.5 mmol·$L^{-1}$, ~1 h after ingestion [15]. Likewise, the elimination half-life of the five-day loading of betaine is ~41 ± 14 h, with <5% of the original dose present in 8.6 days. Thus, a five-day loading protocol of betaine increases blood concentrations 50% more than a single dose and may function nearly three times as long.

### 2.1. Methyl Donation

It is universally accepted that betaine serves two primary roles in mammalian physiology [12,17]. The first is that of a methyl donor. As the name indicates, trimethylglycine (i.e., betaine) has three methyl groups, which can serve as reagents for transmethylation reactions. If this occurs, betaine is converted into dimethylglycine, or further catabolized into sarcosine, ultimately adding to the amino acid pool as glycine [12,18]. Notably, betaine metabolism supplies methyl groups for the conversion of homocysteine to methionine [19,20], and aids in the synthesis of key metabolic proteins such as creatine [21,22] and carnitine [23], especially during periods of hypertonicity [24]. These findings have led to several lines of research that examine betaine's role in health and disease prevention [12,19,25,26,27] as well as human performance [28,29,30,31,32].

### 2.2. Osmolyte

The second role that betaine serves is that of an osmolyte. Osmolytes are organic molecules used in the regulation of intracellular fluid concentrations and cell volume [33,34]. When presented with an external hypertonic stressor, the immediate response of mammalian cells is to decrease cell volume (i.e., fluid loss) and increase inorganic solute concentrations (i.e., electrolytes) in efforts to maintain homeostasis [33]. However, this accumulation of inorganic solutes, if severe enough, can interfere with electrical signaling and protein conformation. Therefore, in order to preserve long-term cellular function, mammalian cells seek to mitigate this problem by exchanging the potentially harmful inorganic solutes for compatible organic osmolytes, such as betaine [**33**,**35**].

Indeed, when presented with hypertonic stress, membrane-bound betaine/$\gamma$-aminobutyric acid transporter 1 (BGT1) mRNA and expression are up-regulated, leading to an increase in intracellular betaine concentration [**16**,**34**]. Interestingly, once the cells are returned to an isotonic (300 mOsm) environment, BGT1 expression remains elevated for at least 24 h [**16**]. This may play an important role for individuals engaging in daily exercise in hot-humid environments creating hypertonic stress. Further supporting the importance of osmolyte accumulation, Alfieri et al. cultured porcine vascular endothelial cells in a hypertonic (500 mOsm) solution with and without osmolytes (0.1 mmol betaine and myo-inositol). Cultures without osmolytes present experienced a 63% mean reduction in cell number after 56 h, however cultures with betaine and inositol experienced only a 32% decrease in cell number during the same time [**16**]. In a separate experiment measuring morphological changes in cell cultures with and without osmolytes, the same group observed that cultures with betaine and myo-inositol grew well and maintained proper morphology, whereas those without osmolytes experienced significant apoptosis, detaching from the plates [**16**]. Thus, it appears that osmolytes, such as betaine, are responsible for decreasing hypertonic stress in mammalian cells, which results in preserved functionality and increased survivability.

Simultaneously, as an osmolyte, betaine acts to retain intracellular fluid and preserve the osmotic balance during hypertonic stress. As such, this has profound impacts on bolstering membrane integrity, which becomes particularly important for enterocytes undergoing heat stress (see the *Gut and Immune Health* section, below).

## 3. HEAT STRESS AND HEAT SHOCK PROTEINS

Training in hot-humid environments can result in several physiological changes. Most notably, during active heat stress, increases in core temperature lead to elevated peripheral blood flow and an increase in skin temperature [**36**,**37**]. If core temperature continues to increase, cholinergic eccrine sweat glands become stimulated and present an electrolyte solution of sweat to the surface of the skin [**38**]. Sweat is generated initially from the extracellular compartment, but cells will attempt to defend plasma volume and osmolality by actively excreting water to counteract the osmotic stress. Therefore, the intracellular compartment is presented with not only a thermal stress, but additionally an osmotic stress. Proteins, when presented with a great enough thermal or osmotic stress, denature and lose functionality [**39**,**40**,**41**].

To combat this loss in functionality, cells express a class of molecular chaperones known as heat shock proteins (HSPs), which are categorized by their molecular weight (i.e., HSP60, HSP70, HSP90, etc.) [**42**,**43**]. HSPs promote correct protein conformation by refolding denatured proteins and thereby reestablishing functionality [**44**]. Despite being constitutively expressed, many HSPs are considered to be stress-induced [**42**]. This suggests that the baseline concentrations of HSPs are adequate to maintain protein homeostasis, until additional cellular stress like that induced from exercise (i.e., hypertonic, thermal, acidic, oxidative, etc.) is applied. Interestingly, beyond the standard role of a molecular chaperone, HSPs have been reported to interact with the plasma membrane and extracellular matrix to signal immune cells [**42**]. This interaction may play an important role, especially in the enterocyte, with regard to the systemic immune response that occurs during heat-related injuries [**45**]. Of note, HSP expression is reactionary, suggesting that the response is not fully engaged until cellular damage has already begun.

However, betaine functions in a similar capacity to molecular chaperones (i.e., attenuating stress-induced protein denaturation), by stabilizing intracellular protein conformation through enhanced hydrogen bonding between aqueous proteins in the folded state [**41,46**]. Indeed, osmolytes have been shown to prevent or delay stress-induced denaturation as well as help refold already denatured proteins [**47,48**]. Further, when osmolytes are present, there is a decreased need for HSP up-regulation during times of cellular stress, indicating osmolytes are filling the role of HSPs, attenuating cellular stress [**16,34,49,50**].

However, a hierarchy may exist for the cellular response to stress. It has been demonstrated that thermal stress alone (42 °C in an isotonic environment for 3 h) resulted in a ~15-fold increase in HSP70 mRNA expression, but no reported change in BGT1 expression in madin-darby canine kidney (MDCK) cells [**34**]. However, hypertonicity alone (515 mOsm in a thermoneutral environment for 3 h) resulted in an up regulation of both HSP70 and BGT1 mRNA expression [**34**]. Additionally, compared to a physiological neutral (7.4 pH), an acidic environment (6.5 pH) has been shown to increase the expression of HSP72 in MDCK cells ~2-fold [**51**]. In the same study, when combining an acidic environment (6.5 pH) with a hypertonic insult (+50 mM NaCl, ~400 mOsm, or +150 mM NaCl, ~600 mOsm), HSP72 expression experienced a ~6-fold and ~9-fold increase, respectively [**51**]. Likewise, incubating MDCK cells in a medium with hyperkalemic insult (20 and 40 mM $K^+$) resulted in a modest but significant ~2-fold increase in HSP72 expression [**51**]. Additionally, using an in vitro CYP2E1 human hepatoblastoma cell line, betaine was shown to reduce the mRNA expression of HSP70 when presented with oxidative stress [**52**]. Taken together, this further supports the idea that mammalian cells rely upon HSPs to defend against many types of cellular stress (i.e., thermal, hypertonic, acidic, oxidative) and that intracellular betaine accumulation may aid in this defense by acting in a similar capacity to HSPs.

Yet, organisms of higher order and complexity may not behave as is observed in cell culture models. Nevertheless, using an animal model, Dangi et al. demonstrated that goats supplemented with betaine and subjected to long-term heat stress (42 °C, 36 ± 2% RH, 6 h per day, for 16 days) produced significantly lower concentrations of HSP60, HSP70, and HSP90 compared to those without betaine [**53**]. Thus, similar to cell culture data, betaine was effective in combating cellular heat stress as evidenced by a reduced need for HSP expression. These data demonstrate that animals consuming betaine were able to withstand the heat stress with reduced cellular responses and could therefore, theoretically, withstand a greater heat load before experiencing detrimental consequences. In human models, Walsh et al. demonstrated that treadmill running (70% $VO_2$ peak for 60 min) at room temperature (20 °C, <40% RH) was a sufficient stimulus to increase serum HSP70 expression [**54**]. However, to our knowledge, there is no research in humans examining the relationship between osmolyte supplementation and HSP expression. More research is needed to further elucidate these findings and to determine if they translate to human models.

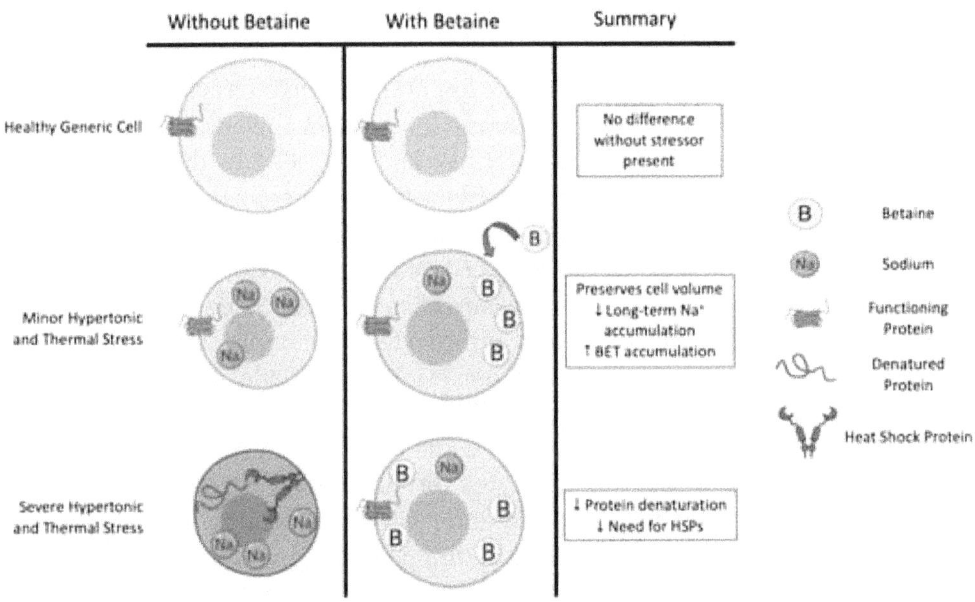


**Figure 1. Betaine's potential role in preserving cell function during increasing severities of hypertonic and thermal stress, as evidenced by data from cell culture models. BET: betaine, HSPs: heat shock proteins, $Na^+$: sodium.**

Thus, it appears that in cell culture and animal models, HSP expression is quite sensitive to many types of cellular stress that may compromise intracellular proteins' shape and function (i.e., hyperthermia, hypertonicity, acidity, hyperkalemia, and oxidative stress). When present in great enough quantity, intracellular osmolytes appear to be the preferred method of combatting many types of cellular stress, insomuch as they attenuate the stressor and thereby delay the onset of HSP expression (**Figure 1**). Although not measured specifically during every type of cellular stress, it appears that hypertonicity is the specific stimulus required to up-regulate the betaine transporter [**34**]. Against the two primary stressors associated with exercising in hot-humid conditions (thermal and hypertonic), betaine attenuated the mRNA expression for HSP70 by >50%, suggesting a greater protection against these types of cellular stress [**34**]. Pre-loading betaine prior to the cellular stress may be important, as it appears that betaine is more effective at stabilizing and preventing the initial denaturation process of proteins compared to the refolding of proteins [**55**]. Further, there may be an additive effect if the cellular stress is too great for either method (HSP expression or pre-loading betaine) alone. If true at a systemic level, this should lead to prolonged cellular function and exercise capacity in humans.

## 4. GUT AND IMMUNE HEALTH

Lipopolysaccharide (LPS) is an endotoxin associated with the cell membrane of Gram-negative bacteria, and is commonly found in the gastrointestinal tract of mammals [**56,57**]. The presentation of toxins (e.g., LPS) and gut bacteria into the blood is termed endotoxemia and is thought to be a primary pathway of heat stroke. Indeed, several studies displayed symptoms of endotoxemia in animals [**58,59**] and humans with heat-related injuries [**58,60,61**].

The mechanism by which LPS is thought to enter systemic circulation is through a breakdown of tight junctions and membrane integrity in the gut, thereby increasing intestinal permeability. As exercise intensity and the need to dissipate body heat increases, functional sympatholysis shunts blood flow away from the viscera and toward the active tissue and periphery. Physical activity has been shown to reduce intestinal blood flow by 40–80% of resting values [**62,63,64,65**], with even greater reductions in blood flow occurring when heat stress accompanies exercise [**58,64,66**]. This significant decrease in intestinal perfusion leaves enterocytes vulnerable to severe stress (i.e., hypoxia-related oxidative stress, ATP depletion, and acidosis), which results in quantifiable injury and increased permeability of the small intestine [**45,67,68,69,70**]. Increased intestinal permeability allows LPS and related bacteria to translocate across the tight junctions or through enterocytes into the blood [**58,71,72,73**]. While not uncommon for small amounts of LPS to enter portal circulation, it is thought to be quickly detoxified and cleared via the liver and never enter systemic circulation [**58**]. However, stressors (e.g., exercise in the heat) can lead to increased concentrations of LPS entering portal circulation, thereby overwhelming hepatic defenses and promoting immune responses and signs of exertional heat stroke [**65,68**].

Indeed, when severe enough, LPS in the blood causes elevated presentation of liver enzymes alanine aminotransferase (ALT) and aspartate aminotransferase (AST) in the serum. Despite these enzymes being non-specific (that is, they are known to be elevated from several stimuli), elevations may indicate the presence of hepatic injury [**65,74,75**]. Demonstrating this, injections of LPS (5 mg·kg$^{-1}$) into the tail vein of rats significantly increased serum expression of ALT (LPS: 805.8 ± 245.0 units·mL$^{-1}$ vs. CON: 38.1 ± 3.8 units·mL$^{-1}$; $p < 0.05$) and AST (LPS: 651.0 ± 101.6 units·mL$^{-1}$ vs. CON: 82.1 ± 3.7 units·mL$^{-1}$; $p < 0.05$) [**75**]. Further, LPS in systemic circulation results in a rise in several markers of inflammation [**45,70,76,77,78**], most notably tumor necrosis factor-α (TNF-α) and interleukin-6 (IL-6) [**74,79**]. In the same study, injections of 5 mg·kg$^{-1}$ LPS into the tail vein of rats significantly increased serum expression of inflammatory cytokine TNF-α (LPS: 20.9 ± 0.7 ng·mL$^{-1}$ vs. CON: <0.01 ng·mL$^{-1}$; $p < 0.05$) [**75**]. Similarly, 90 min after injection with 0.3 ng *E. coli* LPS·kg$^{-1}$, humans display a significant increase in plasma TNF-α (~19-fold, $p < 0.05$) and IL-6 (~17-fold, $p < 0.05$), compared to baseline values [**79**].

Large increases in inflammatory markers, such as the ones evident in this study, can be suggestive of increased gut permeability and heat-related injury as temperature-dependent endotoxemia is known to result in large increases in inflammatory markers [**45,69,71**].

Importantly, betaine may be able to attenuate or prevent symptoms of heat-related injuries at key steps along the proposed pathway. There is some evidence that suggests betaine is able to attenuate or entirely prevent oxidative stress [**52,80**]. If true within the stressed enterocyte, this should minimize exercise-induced cellular damage and may help maintain membrane integrity, thereby preventing the translocation of endotoxins across the gut. In a key study, Ganesan et al., using a rat model, tested the effects of pre-loaded betaine (250 mg·kg·day$^{-1}$ dissolved in distilled water for 30 days) on indicators of oxidative stress with and without additional restraint stress (immobilization for 6 h·day$^{-1}$ for 30 days) [**80**]. Restraint stress alone resulted in significant increases in plasma corticosterone ($p < 0.001$), alongside significant decreases in betaine concentrations within the thymus and spleen ($p < 0.001$). Coinciding with the decrease in betaine concentration in the thymus and spleen, the restraint-stressed rats experienced statistically significant decreases in antioxidant function (glutathione peroxidase activity ($p < 0.001$), glutathione-S-transferase activity ($p < 0.001$), superoxide dismutase activity ($p < 0.001$), and catalase activity ($p < 0.001$)) compared to the non-stressed control group. Conversely, rats that experienced the restraint stress and pre-loaded with betaine for 30 days had a significant increase in betaine within the thymus and spleen ($p < 0.05$). Further, they did not experience a significant decrease, but were able to maintain all antioxidant markers comparable to the non-stressed control group. Interestingly, the non-stressed group that were pre-loaded with betaine did not experience significant changes in any markers of antioxidant function compared to the control group. These results suggest that betaine supplementation alone does not augment natural antioxidant capabilities but acts as another means of defending against stress-induced oxidation.

Moreover, a recent study by Wang et al. described betaine's effect on gut health in high-salt (4.0% NaCl in the diet)-stressed rats with and without supplemental betaine (0.0%, 0.5%, 1.0%) dissolved in the water supply for 28 days [**81**]. Compared to the high-salt-stressed condition without betaine, betaine (0.5% and 1.0%) significantly improved markers of gut health (intestinal villi length and the ratio of villus height to crypt depth) across the duodenum ($p < 0.05$), jejunum ($p < 0.05$), and ileum ($p < 0.05$) [**81**]. However, betaine did not significantly alter plasma, liver, or intestinal osmolarity ($p > 0.05$), suggesting betaine was able to bolster these cells against the hypertonic stress and maintain normal osmolarity in these tissues.

These data demonstrate that betaine may reduce oxidative stress and improve gut health, both of which may attenuate LPS translocation. However, if LPS translocation remains unabated, liver damage and elevated inflammatory responses are known to occur. Yet, even in the presence of 5 mg·kg$^{-1}$ LPS in systemic circulation, 1% betaine supplementation added to the water supply (consumption of ~1.5 g·kg$^{-1}$, for 14 days) resulted in an attenuation of circulating TNF-α, ALT, and AST concentrations ($p < 0.05$) using a rat model [75]. Additionally, betaine supplementation has been shown to reduce total leukocyte count in heat-stressed animal models. Leukocytes are a class of immune cells that aid in the identification or disposal of foreign cells. Non-heat-stressed broiler chickens have a normal total leukocyte count of $1.14–1.17 \times 10^4$ cells·μL$^{-1}$ [**82**] and this value rises when presented with cellular stress [**83**]. Khattak et al. measured markers of immune response in broiler chickens supplemented with or without betaine when exposed to cyclical heat stress (10 h, 32–35 °C, 75–85% RH). The control group experienced a significant increase in total leukocyte count, whereas betaine supplementation was able to attenuate this immune response (BET: $1.5 \times 10^4$ cells·μL$^{-1}$ vs. CON: $3.2 \times 10^4$ cells·μL$^{-1}$; $p < 0.05$) [**84**].

Collectively, these data from cell culture and animal models demonstrate that betaine can independently reduce measures of oxidative damage, improve enterocyte health, as well as attenuate markers of potential liver damage and inflammatory responses to LPS endotoxemia (**Figure 2**). Thus, betaine bolsters cells against several key points in the proposed mechanistic pathway of LPS endotoxemia and may prevent heat-related injuries.

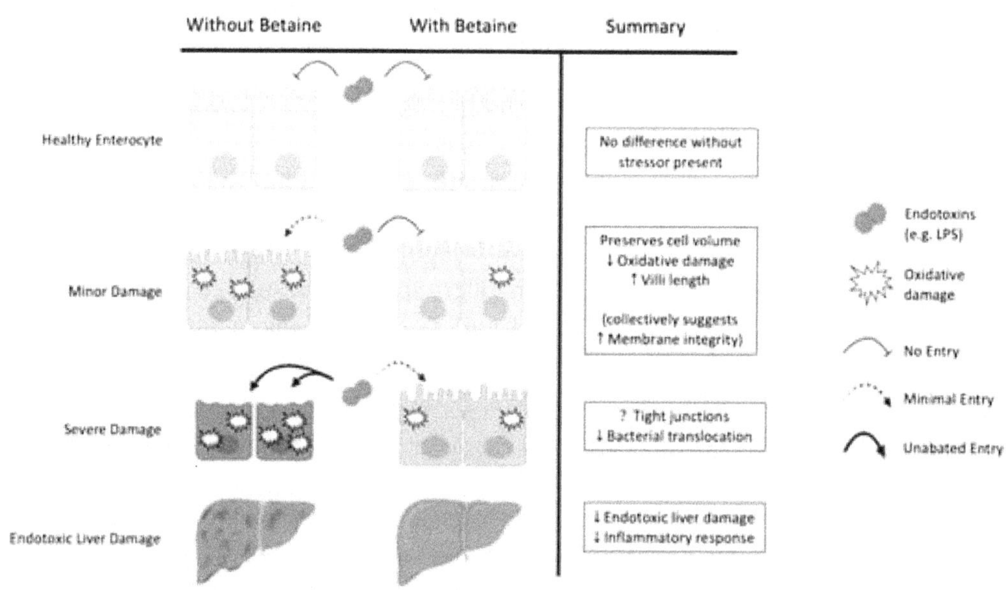


**Figure 2. Betaine's potential role in minimizing gut permeability through the preservation of enterocyte integrity and function during increasing severities of damage, as evidenced by data from cell culture and animal models.**

## 5. ANIMAL MODELS OF HEAT STRESS

As core temperature is a key indicator of exercise-associated GI disturbances [77,78,85,86], if betaine can attenuate the rise in core temperature during exercise in the heat, endotoxemia and thereby heat-related injuries may be preventable. The majority of this work has been performed in animal models (i.e., chickens, cows, ducks, goats, poultry, and sheep) with most demonstrating betaine to effectively combat thermal stress [**84,87,88,89**].

Pre-loading betaine has been shown to effectively reduce core temperature in the short (6 days), medium (21 days), and long term (63 days) in animal models exposed to cyclical heat stress. Specifically, Zulkifli et al. showed that 50 $g{\cdot}kg^{-1}$ betaine supplementation in water reduced rectal temperature (BET: 44.75 ± 0.21 °C vs. CON: 45.61 ± 0.28 °C; $p < 0.05$) in broiler chickens exposed to cyclical heat stress (4 h, 36 ± 1 °C, 75% RH) for six days [**90**]. Likewise, using sheep exposed to cyclical heat stress (43 °C, 49% RH, 8 h/day, 21 days), DiGiacomo et al. demonstrated that BET supplementation (2 $g{\cdot}day^{-1}$ BET in the feed) decreased core (BET: 39.6 °C vs. CON: 40.1 °C; $p < 0.001$) and skin (BET: 38.0 °C vs. CON: 39.3 °C; $p < 0.001$) temperature compared to the heat-stressed control group [**91**]. Moreover, Attia et al. using 1.0 $g{\cdot}kg^{-1}$ BET supplementation in the feed, demonstrated a reduced core temperature during (BET: 41.9 ± 0.50 °C vs. CON: 43.2 ± 0.60 °C; $p < 0.05$) and after (BET: 40.5 ± 0.22 °C vs. CON: 41.3 ± 0.57 °C; $p < 0.05$) exposure to cyclical heat stress (38 °C, 49% RH, 6 $h{\cdot}day^{-1}$, 3 successive $days{\cdot}week^{-1}$, for nine weeks) in slow-growing chicks compared to a heat-stressed control [**92**]. Further, in broiler chickens exposed to natural cyclical heating patterns (10 h, 32–35 °C, 75–85% RH), betaine supplementation has been shown to decrease the mortality rate by 10-fold (BET: 3.3% vs. CON: 33%, $p < 0.05$) [**84**]. Coupling these data with the reduced need for HSP expression in goats exposed to heat stress [**53**], it becomes evident that betaine may play a significant, direct role in managing heat stress.

Additionally, betaine supplementation may play an indirect role in managing heat stress through alterations in cellular metabolism and blood chemistry. Several researchers have demonstrated that broiler chickens without betaine supplementation experienced a reduction in mitochondrial function when exposed to heat stress [**87,93**]. However, betaine supplementation successfully attenuated this loss, restoring function to thermoneutral levels [**87**]. Although the exact mechanism is unclear, mitochondrial function may be improved due to decreased osmotic stress and thereby decreased reactive oxygen species formation [**80,94**]. While an increase in metabolism may seem counter-intuitive to promote heat dissipation, some researchers speculate that the decreases in lean mass and an increased mortality rate associated with heat stress are due to the inability to produce enough ATP to pant (i.e., hyperventilate) effectively [**95**].

In addition to restoring mitochondrial function, betaine has been shown to alter blood chemistry. Indeed, increases in red blood cell count (BET: 2.75 $M{\cdot}\mu L^{-1}$ vs. CON: 2.45 $M{\cdot}\mu L^{-1}$; $p < 0.001$), hemoglobin count (BET: 18.72 $g{\cdot}dL^{-1}$ vs. CON: 15.02 $g{\cdot}dL^{-1}$; $p = 0.005$), and hematocrit percentage (BET: 38.63% vs. CON: 28.63%; $p < 0.001$) have been demonstrated in meat-type ducks supplemented with betaine [**96**]. The changes in blood composition resulted in an increase in the partial pressure of oxygen (BET: 55.03 mmHg vs. CON: 37.34 mmHg; $p < 0.001$) thereby increasing oxygen carrying capacity [**96**]. These adaptations are thought to be a prerequisite to successful aerobic performance, especially in the heat. Therefore, betaine supplementation may not only affect heat tolerance, but perhaps also exercise performance in the heat.

Additionally, betaine supplementation has been shown to alter blood electrolyte concentrations during heat stress [**84,96**]. It is expected that heat-stressed broiler chickens experience a decrease in blood electrolyte concentrations, compared to chickens in a thermoneutral environment [**97**]. Yet, data measuring betaine's effects on electrolyte concentrations are equivocal. In broiler chickens exposed to cyclical heat stress, betaine supplementation significantly lowered serum $Na^+$ (BET: 229.4 g·kg$^{-1}$ vs. CON: 305.8 g·kg$^{-1}$; $p < 0.05$) and $K^+$ (BET: 26.6 g·kg$^{-1}$ vs. CON: 30.0 g·kg$^{-1}$; $p < 0.05$), but did not significantly change serum $Cl^-$ compared to the control [**84**]. Conversely, Park and Kim et al. using whole blood from heat-stressed ducks, found a significant increase in $Na^+$ (BET: 145.52 mEq·kg$^{-1}$ vs. CON: 126.82 mEq·kg$^{-1}$; $p < 0.05$), $K^+$ (BET: 3.17 mEq·kg$^{-1}$ vs. CON: 2.60 mEq·kg$^{-1}$; $p < 0.05$), and $Cl^-$ (BET: 120.53 mEq·kg$^{-1}$ vs. CON: 105.61 mEq·kg$^{-1}$; $p < 0.05$) concentrations with betaine supplementation [**96**]. The mechanisms by which betaine supplementation impacts electrolyte concentrations during heat stress remains unclear.

It is clear, however, that betaine supplementation has decreased core temperature, decreased mortality rate, and altered the composition of blood through direct and indirect means in several animal models when experiencing heat stress (**Table 1**). It is important to note that these results are in animals experiencing passive heat stress and may not accurately reflect humans undergoing active heat stress. Yet, if these data translate to human models well, it is reasonable to expect that many people (e.g., athletes, factory or field workers, military personnel) undergoing work in hot-humid conditions will benefit. More research is needed to determine if the same physiological changes occur when experiencing active vs. passive heat loads in human models.

**Table 1. Animal models successfully using BET to combat passive thermal stress.**

| Author | Population | Supplementation | Thermal Stress | Significant Findings (Compared to Identified CON) |
|---|---|---|---|---|
| **Zulkifli et al., 2004** | Chickens (N = 150) | Ad libitum intake, water supplemented with 0 (CON) or 50 g·kg$^{-1}$ BET | Cyclical heat stress (36 °C, 75% RH) for 4 h·day$^{-1}$, 6 days | BET ↓↓ core temperature immediately post-heat stress |
| **Attia et al., 2009** | Chickens (N = 300) | Ad libitum intake, feed supplemented with 0 (CON) or 1.0 g·kg$^{-1}$ BET | Cyclical heat stress (38 °C, 49% RH) for 6 h·day$^{-1}$, 3 days·week$^{-1}$, 9 weeks | BET ↓↓ core temperature during and after heat stress<br>BET ↑↑ Hgb during and after heat stress<br>BET ↓↓ blood pH during, but not after heat stress |

| Author | Population | Supplementation | Thermal Stress | Significant Findings (Compared to Identified CON) |
|---|---|---|---|---|
| **Khattak et al., 2012** | Chickens (N = 250) | Ad libitum intake, feed supplemented with 0 (CON) or 1.2 $g \cdot kg^{-1}$ BET | Natural daily cyclical heat stress (30–41 °C, 40–93% RH), 35 days | BET ↓↓ total leukocyte count<br>BET ↓↓ mortality 10-fold |
| **Dangi et al., 2015** | Goats (N = 18) | Intramuscular injections of saline (CON) or saline + 0.2 $g \cdot kg^{-1}$ BET immediately prior to heat stress | Cyclical heat stress (42 °C, 36% RH) for 6 $h \cdot day^{-1}$, 16 days | BET ↓↓ HSP60, HSP70, and HSP90 |
| **DiGiacomo et al., 2016** | Sheep (N = 36) | Ad libitum intake, feed supplemented with 0 (CON), 2, or 4 g BET daily in morning feed | Cyclical heat stress (43 °C, 49% RH) for 8 $h \cdot day^{-1}$, 21 days | BET (2 g) + Heat ↓↓ core and skin temperature |
| **Sahebi Ala et al., 2017** | Chickens (N = 1200) | BET as a replacement for 30% methionine needs according to methyl groups | Cyclical heat stress (32 °C, 40% RH) for 6 $h \cdot day^{-1}$, 31 days | BET + Heat ↔↔ mitochondrial Complex-1 function, whereas Heat alone ↓↓ mitochondrial Complex-1 function |
| **Park and Kim, 2017** | Ducks (N = 360) | Ad libitum intake, water supplemented with 0 (CON), 700, 1000, or 1300 ppm BET | Cyclical heat stress (33–43 °C, 70% RH) for 8 $h \cdot day^{-1}$, 20 days | All doses of BET<br>↑↑ RBC count, Hct, and Hgb<br>↑↑ $PO_2$ and $PCO_2$<br>↓↓ blood pH<br>↑↑ Blood electrolyte concentrations ($Na^+$, $K^+$, $Cl^-$) |

BET: betaine, $Cl^-$: chloride, CON: control group, Hct: hematocrit, Hgb: hemoglobin, HSP: heat shock protein, $K^+$: potassium, $Na^+$: sodium, $PCO_2$: partial pressure of carbon dioxide, $PO_2$: partial pressure of oxygen, ppm: parts per million, RBC: red blood cell, RH: relative humidity.

## 6. HUMAN MODELS OF HEAT STRESS

Despite these findings in animals, there is a gap in the knowledge regarding betaine's ability to attenuate thermal stress in humans. In fact, only one study has specifically examined this phenomenon in humans **[98]**. The study examined acute intake of betaine on thermoregulation and rehydration after a dehydrating protocol (2.7% body mass loss) in the heat (31.1 ± 0.7 °C, 34.7 ± 5.5% RH) in 10 male runners (age: 20 ± 2 years, height: 177 ± 6 cm, weight: 70.6 ± 6.8 kg, body fat: 6.2 ± 2.1%, $VO_2$: 63.5 ± 4.1 $mL \cdot kg \cdot min^{-1}$). It is no surprise that these authors report limited data supporting betaine's ability to combat thermal stress, as rehydration after a dehydrating thermal stress effectively bypasses betaine's preventative role in protein stabilization. Specifically, these authors found that 5 g of betaine dissolved in a carbohydrate drink did not significantly affect core or skin temperature during exercise. Yet, participants with betaine supplementation did report a lower perceived thermal sensation prior to (BET: 4.1 ± 0.2 vs. CON: 4.5 ± 0.2; $p < 0.05$) and immediately following (BET: 7.3 ± 0.2 vs. CON: 7.6 ± 0.1; $p < 0.05$) 75 min of treadmill running at 65% $VO_2$ max [**98**]. Additionally, betaine supplementation increased oxygen consumption during the sprinting protocol (84% $VO_2$ max) to exhaustion (BET: 55.0 ± 5.7 mL·kg·min$^{-1}$ vs. CON: 52.3 ± 2.7 mL·kg·min$^{-1}$; $p < 0.05$) [**98**]. Increasing oxygen consumption during exercise is universally considered to be an advantage if it translates to an increase in performance. In this particular study, although betaine significantly increased oxygen consumption, this did not lead to a significant improvement in treadmill sprint duration (BET: 228 ± 173 s vs. CON: 196 ± 119 s; $p = 0.12$). Although not statistically significant, an increase in mean sprint duration of 32 s is physiologically meaningful for athletes.

It is important to highlight that the studies demonstrating improved heat tolerance in animal models supplemented with betaine chronically in the feed or the water supply [**84,87,88,89,91,99,100**]. This strategy provides a daily dose of betaine, thereby loading the compound within the body. However, the human study examining heat tolerance never implemented a loading strategy but examined an acute dosage. Moreover, Armstrong et al. examined rehydration, thereby introducing betaine after the thermal stress was applied. This effectively negates the protein stabilization effects betaine has been shown to demonstrate [**48,55**].

## 7. CONCISE SUMMARY

Osmolytes, including betaine, mitigate hypertonic stress in mammalian cells, hence preserving functionality and enhancing survivability. Betaine has demonstrated the ability to mitigate several forms of cellular stressors, including hyperthermia, hypertonicity, acidity, hyperkalemia, and oxidative stress, which necessitate the assistance of molecular chaperones. Betaine can autonomously diminish indicators of oxidative damage, enhance enterocyte health, and mitigate signs of possible liver damage and inflammatory reactions to LPS endotoxemia. Consequently, betaine fortifies cells against multiple critical aspects of the suggested molecular pathway of LPS endotoxemia and may avert heat-induced damage.

Employing diverse dosage regimens in animal models, dietary pre-loading of betaine has demonstrated a reduction in core temperature, cutaneous temperature, mortality rate, and oxidative damage. Numerous elite and recreational athletes engage in prolonged exercise in hot-humid conditions and experience various stresses, including hyperthermia, hypertonicity, acidity, and oxidative damage. Supplemental pre-loaded betaine may effectively address these difficulties, as demonstrated in animal studies. If accurate on a systemic scale, pre-loading with betaine may enhance heat tolerance and offer athletes, for whom heat stress is a significant constraint, an additional means of safeguarding their training and performance. However, this remains conjectural unless empirical evidence substantiates such effects in humans.

## 8. FURTHER STUDY

This review elucidates various distinct avenues for investigation. Initially, researchers should strive to extrapolate findings from mammalian cell cultures of various species to humans. Future study should specifically assess the effects of betaine on various cellular stressors (e.g., hypertonic, heat, oxidative, acidic, etc.) both in isolation and in combination, utilizing specific tissues or tissue analogs (e.g., human enterocytes, hepatocytes, and skeletal muscle). Secondly, future researchers should investigate the effects of pre-loaded betaine on people under conditions of passive and active heat stress, when both cellular stressors are expected to occur. Future researchers should specifically assess indicators of heat stress, hypertonic stress, and metabolic alterations. Finally, subsequent study should investigate the effects of pre-loaded betaine on immune response during exercise in elevated temperatures to ascertain whether the suggested mechanism for endotoxin translocation may be enhanced by a sequence of exposures and adaptations (i.e., gut training). These considerations will enhance the understanding of how athletes might utilize betaine supplementation to improve safety and performance in conditions when heat and humidity present challenges.

## AT A GLANCE

Betaine has been shown to enhance tolerance to hypertonic and temperature stresses. Intracellular betaine operates at the cellular level akin to molecular chaperones, thereby diminishing the requirement for the expression of inducible heat shock proteins. Besides regulating protein conformations, betaine has been shown to mitigate oxidative damage. In enterocytes, during instances of diminished perfusion and increased oxidative, thermal, and hypertonic stress (such as extended exercise in hot and humid environments), betaine enhances villi length and demonstrates improved membrane integrity. This collectively diminishes exercise-induced intestinal permeability, safeguarding against bacterial translocation and endotoxemia. Chronic betaine consumption at the systemic level has been demonstrated to lower core temperature, decrease all-cause mortality, reduce inflammation markers, and alter blood chemistry in many animal models subjected to heat stress. Notwithstanding compelling research in cell culture and animal models, there is only a single published study investigating betaine's thermoregulatory function in humans. Should the same principle apply to humans, chronic betaine intake may enhance heat tolerance and offer an additional supplements option for individuals who consider heat stress a significant element in their occupational or athletic training. This remains conjectural unless evidence confirms similar effects in humans.

## REFERENCES


1. Kark, J.A.; Burr, P.Q.; Wenger, C.B.; Gastaldo, E.; Gardner, J.W. Exertional heat illness in marine corps recruit training. *Aviat. Space Environ. Med.* **1996**, *67*, 354–360. **[Google Scholar] [PubMed]**
2. Wallace, R.F.; Kriebel, D.; Punnett, L.; Wegman, D.H.; Wenger, C.B.; Gardner, J.W.; Gonzalez, R.R. The effects of continuous hot weather training on risk of exertional heat illness. *Med. Sci. Sports Exerc.* **2005**, *37*, 84–90. **[Google Scholar] [PubMed]**
3. Berko, J.; Ingram, D.D.; Saha, S.; Parker, J.D. Deaths attributed to heat, cold, and other weather events in the United States, 2006–2010. *Natl. Health Stat. Rep.* **2014**, *2014*, 1–15. **[Google Scholar]**
4. Argaud, L.; Ferry, T.; Le, Q.H.; Marfisi, A.; Ciorba, D.; Achache, P.; Ducluzeau, R.; Robert, D. Short- and long-term outcomes of heatstroke following the 2003 heat wave in Lyon, France. *Arch. Intern. Med.* **2007**, *167*, 2177–2183. **[Google Scholar] [PubMed] [Green Version]**
5. Azhar, G.S.; Mavalankar, D.; Nori-Sarma, A.; Rajiva, A.; Dutta, P.; Jaiswal, A.; Sheffield, P.; Knowlton, K.; Hess, J.J. Heat-related mortality in India: Excess all-cause mortality associated with the 2010 Ahmedabad heat wave. *PLoS ONE* **2014**, *9*, e91831. **[Google Scholar]**
6. Hoffmann, B.; Hertel, S.; Boes, T.; Weiland, D.; Jöckel, K.H. Increased cause-specific mortality associated with 2003 heat wave in Essen, Germany. *J. Toxicol. Environ. Health Part A Curr. Issues* **2008**, *71*, 759–765. **[Google Scholar]**
7. Garth, A.K.; Burke, L.M. What do athletes drink during competitive sporting activities? *Sports Med.* **2013**, *43*, 539–564. **[Google Scholar]**
8. McCartney, D.; Desbrow, B.; Irwin, C. The Effect of Fluid Intake Following Dehydration on Subsequent Athletic and Cognitive Performance: A Systematic Review and Meta-analysis. *Sports Med.-Open* **2017**, *3*, 13. **[Google Scholar] [Green Version]**
9. Kenefick, R.W. Drinking Strategies: Planned Drinking Versus Drinking to Thirst. *Sports Med.* **2018**, *48*, 31–37. **[Google Scholar] [Green Version]**
10. McDermott, B.P.; Anderson, S.A.; Armstrong, L.E.; Casa, D.J.; Cheuvront, S.N.; Cooper, L.; Larry Kenney, W.; O'Connor, F.G.; Roberts, W.O. National athletic trainers' association position statement: Fluid replacement for the physically active. *J. Athl. Train.* **2017**, *52*, 877–895. **[Google Scholar] [Green Version]**
11. Casa, D.J.; DeMartini, J.K.; Bergeron, M.F.; Csillan, D.; Eichner, E.R.; Lopez, R.M.; Ferrara, M.S.; Miller, K.C.; O'Connor, F.; Sawka, M.N.; et al. National athletic trainers' association position statement: Exertional heat illnesses. *J. Athl. Train.* **2015**, *50*, 986–1000. **[Google Scholar] [PubMed] [Green Version]**
12. Craig, S.A. Betaine in human nutrition. *Am. J. Clin. Nutr.* **2004**, *80*, 539–549. **[Google Scholar] [PubMed] [Green Version]**
13. Zeisel, S.H.; Mar, M.H.; Howe, J.C.; Holden, J.M. Concentrations of choline-containing compounds and betaine in common foods. *J. Nutr.* **2003**, *133*, 1302–1307. **[Google Scholar] [PubMed]**
14. Lever, M.; Sizeland, P.C.B.; Bason, L.M.; Hayman, C.M.; Chambers, S.T. Glycine betaine and proline betaine in human blood and urine. *BBA-Gen. Subj.* **1994**, *1200*, 259–264. **[Google Scholar]**
15. Schwahn, B.C.; Hafner, D.; Hohlfeld, T.; Balkenhol, N.; Laryea, M.D.; Wendel, U. Pharmacokinetics of oral betaine in healthy subjects and patients with homocystinuria. *Br. J. Clin. Pharmacol.* **2003**, *55*, 6–13. **[Google Scholar] [PubMed] [Green Version]**
16. Alfieri, R.R.; Cavazzoni, A.; Petronini, P.G.; Bonelli, M.A.; Caccamo, A.E.; Borghetti, A.F.; Wheeler, K.P. Compatible osmolytes modulate the response of porcine endothelial cells to hypertonicity and protect them from apoptosis. *J. Physiol.* **2002**, *540*, 499–508. **[Google Scholar]**
17. Ueland, P.M. Choline and betaine in health and disease. *J. Inherit. Metab. Dis.* **2011**, *34*, 3–15. **[Google Scholar] [PubMed]**

18. Anioła, M.; Dega-Szafran, Z.; Katrusiak, A.; Szafran, M. NH···O and OH···O interactions of glycine derivatives with squaric acid. *New J. Chem.* **2014**, *38*, 3556–3568. **[Google Scholar] [Green Version]**

19. Finkelstein, J.D.; Harris, B.J.; Kyle, W.E. Methionine metabolism in mammals: Kinetic study of betaine-homocysteine methyltransferase. *Arch. Biochem. Biophys.* **1972**, *153*, 320–324. **[Google Scholar]**

20. Zeisel, S.H.; Blusztajn, J.K. Choline and human nutrition. *Annu. Rev. Nutr.* **1994**, *14*, 269–296. **[Google Scholar]**

21. Borsook, H.; Borsook, M.E. The biochemical basis of betaine-glycocyamine therapy. *Ann. West. Med. Surg.* **1951**, *5*, 825–829. **[Google Scholar] [PubMed]**

22. Da Silva, R.P.; Nissim, I.; Brosnan, M.E.; Brosnan, J.T. Creatine synthesis: Hepatic metabolism of guanidinoacetate and creatine in the rat In Vitro and In Vivo. *Am. J. Physiol.-Endocrinol. Metab.* **2009**, *296*, E256–E261. **[Google Scholar] [PubMed]**

23. Pekkinen, J.; Olli, K.; Huotari, A.; Tiihonen, K.; Keski-Rahkonen, P.; Lehtonen, M.; Auriola, S.; Kolehmainen, M.; Mykkänen, H.; Poutanen, K.; et al. Betaine supplementation causes increase in carnitine metabolites in the muscle and liver of mice fed a high-fat diet as studied by nontargeted LC-MS metabolomics approach. *Mol. Nutr. Food Res.* **2013**, *57*, 1959–1968. **[Google Scholar]**

24. Carnicelli, D.; Arfilli, V.; Onofrillo, C.; Alfieri, R.R.; Petronini, P.G.; Montanaro, L.; Brigotti, M. Cap-independent protein synthesis is enhanced by betaine under hypertonic conditions. *Biochem. Biophys. Res. Commun.* **2017**, *483*, 936–940. **[Google Scholar] [PubMed]**

25. Best, C.H.; Ridout, J.H.; Lucas, C.C. Alleviation of dietary cirrhosis by betaine and other lipotrophic agents. *Nutr. Rev.* **1969**, *27*, 269–271. **[Google Scholar]**

26. Schwab, U.; Törrönen, A.; Toppinen, L.; Alfthan, G.; Saarinen, M.; Aro, A.; Uusitupa, M. Betaine supplementation decreases plasma homocysteine concentrations but does not affect body weight, body composition, or resting energy expenditure in human subjects. *Am. J. Clin. Nutr.* **2002**, *76*, 961–967. **[Google Scholar] [Green Version]**

27. Abdelmalek, M.F.; Sanderson, S.O.; Angulo, P.; Soldevila-Pico, C.; Liu, C.; Peter, J.; Keach, J.; Cave, M.; Chen, T.; McClain, C.J.; et al. Betaine for nonalcoholic fatty liver disease: Results of a randomized placebo-controlled trial. *Hepatology* **2009**, *50*, 1818–1826. **[Google Scholar]**

28. Lee, E.C.; Maresh, C.M.; Kraemer, W.J.; Yamamoto, L.M.; Hatfield, D.L.; Bailey, B.L.; Armstrong, L.E.; Volek, J.S.; McDermott, B.P.; Craig, S.A. Ergogenic effects of betaine supplementation on strength and power performance. *J. Int. Soc. Sports Nutr.* **2010**, *7*, 27. **[Google Scholar] [Green Version]**

29. Hoffman, J.R.; Ratamess, N.A.; Kang, J.; Gonzalez, A.M.; Beller, N.A.; Craig, S.A.S. Effect of 15 days of betaine ingestion on concentric and eccentric force outputs during isokinetic exercise. *J. Strength Cond. Res.* **2011**, *25*, 2235–2241. **[Google Scholar]**

30. Pryor, J.L.; Craig, S.A.; Swensen, T. Effect of betaine supplementation on cycling sprint performance. *J. Int. Soc. Sports Nutr.* **2012**, *9*, 12. **[Google Scholar]**

31. Cholewa, J.M.; Guimarães-Ferreira, L.; Zanchi, N.E. Effects of betaine on performance and body composition: A review of recent findings and potential mechanisms. *Amino Acids* **2014**, *46*, 1785–1793. **[Google Scholar] [PubMed]**

32. Ismaeel, A. Effects of Betaine Supplementation on Muscle Strength and Power: A Systematic Review. *J. Strength Cond. Res.* **2017**, *31*, 2338–2346. **[Google Scholar] [PubMed]**

33. Burg, M.B. Molecular basis of osmotic regulation. *Am. J. Physiol.-Ren. Fluid Electrolyte Physiol.* **1995**, *268*, F983–F996. **[Google Scholar] [PubMed]**

34. Sheikh-Hamad, D.; Garcia-Perez, A.; Ferraris, J.D.; Peters, E.M.; Burg, M.B. Induction of Gene Expression by Heat Shock Versus Osmotic Stress. *Am. J. Physiol.-Ren. Fluid Electrolyte Physiol.* **1994**, *267*, F28–F34. **[Google Scholar]**

35. Garcia-Perez, A.; Burg, M.B. Renal medullary organic osmolytes. *Physiol. Rev.* **1991**, *71*, 1081–1115. **[Google Scholar]**

36. Kenefick, R.W.; Cheuvront, S.N.; Sawka, M.N. Thermoregulatory function during the marathon. *Sports Med.* **2007**, *37*, 312–315. **[Google Scholar]**

37. Rowell, L.B. Human cardiovascular adjustments to exercise and thermal stress. *Physiol. Rev.* **1974**, *54*, 75–159. **[Google Scholar]**

38. Taylor, N.A. Eccrine sweat glands. Adaptations to Physical Training and Heat Acclimation. *Sports Med.* **1986**, *3*, 387–397. **[Google Scholar]**

39. Baskakov, I.; Bolen, D.W. Forcing thermodynamically unfolded proteins to fold. *J. Biol. Chem.* **1998**, *273*, 4831–4834. **[Google Scholar]** **[Green Version]**

40. Yancey, P.H.; Clark, M.E.; Hand, S.C.; Bowlus, R.D.; Somero, G.N. Living with water stress: Evolution of osmolyte systems. *Science* **1982**, *217*, 1214–1222. **[Google Scholar]**

41. Street, T.O.; Krukenberg, K.A.; Rosgen, J.; Bolen, D.W.; Agard, D.A. Osmolyte-Induced Conformational Changes in the Hsp90 Molecular Chaperone. *Protein Sci.* **2010**, *19*, 57–65. **[Google Scholar]** **[PubMed]** **[Green Version]**

42. Zininga, T.; Ramatsui, L.; Shonhai, A. Heat shock proteins as immunomodulants. *Molecules* **2018**, *23*, 2846. **[Google Scholar]** **[PubMed]** **[Green Version]**

43. Fernández-Fernández, M.R.; Valpuesta, J.M. Hsp70 chaperone: A master player in protein homeostasis. *F1000Research* **2018**, *7*, 1497. **[Google Scholar]**

44. Young, J.C.; Moarefi, I.; Ulrich Hartl, F. Hsp90: A specialized but essential protein-folding tool. *J. Cell Biol.* **2001**, *154*, 267–273. **[Google Scholar]**

45. Pires, W.; Veneroso, C.E.; Wanner, S.P.; Pacheco, D.A.S.; Vaz, G.C.; Amorim, F.T.; Tonoli, C.; Soares, D.D.; Coimbra, C.C. Association Between Exercise-Induced Hyperthermia and Intestinal Permeability: A Systematic Review. *Sports Med.* **2017**, *47*, 1389–1403. **[Google Scholar]**

46. Street, T.O.; Bolen, D.W.; Rose, G.D. A molecular mechanism for osmolyte-induced protein stability. *Proc. Natl. Acad. Sci. USA* **2006**, *103*, 13997–14002. **[Google Scholar]** **[Green Version]**

47. Seeliger, J.; Estel, K.; Erwin, N.; Winter, R. Cosolvent effects on the fibrillation reaction of human IAPP. *Phys. Chem. Chem. Phys.* **2013**, *15*, 8902–8907. **[Google Scholar]**

48. Fan, Y.Q.; Lee, J.; Oh, S.; Liu, H.J.; Li, C.; Luan, Y.S.; Yang, J.M.; Zhou, H.M.; Lü, Z.R.; Wang, Y.L. Effects of osmolytes on human brain-type creatine kinase folding in dilute solutions and crowding systems. *Int. J. Biol. Macromol.* **2012**, *51*, 845–858. **[Google Scholar]**

49. Beck, F.X.; Grünbein, R.; Lugmayr, K.; Neuhofer, W. Heat shock proteins and the cellular response to osmotic stress. *Cell. Physiol. Biochem.* **2000**, *10*, 303–306. **[Google Scholar]** **[Green Version]**

50. Alfieri, R.R.; Petronini, P.G.; Bonelli, M.A.; Desenzani, S.; Cavazzoni, A.; Borghetti, A.F.; Wheeler, K.P. Roles of compatible osmolytes and heat shock protein 70 in the induction of tolerance to stresses in porcine endothelial cells. *J. Physiol.* **2004**, *555*, 757–767. **[Google Scholar]**

51. Neuhofer, W.; Müller, E.; Grünbein, R.; Thurau, K.; Beck, F.-X. Influence of NaCl, urea, potassium and pH on HSP72 expression in MDCK cells. *Pflügers Arch.-Eur. J. Physiol.* **1999**, *439*, 195–200. **[Google Scholar]**

52. Oliva, J.; Bardag-Gorce, F.; Tillman, B.; French, S.W. Protective effect of quercetin, EGCG, catechin and betaine against oxidative stress induced by ethanol in vitro. *Exp. Mol. Pathol.* **2011**, *90*, 295–299. **[Google Scholar]** **[PubMed]** **[Green Version]**

53. Dangi, S.S.; Dangi, S.K.; Chouhan, V.S.; Verma, M.R.; Kumar, P.; Singh, G.; Sarkar, M. Modulatory effect of betaine on expression dynamics of HSPs during heat stress acclimation in goat (Capra hircus). *Gene* **2016**, *575*, 543–550. **[Google Scholar]** **[PubMed]**

54. Walsh, R.C.; Koukoulas, I.; Garnham, A.; Moseley, P.L.; Hargreaves, M.; Febbraio, M.A. Exercise increases serum Hsp72 in humans. *Cell Stress Chaperones* **2001**, *6*, 386–393. **[Google Scholar] [PubMed] [Green Version]**

55. Bruzdźiak, P.; Panuszko, A.; Jourdan, M.; Stangret, J. Protein thermal stabilization in aqueous solutions of osmolytes. *Acta Biochim. Pol.* **2016**, *63*, 65–70. **[Google Scholar] [PubMed]**

56. Stewart, I.; Schluter, P.J.; Shaw, G.R. Cyanobacterial lipopolysaccharides and human health—A review. *Environ. Health A Glob. Access Sci. Source* **2006**, *5*, 7. **[Google Scholar]**

57. Zuhl, M.; Schneider, S.; Lanphere, K.; Conn, C.; Dokladny, K.; Moseley, P. Exercise regulation of intestinal tight junction proteins. *Br. J. Sports Med.* **2012**, *48*, 980–986. **[Google Scholar]**

58. Lim, C.L.; Mackinnon, L.T. The roles of exercise-induced immune system disturbances in the pathology of heat stroke: The dual pathway model of heat stroke. *Sports Med.* **2006**, *36*, 39–64. **[Google Scholar]**

59. Brock-Utne, J.G.; Gaffin, S.L.; Wells, M.T.; Gathiram, P.; Sohar, E.; James, M.F.; Morrell, D.F.; Norman, R.J. Endotoxaemia in exhausted runners after a long-distance race. *S. Afr. Med. J.* **1988**, *73*, 533–536. **[Google Scholar]**

60. Chao, T.C.; Sinniah, R.; Pakiam, J.E. Acute heat stroke deaths. *Pathology* **1981**, *13*, 145–156. **[Google Scholar]**

61. Shapiro, Y.; Seidman, D.S. Field and clinical observations of exertional heat stroke patients. *Med. Sci. Sports Exerc.* **1990**, *22*, 6–14. **[Google Scholar]**

62. Clausen, J.P. Effect of physical training on cardiovascular adjustments to exercise in man. *Physiol. Rev.* **1977**, *57*, 779–815. **[Google Scholar] [PubMed]**

63. Granger, D.N.; Kvietys, P.R. The Splanchnic Circulation: Intrinsic Regulation. *Annu. Rev. Physiol.* **1981**, *43*, 409–418. **[Google Scholar] [PubMed]**

64. Sakurada, S.; Hales, J.R.S. A Role for Gastrointestinal Endotoxins in Enhancement of Heat Tolerance by Physical Fitness. *J. Appl. Physiol.* **1998**, *84*, 207–214. **[Google Scholar] [PubMed] [Green Version]**

65. Van Wijck, K.; Lenaerts, K.; van Loon, L.J.C.; Peters, W.H.M.; Buurman, W.A.; Dejong, C.H.C. Exercise-Induced splanchnic hypoperfusion results in gut dysfunction in healthy men. *PLoS ONE* **2011**, *6*, e22366. **[Google Scholar] [Green Version]**

66. Moseley, P.L.; Gisolfi, C.V. New Frontiers in Thermoregulation and Exercise. *Sports Med.* **1993**, *16*, 163–167. **[Google Scholar]**

67. Hall, D.M.; Baumgardner, K.R.; Oberley, T.D.; Gisolfi, C.V. Splanchnic tissues undergo hypoxic stress during whole body hyperthermia. *Am. J. Physiol.-Gastrointest. Liver Physiol.* **1999**, *276*, G1195. **[Google Scholar]**

68. Walsh, N.P.; Gleeson, M.; Pyne, D.B.; Nieman, D.C.; Dhabhar, S.; Shephard, R.J.; Oliver, S.J.; Bermon, S.; Kajeniene, A. Position Statement. Part two: Maintaining immune health. *Exerc. Immunol. Rev.* **2011**, *17*, 64–103. **[Google Scholar]**

69. Hall, D.M.; Buettner, G.R.; Oberley, L.W.; Xu, L.; Matthes, R.D.; Gisolfi, C.V. Mechanisms of Circulatory and Intestinal Barrier Dysfunction during Whole Body Hyperthermia. *Am. J. Physiol.-Hear. Circ. Physiol.* **2001**, *280*, H509–H521. **[Google Scholar] [Green Version]**

70. Lambert, G.P. Stress-Induced Gastrointestinal Barrier Dysfunction and its Inflammatory Effects. *J. Anim. Sci.* **2009**, *87*, E101–E108. **[Google Scholar] [Green Version]**

71. Selkirk, G.A.; McLellan, T.M.; Wright, H.E.; Rhind, S.G. Mild endotoxemia, NF-κB translocation, and cytokine increase during exertional heat stress in trained and untrained individuals. *Am. J. Physiol.-Regul. Integr. Comp. Physiol.* **2008**, *295*. **[Google Scholar] [PubMed]**

72. Vargas, N.; Marino, F. Heat stress, gastrointestinal permeability and interleukin-6 signaling—Implications for exercise performance and fatigue. *Temperature* **2016**, 3, 240–251. **[Google Scholar]** **[PubMed]** **[Green Version]**

73. Alhenaky, A.; Abdelqader, A.; Abuajamieh, M.; Al-Fataftah, A.R. The effect of heat stress on intestinal integrity and Salmonella invasion in broiler birds. *J. Therm. Biol.* **2017**, *70*, 9–14. **[Google Scholar]** **[PubMed]**

74. Hamesch, K.; Borkham-Kamphorst, E.; Strnad, P.; Weiskirchen, R. Lipopolysaccharide-induced inflammatory liver injury in mice. *Lab. Anim.* **2015**, *49*, 37–46. **[Google Scholar]** **[PubMed]**

75. Kim, S.K.; Kim, Y.C. Attenuation of bacterial lipopolysaccharide-induced hepatotoxicity by betaine or taurine in rats. *Food Chem. Toxicol.* **2002**, *40*, 545–549. **[Google Scholar]**

76. Jirik, F.R.; Podor, T.J.; Hirano, T.; Kishimoto, T.; Loskutoff, D.J.; Carson, D.A.; Lotz, M. Bacterial lipopolysaccharide and inflammatory mediators augment IL-6 secretion by human endothelial cells. *J. Immunol.* **1989**, *142*, 144–147. **[Google Scholar]**

77. Snipe, R.M.J.; Costa, R.J.S. Does the temperature of water ingested during exertional-heat stress influence gastrointestinal injury, symptoms, and systemic inflammatory profile? *J. Sci. Med. Sport* **2018**, *21*, 771–776. **[Google Scholar]**

78. Costa, R.J.S.; Camões-Costa, V.; Snipe, R.M.J.; Dixon, D.; Russo, I.; Huschtscha, Z. Impact of Exercise-Induced Hypohydration on Gastrointestinal Integrity, Function, Symptoms, and Systemic Endotoxin and Inflammatory Profile. *J. Appl. Physiol.* **2019**, *126*, 1281–1291. **[Google Scholar]**

79. Olesen, J.; Biensø, R.S.; Meinertz, S.; Van Hauen, L.; Rasmussen, S.M.; Gliemann, L.; Plomgaard, P.; Pilegaard, H. Impact of training status on LPS-induced acute inflammation in humans. *J. Appl. Physiol.* **2015**, *118*, 818–829. **[Google Scholar]** **[Green Version]**

80. Ganesan, B.; Anandan, R.; Lakshmanan, P.T. Studies on the protective effects of betaine against oxidative damage during experimentally induced restraint Stress in Wistar albino rats. *Cell Stress Chaperones* **2011**, *16*, 641–652. **[Google Scholar]** **[Green Version]**

81. Wang, H.; Li, S.; Fang, S.; Yang, X.; Feng, J. Betaine improves intestinal functions by enhancing digestive enzymes, ameliorating intestinal morphology, and enriching intestinal microbiota in high-salt stressed rats. *Nutrients* **2018**, *10*, 907. **[Google Scholar]**

82. Orawan, C.; Aengwanich, W. Blood cell characteristics, hematological values and average daily gained weight of Thai indigenous, Thai indigenous crossbred and broiler chickens. *Pakistan J. Biol. Sci.* **2007**, *10*, 302–309. **[Google Scholar]** **[PubMed]**

83. Cui, Y.; Hao, Y.; Li, J.; Bao, W.; Li, G.; Gao, Y.; Gu, X. Chronic heat stress induces immune response, oxidative stress response, and apoptosis of finishing pig liver: A proteomic approach. *Int. J. Mol. Sci.* **2016**, *17*, 393. **[Google Scholar]** **[PubMed]** **[Green Version]**

84. Khattak, F.M.; Acamovic, T.; Sparks, N.; Pasha, T.N.; Joiya, M.H.; Hayat, Z.; Ali, Z. Comparative efficacy of different supplements used to reduce heat stress in broilers. *Pak. J. Zool.* **2012**, *44*, 31–41. **[Google Scholar]**

85. Costa, R.J.S.; Crockford, M.J.; Moore, J.P.; Walsh, N.P. Heat acclimation responses of an ultra-endurance running group preparing for hot desert-based competition. *Eur. J. Sport Sci.* **2014**, *14*, 131–141. **[Google Scholar]**

86. Snipe, R.M.J.; Khoo, A.; Kitic, C.M.; Gibson, P.R.; Costa, R.J.S. Carbohydrate and protein intake during exertional heat stress ameliorates intestinal epithelial injury and small intestine permeability. *Appl. Physiol. Nutr. Metab.* **2017**, *42*, 1283–1292. **[Google Scholar]**

87. Sahebi Ala, F.; Hassanabadi, A.; Golian, A. Effects of dietary supplemental methionine source and betaine replacement on the growth performance and activity of mitochondrial respiratory chain enzymes in normal and heat-stressed broiler chickens. *J. Anim. Physiol. Anim. Nutr. (Berl.)* **2019**, *103*, 87–99. **[Google Scholar]** **[Green Version]**

88. Zhang, L.; An, W.J.; Lian, H.; Zhou, G.B.; Han, Z.Y.; Ying, S.J. Effects of dietary betaine supplementation subjected to heat stress on milk performances and physiology indices in dairy cow. *Genet. Mol. Res.* **2014**, *13*, 7577–7586. **[Google Scholar]**

89. Ratriyanto, A.; Mosenthin, R. Osmoregulatory function of betaine in alleviating heat stress in poultry. *J. Anim. Physiol. Anim. Nutr. (Berl.)* **2018**, *102*, 1634–1650. **[Google Scholar]**

90. Zulkifli, I.; Mysahra, S.A.; Jin, L.Z. Dietary Supplementation of Betaine (Betafin®) and Response to High Temperature Stress in Male Broiler Chickens. *Asian-Australasian J. Anim. Sci.* **2004**, *17*, 244–249. **[Google Scholar]**

91. DiGiacomo, K.; Simpson, S.; Leury, B.J.; Dunshea, F.R. Dietary betaine impacts the physiological responses to moderate heat conditions in a dose dependent manner in sheep. *Animals* **2016**, *6*, 51. **[Google Scholar] [PubMed] [Green Version]**

92. Attia, Y.A.; Hassan, R.A.; Qota, E.M.A. Recovery from adverse effects of heat stress on slow-growing chicks in the tropics 1: Effect of ascorbic acid and different levels of betaine. *Trop. Anim. Health Prod.* **2009**, *41*, 807–818. **[Google Scholar] [PubMed]**

93. Huang, C.; Jiao, H.; Song, Z.; Zhao, J.; Wang, X.; Lin, H. Heat stress impairs mitochondria functions and induces oxidative injury in broiler chickens. *J. Anim. Sci.* **2015**, *93*, 2144–2153. **[Google Scholar] [PubMed]**

94. Garrett, Q.; Khandekar, N.; Shih, S.; Flanagan, J.L.; Simmons, P.; Vehige, J.; Willcox, M.D.P. Betaine stabilizes cell volume and protects against apoptosis in human corneal epithelial cells under hyperosmotic stress. *Exp. Eye Res.* **2013**, *108*, 33–41. **[Google Scholar] [PubMed]**

95. Zhou, W.T.; Fujita, M.; Yamamoto, S.; Iwasaki, K.; Ikawa, R.; Oyama, H.; Horikawa, H. Effects of Glucose in Drinking Water on the Changes in Whole Blood Viscosity and Plasma Osmolality of Broiler Chickens during High Temperature Exposure. *Poult. Sci.* **1998**, *77*, 644–647. **[Google Scholar] [PubMed]**

96. Park, S.O.; Kim, W.K. Effects of betaine on biological functions in meat-type ducks exposed to heat stress. *Poult. Sci.* **2017**, *96*, 1212–1218. **[Google Scholar]**

97. Borges, S.A.; Fischer Da Silva, A.V.; Majorka, A.; Hooge, D.M.; Cummings, K.R. Physiological responses of broiler chickens to heat stress and dietary electrolyte balance (sodium plus potassium minus chloride, milliequivalents per kilogram). *Poult. Sci.* **2004**, *83*, 1551–1558. **[Google Scholar]**

98. Armstrong, L.E.; Casa, D.J.; Roti, M.W.; Lee, E.C.; Craig, S.A.S.; Sutherland, J.W.; Fiala, K.A.; Maresh, C.M. Influence of betaine consumption on strenuous running and sprinting in a hot environment. *J. Strength Cond. Res.* **2008**, *22*, 851–860. **[Google Scholar]**

99. Shakeri, M.; Cottrell, J.J.; Wilkinson, S.; Ringuet, M.; Furness, J.B.; Dunshea, F.R. Betaine and antioxidants improve growth performance, breast muscle development and ameliorate thermoregulatory responses to cyclic heat exposure in broiler chickens. *Animals* **2018**, *8*, 162. **[Google Scholar] [Green Version]**

100. Egbuniwe, I.C.; Ayo, J.O.; Ocheja, O.B. Betaine and ascorbic acid modulate indoor behavior and some performance indicators of broiler chickens in response to hot-dry season. *J. Therm. Biol.* **2018**, *76*, 38–44. **[Google Scholar]**

13

Chapter

# DOES PROTEIN SUPPLEMENTATION FACILITATE ADAPTATIONS TO STRENUOUS CONCURRENT EXERCISE TRAINING?

## A SYSTEMATIC REVIEW AND META-ANALYSIS FOCUSED ON MILITARY APPLICATIONS

## 1. INTRODUCTION: AN OVERVIEW

Concurrent training is characterized as the integration of resistance and endurance training within a periodized physical training framework [1]. The concurrent enhancement of strength, power, and endurance is essential for several athletic and exercise populations to fulfill the physical requirements of their selected sports (e.g., soccer, rugby, hockey) or exercise regimens (e.g., circuits, cross-fit training) [2,3,4,5,6]. Recruits undertaking rigorous military training frequently participate in concurrent training to fulfill the training and operational requirements of military life [7,8,9,10,11,12,13]. Military recruit training programs aim to convert civilians into proficient soldiers; hence, physical training is inherently rigorous, encompassing aerobic exercises, strength and conditioning, obstacle courses, swimming, circuit training, and loaded marching. Although concurrent training is essential for athletic and military recruits, and protein supplementation may enhance training results, most systematic reviews and meta-analyses have primarily examined the effects of protein supplementation in isolation with either resistance or endurance training, without focusing on any specific population.In untrained individuals, a session of endurance exercise enhances muscle protein synthesis (MPS) in both mitochondrial and myofibrillar proteins, but a session of resistance training predominantly stimulates myofibrillar protein synthesis. Furthermore, a duration of chronic (10 weeks) endurance or resistance training enhances the muscle protein synthesis (MPS) response post-exercise in proteins particular to each training modality. Consequently, persistent endurance training enhances the oxidative capacity of muscle, hence augmenting whole-body oxygen intake and resulting in more fatigue-resistant muscle, while resistance training increases muscle strength [21]. Both exercise modalities have demonstrated an enhancement in the phosphorylation of proteins within the protein kinase B-mammalian target of rapamycin-p70 ribosomal protein S6 kinase (Akt-mTOR-p70S6K) pathway, resulting in an elevation of muscle protein synthesis (MPS) [20]. Research indicates a potential interference impact when both training modalities are implemented simultaneously within the same program [22,23,24,25,26,27,28]; nevertheless, this interaction has been contested by other studies [29,30,31]. Endurance exercise mechanistically induces an increase in adenosine monophosphate-activated protein kinase (AMPK) [32], which may suppress mTOR via the activation of the tuberous sclerosis complex (TSC) [2]. This may diminish the post-exercise muscle protein synthesis response, hence reducing muscle strength gains when individuals engage in concurrent endurance training.

Muscle protein synthesis (MPS) is optimized when protein is ingested in 20–40 g increments immediately following resistance training [33]. Research indicates that simultaneous resistance and aerobic training promotes myofibrillar protein production to a comparable extent as resistance training conducted in isolation [34]. This response is enhanced when 25 g of protein is consumed immediately after exercise [35]. Increased concentrations of amino acids in the bloodstream enhance the localization and activation of mTOR via inhibiting the TSC. The notion of "nutrient sensing" has been proposed, indicating that proteins like VPS34 may play a crucial role in activating the mTOR pathway and promoting myofibrillar protein synthesis in reaction to increased blood amino acid levels [27,36,37]. An increased protein intake during strenuous concurrent training may effectively mitigate the interference effect of endurance exercise by optimizing mTOR activity and the muscle protein synthesis response to resistance training, thereby facilitating muscle strength adaptations. Furthermore, individuals engaged in strenuous concurrent training with insufficient recovery time between sessions (e.g., military recruit training) may derive additional advantages from dietary methods that increase energy and protein intake to facilitate muscle adaptations [44]. Alongside muscle endurance, military trainees must successfully complete strength-based assessments throughout basic training [7,8]. Consequently, measures that enhance muscle strength and/or mitigate the interference effect are likely beneficial, especially given that strength is a crucial factor in occupational performance [7].To our knowledge, no research has thoroughly assessed the literature to determine the impact of protein supplementation on training adaptations during strenuous concurrent training. The objective of this systematic review and meta-analysis was to assess the literature regarding protein supplementation and its impact on adaptations to strenuous concurrent exercise training in healthy individuals, with possible implications for recruits in military training.

## 2. MATERIALS AND METHODS

This systematic review was conducted in compliance with the Preferred Reporting Items for Systematic Reviews and Meta-Analyses (PRISMA) guideline [45].

## 2.1. Eligibility Criteria

This review sought peer-reviewed papers with human participants published in English with the following Population, Intervention, Comparison and Outcome (PICO) criteria being implemented to identify eligible studies [**46**]. The PICO was designed with the aim of the findings of this review being applied to military recruits undertaking military training. Military recruits are typically aged between 16–35 years [**47**], and are required to meet aerobic fitness and muscular strength test standards such as maximal strength and muscular endurance tests [**8**]. Studies that did not meet all the PICO were excluded from this review.

Population: (a) stated as healthy active male or females; (b) aged between 16–35 years.

Intervention: (c) include both endurance/aerobic training and resistance/weight training, circuit training, cross-fit training, military training but not high-intensity interval training (HIIT); (d) daily protein supplementation included but not with vitamins and/or antioxidants or through an increased intake of whole-food protein sources in the diet; (e) studies assessing body composition and/or performance were required to have ≥two sessions per week and be ≥four weeks in duration; (f) studies assessing muscle recovery were required to be <one week in duration; (g) training sessions performed at moderate or vigorous intensity (e.g., jogging, running, cycling, weight training) [**17**].

Comparison: (h) changes in outcome measures across repeated timepoints; (i) participants grouped by supplement condition.

Outcome: (j) change in primary variable(s): maximal oxygen uptake ($\dot{V}\dot{V}O_{2max}$), time trial (TT), one-repetition maximum (1RM), fat-free mass (FFM), fat mass, musculoskeletal injury (MSKI) incidence, muscle function/soreness/damage.

## 2.2. Search Strategy and Study Selection

The final electronic database searches were completed in February 2021 in three databases (PubMed, Web of science and SPORTDiscus) using the terms “protein” or “protein supplementation”, “training”, and “concurrent training”” either alone or concurrently. The reference lists of all papers that met the inclusion criteria were interrogated to identify additional studies not found in the electronic search, until no further studies could be identified [**48**]. First, the study title and abstract were screened by one reviewer (SC) followed by the full text by the same reviewer. The characteristics that were extracted from each study included: author, participant sample, total protein intake ($g{\cdot}kg^{-1}{\cdot}day^{-1}$), training intervention, protein timing and dose. The study selection process is outlined in **Figure 1**.

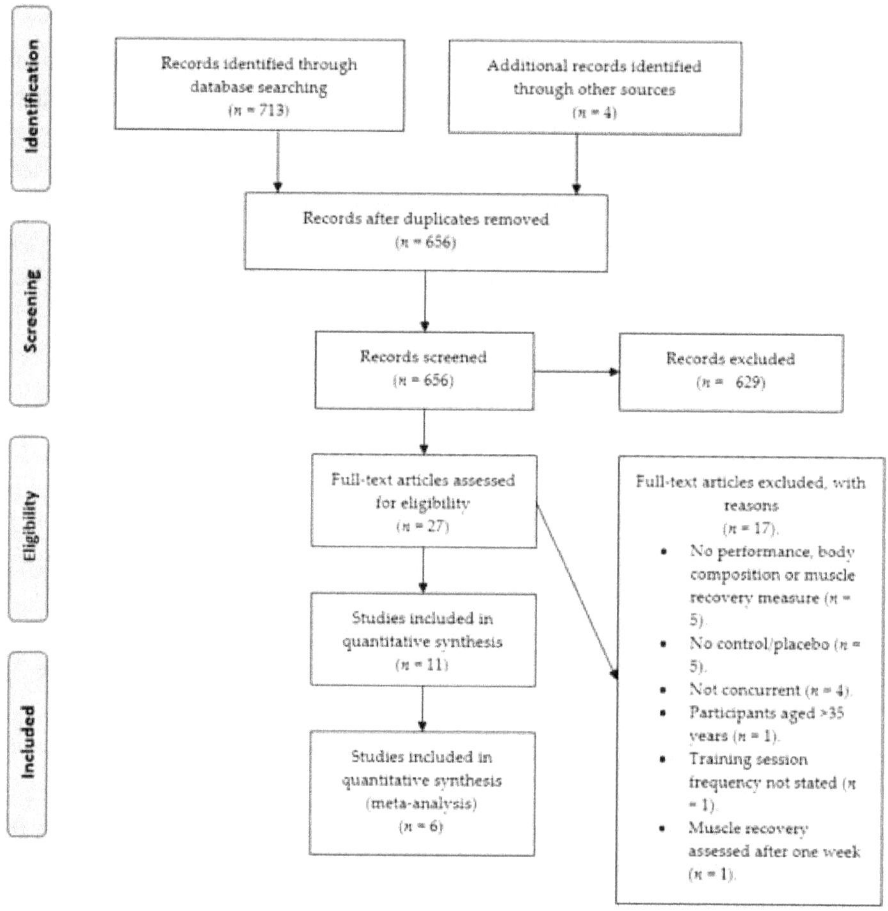


**Figure 1. Flow chart of study retrieval process.**

## 2.3. Risk of Bias Assessment

Studies were evaluated for methodological quality according to the COnsensus based standards for the selection of health status measurement instruments (COSMIN) checklist by two separate reviewers (SC and HC) (Table 1). This review used the recommended "worst score counts" method to obtain a total score for study quality. This was done by obtaining a quality score per measurement by taking the lowest rating of any item in a criteria box [**49**]. Each COSMIN item for all categories were scored from 4–1, where 4 was low risk and 1 was high risk. Each study needed a mean score of ≥ 3 to be included in this review [**49**].

## 2.4. Data Synthesis and Analyses

The analysis was conducted by first extracting the relevant information from all study groups at baseline and at the end of the intervention. This included the number of participants (*n*), *p* values, mean, standard deviation (SD) and 95% confidence intervals (if available). To compare the effects of protein supplementation against placebo conditions, pooling was used of the continuous data as standardized mean difference

(SMD) represented as Cohen's d effect sizes (ES), standard error (SE) and 95% confidence intervals calculated for each main outcome using the reported mean change differences (delta scores), *n* and corresponding SDs [**17,19**]. If the mean change difference was not reported this was calculated based on the reported pre-and-post mean and SDs in each study. If a study used multiple protein-supplemented groups, we combined the data into an overall protein-supplemented group for subsequent analyses [**17**]. When a study used multiple performance outcome measures, the relative $V'V'O_{2peak}$ and lower body 1RM were prioritised for muscle strength and aerobic endurance [**17**]. Effect sizes were classed as small (0.2), medium (0.5), and large effects (0.8) [**50**]. Effect size was calculated using the following equations:

$$E1: \text{Cohen's } d = (M2 - M1)/SD_{pooled}$$

$$E2: SD_{pooled} = \sqrt{((SD_1^2 + SD_2^2)/2)}$$

A random-effects model was applied with heterogeneity across studies tested using $I^2$ test. $I^2$ values of 25%, 50%, and 75% were considered low, moderate and high, respectively [**17**]. Each study was weighted (%) based on its inverse within study variance and between study variance using the Meta-Essentials spreadsheet 1.4 (Microsoft Excel 2016, Washington, DC, USA). Meta-Essentials was used for the meta-analysis, creation of forest and Egger's funnel plots (including the trim and fill method) and running statistical analysis, with alpha set at $p \leq 0.05$.

## 3. RESULTS

### 3.1. Study Quality and Risk of Bias Assessment

**Table 1** outlines the quality assessment scores for each study. All 11 studies were considered eligible for this review based on their COSMIN quality assessments scores.

**Table 1. The individual and mean reviewer quality assessment scores for each study.**

| Study | Reviewer 1 | Reviewer 2 | Mean | Included |
|---|---|---|---|---|
| McAdam et al. [**51**] | 4.00 | 3.70 | 3.85 | Y |
| Eddens et al. [**52**] | 3.60 | 3.30 | 3.45 | Y |
| Crowe, Weatherson and Bowden [**53**] | 4.00 | 3.40 | 3.70 | Y |
| Forbes and Bell [**54**] | 3.80 | 3.20 | 3.50 | Y |
| Ormsbee et al. [**55**] | 3.80 | 3.40 | 3.60 | Y |
| Taylor et al. [**56**] | 4.00 | 4.00 | 4.00 | Y |
| Longland et al. [**57**] | 4.00 | 3.50 | 3.75 | Y |
| Walker et al. [**58**] | 4.00 | 3.90 | 3.95 | Y |
| Jimenez-Flores et al. [**59**] | 3.30 | 2.90 | 3.10 | Y |
| Blacker et al. [**60**] | 3.40 | 3.00 | 3.20 | Y |
| Flakoll et al. [**61**] | 4.00 | 3.80 | 3.90 | Y |

Yes = Y; 1 = poor, 2 = fair,3 = good,4 = excellent.

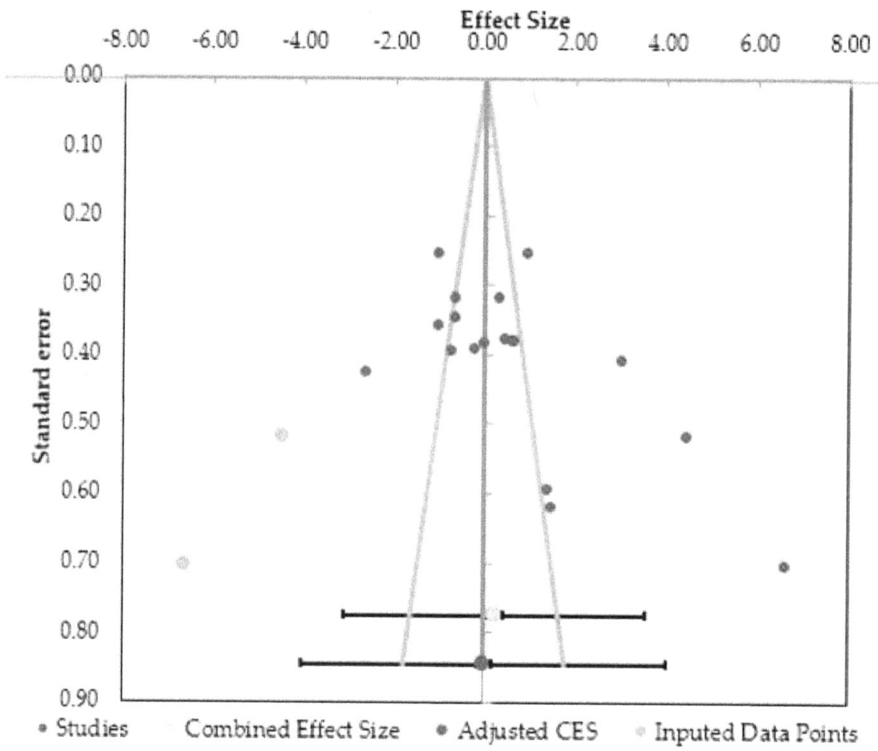


**Figure 2. Funnel plot of the comparison of the effect of protein supplementation vs. placebo on muscle strength, aerobic endurance, fat-free mass (FFM) and fat-mass (FM) adaptations. CES = combined effect size.**

Egger's regression analysis found asymmetries in the funnel plot (**Figure 2**) suggesting that results might be influenced by biasing factors such as publication bias. One study was particularly responsible for this asymmetry [**57**] as they showed the strongest beneficial effects of the treatment group when compared with the placebo group. When this outlier was removed the funnel plot was symmetric ($p > 0.05$). The funnel plot with this outlier included can be seen in **Supplementary Figure 1**.

## 3.2. Participant Characteristics and Study Interventions

Details of the studies' characteristics are provided in **Table 2** and **Table 3**. The sample sizes ranged from 10 to 387 with a total participant sample size of 681 (645 men, 61 women) for all studies. The reported mean age of participants ranged between 18 and 31 years. Intervention durations ranged from one day to six months with seven studies using a standardised concurrent endurance and resistance training programme [**53,54,55,56,57,58**], two studies using a military training programme [**51,58**] and two studies using an acute loaded march protocol [**59,60,61**].

**Table 2. The impact of protein on performance and body composition during concurrent exercise training.**

| Study | Sample | Age | Total Protein Intake | Intervention | Supplement Type & Dose |
|---|---|---|---|---|---|
| McAdam et al. [51] | 69 male U.S. Army recruits. | 19 ± 1 years | 2.8 ± 0.5 & 1.6 ± 0.4 $g{\cdot}kg^{-1}{\cdot}d^{-1}$ in PRO and PLA. | 8-week U.S. Army Initial Entry Training. | 38.6 g WP or isocaloric PLA post-exercise in AM & prior to sleep. |
| Crowe, Weatherson and Bowden [53] | 10 male, 3 female trained canoeists. | 32 ± 2 years | 0.85 ± 0.06 & 0.85 ± 0.05 $g{\cdot}kg^{-1}{\cdot}day^{-1}$ in PRO & PLA. | 6-weeks endurance & resistance training. | 45 $mg{\cdot}kg^{-1}{\cdot}day^{-1}$ leucine or PLA. |
| Ormsbee et al. [55] | 26 sedentary men and 25 sedentary women. | 21± 1 years & 20 ± 1 years in PRO & PLA. | 2.2 ± 0.1 & 1.1 ± 0.1 $g{\cdot}kg^{-1}{\cdot}day^{-1}$ for the PRO & PLA groups. | 6-month endurance & resistance training. | 42 g PRO or isocaloric PLA consumed immediately post-exercise & 8–12 h later. |
| Taylor et al. [56] | 16 female intermittent sport athletes. | 20 ± 2 years | Not measured. | 8-week endurance & resistance training. | 24 g pre-and-post-exercise. |
| Longland et al. [57] | 40 recreationally active men. | 23 ± 2 years | 2.4 & 1.2 $g{\cdot}kg^{-1}{\cdot}day^{-1}$ for the PRO & PLA groups. | 4-weeks endurance & resistance training with an energy deficit | 50 g WP or CHO drink given post-exercise to PRO & PLA groups. |
| Walker et al. [56] | 30 U.S. Air force men. | 26 ± 9 years | Not measured. | 8-week U.S. Air force training. | 20 g WP or isocaloric PLA post-exercise. |
| Forbes and Bell [54] | 15 healthy women & 16 men. | Women: 27 ± 4 years, men: 26 ± 3 years | PLA (men = 1.4 ± 0.4 $g{\cdot}kg^{-1}{\cdot}day^{-1}$, women= 1.2 ± 0.2 $g{\cdot}kg^{-1}{\cdot}day^{-1}$), PRO (men = 3.8 ± 0.4 $g{\cdot}kg^{-1}{\cdot}day^{-1}$, women= 3.2 ± 0.3 $g{\cdot}kg^{-1}{\cdot}day^{-1}$). | 6-weeks endurance & resistance training. | 2.0 and 2.4 $g{\cdot}kg^{-1}{\cdot}day^{-1}$ WP for women & men. |

**Data reported as mean ± standard deviation where possible. U.S. = United states, $g{\cdot}kg^{-1}{\cdot}day^{-1}$ = grams per kilogram of body mass per day, PLA = placebo, PRO = protein, WP = whey protein, CHO = carbohydrate, CON = control, AM = morning.**

**Table 3. Concurrent exercise training and the impact of protein on muscle recovery.**

| Study | Sample | Age | Total Protein Intake | Intervention | Supplement Type & Dose |
|---|---|---|---|---|---|
| Eddens et al. [52] | 24 male cyclists. | PRO = 27 ± 3 years; PLA = 28 ± 5 years; CHO = 26 ± 5 years | PRO = 1.2 ± 0.6 $g{\cdot}kg^{-1}{\cdot}day^{-1}$; PLA = 1.2 ± 0.6 $g{\cdot}kg^{-1}{\cdot}day^{-1}$; CHO = 1.2 ± 0.7 $g{\cdot}kg^{-1}{\cdot}day^{-1}$ | Single concurrent exercise event (high-intensity cycling followed by 100 box jumps). | 20 g WP, isocaloric CHO or low-calorific PLA post-exercise. |
| Jimenez-Flores et al. [59] | 33 healthy men and 2 healthy women. | 21 ± 1 years & 21 ± 1 years in PLA & PRO groups | Not measured. | 4-day loaded (13.2–26.4 kg) mountain skirmish. | 25 g protein bar or isocaloric CHO bar post-exercise. |
| Blacker et al. [60] | 10 healthy men. | 28 ± 9 years | * 0.9 ± 0.3 $g{\cdot}kg^{-1}{\cdot}day^{-1}$, in the PLA, CHO & PRO. | 3 days post-load (25 kg) carriage exercise. | 36 g PRO, 32 g CHO or low-calorie PLA post-exercise. |
| Flakoll et al. [61] | 387 male U.S. Marine recruits. | 19 ± 1 years | Not measured. | Single day loaded march hike. | PLA = 0 g CHO, 0 g PRO, 0 g fat; CON = 0 g PRO, 8 g CHO and 3 g fat; PRO = 10 g PRO, 8 g CHO and 3 g fat. Participants who weighed <81.8 kg received one portion and those weighing >81.8 kg received two portions post-exercise. |

Data reported as mean ± standard deviation. U.S. = United States, $g{\cdot}kg^{-1}{\cdot}day^{-1}$ = grams per kilogram of body mass per day, PLA = placebo, PRO = protein, WP = whey protein, CHO = carbohydrate, CON = control. * maximum across three timepoints.

## 3.3. Protein Dose and Timing

The majority of studies supplemented participants with whey protein in the form of a beverage, except one which used a protein bar [59], with the most common strategy being to provide an absolute bolus dose of protein ranging between 20–50 g. One study provided an additional dose of whey protein relative to body mass (2.4 $g{\cdot}kg^{-1}{\cdot}day^{-1}$) [54]. Crowe et al. [53] provided participants with a leucine supplement (45 $mg{\cdot}kg^{-1}{\cdot}day^{-1}$).

In terms of timing, the majority of studies provided protein immediately (<1 h) post-exercise [**52,55,56,57,58,59,60,61**]. Others also provided protein at breakfast [**54**] and some provided protein both prior to sleep and immediately post-exercise [**51**]. Seven studies assessed and reported total daily protein intake [**51,52,53,54,55,57,60**], whereas four studies did not [**56,58,59,61**].

## 3.4. Synthesis of Results

This review identified 11 individual studies; one focused only on performance [**55**], six on performance and body composition [**51,53,55,56,57,58**] and four on muscle recovery adaptations only [**52,59,60,61**]. Four studies found a benefit on muscle strength, five studies reported a benefit on body composition changes such as increasing FFM, reducing fat-mass or both, and one study reported a benefit on muscle recovery. The characteristics of these studies are outlined in **Table 2** and **Table 3**.

### 3.4.1. Performance Adaptations

McAdam et al. [**51**] observed a greater increase in muscle strength (push-up repetition performance) with protein supplementation (+6.8, 95%CI: 2.9–10.7) compared to a placebo (+2.6, -0.7–6.0 95% CI) during a two-minute maximal push-up test. There was no effect on run time performance (protein: -48.3 s, -63.0–33.6 s 95%; placebo: -74.2 s, -95.5–51.9 95% CI) during a two-minute maximal time trial. Similarly, Ormsbee et al. [**55**] found a greater increase in 1 RM bench press after six-months of concurrent training with protein supplementation (+27.4 ± 2.4 kg vs. +15.9 ± 2.8 kg, $p = 0.003$) but not 1 RM hip sled performance (protein: 72.3 ± 7.8 kg; placebo: 73.6 ± 9.0 kg). Both groups had a statistically significant increase in V'V'O$_{2peak}$ at six months compared to baseline but no differences between groups were reported. Taylor et al. [**56**] reported a statistically significant change in 1 RM bench press performance with additional protein in female basketball players over an eight-week period (protein = +4.9 ± 2.1 kg vs. placebo = +2.3 ± 1.4 kg, $p = 0.046$). Walker et al. [**58**] reported a statistically significant increase in 1 RM bench press performance (protein: +3.5 ± 5.2 kg; placebo: +1.3 ± 4.4 kg, $p < 0.05$) and the number of push-ups (protein: +5.4 ± 6.8; placebo: +3.2 ± 6.8, $p < 0.05$) performed with protein supplementation over eight weeks of recruit military training. There was, however, no effect of protein on run time performance during a maximal three-mile time-trial (protein: -1.4 ± 0.4 s; placebo: -0.9 ± 3.3 s, $p > 0.05$). The remaining study also observed a greater increase in rowing time to exhaustion with leucine supplementation compared to a placebo ($p = 0.008$) [**53**]. The remaining three studies reported no statistical effects on exercise performance with protein supplementation compared to a placebo or control condition [**54,57**]. For instance, Longland et al. [**57**] reported no impact of protein supplementation on leg and bench press 1 RM or cycling time trial performance. Similarly, no differences in men or women were reported between groups for changes in V'V'O$_{2peak}$, 2000 m rowing time trial, leg and bench press 1 RM performance [**54**]. It was possible to include five and three studies in the meta-analyses for muscle strength [**54,55,56,57,58**] and aerobic endurance adaptations [**54,55,57**], respectively. One study was not included in the muscle strength analysis [**51**] whilst two studies were not included in the aerobic endurance adaptations [**51,53**] due to no SD being reported. Additionally, another study was removed from the $V'V'O_{2peak}$ meta-analysis due to assessing time trial performance [**58**]. The results of the meta-analysis are reported as SMD and showed that protein supplementation improved performance outcomes when muscle strength and aerobic endurance parameters were analysed together (SMD = 0.89, 95% CI = 0.08–1.70). When performance outcomes were analysed independently, protein supplementation was found to enhance muscle strength adaptations during concurrent training compared to placebo (ES = 1.18, SMD = +4.92 kg, 95% CI = -2.70–12.54 kg) (**Figure 3**). However, the meta-analysis found protein supplementation to not enhance aerobic endurance adaptations ($V'V'O_{2peak}$) with the analysis favoring placebo (ES = 0.79, SMD = −0.37 ml·kg$^{-1}$·min$^{-1}$, 95% CI = −1.45–0.71) (**Figure 4**). The individual study effect sizes for muscle strength and aerobic endurance adaptations can be found in **Supplementary Figures S2 and S3**. There was substantial heterogeneity between studies for muscle strength ($I^2$ = 94%) and aerobic endurance adaptations ($I^2$ = 95%).

| Study | Protein Mean | SD | N | Placebo Mean | SD | N | ES | SMD | 95% CI Lower | 95% CI Upper | Weight |
|---|---|---|---|---|---|---|---|---|---|---|---|
| Ormsbee et al. 2018 [55] | 27.40 | 2.40 | 29 | 15.90 | 2.60 | 22 | 4.46 | 11.50 | 10.03 | 12.97 | 19.5% |
| Taylor et al. 2016 [56] | 4.90 | 2.10 | 5 | 2.30 | 1.40 | 6 | 1.41 | 2.60 | 0.43 | 4.77 | 19.4% |
| Walker et al. 2010 [55] | 3.50 | 5.20 | 15 | 1.30 | 4.40 | 12 | 0.45 | 2.20 | -1.54 | 5.94 | 20.3% |
| Longland et al. 2016 [57] | 169.00 | 47.00 | 20 | 156.00 | 32.00 | 20 | 0.32 | 13.00 | -12.74 | 38.74 | 20.6% |
| Forbes and Bell 2020 [59] | 28.70 | 5.30 | 21 | 33.40 | 5.20 | 10 | -0.74 | -4.70 | -9.68 | 0.28 | 20.2% |
| Average | | | | | | | 1.18 | 4.92 | -2.70 | 12.54 | |

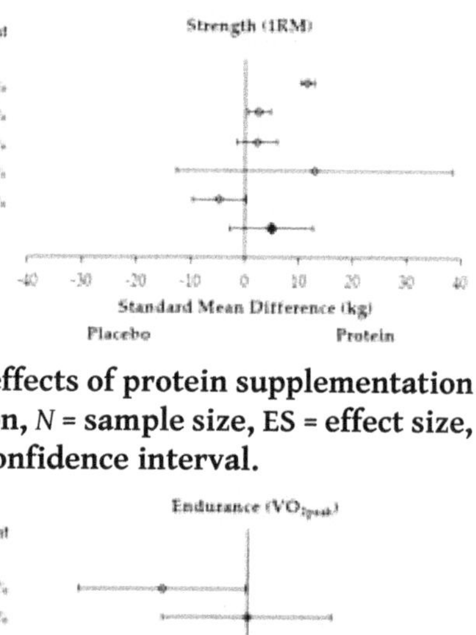


**Figure 3. Forest plot of the studies which assessed the effects of protein supplementation on muscle strength adaptations. SD = standard deviation, *N* = sample size, ES = effect size, SMD = standard mean difference, CI = confidence interval.**

| Study | Protein Mean | SD | N | Placebo Mean | SD | N | ES | SMD | 95% CI Lower | 95% CI Upper | Weight |
|---|---|---|---|---|---|---|---|---|---|---|---|
| Longland et al. 2016 [57] | 5.3 | 2.80 | 20 | 6.90 | 2.00 | 20 | -0.66 | -1.60 | -3.16 | -0.04 | 33.7% |
| Forbes and Bell 2020 [59] | 3.40 | 1.20 | 21 | 3.40 | 3.15 | 10 | 0.00 | 0.00 | -1.59 | 1.59 | 33.3% |
| Ormsbee et al. 2018 [55] | 3.40 | 0.20 | 29 | 2.90 | 0.10 | 22 | 3.03 | 0.50 | 0.41 | 0.59 | 33.1% |
| Average | | | | | | | 0.79 | -0.37 | -1.45 | 0.71 | |

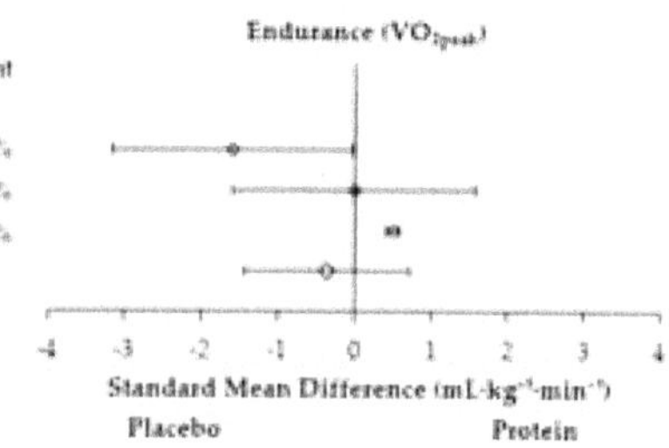


**Figure 4. Forest plot of the studies which assessed the effects of protein supplementation on aerobic endurance adaptations. SD = standard deviation, *N* = sample size, ES = effect size, SMD = standard mean difference, CI = confidence interval.**

### 3.4.2. Body Composition Adaptations

Fat-free mass (FFM) was shown to increase to a greater extent with protein supplementation over an eight-week training period in military recruits (protein: +0.7 ± 1.2 kg; placebo 0.0 ± 0.9 kg, $p < 0.05$) [**58**]. Similarly, FFM was also shown to increase to a greater extent in female basketball players over an eight-week period (protein:

+1.4 kg; placebo: +0.4 kg, $p$ = 0.025) **[56]**. McAdam et al. [51] also observed greater reductions in fat-mass over an eight-week period in military recruits with protein supplementation compared to a placebo (protein: −4.5 kg; placebo: −2.7 kg, $p$ = 0.04) after controlling for initial fat-mass **[51]**. A trend for greater reductions in fat-mass (protein: -1.0 ± 0.3 kg; placebo: −0.3 ± 0.4 kg, $p > 0.05$) and gains in FFM (protein: +2.4 ± 0.3 kg; placebo: +1.9 ± 0.3 kg, $p > 0.05$) were reported by Ormsbee et al. **[55]**. However, significant differences were observed only at three months into the six-month concurrent training intervention for gains in FFM (protein:+2.6 ± 0.2 kg; placebo: 1.7 ± 0.3 kg, $p$ = 0.02) in sedentary men and women. Longland et al. **[57]** reported greater reductions in fat-mass (protein: −4.8 ± 1.6 kg; placebo: −3.5 ± 1.4 kg, $p < 0.05$) and gains in FFM (+1.2 ± 1.0 vs. +0.1 ± 1.0 kg, $p < 0.05$) with protein supplementation compared to a placebo over a four-week period. Conversely, no effect of leucine supplementation was reported after six-weeks on fat mass (body fat percentage) changes **[53]**. In total, five out of six studies reported a beneficial impact of protein supplementation on body composition adaptations. Four studies were included in the meta-analysis for changes in FFM **[51,55,57,58,59]** whereas three studies were included in the meta-analysis for fat-mass **[51,57,58]**. One study was excluded from the FFM adaptations analysis due to no SD being reported **[56]** and one study was excluded from the fat-mass adaptations analysis due to body fat percentage being reported **[53]**. The meta-analysis found that protein supplementation enhanced gains in FFM (ES = 6.29, SMD = +0.75 kg, 95% CI = 0.44–1.06 kg) (**Figure 5**). The meta-analysis also found protein supplementation to enhance reductions in fat-mass compared to placebo (ES = -0.99, SMD = 0.60 kg, 95% CI = −1.20–0.45 kg) (**Figure 6**). The individual study effect sizes for FFM and fat-mass adaptations can be found in **Supplementary Figures S4 and S5**, respectively. There was considerable heterogeneity between studies for FFM ($I^2$ = 98%) and fat-mass adaptations ($I^2$ = 91%).

| Study | Protein Mean | SD | N | Placebo Mean | SD | N | ES | SMD | 95% CI Lower | 95% CI Upper | Weight |
|---|---|---|---|---|---|---|---|---|---|---|---|
| McAdam et al. 2018 [51] | 4.20 | 0.40 | 34 | 3.60 | 0.50 | 35 | 0.94 | 0.60 | 0.29 | 0.91 | 21.7% |
| Ormsbee et al. 2018 [55] | 2.40 | 0.10 | 29 | 1.90 | 0.00 | 22 | 6.61 | 0.50 | 0.46 | 0.54 | 20.5% |
| Longland et al. 2016 [57] | 1.20 | 0.10 | 20 | 0.00 | 0.00 | 20 | 16.97 | 1.20 | 1.15 | 1.25 | 14.9% |
| Walker et al. 2010 [58] | 0.70 | 1.20 | 16 | 0.00 | 0.90 | 12 | 0.64 | 0.70 | -0.13 | 1.53 | 21.4% |
| Average | | | | | | | 6.29 | 0.75 | 0.44 | 1.06 | |

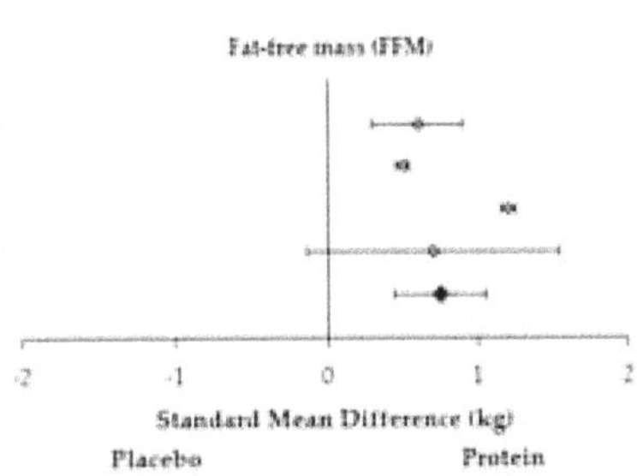


**Figure 5. Forest plot of the studies which assessed the effects of protein supplementation on fat-free mass (FFM) changes in response to concurrent training. SD = standard deviation, $N$ = sample size, ES = effect size, SMD = standard mean difference, CI = confidence interval.**

| Study | Protein Mean | SD | N | Placebo Mean | SD | N | ES | SMD | 95% CI Lower | 95% CI Upper | Weight |
|---|---|---|---|---|---|---|---|---|---|---|---|
| McAdam et al. 2018 [51] | -4.50 | 1.90 | 34 | -2.70 | 1.70 | 35 | -1.00 | -1.80 | -2.67 | -0.93 | 34.5% |
| Longland et al. 2016 [57] | -4.80 | 0.60 | 20 | -3.70 | 0.00 | 20 | -2.59 | -1.10 | -1.37 | -0.83 | 32.5% |
| Walker et al. 2010 [58] | 0.30 | 1.70 | 18 | -0.80 | 1.90 | 12 | 0.62 | 1.10 | -0.26 | 2.46 | 33.1% |
| Average | | | | | | | -0.99 | -0.60 | -1.43 | 0.23 | |

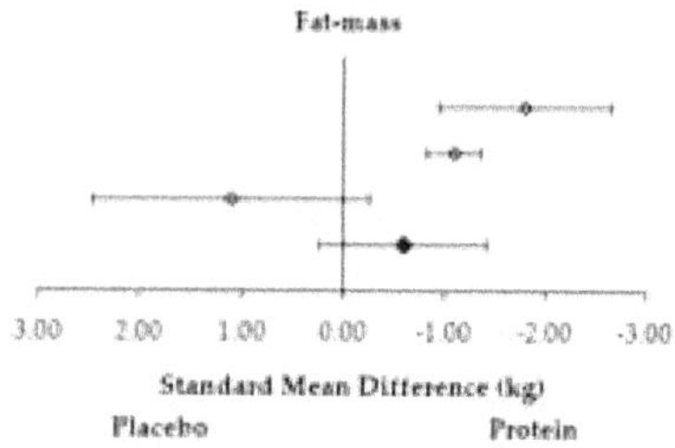


**Figure 6. Forest plot of the studies which assessed the effects of protein supplementation on fat-mass changes in response to concurrent training. SD = standard deviation, *N* = sample size, ES = effect size, SMD = standard mean difference, CI = confidence interval.**

### 3.4.3. Muscle Recovery Adaptations

Perceived muscle soreness after a six-mile hike was reduced by 7% with post-exercise protein supplementation compared to increases of 10% and 16% in the placebo and control conditions, respectively ($p < 0.05$) [**61**]. The remaining studies found no significant difference between protein and placebo conditions for the recovery of muscle function [**60**], muscle damage [**59**] or both [**52**]. Blacker et al. [**60**] reported no effect of protein compared to CHO on muscle function recovery. At 48 hours post-exercise, knee extensor isometric force was reduced by 10 ± 10% for the low caloric placebo condition ($p = 0.008$) but had returned to baseline in the CHO ($p = 0.199$) and protein condition ($p = 0.099$). At 72 h post-exercise, participants in the placebo condition returned to baseline ($p = 0.145$), whereas both the CHO ($p = 0.457$) and protein conditions ($p = 0.731$) remained at baseline at 48 h post-exercise. Only one study assessed the impact of protein supplementation on markers of exercise induced muscle damage and inflammation [**59**]. It was found that there were no differences between protein and isocaloric placebo conditions for changes in blood concentrations of cortisol (placebo: -0.79 ± 0.89; protein: 1.39 ± 1.08 $\mu g{\cdot}dL^{-1}$, $p = 0.160$), C-reactive protein (placebo: 0.13 ± 0.77; protein: 0.99 ± 0.16 $mg{\cdot}L^{-1}$, $p = 0.305$), creatine kinase (placebo: 278.65 ± 50.23; protein: 422.18 ± 149.87 $U{\cdot}L^{-1}$, $p = 0.722$) or aldolase (placebo: 2.06 ± 0.46; protein: 1.98 ± 0.91 $U{\cdot}L^{-1}$, $p = 0.704$). Based on the limited number of studies and available data, it was not possible to complete a meta-analysis of studies assessing the effect of protein supplementation on muscle recovery adaptations. These limitations include the SD not being reported [**61**] and different outcome measures, such as muscle damage [**59**], muscle function [**52,60**] and muscle soreness [**61**].

## 4. DISCUSSION

This review identified 11 studies which investigated the effects of protein supplementation on exercise performance, body composition and muscle recovery adaptations to concurrent exercise training compared to a placebo in healthy adults, confirming the need for more work in this area. The key findings from the literature that met our inclusion criteria demonstrated that protein supplementation had a large effect on muscle strength and FFM adaptations to concurrent exercise training. There was limited evidence to suggest that protein supplementation can support aerobic endurance and muscle recovery adaptations.

## 4.1. Muscle Strength and Body Composition Adaptations

Longland et al. [57] reported no impact of protein supplementation on muscle strength adaptations despite a greater increase in FFM compared to a placebo condition. This was the only study to purposely induce a negative energy balance while participants consumed a total protein intake of 2.4 g·kg$^{-1}$·day$^{-1}$. The study duration (four weeks) may have been too short for differences in strength development to be detected, particularly as protein supplementation is suggested to promote gains in FFM and muscle strength as the duration of training increases [62]. Forbes and Bell [54] also reported no effect of an additional 2.0–2.4 g·kg$^{-1}$·day$^{-1}$ of protein on muscle strength and body composition adaptations over a six-week period (**Table 2**). It may be that the findings were also confounded by the intervention duration, given that it was shorter than each study reporting a positive effect of protein supplementation. The results were analysed by sex and the small sample size (15 women and 16 men) may have also limited the statistical findings as acknowledged by the study authors. Furthermore, the participants in the control condition consumed 1.2–1.4 g·kg$^{-1}$·day$^{-1}$ of protein, which may have been adequate to meet the demands of training, however, with no measure of nitrogen balance or protein turnover, this cannot be confirmed. The final study which observed no effect of protein supplementation on body composition adaptations may have had low total daily protein intakes (0.85 g·kg$^{-1}$·day$^{-1}$) [53].

The studies that reported a positive effect of protein supplementation on muscle strength and body composition adaptations provided protein to participants immediately post-exercise [51,55,56,57,58]. This likely maximised myofibrillar protein synthesis in response to concurrent training [33,35,38,39] and modulated muscle strength and FFM adaptations [63,64]. Promoting MPS post-exercise is an important factor at enhancing skeletal muscle remodelling and adaptation [39,42,64,65]. Subsequently, this could have attenuated the interference effect of endurance training on strength adaptations [35,66] by promoting the activation of mTOR and inhibiting the activation of the tuberous sclerosis complex [27,28]. Skeletal muscle is sensitive to protein feeding for 24 hours post-exercise and thus, consuming protein in 20–40 g doses evenly throughout the day is recommended [64,67,68]. More recently, it has been shown that consuming protein prior to sleep also augments MPS throughout the night [69]. Consuming protein prior to sleep, and subsequently increasing total daily protein intake may be advantageous at optimising MPS responses and supporting muscle strength and body composition adaptations when undertaking concurrent training [70].Nevertheless, it should be acknowledged that acute changes in MPS does not necessarily predict changes in muscle strength and FFM [71]. Instead it is likely the chronic and repetitive changes in MPS and muscle protein breakdown (MPB) which contribute to these [65]. Two studies that reported a greater increase in muscle strength reported a larger reduction in fat-mass with protein intakes ≥2.2 g·kg$^{-1}$·day$^{-1}$ compared to a placebo [51,55]. This suggests that individuals undergoing arduous concurrent training may benefit from protein intakes higher than the current recommendation of 1.8–2.2 g·kg$^{-1}$·day$^{-1}$ [**72**]. Mechanistically, it is speculative as to how an elevated protein intake promoted a greater loss in fat-mass, but previous work suggests that the greater thermic effect of protein may play a key role [**73**]. However, despite similar daily energy intakes between groups in both studies, neither included a measure of energy expenditure, and therefore, it is unclear if participants were in energy balance. Consuming a protein intake >2.2 g·kg$^{-1}$·day$^{-1}$ and possibly higher than 3.0 g·kg$^{-1}$·day$^{-1}$ while restricting energy intake has been suggested to maximise the loss of fat-mass and promote the maintenance of FFM [**72**]. It is unclear if the greater reduction of fat-mass promoted greater improvements in muscle strength performance in studies included in this review [**51,55**]. More work is needed to better determine the impact of protein intakes higher than the current recommendations (1.7–2.2 g·kg$^{-1}$·day$^{-1}$) on body composition adaptations, and how this may influence exercise performance in individuals undergoing arduous concurrent training. The studies identified in this review suggest that protein supplementation may be an effective strategy at augmenting muscle strength and body composition adaptations in healthy adults undertaking concurrent training. It is likely that this effect is facilitated by maximising the MPS post-exercise and attenuating the potential interference effect of endurance training on muscle strength and FFM adaptations. However, more work which includes measures of nitrogen balance or protein turnover are needed to confirm this. Furthermore, future work should also consider factors such as the timing of protein intake around exercise, energy intake/expenditure, and the duration of the training intervention.

## 4.2. Aerobic Adaptations

Protein requirements are elevated in endurance athletes to 1.6–1.8 g·kg$^{-1}$·day$^{-1}$ [**74**] but may be higher (1.7–2.2 g·kg$^{-1}$·day$^{-1}$) during periods of intense and/or high volume training [**72**]. Protein feeding has been shown to facilitate recovery and performance adaptations to endurance training [**17,64**]. Nonetheless, the effects of protein supplementation on aerobic performance adaptations during an arduous concurrent training programme are unknown. Similar improvements in run time performance was observed in military recruits with total daily protein intake of 2.8 ± 0.5 and 1.6 ± 0.4 g·kg$^{-1}$·day$^{-1}$ in the protein and placebo conditions, respectively [**51**]. As such, the dietary protein requirements to facilitate endurance-based adaptations were likely met in both groups, therefore, between groups differences were not observed. This suggests that to promote endurance-based performance adaptations, additional protein intake is not warranted when total habitual intake is ≥1.6 g·kg$^{-1}$·day$^{-1}$. Walker et al. [**58**] also observed no between group differences in run time performance in military recruits supplemented with whey protein or CHO for eight-weeks. However, the total daily protein intakes were not reported, and it is unknown if protein requirements were met. In contrast, one study found leucine supplementation (45 mg·kg$^{-1}$·day$^{-1}$) for six-weeks improved exercise time to exhaustion in canoeists [**53**]. The reported total daily protein intake was 0.85 ± 0.06 g·kg$^{-1}$·day$^{-1}$ and 0.85 ± 0.05 g·kg$^{-1}$·day$^{-1}$ in the protein and placebo groups, therefore, participants likely benefited from the elevated leucine intake given that this amount of protein per day is much lower than the recommended amount [**72**,**74**]. Leucine is the key amino acid which stimulates MPS through the mTOR pathway [**39**,**75**], but given that the other essential amino acids are required to support this process [**36**,**39**], it is unclear how leucine supplementation improved exercise time to exhaustion. The results of the meta-analysis suggest that there is limited evidence to support the use of protein supplementation for aerobic endurance adaptations in response to concurrent training compared to placebo. However, based on the limited number of studies identified, more work is needed to confirm this.

## 4.3. Muscle Recovery Adaptations

Protein supplementation has been shown to improve muscle function recovery following resistance training [**19**] and other modes of exercise including cycling, running, eccentric exercise and resistance training [**62**], yet no review has evaluated the effects following arduous concurrent exercise training specifically. Protein consumption in close proximity to exercise prevents a decrease in myogenin messenger RNA expression, which can accelerate the remodelling and recovery of skeletal muscle [**76**]. Specifically, leucine may be a key component at initiating this process post-exercise through the activation of mTOR and MPS [**39**,**75**]. One study found post-exercise protein ingestion reduced muscle soreness in U.S. Marines following a loaded march [**61**]. However, Flakoll et al. [**61**] failed to provide the total daily protein intake, which therefore, limits our understanding of the impact of protein supplementation specifically on recovery adaptations [**77**]. The remaining studies all failed to find an effect of protein supplementation on muscle recovery in the days following arduous concurrent exercise [**52**,**59**,**60**]. Specifically, no impact was observed on markers of muscle damage [**59**], soreness [**52**] or function [**52**,**60**]. Jimenez-Flores et al. [**59**] observed no differences in markers of muscle inflammation or damage between protein and placebo conditions. However, some of the markers which were chosen may be questionable. For example, cortisol is a stress hormone [**78**,**79**] which can indicate changes in whole-body catabolism [**79**]. C-reactive protein is a marker of whole-body inflammation and is not necessarily specific to skeletal muscle [**78**]. The data also suggest a large inter-participant variability, which is a known limitation of such markers, particularly creatine kinase [**79**].

Eccentric exercise initiates a chain of events which leads to myofibrillar damage, degradation of structural proteins and membrane damage, thus inhibiting muscle function especially if individuals are unaccustomed to the exercise bout [**80**]. The participants in the study by Eddens et al. [**52**] completed a bout of concurrent endurance and eccentric exercise. The participants consumed a similar total daily protein intake, which corresponds to current recommendations [**64**]. As such, it is possible that the additional protein consumed post-exercise in the experimental group did not accelerate muscle recovery, due to protein requirements already being met by the participants. It was acknowledged by Eddens et al. [**52**] that the decrement in muscle function over the 24 h post-exercise was ~15%, which is lower than that observed with other eccentric exercise protocols, with decrements of between 10–65% reported elsewhere [**81**]. Therefore, it cannot be excluded that the muscle damaging protocol may not have been arduous enough, which might explain the lack of statistical difference between conditions [**52**]. Blacker et al. [**60**] found no statistically significant difference between protein and placebo conditions on acute muscle function recovery following arduous concurrent exercise. However, both supplement conditions accelerated recovery of muscle function compared to the control condition. Similarly, participants consumed a standardised total daily amount of protein (0.9 ± 0.3 $g{\cdot}kg^{-1}{\cdot}day^{-1}$) across conditions. Although the amount of protein is lower than the current general recommendations (1.2–2.0 $g{\cdot}kg^{-1}{\cdot}day^{-1}$) [**64**], no effect of protein supplementation post-exercise was observed by Blacker et al. [**60**] when compared to an isocaloric placebo [**60**]. Jimenez-Flores et al. [**59**] found no impact of protein supplementation compared to an isocaloric placebo on markers of muscle damage following arduous concurrent exercise, however, high-variability between study participants was observed and likely influenced the ability to detect statistical differences [**59**]. However, unlike Blacker et al. [**60**], there was no control group, therefore, it is unknown if the additional energy intake accelerated muscle recovery [**59**]. The limited number of studies and the differences between methodologies and outcome measures make it difficult to determine whether protein supplementation does improve muscle recovery, thus warranting further research. Additionally, due to the lack of women included in studies to date, future research is needed in women to examine the impact of protein on muscle recovery, particularly given the known difference in the rate of muscle function recovery post-exercise between men and women [**82**].

## 4.4. Limitations

Only one study identified in this review included a measure of protein balance or turnover [**57**]. Therefore, it is unknown if participants were in a positive protein balance before, during or after the interventions in the remaining studies. Including a measure of protein requirements in future studies can allow for a better understanding of how much additional protein is potentially needed during arduous concurrent training by estimating changes in MPS and whole-body protein balance. The majority of studies failed to include markers of skeletal muscle damage or inflammation when focusing on muscle recovery and therefore, the mechanisms of the effects observed are speculative. The control of dietary intake is critical for comparison between studies involving nutritional interventions. Four studies failed to report the total daily protein intake during the intervention [**56,58,59,61**], making the comparisons between studies even more challenging, given that this is considered more important than the timing of protein intake [**71,83**]. It is recommended that these methodological considerations be factored into future studies aimed at investigating the influence of protein supplementation on arduous concurrent training adaptations. The heterogeneity of the meta-analysis results should be acknowledged as this may make it difficult to apply these findings to a specific population. Nonetheless, the findings of this review infer that protein supplementation can support muscle strength, aerobic endurance, and body composition adaptations during concurrent training. However, more population specific randomised controlled trials (RCTs) are needed to build upon these findings.

### 4.5. Military Research Applications

Five of the eleven studies included in this review quantified the effects of protein supplementation in those during military training, or in response to a military training-based activity [**51,58,59,60,61**]. Given the potential for concurrent endurance training to inhibit muscle strength adaptations [**27,28**], military recruits may be one population who can benefit from strategies which aim to promote gains in FFM and muscle strength during arduous concurrent military training. The findings of this systematic review suggest that protein supplementation may be an effective strategy to support body composition and muscle strength development. However, to better understand the effects protein supplementation has on adaptation and performance outcomes of military recruits, additional population specific RCTs are needed. Future RCTs should consider investigating the effects of elevated protein intakes on training adaptations during arduous military training, including muscle strength, body composition and muscle recovery. Additionally, future work may want to consider adaptations not included in this review, such as bone adaptations, given that bone health and stress fracture incidence are important areas of military research [**84,85,86**] and which protein supplementation may be able to support [**70,87**]. The lack of women studied to date in this area also highlights a gap in the current literature. Therefore, future work should aim to include data in women since they now take-up more arduous (ground close combat) roles in the military [**88**]. Furthermore, including measures of protein metabolism, such as nitrogen balance and protein turnover, in future work should be considered as a means of better understanding the effects of protein supplementation during military recruit training.

## 5. CONCISE SUMMARY

This is the inaugural systematic study and meta-analysis examining the impact of protein supplements on adaptations to strenuous concurrent exercise. The limited number of identified studies indicates an obvious need for more research, especially considering the significance of concurrently building aerobic fitness and muscle strength in various exercising populations. This review indicates that protein supplementation may effectively promote lean mass gain and muscle strength improvements in healthy adults, while also accounting for the influence of training program duration, total energy, and protein intake on outcome measures. Based on the current literature, it is advisable for individuals to target total daily protein intakes of 1.7 to 2.2 $g{\cdot}kg^{-1}{\cdot}day^{-1}$, while consuming 20–40 g of protein immediately after exercise to optimize muscle protein synthesis and enhance muscle strength and fat-free mass adaptations. Nonetheless, the distinction between MPS and chronic physiological adaptations must be recognized. This study suggests that future studies should explore the possible advantages of increased total daily protein consumption during strenuous concurrent training on adaption and performance results.

## AT A GLANCE

We assessed the effects of protein supplementation on adaptations to strenuous concurrent training in healthy adults, with possible implications for those in military training. English-language peer-reviewed articles that satisfied the population, intervention, comparison, and outcome criteria were included. Database searches were conducted in PubMed, Web of Science, and SPORTDiscus. The quality of the study was assessed utilizing the COnsensus-based Standards for the Selection of Health Status Measurement Instruments checklist. Among the 11 studies included, nine concentrated on performance, six on body composition, and four on muscle recovery. Cohen's d effect sizes showed that protein supplementation improved performance outcomes in response to concurrent training (ES = 0.89, 95% CI = 0.08–1.70). When analysed separately, improvements in muscle strength (SMD = +4.92 kg, 95% CI = -2.70–12.54 kg) were found, but not in aerobic endurance. Gains in fat-free mass (SMD = +0.75 kg, 95% CI = 0.44–1.06 kg) and reductions in fat-mass (SMD = -0.99, 95% CI = -1.43–0.23 kg) were greater with protein supplementation.Most studies failed to describe protein turnover, nitrogen balance, and/or total daily protein intake. Consequently, additional investigation is necessary.Our data suggest that protein supplementation may enhance Most studies failed to describe protein turnover, nitrogen balance, and/or total daily protein intake. Consequently, additional investigation is necessary. Our data suggest that protein supplementation may enhance lean mass accumulation and strength improvements during intense concurrent training in physically active groups, including militaryrecruits. lean mass accumulation and strength improvements during intense concurrent training in physically active groups, including military recruits.

## REFERENCES


1. Wilson, J.M.; Marin, P.J.; Rhea, M.R.; Wilson, S.M.; Loenneke, J.P.; Anderson, J.C. Concurrent Training. *J. Strength Cond. Res.* **2012**, *26*, 2293–2307. **[Google Scholar]**
2. Nader, G.A. Concurrent Strength and Endurance Training. *Med. Sci. Sports Exerc.* **2006**, *38*, 1965–1970. **[Google Scholar]** **[Green Version]**
3. Claudino, J.G.; Gabbett, T.J.; Bourgeois, F.; Souza, H.D.S.; Miranda, R.C.; Mezêncio, B.; Soncin, R.; Filho, C.A.C.; Bottaro, M.; Hernandez, A.J.; et al. CrossFit Overview: Systematic Review and Meta-analysis. *Sports Med.-Open* **2018**, *4*, 1–14. **[Google Scholar]**
4. Bonnici, D.C.; Greig, M.; Akubat, I.; Sparks, S.A.; Bentley, D.; Mc Naughton, L.R. Nutrition in Soccer: A Brief Review of the Issues and Solutions. *J. Sci. Sport Exerc.* **2019**, *1*, 3–12. **[Google Scholar]** **[Green Version]**
5. Bradley, W.; Cavanagh, B.; Douglas, W.; Donovan, T.F.; Morton, J.P.; Close, G.L. Quantification of Training Load, Energy Intake, and Physiological Adaptations during a Rugby Preseason: A Case Study from an Elite European Rugby Union Squad. *J. Strength Cond. Res.* **2014**, *12*, 1–12. **[Google Scholar]**
6. Calleja-González, J.; Mielgo-Ayuso, J.; Sampaio, J.; Delextrat, A.; Ostojic, S.M.; Marques-Jiménez, D.; Arratibel, I.; Sánchez-Ureña, B.; Dupont, G.; Schelling, X.; et al. Brief ideas about evidence-based recovery in team sports. *J. Exerc. Rehabil.* **2018**, *14*, 545–550. **[Google Scholar]** **[PubMed]**
7. O'Leary, T.; Saunders, S.; McGuire, S.; Kefyalew, S.; Venables, M.; Izard, R. Sex differences in physical performance and body composition adaptations to British Army basic military training. *J. Sci. Med. Sport* **2017**, *20*, S80. **[Google Scholar]**

8. Drain, J.R.; Sampson, J.A.; Billing, D.C.; Burley, S.D.; Linnane, D.M.; Groeller, H. The Effectiveness of Basic Military Training to Improve Functional Lifting Strength in New Recruits. *J. Strength Cond. Res.* **2015**, *29*, S173–S177. **[Google Scholar] [PubMed]**

9. Richmond, V.L.; Carter, J.M.; Wilkinson, D.M.; Horner, F.E.; Rayson, M.P.; Wright, A.; Bilzon, J.L. Comparison of the Physical Demands of Single-Sex Training for Male and Female Recruits in the British Army. *Mil. Med.* **2012**, *177*, 709–715. **[Google Scholar] [PubMed] [Green Version]**

10. Richmond, V.L.; Horner, F.E.; Wilkinson, D.M.; Rayson, M.P.; Wright, A.; Izard, R. Energy Balance and Physical Demands During an 8-Week Arduous Military Training Course. *Mil. Med.* **2014**, *179*, 421–427. **[Google Scholar] [Green Version]**

11. Blacker, S.D.; Wilkinson, D.M.; Rayson, M.P. Gender Differences in the Physical Demands of British Army Recruit Training. *Mil. Med.* **2009**, *174*, 811–816. **[Google Scholar] [PubMed] [Green Version]**

12. Sharma, J.; Heagerty, R.; Dalal, S.; Banerjee, B.; Booker, T. Risk Factors Associated With Musculoskeletal Injury: A Prospective Study of British Infantry Recruits. *Curr. Rheumatol. Rev.* **2018**, *15*, 50–58. **[Google Scholar]**

13. Wardle, S.L.; Greeves, J.P. Mitigating the risk of musculoskeletal injury: A systematic review of the most effective injury prevention strategies for military personnel. *J. Sci. Med. Sport* **2017**, *20*, S3–S10. **[Google Scholar] [PubMed]**

14. O'Leary, T.J.; Wardle, S.L.; Greeves, J.P. Energy Deficiency in Soldiers: The Risk of the Athlete Triad and Relative Energy Deficiency in Sport Syndromes in the Military. *Front. Nutr.* **2020**, 7, 1–19. **[Google Scholar] [PubMed]**

15. Chapman, S.; Rawcliffe, A.J.; Izard, R.; Jacka, K.; Tyson, H.; Smith, L.; Roberts, J. Dietary Intake and Nitrogen Balance in British Army Infantry Recruits Undergoing Basic Training. *Nutrients* **2020**, *12*, 2125. **[Google Scholar]**

16. Cermak, N.M.; Res, P.T.; De Groot, L.C.P.G.M.; Saris, W.H.M.; Van Loon, L.J.C. Protein supplementation augments the adaptive response of skeletal muscle to resistance-type exercise training: A meta-analysis. *Am. J. Clin. Nutr.* **2012**, *96*, 1454–1464. **[Google Scholar] [Green Version]**

17. Lin, Y.-N.; Tseng, T.-T.; Knuiman, P.; Chan, W.P.; Wu, S.-H.; Tsai, C.-L.; Hsu, C.-Y. Protein supplementation increases adaptations to endurance training: A systematic review and meta-analysis. *Clin. Nutr.* **2020**, 1–10. **[Google Scholar]**

18. Morton, R.W.; Murphy, K.T.; McKellar, S.R.; Schoenfeld, B.J.; Henselmans, M.; Helms, E.; Aragon, A.; Devries, M.C.; Banfield, L.; Krieger, J.W.; et al. A systematic review, meta-analysis and meta-regression of the effect of protein supplementation on resistance training-induced gains in muscle mass and strength in healthy adults. *Br. J. Sports Med.* **2018**, *52*, 376–384. **[Google Scholar]**

19. Davies, R.W.; Carson, B.P.; Jakeman, P.M. The Effect of Whey Protein Supplementation on the Temporal Recovery of Muscle Function Following Resistance Training: A Systematic Review and Meta-Analysis. *Nutrients* **2018**, *10*, 221. **[Google Scholar] [Green Version]**

20. Wilkinson, S.B.; Phillips, S.M.; Atherton, P.J.; Patel, R.; Yarasheski, K.E.; Tarnopolsky, M.A.; Rennie, M.J. Differential effects of resistance and endurance exercise in the fed state on signalling molecule phosphorylation and protein synthesis in human muscle. *J. Physiol.* **2008**, *586*, 3701–3717. **[Google Scholar]**

21. Egan, B.; Zierath, J.R. Exercise Metabolism and the Molecular Regulation of Skeletal Muscle Adaptation. *Cell Metab.* **2013**, *17*, 162–184. **[Google Scholar] [Green Version]**

22. Craig, B.W.; Lucas, J.; Pohlman, R.; Stelling, H. The Effects of Running, Weightlifting and a Combination of Both on Growth Hormone Release. *J. Strength Cond. Res.* **1991**, *5*, 198–203. **[Google Scholar]**

23. Hennessy, L.C.; Watson, A.W.S. The Interference Effects of Training for Strength and Endurance Simultaneously. *J. Strength Cond. Res.* **1994**, *8*, 12–19. **[Google Scholar]**

24. Kraemer, W.J.; Patton, J.F.; Gordon, S.E.; Harman, E.A.; Deschenes, M.R.; Reynolds, K.; Newton, R.U.; Triplett, N.T.; Dziados, J.E. Compatibility of high-intensity strength and endurance training on hormonal and skeletal muscle adaptations. *J. Appl. Physiol.* **1995**, *78*, 976–989. **[Google Scholar]** **[PubMed]**

25. Fyfe, J.J.; Bishop, D.J.; Bartlett, J.D.; Hanson, E.D.; Anderson, M.J.; Garnham, A.P.; Stepto, N.K. Enhanced skeletal muscle ribosome biogenesis, yet attenuated mTORC1 and ribosome biogenesis-related signalling, following short-term concurrent versus single-mode resistance training. *Sci. Rep.* **2018**, *8*, 560. **[Google Scholar]** **[PubMed]** **[Green Version]**

26. Fyfe, J.J.; Bartlett, J.D.; Hanson, E.D.; Stepto, N.K.; Bishop, D.J. Endurance Training Intensity Does Not Mediate Interference to Maximal Lower-Body Strength Gain during Short-Term Concurrent Training. *Front. Physiol.* **2016**, *7*, 1–16. **[Google Scholar]** **[PubMed]** **[Green Version]**

27. Baar, K. Training for Endurance and Strength: Lessons from Cell Signaling. *Med. Sci. Sport Exerc.* **2006**, *7*, 1–7. **[Google Scholar]** **[PubMed]** **[Green Version]**

28. Baar, K. Using molecular biology to maximize concurrent training. *Sports Med.* **2014**, *44*, S117–S125. **[Google Scholar]** **[PubMed]** **[Green Version]**

29. Lundberg, T.R.; Fernandez-Gonzalo, R.; Gustafsson, T.; Tesch, P.A. Aerobic exercise does not compromise muscle hypertrophy response to short-term resistance training. *J. Appl. Physiol.* **2013**, *114*, 81–89. **[Google Scholar]** **[Green Version]**

30. De Souza, E.O.; Roschel, H.; Brum, P.C.; Bacurau, A.N.; Ferreira, J.B.; Aoki, M.S.; Neves, M., Jr.; Aihara, A.Y.; Ugrinowitsch, C.; Tricoli, V.; et al. Molecular Adaptations to Concurrent Training. *Int. J. Sports Med.* **2012**, *34*, 207–213. **[Google Scholar]** **[Green Version]**

31. Lundberg, T.R.; Fernandez-Gonzalo, R.; Tesch, P.A. Exercise-induced AMPK activation does not interfere with muscle hypertrophy in response to resistance training in men. *J. Appl. Physiol.* **2014**, *116*, 611–620. **[Google Scholar]** **[Green Version]**

32. Lantier, L.; Fentz, J.; Mounier, R.; Leclerc, J.; Treebak, J.T.; Pehmøller, C.; Sanz, N.; Sakakibara, I.; Saint-Amand, E.; Rimbaud, S.; et al. AMPK controls exercise endurance, mitochondrial oxidative capacity, and skeletal muscle integrity. *FASEB J.* **2014**, *28*, 3211–3224. **[Google Scholar]**

33. Macnaughton, L.S.; Wardle, S.L.; Witard, O.C.; McGlory, C.; Hamilton, D.L.; Jeromson, S.; Lawrence, C.E.; Wallis, G.A.; Tipton, K.D. The response of muscle protein synthesis following whole-body resistance exercise is greater following 40 g than 20 g of ingested whey protein. *Physiol. Rep.* **2016**, *4*, e12893. **[Google Scholar]**

34. Donges, C.E.; Burd, N.A.; Duffield, R.; Smith, G.C.; West, D.W.D.; Short, M.J.; MacKenzie, R.; Plank, L.D.; Shepherd, P.R.; Phillips, S.M.; et al. Concurrent resistance and aerobic exercise stimulates both myofibrillar and mitochondrial protein synthesis in sedentary middle-aged men. *J. Appl. Physiol.* **2012**, *112*, 1992–2001. **[Google Scholar]**

35. Camera, D.M.; West, D.W.D.; Phillips, S.M.; Rerecich, T.; Stellingwerff, T.; Hawley, J.A.; Coffey, V.G. Protein Ingestion Increases Myofibrillar Protein Synthesis after Concurrent Exercise. *Med. Sci. Sports Exerc.* **2015**, *47*, 82–91. **[Google Scholar]** **[PubMed]**

36. Pasiakos, S.M. Exercise and Amino Acid Anabolic Cell Signaling and the Regulation of Skeletal Muscle Mass. *Nutrients* **2012**, *4*, 740–758. **[Google Scholar]** **[PubMed]**

37. Roberts, J.; Zinchenko, A.; Suckling, C.; Smith, L.; Johnstone, J.; Henselmans, M. The short-term effect of high versus moderate protein intake on recovery after strength training in resistance-trained individuals. *J. Int. Soc. Sports Nutr.* **2017**, *14*, 44. **[Google Scholar]** **[Green Version]**

38. Tipton, K.D. Protein for adaptations to exercise training. *Eur. J. Sport Sci.* **2008**, *8*, 107–118. **[Google Scholar]**

39. Witard, O.C.; Wardle, S.L.; Macnaughton, L.S.; Hodgson, A.B.; Tipton, K.D. Protein Considerations for Optimising Skeletal Muscle Mass in Healthy Young and Older Adults. *Nutrients* **2016**, *8*, 181. **[Google Scholar]** **[PubMed]**

40. Tipton, K.D.; Sharp, C.P. The response of intracellular signaling and muscle-protein metabolism to nutrition and exercise. *Eur. J. Sport Sci.* **2005**, *5*, 107–121. **[Google Scholar]**

41. Tipton, K.D.; Wolfe, R.R. Protein and amino acids for athletes. *J. Sports Sci.* **2004**, *22*, 65–79. **[Google Scholar]**

42. Phillips, S.M.; Hartman, J.W.; Wilkinson, S.B. Dietary Protein to Support Anabolism with Resistance Exercise in Young Men. *J. Am. Coll. Nutr.* **2005**, *24*, 134S–139S. **[Google Scholar]**

43. Phillips, S.M.; Van Loon, L.J. Dietary protein for athletes: From requirements to optimum adaptation. *J. Sports Sci.* **2011**, *29*, S29–S38. **[Google Scholar]**

44. McLellan, T.M. Protein Supplementation for Military Personnel: A Review of the Mechanisms and Performance Outcomes. *J. Nutr.* **2013**, *143*, 1820S–1833S. **[Google Scholar] [PubMed] [Green Version]**

45. Moher, D.; Liberati, A.; Tetzlaff, J.; Altman, D.G.; The PRISMA Group. Preferred reporting items for systematic reviews and meta-analyses: The PRISMA statement. *PLoS Med.* **2009**, *6*, e1000097. **[Google Scholar] [Green Version]**

46. Methley, A.M.; Campbell, S.; Chew-Graham, C.; McNally, R.; Cheraghi-Sohi, S. PICO, PICOS and SPIDER: A comparison study of specificity and sensitivity in three search tools for qualitative systematic reviews. *BMC Health Serv. Res.* **2014**, *14*, 1–10. **[Google Scholar] [Green Version]**

47. Blacker, S.D.; Wilkinson, D.M.; Bilzon, J.L.; Rayson, M.P. Risk Factors for Training Injuries among British Army Recruits. *Mil. Med.* **2008**, *173*, 278–286. **[Google Scholar] [Green Version]**

48. Needleman, I.G. A guide to systematic reviews. *J. Clin. Periodontol.* **2002**, *29*, 6–9. **[Google Scholar] [PubMed]**

49. Terwee, C.B.; Mokkink, L.B.; Knol, D.L.; Ostelo, R.W.J.G.; Bouter, L.M.; De Vet, H.C.W. Rating the methodological quality in systematic reviews of studies on measurement properties: A scoring system for the COSMIN checklist. *Qual. Life Res.* **2011**, *21*, 651–657. **[Google Scholar] [PubMed] [Green Version]**

50. Cohen, J. A power primer. *Tutor. Quant. Methods Psychol.* **2007**, *3*, 79. **[Google Scholar] [Green Version]**

51. McAdam, J.S.; McGinnis, K.D.; Beck, D.T.; Haun, C.T.; Romero, M.A.; Mumford, P.W.; Roberson, P.A.; Young, K.C.; Lohse, K.R.; Lockwood, C.M.; et al. Effect of Whey Protein Supplementation on Physical Performance and Body Composition in Army Initial Entry Training Soldiers. *Nutrients* **2018**, *10*, 1248. **[Google Scholar] [Green Version]**

52. Eddens, L.; Browne, S.; Stevenson, E.J.; Sanderson, B.; Van Someren, K.; Howatson, G. The efficacy of protein supplementation during recovery from muscle-damaging concurrent exercise. *Appl. Physiol. Nutr. Metab.* **2017**, *42*, 716–724. **[Google Scholar]**

53. Crowe, M.J.; Weatherson, J.N.; Bowden, B.F. Effects of dietary leucine supplementation on exercise performance. *Graefe's Arch. Clin. Exp. Ophthalmol.* **2005**, *97*, 664–672. **[Google Scholar]**

54. Forbes, S.C.; Bell, G.J. Whey protein isolate or concentrate combined with concurrent training does not augment performance, cardiorespiratory fitness, or strength adaptations. *J. Sports Med. Phys. Fit.* **2020**, *60*, 1–9. **[Google Scholar]**

55. Ormsbee, M.J.; Willingham, B.D.; Marchant, T.; Binkley, T.L.; Specker, B.L.; Vukovich, M.D. Protein Supplementation During a 6-Month Concurrent Training Program: Effect on Body Composition and Muscular Strength in Sedentary Individuals. *Int. J. Sport Nutr. Exerc. Metab.* **2018**, *28*, 619–628. **[Google Scholar]**

56. Taylor, L.W.; Wilborn, C.; Roberts, M.D.; White, A.J.P.; Dugan, M.K. Eight weeks of pre- and postexercise whey protein supplementation increases lean body mass and improves performance in Division III collegiate female basketball players. *Appl. Physiol. Nutr. Metab.* **2016**, *41*, 249–254. **[Google Scholar]**

57. Longland, T.M.; Oikawa, S.Y.; Mitchell, C.J.; Devries, M.C.; Phillips, S.M. Higher compared with lower dietary protein during an energy deficit combined with intense exercise promotes greater lean mass gain and fat mass loss: A randomized trial. *Am. J. Clin. Nutr.* **2016**, *103*, 738–746. **[Google Scholar]**

58. Walker, T.B.; Smith, J.; Herrera, M.; Lebegue, B.; Pinchak, A.; Fischer, J. The Influence of 8 Weeks of Whey-Protein and Leucine Supplementation on Physical and Cognitive Performance. *Int. J. Sport Nutr. Exerc. Metab.* **2010**, *20*, 409–417. **[Google Scholar]**

59. Jimenez-Flores, R.; Heick, J.; Davis, S.C.; Hall, K.G.; Schaffner, A. A Comparison of the Effects of a High Carbohydrate vs. a Higher Protein Milk Supplement Following Simulated Mountain Skirmishes. *Mil. Med.* **2012**, *177*, 723–731. **[Google Scholar]** **[Green Version]**

60. Blacker, S.D.; Williams, N.C.; Fallowfield, J.L.; Bilzon, J.L.; Willems, M.E. Carbohydrate vs protein supplementation for recovery of neuromuscular function following prolonged load carriage. *J. Int. Soc. Sports Nutr.* **2010**, *7*, 2. **[Google Scholar]** **[Green Version]**

61. Flakoll, P.J.; Judy, T.; Flinn, K.; Carr, C.; Flinn, S. Postexercise protein supplementation improves health and muscle soreness during basic military training in marine recruits. *J. Appl. Physiol.* **2004**, *96*, 951–956. **[Google Scholar]** **[PubMed]**

62. Pasiakos, S.M.; McLellan, T.M.; Lieberman, H.R. The Effects of Protein Supplements on Muscle Mass, Strength, and Aerobic and Anaerobic Power in Healthy Adults: A Systematic Review. *Sports Med.* **2015**, *45*, 111–131. **[Google Scholar]** **[PubMed]**

63. Witard, O.C.; Garthe, I.; Phillips, S.M.; Philips, S.M. Dietary Protein for Training Adaptation and Body Composition Manipulation in Track and Field Athletes. *Int. J. Sport Nutr. Exerc. Metab.* **2019**, *29*, 165–174. **[Google Scholar]** **[PubMed]** **[Green Version]**

64. Jäger, R.; Kerksick, C.M.; Campbell, B.I.; Cribb, P.J.; Wells, S.D.; Skwiat, T.M.; Purpura, M.; Ziegenfuss, T.N.; Ferrando, A.A.; Arent, S.M.; et al. International Society of Sports Nutrition Position Stand: Protein and exercise. *J. Int. Soc. Sports Nutr.* **2017**, *14*, 20. **[Google Scholar]** **[Green Version]**

65. Damas, F.; Phillips, S.M.; Libardi, C.A.; Vechin, F.C.; Lixandrão, M.E.; Jannig, P.R.; Costa, L.A.R.; Bacurau, A.V.; Snijders, T.; Parise, G.; et al. Resistance training-induced changes in integrated myofibrillar protein synthesis are related to hypertrophy only after attenuation of muscle damage. *J. Physiol.* **2016**, *594*, 5209–5222. **[Google Scholar]** **[Green Version]**

66. Pérez-Schindler, J.; Hamilton, D.L.; Moore, D.R.; Baar, K.; Philp, A. Nutritional strategies to support concurrent training. *Eur. J. Sport Sci.* **2015**, *15*, 41–52. **[Google Scholar]**

67. Areta, J.L.; Burke, L.M.; Ross, M.L.; Camera, D.M.; West, D.W.D.; Broad, E.M.; Jeacocke, N.A.; Moore, D.R.; Stellingwerff, T.; Phillips, S.M.; et al. Timing and distribution of protein ingestion during prolonged recovery from resistance exercise alters myofibrillar protein synthesis. *J. Physiol.* **2013**, *591*, 2319–2331. **[Google Scholar]**

68. Mamerow, M.M.; Mettler, J.A.; English, K.L.; Casperson, S.L.; Arentson-Lantz, E.; Sheffield-Moore, M.; Layman, D.K.; Paddon-Jones, D. Dietary Protein Distribution Positively Influences 24-h Muscle Protein Synthesis in Healthy Adults. *J. Nutr.* **2014**, *144*, 876–880. **[Google Scholar]** **[Green Version]**

69. Trommelen, J.; Van Loon, L.J.C. Pre-Sleep Protein Ingestion to Improve the Skeletal Muscle Adaptive Response to Exercise Training. *Nutrients* **2016**, *8*, 763. **[Google Scholar]** **[Green Version]**

70. Antonio, J.; Candow, D.G.; Forbes, S.C.; Ormsbee, M.J.; Saracino, P.G.; Roberts, J. Effects of Dietary Protein on Body Composition in Exercising Individuals. *Nutrients* **2020**, *12*, 1890. **[Google Scholar]**

71. Reidy, P.T.; Rasmussen, B.B. Role of Ingested Amino Acids and Protein in the Promotion of Resistance Exercise-Induced Muscle Protein Anabolism. *J. Nutr.* **2016**, *146*, 155–183. **[Google Scholar]**

72. Kerksick, C.M.; Wilborn, C.D.; Roberts, M.D.; Smith-Ryan, A.E.; Kleiner, S.M.; Jäger, R.; Collins, R.; Cooke, M.; Davis, J.N.; Galvan, E.; et al. ISSN exercise & sports nutrition review update: Research & recommendations. *J. Int. Soc. Sports Nutr.* **2018**, *15*, 38. **[Google Scholar]** **[Green Version]**

73. Aragon, A.A.; Schoenfeld, B.J.; Wildman, R.; Kleiner, S.; VanDusseldorp, T.; Taylor, L.; Earnest, C.P.;

Arciero, P.J.; Wilborn, C.; Kalman, D.S.; et al. International society of sports nutrition position stand: Diets and body composition. *J. Int. Soc. Sports Nutr.* **2017**, *14*, 1–19. **[Google Scholar] [Green Version]**

74. Kato, H.; Suzuki, K.; Bannai, M.; Moore, D.R. Protein Requirements Are Elevated in Endurance Athletes after Exercise as Determined by the Indicator Amino Acid Oxidation Method. *PLoS ONE* **2016**, *11*, e0157406. **[Google Scholar] [Green Version]**
75. Aguirre, N.; Baar, K. The Role of Amino Acids in Skeletal Muscle Adaptation to Exercise. *Issues Complementary Feed.* **2013**, *76*, 85–102. **[Google Scholar] [Green Version]**
76. Hulmi, J.J.; Kovanen, V.; Selänne, H.; Kraemer, W.J.; Häkkinen, K.; Mero, A.A. Acute and long-term effects of resistance exercise with or without protein ingestion on muscle hypertrophy and gene expression. *Amino Acids* **2008**, *37*, 297–308. **[Google Scholar]**
77. Huecker, M.; Sarav, M.; Pearlman, M.; Laster, J. Protein Supplementation in Sport: Source, Timing, and Intended Benefits. *Curr. Nutr. Rep.* **2019**, *8*, 382–396. **[Google Scholar] [PubMed]**
78. Lindsay, A.; Costello, J.T. Realising the Potential of Urine and Saliva as Diagnostic Tools in Sport and Exercise Medicine. *Sports Med.* **2017**, *47*, 11–31. **[Google Scholar] [PubMed] [Green Version]**
79. Lee, E.C.; Fragala, M.S.; Kavouras, S.A.; Queen, R.M.; Pryor, J.L.; Casa, D.J. Biomarkers in Sports and Exercise: Tracking Health, Performance, and Recovery in Athletes. *J. Strength Cond. Res.* **2017**, *31*, 2920–2937. **[Google Scholar] [PubMed] [Green Version]**
80. Markus, I.; Constantini, K.; Hoffman, J.R.; Bartolomei, S.; Gepner, Y. Exercise-induced muscle damage: Mechanism, assessment and nutritional factors to accelerate recovery. *Graefe's Arch. Clin. Exp. Ophthalmol.* **2021**, *121*, 969–992. **[Google Scholar]**
81. Clarkson, P.M.; Hubal, M.J. Exercise-Induced Muscle Damage in Humans. *Am. J. Phys. Med. Rehabil.* **2002**, *81*, S52–S69. **[Google Scholar]**
82. O'Leary, T.J.; Saunders, S.C.; McGuire, S.J.; Izard, R.M. Sex differences in neuromuscular fatigability in response to load carriage in the field in British Army recruits. *J. Sci. Med. Sport* **2018**, *21*, 591–595. **[Google Scholar] [PubMed]**
83. Schoenfeld, B.B.; Aragon, A.A.; Krieger, J.W. The effect of protein timing on muscle strength and hypertrophy: A meta-analysis. *J. Int. Soc. Sports Nutr.* **2013**, *10*, 53. **[Google Scholar] [PubMed] [Green Version]**
84. Moran, D.S.; Heled, Y.; Arbel, Y.; Israeli, E.; Finestone, A.S.; Evans, R.K.; Yanovich, R. Dietary intake and stress fractures among elite male combat recruits. *J. Int. Soc. Sports Nutr.* **2012**, *9*, 6. **[Google Scholar] [PubMed] [Green Version]**
85. Wentz, L.; Liu, P.-Y.; Haymes, E.; Ilich, J.Z. Females Have a Greater Incidence of Stress Fractures Than Males in Both Military and Athletic Populations: A Systemic Review. *Mil. Med.* **2011**, *176*, 420–430. **[Google Scholar] [PubMed] [Green Version]**
86. O'Leary, T.J.; Walsh, N.P.; Casey, A.; Izard, R.M.; Tang, J.C.Y.; Fraser, W.D.; Greeves, J.P. Supplementary Energy Increases Bone Formation during Arduous Military Training. *Med. Sci. Sports Exerc.* **2021**, *53*, 394–403. **[Google Scholar]**
87. Sale, C.; Elliott-Sale, K.J. Nutrition and Athlete Bone Health. *Sports Med.* **2019**, *49*, 139–151. **[Google Scholar] [Green Version]**
88. O'Leary, T.J.; Wardle, S.L.; Rawcliffe, A.J.; Chapman, S.; Mole, J.; Greeves, J.P. Understanding the musculoskeletal injury risk of women in combat: The effect of infantry training and sex on musculoskeletal injury incidence during British Army basic training. *BMJ Mil. Health* **2020**, 1–5. **[Google Scholar]**

# INDEX

www.ingramcontent.com/pod-product-compliance
Lightning Source LLC
LaVergne TN
LVHW062114200926
848484LV00007B/1663
* 9 7 8 1 7 8 7 1 5 4 1 6 2 *